D0793436

Textbook of
SYSTEMIC VASCULITIS

Textbook of
SYSTEMIC VASCULITIS

Editor

Aman Sharma

MD MAMS FIACM FICP FRCP (London)

Associate Professor
Rheumatology and HIV Wing
Department of Internal Medicine
Postgraduate Institute of Medical Education and Research (PGIMER)
Chandigarh, India

Deputy Program Director
Centers of Excellence (COE) in HIV Care
PGIMER, Chandigarh, India

Foreword

Paul Bacon

CLARKSTON CENTER

WALLA WALLA COMMUNITY
COLLEGE LIBRARY

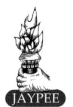

The Health Sciences Publisher

New Delhi | London | Philadelphia | Panama

Jaypee Brothers Medical Publishers (P) Ltd.

Headquarters
Jaypee Brothers Medical Publishers (P) Ltd.
4838/24, Ansari Road, Daryaganj
New Delhi 110 002, India
Phone: +91-11-43574357
Fax: +91-11-43574314
E-mail: jaypee@jaypeebrothers.com

Overseas Offices

J.P. Medical Ltd.
83, Victoria Street, London
SW1H 0HW (UK)
Phone: +44-20 3170 8910
Fax: +44(0) 20 3008 6180
E-mail: info@jpmedpub.com

Jaypee-Highlights Medical Publishers Inc.
City of Knowledge, Bld. 237, Clayton
Panama City, Panama
Phone: +1 507-301-0496
Fax: +1 507-301-0499
E-mail: cservice@jphmedical.com

Jaypee Medical Inc.
The Bourse
111, South Independence Mall East
Suite 835, Philadelphia, PA 19106, USA
Phone: +1 267-519-9789
E-mail: jpmed.us@gmail.com

Jaypee Brothers Medical Publishers (P) Ltd.
17/1-B, Babar Road, Block-B, Shaymali
Mohammadpur, Dhaka-1207
Bangladesh
Mobile: +08801912003485
E-mail: jaypeedhaka@gmail.com

Jaypee Brothers Medical Publishers (P) Ltd.
Bhotahity, Kathmandu, Nepal
Phone: +977-9741283608
E-mail: kathmandu@jaypeebrothers.com

Website: www.jaypeebrothers.com
Website: www.jaypeedigital.com

© 2015, Jaypee Brothers Medical Publishers

The views and opinions expressed in this book are solely those of the original contributor(s)/author(s) and do not necessarily represent those of editor(s) of the book.

All rights reserved. No part of this publication may be reproduced, stored or transmitted in any form or by any means, electronic, mechanical, photocopying, recording or otherwise, without the prior permission in writing of the publishers.

All brand names and product names used in this book are trade names, service marks, trademarks or registered trademarks of their respective owners. The publisher is not associated with any product or vendor mentioned in this book.

Medical knowledge and practice change constantly. This book is designed to provide accurate, authoritative information about the subject matter in question. However, readers are advised to check the most current information available on procedures included and check information from the manufacturer of each product to be administered, to verify the recommended dose, formula, method and duration of administration, adverse effects and contraindications. It is the responsibility of the practitioner to take all appropriate safety precautions. Neither the publisher nor the author(s)/editor(s) assume any liability for any injury and/or damage to persons or property arising from or related to use of material in this book.

This book is sold on the understanding that the publisher is not engaged in providing professional medical services. If such advice or services are required, the services of a competent medical professional should be sought.

Every effort has been made where necessary to contact holders of copyright to obtain permission to reproduce copyright material. If any have been inadvertently overlooked, the publisher will be pleased to make the necessary arrangements at the first opportunity.

Inquiries for bulk sales may be solicited at: jaypee@jaypeebrothers.com

Textbook of Systemic Vasculitis

First Edition: **2015**

ISBN: 978-93-5152-652-0

Printed at Replika Press Pvt. Ltd.

Dedicated to

My father, Shri Balbir Parkash Sharma, the guiding light of my life
My mother, Smt Sudesh Sharma, my pillar of strength
Kusum, my sister, who believes that her brother can do anything
Sushmita, my caring wife, who always stood by me
and dealt with all of my absence without any complaints
and
my loving daughters Ananya and Sharanya

Contributors

Ajay Wanchu
Division of Arthritis and Rheumatic Diseases
Oregon Health and Science University
Portland, Oregon, USA

Alice Coughlan
Trinity College Dublin/Tallaght and Beaumont Hospitals
Trinity Health Kidney Center
Institute of Molecular Medicine
St James's Hospital Campus
Dublin, Ireland

Amanjit Bal
Department of Histopathology
Postgraduate Institute of Medical Education and Research
Chandigarh, India

Aman Sharma
Associate Professor
Rheumatology and HIV Wing
Department of Internal Medicine
Postgraduate Institute of Medical Education and Research
(PGIMER)
Chandigarh, India
Deputy Program Director
Centers of Excellence (COE) in HIV Care
PGIMER, Chandigarh, India

Amita Aggarwal
Department of Clinical Immunology
Sanjay Gandhi Postgraduate Institute of Medical Sciences
Lucknow, Uttar Pradesh, India

Amod Gupta
Advance Eye Center
Postgraduate Institute of Medical Education and Research
Chandigarh, India

Anuj Shukla
Department of Clinical Immunology
Sanjay Gandhi Postgraduate Institute of Medical Sciences
Lucknow, Uttar Pradesh, India

Anupam Wakhlu
Department of Rheumatology
King George's Medical University
Lucknow, Uttar Pradesh, India

Aravind G Hegde
Clinical Immunology and Rheumatology
Christian Medical College
Vellore, Tamil Nadu, India

Arjun D Law
Department of Internal Medicine
Postgraduate Institute of Medical Education and Research
Chandigarh, India

Arnaud Roccabianca
INSERM U1016; Institut Cochin
Université Paris Descartes
CNRS-UMR 8104
Université Sorbonne Paris Cité
Laboratoire d'excellence INFLAMEX Paris
France

Ashim Das
Department of Histopathology
Postgraduate Institute of Medical Education and Research
Chandigarh, India

Ashish Aggarwal
Center of Excellence in HIV Care
Department of Internal Medicine
Postgraduate Institute of Medical Education and Research
Chandigarh, India

Atul Khasnis
Center for Vasculitis Care and Research
Cleveland Clinic
Cleveland, OH, USA

BD Radotra
Department of Histopathology
Postgraduate Institute of Medical Education and Research
Chandigarh, India

Chetan Mukhtyar
Norfolk and Norwich University Hospital
Norwich, UK

Chirag Ahuja
Department of Radiodiagnosis and Imaging
Postgraduate Institute of Medical Education and Research
Chandigarh, India

Christian Pagnoux
Mount Sinai Hospital
Division of Rheumatology—Vasculitis Clinic
Toronto, Canada

Cloé Comarmond
Departement Hospitalo-Universitaire I2B
UPMC Univ Paris 06
UMR 7211, F-75005
Paris, France

Corisande Baldwin
Division of Rheumatology
Vancouver General and St Paul's Hospitals
University of British Columbia
Vancouver, British Columbia, Canada

David GI Scott
Honorary Professor
Norwich Medical School
Norwich, UK

David Jayne
Department of Medicine
University of Cambridge
UK

Debashish Danda
Clinical Immunology and Rheumatology
Christian Medical College
Vellore, Tamil Nadu, India

Deepti Suri
Department of Pediatrics
Postgraduate Institute of Medical Education and Research
Chandigarh, India

Durga Prasanna Misra
Department of Clinical Immunology
Sanjay Gandhi Postgraduate Institute of Medical Sciences
Lucknow, Uttar Pradesh, India

Enrico Tombetti
Unità di Medicina ad Indirizzo Immunologico
San Raffaele Scientific Institute
Milan, Italy

Fatma Alibaz-Oner
Division of Rheumatology
Marmara University Hospital
Fevzi Çakmak Mahallesi
Mimar Sinan Cad
Istanbul, Turkey

Gaurav Prakash
Department of Internal Medicine
Postgraduate Institute of Medical Education and Research
Chandigarh, India

George Joseph
Department of Cardiology
Christian Medical College
Vellore, Tamil Nadu, India

Haner Direskeneli
Division of Rheumatology
Marmara University Hospital
Fevzi Çakmak Mahallesi
Mimar Sinan Cad
Istanbul, Turkey

J Charles Jennette
Department of Pathology and Laboratory Medicine
School of Medicine
University of North Carolina at Chapel Hill
North Carolina, USA

John Mathew
Department of Clinical Immunology and Rheumatology
Christian Medical College
Vellore, Tamil Nadu, India

Justin C Mason
Vascular Sciences and Rheumatology
National Heart and Lung Institute
Imperial College
London, UK

Kusum Sharma
Department of Medical Microbiology
Postgraduate Institute of Medical Education and Research
Chandigarh, India

Leonard Calabrese
Center for Vasculitis Care and Research
Cleveland Clinic
Cleveland, OH, USA

Loïc Guillevin
Department of Internal Medicine
National Reference Center for Rare
Autoimmune and Systemic Diseases
INSERM U1060, Hôpital Cochin
Assistance Publique–Hôpitaux de Paris
University of Paris 5-René-Descartes
27, rue du Faubourg Saint-Jacques
75679 Paris Cedex 14, France

Luc Mouthon
INSERM U1016; Institut Cochin
Université Paris Descartes
CNRS-UMR 8104, Université Sorbonne Paris Cité
Laboratoire d'excellence INFLAMEX
Paris, France

Manish Modi
Department of Neurology
Postgraduate Institute of Medical Education and Research
Chandigarh, India

Manish Rathi
Department of Nephrology
Postgraduate Institute of Medical Education and Research
Chandigarh, India

Manoj Goyal
Department of Neurology
Postgraduate Institute of Medical Education and Research
Chandigarh, India

Mark Little
Trinity College Dublin/Tallaght and Beaumont Hospitals
Trinity Health Kidney Center
Institute of Molecular Medicine
St James's Hospital Campus
Dublin, Ireland

Mohit Dogra
Advance Eye Center
Postgraduate Institute of Medical Education and Research
Chandigarh, India

M Vishnu Vardhan Reddy
Vizag Rheumatology and Immunology Center
Visakhapatnam, Andhra Pradesh, India

Narendra Kumar
Department of Radiotherapy and Regional Cancer Center
Postgraduate Institute of Medical Education and Research
Chandigarh, India

Naresh K Panda
Department of Otolaryngology
Postgraduate Institute of Medical Education and Research
Chandigarh, India

Neha Garg
Division of Arthritis and Rheumatic Diseases
Oregon Health and Science University
Portland, Oregon, USA

NK Khandelwal
Department of Radiodiagnosis and Imaging
Postgraduate Institute of Medical Education and Research
Chandigarh, India

Pankaj Kumar
Department of Radiotherapy and Regional Cancer Center
Postgraduate Institute of Medical Education and Research
Chandigarh, India

Pankaj Malhotra
Department of Internal Medicine
Postgraduate Institute of Medical Education and Research
Chandigarh, India

Patrice Cacoub
Departement Hospitalo-Universitaire I2B
UPMC Univ Paris 06, UMR 7211
F-75005, Paris, France

Paul Bacon
Professor Emeritus
Division of Immunity and Infection
College of Medicine
University of Birmingham
UK

Pradeep Bambery
Bundaberg Base Hospital
Bundaberg, QLD
Australia

Poonam Sharma
Norfolk and Norwich University Hospital
Norwich, UK

Raghavendra Prasada
Department of Gastroenterology
Postgraduate Institute of Medical Education and Research
Chandigarh, India

Rajesh Vijayvergiya
Department of Cardiology
Advanced Cardiac Center
Postgraduate Institute of Medical Education and Research
Chandigarh, India

Rakesh Kochhar
Department of Gastroenterology
Postgraduate Institute of Medical Education and Research
Chandigarh, India

Ram Nath Misra
Department of Clinical Immunology
Sanjay Gandhi Postgraduate Institute of Medical Sciences
Lucknow, Uttar Pradesh, India

Ramya J
Department of Clinical Immunology and Rheumatology
Christian Medical College
Vellore, Tamil Nadu, India

Reema Bansal
Advance Eye Center
Postgraduate Institute of Medical Education and Research
Chandigarh, India

Richard Watts
Consultant Rheumatologist
Ipswich Hospital
Senior Lecturer
Norwich Medical School
Norwich, UK

Ritambhra Nada
Department of Histopathology
Postgraduate Institute of Medical Education and Research
Chandigarh, India

RK Vasishta
Department of Histopathology
Postgraduate Institute of Medical Education and Research
Chandigarh, India

Rohini Handa
Apollo Indraprastha Hospitals
New Delhi, India

Roshan K Verma
Department of Otolaryngology
Postgraduate Institute of Medical Education and Research
Chandigarh, India

Ruchika Goel
Clinical Immunology and Rheumatology
Christian Medical College
Vellore, Tamil Nadu, India

Rupali Agarwal
Department of Radiotherapy and Regional Cancer Center
Postgraduate Institute of Medical Education and Research
Chandigarh, India

Saroj K Sinha
Department of Gastroenterology
Postgraduate Institute of Medical Education and Research
Chandigarh, India

Saujatya Chakraborty
Department of Cardiology
Advanced Cardiac Center
Postgraduate Institute of Medical Education and Research
Chandigarh, India

Shabab Lalit Angurana
Department of Radiotherapy and Regional Cancer Center
Postgraduate Institute of Medical Education and Research
Chandigarh, India

Shankar Naidu
Department of Internal Medicine
Postgraduate Institute of Medical Education and Research
Chandigarh, India

SK Jindal
Department of Pulmonary and Critical Care Medicine
Postgraduate Institute of Medical Education and Research
Chandigarh, India

S Madhusudan
Pediatric Allergy Immunology Unit
Advanced Pediatrics Center
Postgraduate Institute of Medical Education and Research
Chandigarh, India

Subhash Varma
Department of Internal Medicine
Postgraduate Institute of Medical Education and Research
Chandigarh, India

Subramanian Ramaswamy
Department of Rheumatology and Immunology
JSS Medical College
Mysuru, Karnataka, India

Sunil Dogra
Department of Dermatology, Venereology and Leprology
Postgraduate Institute of Medical Education and Research
Chandigarh, India

Surjit Singh
Clinical Immunology and Rheumatology Services
Department of Internal Medicine
Pediatric Allergy Immunology Unit
Advanced Pediatrics Center
Postgraduate Institute of Medical Education and Research
Chandigarh, India

Susmita Sharma
Gian Sagar Medical College and Hospital
Banur, Punjab, India

Tanaz A Kermani
UCLA Med-Rheum
BOX 951670, 2020 Santa Monica Blvd.
Suite 540, Santa Monica,
CA 90404, USA

Tommy CY Chan
Department of Ophthalmology and Visual Sciences
The Chinese University of Hong Kong
Hong Kong

Varun Dhir
Clinical Immunology and Rheumatology Services
Internal Medicine
Postgraduate Institute of Medical Education and Research
Chandigarh, India

Vikas Agarwal
Department of Clinical Immunology
Sanjay Gandhi Postgraduate Institute of Medical Sciences
Lucknow, Uttar Pradesh, India

Vikas Suri
Department of Internal Medicine
Postgraduate Institute of Medical Education and Research
Chandigarh, India

Vinay Keshavamurthy
Department of Dermatology, Venereology and Leprology
Postgraduate Institute of Medical Education and Research
Chandigarh, India

Vinay Sagar
Internal Medicine
Postgraduate Institute of Medical Education and Research
Chandigarh, India

Vinod Ravindran
Department of Rheumatology
MES Medical College
Perinthalmanna, Kerala, India

Vishal Jhanji
Department of Ophthalmology and Visual Sciences
The Chinese University of Hong Kong
Hong Kong

Véronique Witko-Sarsat
INSERM U1016, Institut Cochin
27bis rue du faubourg St Jacques
75014 Paris, France

Wolfgang L Gross
Senior Professor
Department of Rheumatology
University of Luebeck
Germany

Foreword

This unique tome is the first textbook entirely devoted to systemic vasculitis (SV) edited in country by a multinational team of contributors. It will be a boon for colleagues not only in India but also across Asia and the Middle East. It can be whole-heartedly recommended to both; to those physicians who think SV is so rare, they need not bother with it and to those who see themselves as experts in the field and so do not need this new text. All rheumatologists should read it, while physicians across the many fields where multisystem disease can present, should consult it. Systemic vasculitis can involve virtually any organ; and although it may present as pulmonary, renal, or cardiac disease, etc., it is rarely confined to a single system. Awareness of the systemic nature of SV stimulates the need for the collaboration in management which is a major feature of the modern approach to these diseases.

The book is full of detailed guidance for the clinician seeing SV. The in-depth reviews do not just cover the range of individual vasculitic syndromes. A section also addresses the ways in which vasculitis can manifest itself across the spectrum of organs that can be involved; and hence, it may present to different medical specialties. This is an important knowledge needed to adequately assess the extent and severity of individual cases and is the basis of standardized disease activity and disease damage scores. In the absence of suitable laboratory markers, these clinical scores are basic to selecting suitable therapy for individual patients and grading their response to treatment, as discussed here.

For those seeking a deeper understanding of the complex field of vasculitis, the book starts with chapters on the science of inflammation in blood vessels. The histological patterns of involvement in various organs are covered in detail, reflecting the importance of a positive biopsy in the diagnosis of SV. It is pertinent to note the chapter on renal histology, a good example of the benefit of collaboration across specialties. This is often the best site for diagnosis, particularly in antineutrophil cytoplasmic antibody (ANCA)-related vasculitis. In addition, the presence of scarring provides a better guide to long-term renal function than does clinical activity. I have been surprised at the relative reluctance of rheumatologists in Asia to make use of this technique compared to the European or the US practice.

The clinical science of assessing individual patients is included in the section on principles of management along with contributions on the approach to both adults and children with SV. The stimulating chapter on therapy looks at potential future developments as well as the huge advances that treatment has made over the past half-century. Good control of acute flares can be achieved in the large majority of cases but these are not cures and relapse remains a significant feature, so the 10-year prognosis still leaves a lot to be desired.

The cynic may ask whether rare disease warrants a book with this in-depth coverage aimed at all rheumatologists and the wider group of physicians who see SV. The answer must be yes for two reasons. Firstly, systemic vasculitis is a set of severe diseases which can be lethal. Thus, they need aggressive treatment which itself can have problems. Therapy is now directed at the severity of the individual case, as assessed by standardized techniques, rather than at the diagnostic label. Thus, a wider understanding of these syndromes is needed, then it is required, for example, to prescribe antibiotics for a classified infection. The second problem is that the majority of cases present first to generalists—not to the rather small group of vasculitis specialists. The comprehensive coverage of the book will bring sufficient expertise within the range of all to recognize and manage the initial presentation—as well as learning when to refer on.

The book should also open-up future opportunities to readers keen to see the field develop further. The more doctors see and recognize SV; the more opportunities, they have to learn about these syndromes. There are multiple unanswered questions about SV in the underdeveloped world that could be addressed by groups of educated physicians such as Asia-Pacific Leagues of Associations for Rheumatology (APLAR) acting together in collaborative exercises. The most obvious opportunity is in epidemiology. The accepted paradigm is that these are rare disorders and certainly there is a dearth of published scientific papers. One recent review found only a thousand odd cases reported in the Indian literature. However, wherever I have visited, colleagues have shown me their collections of cases suggesting there is a huge range of material seen across that country. There have been no real epidemiological studies to document this. Most series are unreported but some reach the gray literature of unreviewed material. This includes two major series of Takayasu's arteritis, one with 600 cases, described in locally-published monographs. Another problem is that it has come from major referral centers so it is impossible to know the population base that supplies such material. A central disease registry collecting data in a standardized approach across the country would be ideal. An alternative would be regional groups collecting standardized case material in a defined area. It would be more likely to engage a high percentage of local physicians through active feedback and thus to collect more rigorous data. A clear picture of the pattern of disease prevalence in a single area would be a major step forward. As a well-known epidemiologist said to me recently, any data is an important advance in a situation where there is currently no real data.

Outcome studies, using the therapy regimes possible in these diseases on the restricted budgets available, where there is no universal health system, would also be immensely valuable. The result of treatment in real-life practice rarely reflects closely the response to new therapeutic regimes documented in short-term controlled trials with restricted entry criteria. How much this influences the long-term prognosis needs to be examined? There is a particular need to pursue this in Asia where genetic differences, individual reluctance to pursue a long-term drug regime and expense may all play a part in the long-term outcome. Better assessment of disease progression will help this and newer approaches such as ultrasound are getting nearer to the clinical need to incorporate risk-free imaging into routine assessment on follow-up. This is particularly important in Takayasu's arteritis where vessel narrowing and blockage are central features—and, of course, the Indian experience with this disease is so much greater than that of Western nations. This is recognized here by the inclusion of two chapters on imaging SV. One covers the spectrum of conventional imaging from angiography to ultrasonography. The other focuses on the developing field of positron emission tomography-computed tomography (PET-CT).

Any textbook will have some omissions, particularly one that attempts as much as this does. Clearly, there will be some known facets which have not found their way in despite the comprehensive coverage. More importantly, there are many known unknowns, which could be addressed by readers stimulated by the book, to add their experiences to the published literature so as to expand the database of SV available for the next edition. Dr Aman Sharma is to be congratulated on taking on this major effort which should stimulate and empower a new generation of clinicians seeking to provide an accurate future picture of vasculitis as it is seen outside major Western centers.

Paul Bacon
Professor Emeritus
Division of Immunity and Infection
College of Medicine
University of Birmingham, UK

Preface

Vasculitides are enigmatic diseases having the prowess to test the skills of even the most astute clinicians. Since the first description more than two centuries ago, a lot has been written about these diseases, and rapid strides have been taken in various areas of vasculitis research in recent times. These include the areas of genetics, epidemiology, basic sciences including animal models, revised nomenclature systems, imaging modalities such as positron emission tomography (PET) scanning, disease activity assessment tools and some promising newer therapies which are raising the questions of changing the standard of care of some of these diseases.

The book is not an attempt to replace but to complement the existing texts. The contributors have been chosen due to their standing in the field or rich individual experience in a particular aspect.

The book has six sections. The first section deals with epidemiology, genetics, and classification of vasculitis syndrome. There are likely to be changes in the classification system once the results of some of the ongoing studies become available, and these can be incorporated in the subsequent editions of the book. The second section deals with basic sciences and discusses the role of neutrophils, antineutrophil cytoplasmic antibodies, and details skin, nerves and brain, lungs and kidney pathology. The understanding of vasculitis can never be complete without the knowledge of pathology, and hence a special emphasis has been laid down on the details of pathological changes in the areas most commonly inflicted by these diseases. These sections contain innumerable illustrative microphotographs of various pathological changes in different organs and would be of interest to both the clinicians and pathologists. The third section deals with imaging modalities as they have assumed a significant role in diagnosing and assessing disease activity.

The fourth section deals with the clinical manifestations based upon organ system. The fifth section has chapters detailing the approach to children and adults with vasculitis and assessing disease activity and damage. Newer therapies have been shown great promise in management of these disorders, thus newer and future modalities have been discussed in this section. The last section deals with the individual vasculitis syndromes. Management of these diseases is a challenge.

As is true for other areas of Medicine, a lot is still to be learnt about these diseases. I sincerely hope that the book, with the comprehensive outline can help in 'bridging the gap' and would meet the needs of practicing and academic rheumatologists, pathologists, internists and other clinicians involved in management of patients with systemic vasculitides.

Aman Sharma

Acknowledgments

I would like to put on record, my acknowledgment to Professor Pradeep Bambery, who taught me to think out of the book while dealing with these diseases, Professor Subhash Chander Varma for being a role model teacher, Professor SK Jindal for guiding me from the very beginning of this project and Professor Amod Gupta for being instrumental in making the idea of this book a reality. I would like to thank all the international and national contributors, who accepted my request to contribute to the book. Dr Ashwani Jha and Dr Ashish Aggarwal need a special mention for painstakingly proofreading the draft manuscripts. I would also like to thank Shri Jitendar P Vij (Group Chairman), Mr Ankit Vij (Group President) and Mr Tarun Duneja (Director–Publishing) of M/s Jaypee Brothers Medical Publishers (P) Ltd, New Delhi, India, for making this project a success.

Contents

SECTION 6 Individual Vasculitis Syndromes

Introduction

- Epidemiology of Systemic Vasculitis
- Genetics of Vasculitis
- Classification of Vasculitis

CHAPTER 1

Epidemiology of Systemic Vasculitis

David GI Scott, Paul Bacon

INTRODUCTION

The vasculitides are relatively uncommon conditions whose etiology is still poorly understood, and this has made detailed epidemiology studies difficult. They can affect any age. Two diseases predominate in children—Kawasaki's disease (KD) and Henoch-Schönlein Purpura (HSP), while the other more common systemic vasculitides occur with increasing age. Changing definitions and understanding of these diseases have led to epidemiology studies being relatively recent, but the development of prospective population-based registers has been an important emerging database for comparative studies in recent years. Hopefully, this trend will be extended across the less-developed world as interest in these diseases extends.

Epidemiology studies require a sound basis for classification and that has also evolved over recent years. Of particular importance have been the American College of Rheumatology (ACR) classification criteria 1990 and the two Chapel Hill Consensus Conference (CHCC) definitions for vasculitis proposing criteria for classifying vasculitides with a variety of sensitivities and specificities. The most sensitive and specific of the seven ACR criteria were found in Churg–Strauss syndrome (now called eosinophilic granulomatosis with polyangiitis [EGPA]), giant cell arteritis (GCA), and Takayasu's arteritis (TAK). That study also identified a condition called hypersensitivity vasculitis which has disappeared (no longer recognized) from current definitions, as it has been replaced mainly by HSP and microscopic polyangiitis (MPA). The next development was the first CHCC in 1994 which included MPA but did not consider the role of antineutrophil cytoplasmic antibodies (ANCAs). Because of this and further developments in understanding pathogenesis, a further consensus conference was called in 2011 and this led to the current classification shown in Table 1.1. This recognizes the

importance of ANCA in separating small-vessel vasculitis into ANCA-associated vasculitis (AAV) or immune complex-associated vasculitis, and also recognizes potential probable etiologies, as shown in the Table. It also reflects the fact that some vasculitides are restricted to a single organ and others associated with systemic disease. Furthermore, it recognizes the fact that some vasculitides can affect a wide variety of blood vessels, particularly Behçet's syndrome and Cogan's syndrome. The consensus also introduced different nomenclature, particularly for HSP—now known as immunoglobulin A (IgA) vasculitis, Churg-Strauss syndrome (now known as eosinophilic granulomatosis with polyangiitis)—and confirmed the move away from Wegener's granulomatosis to the term granulomatosis with polyangiitis. Currently, the eponyms are still included after the descriptive terms to avoid confusion, but it is expected that these will disappear with time.

It is important to recognize that the definitions of the different vasculitic diseases did not change dramatically between 1994 and 2011, and so the original criteria are still used in epidemiology studies. The problem has been that the original CHCC (1994) and ACR criteria did not have any classification criteria for MPA and polyarteritis nodosa (PAN) which has made epidemiological studies in those diseases more difficult. What follows is a brief description of current epidemiological data for the commoner types of vasculitis based on the classification system shown in Table 1.1, i.e. large-, medium-, and small-vessel disease.

LARGE-VESSEL VASCULITIS

Giant Cell Arteritis

Giant cell arteritis (GCA) is defined in CHCC 2012 as "arteritis, often granulomatous, usually affecting the aorta or

Table 1.1 Classification of the vasculitides[*]

Dominant vessel	Idiopathic (primary)	Probable etiology (secondary)
Large	Takayasu's arteritis Giant cell arteritis	Aortitis associated with tuberculosis, syphilis, RA, AS
Medium	Polyarteritis nodosa Kawasaki's disease	Polyarteritis nodosa (HBV associated)
Small ANCA	Microscopic polyangiitis Granulomatosis with polyangiitis (Wegener's) Eosinophilic granulomatosis with polyangiitis (Churg-Strauss)	Drugs Propylthiouracil[a] Hydralazine[a]
Immune complex	Cryoglobulinemic vasculitis (non-HCV) Anti-GBM disease IgA vasculitis (Henoch-Schönlein) Hypocomplementemic vasculitis	Cryoglobulinemic vasculitis (HCV associated) Vasculitis associated with RA, SLE, Sjögren's syndrome, and many drugs[b]
Variable	Behçet's syndrome Cogan's syndrome	

Source: Epidemiology of Vasculitis, Richard A Watts & David GI Scott, Oxford Textbook of Vasculitis, 3rd Edition, page 7
[a] Most commonly induce MPO-ANCA
[b] For example, sulfonamides, penicillins, thiazide diuretics, and many others.
Abbreviations: RA, Rheumatoid arthritis; AS, Ankylosing spondylitis; SLE, Systemic lupus erythematosus; HBV, Hepatitis B virus; HCV, Hepatitis C virus

its major branches with a predilection for the branches of the carotid and vertebral arteritis. Often involves the temporal artery. Onset usually in patients older than 50 and often associated with polymyalgia rheumatica (PMR)."[1] Difficulties in reviewing epidemiology studies relate particularly to the presence or absence of biopsy. Most older studies include only biopsy-positive cases. Biopsy rates and the intensity of the histological search for evidence of arteritis will therefore have a profound effect on any reported incidence. Giant cell arteritis is also closely related to polymyalgia and there are different epidemiology studies for polymyalgia and for GCA. It is reckoned that about 20% of patients with polymyalgia have biopsy-proven GCA, and conversely more than 40% of patients with GCA have polymyalgic symptoms.

A summary of the extensive current data on this suggests that the annual incidence is particularly high in Scandinavia, with an annual rate between 15 and 35 per 100,000 individuals over 50. Similar rates have been described in the United States and in a community study in the United Kingdom. There is an increasing incidence with age which peaks in those 80 years or more. It is very rare under the age of 50 (summarized in Ref. 2).

Time Trends

Over the last six or seven decades, incidence of GCA appears to have increased, certainly in those reported from Olmstead County (Minnesota, USA). Between 1950–1954 and 1980–1984, the annual incidence increased from 6.7 to 28.5 per year per 100,000 individual over 50. Since then, the rate appears to have stabilized. Similar changes over time were noted in Sweden and Spain. Some of this increase may reflect improved recognition of cases as well as an aging population.

Giant cell arteritis appears to be more common in higher latitudes such as Scandinavia, whereas studies from southern Europe consistently reported low incidence rates than those from Scandinavia. Similar findings have been reported within North America where the lowest incidence is reported in the south.

Ethnic Differences

Giant cell arteritis appears to be most common in Caucasians and is uncommon in non-Caucasians. The incidence is highest in Scandinavians and in populations descended from them (e.g., the population from Olmstead County). Within America, there appears to be a particularly low incidence in African Americans (0.36 per 100,000 over the age of 50) compared with 2.24 in the white population in Tennessee.[2] A study from California also suggested that GCA is much less common in Asians than Caucasians. There is also a particularly low incidence in Japan compared with Europe[3] but this has not been studied elsewhere in Asia.

Genetic Factors

These have been linked particularly to the human leukocyte antigen (HLA) DR4 and HLA DRB1*0401 genes. It is interesting that these genes are much less common in the normal Japanese population, which may explain why GCA is seen much less commonly in Japan.

Environmental Factors

The latitude effect on incidence is also seen in multiple sclerosis and rheumatoid arthritis (RA), and possibilities to explain this have included the effects of exposure to UV light and its potential effect on vitamin D synthesis. In the Olmstead County cohort, they describe peaks in incidence every 7 years, which suggests a possible infectious etiology, and some studies have suggested an association with *mycoplasma pneumoniae* but this has never been confirmed. Some, but not all studies, have suggested a season of maximum occurrence with GCA more likely to be diagnosed in warmer summer months in the United Kingdom.

Takayasu's Arteritis

Takayasu's arteritis was described in Japan in 1908, although older case reports indicate that it was not a new disease. The 2012 CHCC definition describes TAK as "arteritis, often granulomatous, predominately effecting the aorta and/or its major branches. Onset is usually in patients younger than 50."[1] It is thought to be much more common in Asia than in the United Kingdom, with an incidence somewhere between 0.5 and 3 per million. The peak age of onset is in the third decade and it is more common in women.

Takayasu's arteritis has been described in most ethnic groups, including Africans and Asians, and may be particularly common in India. Some reports suggest a high incidence in India, with as many as 500 patients with TAK attending vasculitis clinics in Mumbai or cardiology clinics in Kolkata. Takayasu's arteritis also has a higher prevalence in Japan (40 per million) compared with Europe (4–7 per million) and is also more common in Turkey (15 per million). Different subtypes of TAK are recognized depending on the site of major vessel involvement at arteriography. In India and other South Asian countries, the renal arteritis are affected the majority of patients, leading to a high number presenting with hypertension at a young age. In South African patients, lower abdominal aorta involvement is more common than in Japan. Aneurysmal disease is also more common in Africa compared with Japan.

The etiology of TAK is unknown. The granulomatous nature has suggested links to mycobacterial disease but that has never been proven. Genetic susceptibility may be important, as it has been recorded in monozygotic twins, and about 1% of Japanese patients with TAK have an affected relative.

MEDIUM-VESSEL VASCULITIS

Kawasaki's Disease

The CHCC 2012 defined Kawasaki's disease (KD) as "arteritis associated with mucocutaneous lymph node syndrome and predominantly affecting medium and small arteries. Coronary arteries are often involved. Aorta and large arteries may be involved. Usually occurs in infants and children."[1] The most obvious difference between KD and other vasculitides is its predilection for infants and young children. It was first recognized in Japan, which still has the highest incidence of over 200 per 100,000 per year in children aged under 5.

Geographical variations and ethnic factors are important. Kawasaki's disease is for example rare in the United Kingdom but much more common in individuals from southeast Asia. A study from Birmingham showed an incidence of 14.6 per 100,000 per year in children aged under 5 in Asians from the Indian subcontinent as compared with 5.9 per 100,000 per year in black Afro-Caribbeans and 4.6 per 100,000 per year in Caucasians.[4] A large case series has been recently described from Chandigarh.[5] Similarly in the United States, the incidence is highest amongst southeast Asians and Pacific islanders (2.4 times more common than in the white population). Interestingly, in Hawaii, the state with the highest proportion of southeast Asians or Pacific islanders, the incidence amongst Japanese Americans is very similar to that in native Japanese and twice that in native Hawaiians or Chinese Americans. Kawasaki's disease is also slightly more common in boys and the age-specific incidence is greatest in children aged 6–11 months, with nearly 90% of cases aged <5 years.

Other Factors

A lot of research has gone into possible infectious etiology because of the predominance of the disease in young children. It is rare before 6 months, suggesting that passively acquired maternal immunity may prevent the disease and the low frequency after the age of 5 suggests a possible early exposure to a common pathogen against which children mount an appropriate protective immune response. There have also been "epidemics" described in Japan and a seasonal variation with a peak incidence in winter and summer. However, there has been no convincing organism detected as a possible cause.

Polyarteritis Nodosa

This was the disease originally described by Kussmaul and Maier in 1866. The CHCC 2010 definition of PAN is "necrotising arteritis with medium or small arteries without glomerulonephritis or vasculitis in arterials, capillaries or venules and not associated with ANCA."[1] One of the clinical features that differentiate PAN from the smaller vessel vasculitides is its ability to cause major organ infarction and/or hemorrhage (the latter due to ruptured aneurysms). It is important to recognize that before the 1980s there was a significant overlap between cases labelled as PAN and MPA, and it was really only the development of the CHCC definitions in 1994 that helped to distinguish it followed by the introduction of ANCA. Microscopic polyangiitis is typically associated with myeloperoxidase (MPO) ANCA, and although patients with this disease can occasionally have larger artery involvement similar to that seen in PAN, the converse is not true, i.e., PAN is defined as having an absence of involvement of smaller vessels, as defined above, and is virtually always ANCA negative.

The estimated annual incidence is therefore difficult to interpret, making an exact figure unrealistic. The impression from our local studies is that PAN is much rarer than the smaller vessel vasculitides, probably with an incidence of less than 1 per million per year. It is also apparent from studies in France that the incidence is falling as the public health impact on controlling hepatitis B virus infection by vaccination takes effect. Personal experience suggests that it is still seen regularly in India but cases are predominantly hepatitis B negative.

Ethnic Differences

A particularly high incidence of PAN was recorded in Alaskan Indians in the 1980s, but this was in a very small population and all were positive for hepatitis B infection (PAN incidence 77 per million per year). The only other studies with high incidence rates are also in populations with a high hepatitis B infection including one French series (30 per million per year) and a Swedish study (31 per million per year).

SMALL-VESSEL VASCULITIS ANCA-ASSOCIATED VASCULITIS

The CHCC 2012 split small-vessel vasculitides into those associated with ANCA and those associated with immune complexes. Some older series include patients who fulfil more than one set of criteria, particularly in the ANCA-associated group (i.e., MPA and GPA). Clearly, accurate epidemiology requires a diagnosis without any overlap and an algorithm developed to sort this has been applied to many of the populations discussed.[6,7]

Granulomatosis with Polyangiitis (Wegener's Granulomatosis)

Granulomatosis with polyangiitis was first described in the 1930s (by Klinger as well as Wegener) and is defined by the CHCC 2012 as "necrotizing granulomatous inflammation usually involving the upper and lower respiratory tract and necrotising vasculitis involving predominantly small vessels (e.g. capillaries, venules, arterioles). Necrotising glomerulonephritis is common."[1]

Time Trends

The incidence of GPA appeared to increase in the 1980s following the introduction of ANCA. Other studies since then have suggested a relatively stable incidence and we have not seen any significant change during the 22-year period of the Norwich Vasculitis Cohort.[8] However, we did see a periodicity with peaks every 7.7 years (not seen in MPA), suggesting a possible infectious etiology.

The prevalence, however, has increased over time, but this probably reflects better treatment leading to improved mortality. The recent estimates for Norwich record a prevalence of 146 per million in 2008 similar to a study from Lund with a rate of 160 per million in 2003.[8, 9]

Geographical Factors

The incidence of GPA appears to be higher in northern Europe as compared with southern Europe and is much more common in northern Europe than in Japan where GPA is relatively rare. Studies from India suggest that some patients with GPA may be misdiagnosed because of similarities in pulmonary presentation.

Ethnic Factors

The incidence rates are similar in most Caucasian populations, but the incidence is lower (approximately halved) in nonwhite Caucasian populations in Europe.[10] Similarly in New Zealand, GPA is twice as common in Europeans as compared with Maoris or Asians.[11] In Japan, GPA is much less common than MPA and also the incidence of the associated antibody cANCA or PR3 ANCA is much rarer in Japan than pANCA or MPO ANCA. Similar findings have been reported from China.

Genetic Factors

Various HLA associations have been studied but often in too small populations, but a recent genome-wide association study has shown significant associations. PR3 ANCA was associated with three specific genes—HLA DP, SERPINA 2, and PRTN3. SERPINA 1 encodes alpha-1 antitrypsin which may also be important.

Environmental Factors

A variety of environmental factors have been suggested. Seasonal differences have been described by some but not others; infection may be important, particularly upper respiratory infection with or nasal carriage of *Staphylococcus*. The presence of *Staph aureus* has been associated particularly with an increased risk of relapse. The predominance of GPA in northern versus southern European populations has led to a suggestion that UV radiation might be important (as was mentioned previously in association with GPA).

There have been extensive studies looking at potential occupational exposure. Of note has been an association with silica but that is perhaps more closely linked to MPA than GPA. There are also some data reporting links with occupational exposure to hydrocarbons such as paints and glues, and our own study showed an association with farming. It was not possible to distinguish what type of farming was important although the association appeared stronger in livestock than crops.[12]

Microscopic Polyangiitis

The first description of the disease we now call MPA, in 1948 by Davson and colleagues, used the term microscopic polyarteritis. MPA became the preferred term with the description of the association of this disease with MPO ANCA

and at the time of the 1994 Chapel Hill Conference. Chapel Hill Consensus Conference 2012 defines MPA as "necrotising vasculitis with few or no immune deposits, predominantly affecting small vessels (i.e. capillaries, venules, arterioles). Necrotising arteritis involving small or medium arteries may be present. Necrotising glomerulonephritis is very common. Pulmonary capillaritis often occurs. Granulomatous inflammation is absent."[1] As previously described in the section on PAN, the literature regarding epidemiology has to be carefully interpreted because of the overlapping features of these two diseases prior to the introduction of CHCC definitions.

Time Trends

The incidence of MPA appeared to increase in the 1980s following the introduction of ANCA and our most recent studies suggest an annual incidence of 5.9 per million per year. Other studies from Stockholm also showed an increasing incidence between 1986 and 1992 although we have seen no obvious change in incidence since then. It seems likely that some of the increase in incidence was due to better recognition and changing ideas regarding diagnosis and classification.

Geographical Factors

The north/south gradient relating to the incidence of MPA is the inverse of that seen in GPA. Microscopic polyangiitis is more common in southern Europe (e.g., Lugo, Spain) as compared with Tromsø in northern Norway.[13] The two geographical regions with an apparently high incidence of MPA and PAN are Japan and Kuwait, but the reasons for this are unclear.

Ethnic Differences

The Kuwait study reported only Kuwaitis with vasculitis. In Japan, studies from the Miyazaki prefecture showed an incidence of MPA much higher than European Caucasian populations and as outlined above, MPO ANCA much more frequent than PR3 ANCA-associated disease.

Environmental Factors

Microscopic polyangiitis has been associated with a number of environmental factors, particularly silica, hydrocarbons, drugs, and infections. Drug-associated vasculitis appears to be particularly associated with MPO ANCA and most commonly mimics MPA. The drugs most commonly associated with this are propylthiouracil and hydralazine although others have been implicated.

Case reports have described vasculitis in association with pulmonary silicosis, and as described for GPA, there has been a significant association with silica in many studies, more associated with MPA than GPA. An interesting study after a major earthquake in Kobe, Japan, in 1995 showed a trebling of the incidence of MPO ANCA-associated vasculitis, thought possibly to relate to high levels of silica dust caused by the earthquake. Studies in Norwich showed no significant association between MPA alone and occupational silica exposure, but there was an association overall with the whole range of AAVs.

Eosinophilic Granulomatosis with Polyangiitis (Churg-Strauss)

Eosinophilic granulomatosis with polyangiitis was first described in 1951 by two American pathologists who described features of patients at postmortem.[14] The CHCC 2012 defined EGPA as "eosinophil rich and necrotising granulomatous inflammation often involving the respiratory tract and necrotising vasculitis affecting predominantly small to medium vessels and associated with asthma and eosinophilia. ANCA is more frequent when glomerulonephritis is present."[1] The incidence of EGPA appears broadly similar in all populations and is less common than GPA or MPA, with an incidence of between 0.5 and 2 million per year. Prevalence data show that EGPA is rarer than GPA or MPA in all countries studied, including the United Kingdom, New Zealand, and France (range 10–20 per million).

Environmental Factors

The cause of EGPA is unknown but the strong association with asthma suggests that inhaled antigens may be important. Eosinophilic granulomatosis with polyangiitis has also been described in association with vaccination and desensitization and with some drugs including sulfonamides. It has also been linked to the use of leukotriene inhibitors. Initial studies suggested that this was due to a masking of disease and steroid reduction, but a study from New Zealand showed that the drug may actually act as a trigger for the development of EGPA.

SMALL-VESSEL VASCULITIS-IMMUNE COMPLEX

IgA Vasculitis (Henoch-Schönlein Purpura)

This disease was first described by Heberden in the late 18th century but is attributed to Schönlein (1837), who described the purpura and arthritis, and Henoch (1874), who described the additional features of abdominal pain and kidney involvement. The importance of IgA has been recognized over recent decades, and it is clear that the original ACR studies included patients who we would now define as HSP but who were then classified as hypersensitivity vasculitis. There has therefore been a change in the definition of IgA vasculitis/HSP such that the CHCC 2012 defined IgA vasculitis as "vasculitis with IgA 1 dominant immune deposits, affecting small vessels (predominantly capillaries, venules or arterioles). Often involves skin and gut and frequently causes arthritis. Glomerulonephritis indistinguishable from IgA nephropathy may occur."[1] IgA vasculitis occurs predominantly in children, the peak onset at 5-6 years. It is relatively rare in adults with an incidence of 3 per million per year in adults as compared to 10–20 per 100,000 per year in children <17.

IgA vasculitis is slightly more common in Asians from the Indian subcontinent as compared with white Caucasians and blacks—24 per 100,000 per year in Asians, 17 per 100,000 per year in Caucasians, and 6 per 100,000 per year in blacks, all aged less than 17 years. Drugs have often been implicated in the etiology of IgA vasculitis (these include antibiotics, beta-lactams, analgesics, and nonsteroidal anti-inflammatory drugs).

Vasculitis Associated with Specific Conditions

Vasculitis has been described for many years associated with diseases such as RA, systemic lupus erythematosus, and Sjogren's syndrome. There are few classification criteria for these and less data than in the primary vasculitides.

Systemic Rheumatoid Vasculitis

A histological description of vasculitis in a patient with RA goes back to 1898, but the clinical studies really appeared in the 1940s and 1950s when patients presented with peripheral gangrene, mononeuritis multiplex and a variety of other systemic involvement.[15,16] All types of blood vessels can be involved, with small-vessel vasculitis being more common. This can manifest as a relatively benign nail fold or nail edge infarcts, but this may also be associated with more widespread systemic disease. Systemic rheumatoid vasculitis is most commonly seen in patients with long-standing seropositive erosive RA and more common comparatively in males than females.

There was a strong association between the onset of rheumatoid vasculitis and unrestrained glucocorticoid use in the 1950s and 1960s, suggesting that it may be an important causative factor. It is clear that rheumatoid vasculitis has become less common with the reducing use of glucocorticoids, but even in the original studies, patients were seen who had never been treated with these drugs. The incidence peaked at over 10 per million in the 1970s and 1980s but has now fallen to <4 per million per year in our studies. The relative rarity of rheumatoid vasculitis was first noted in North America and appeared to occur in the United Kingdom in the 1990s so is probably related to better controlled disease with drugs such as methotrexate but not linked to the introduction of biologic agents.

Other Vasculitides

The list of vasculitides shown in Table 1.1 indicates that we have not covered disease such as Cogan's, Behçet's, cryoglobulinemia, or anti-GBM disease. Behçet's disease is more difficult because the clinical features of Behçet's disease are not always due to vasculitis, and the epidemiology of that disease is outside the remit of this chapter. The other diseases have not been well studied in terms of epidemiology. Here, as indicated in the major syndromes discussed above, there is a tremendous need for prospective population-based studies such as disease registers. The increasing interest in systemic vasculitis needs to be accompanied by a strong move away from individual stamp collecting of rarities to organized collaborative systemic studies.

This chapter was adapted from Epidemiology of Vasculitis by Watts and Scott 2014[17] (see references therein).

KEY POINTS

- Epidemiology studies are limited by insufficient detailed studies in vasculitis.
- Standardized definitions and improved classification should stimulate population-based disease registers and prospective studies.

REFERENCES

1. Jennette JC, Falk RJ, Bacon PA, et al. 2012 revised International Chapel Hill Consensus Conference Nomenclature of Vasculitides. Arthritis Rheum. 2013;65:1-11.
2. Smith CA, Fidler WJ, Pinals RS. The epidemiology of giant cell arteritis. Report of a ten-year study in Shelby county, Tennessee. Arthritis Rheum. 1983;26:1214-9.
3. Kobayashi S, Yano T, Matsumoto Y, et al. Clinical and epidemiologic analysis of giant cell (temporal) arteritis from a nationwide survey in 1998 in Japan: the first government-supported nationwide survey. Arthritis Rheum. 2003;49:594-8.
4. Gardner-Medwin JM, Dolezalova P, Cummins C, et al. Incidence of Henoch–Schonlein purpura, Kawasaki disease, and rare vasculitides in children of different ethnic origins. Lancet. 2002;360:1197-202.
5. Singh S, Aulakh R, Bhalla AK, et al. Is Kawasaki disease incidence rising in Chandigarh, north India? Arch Dis Child. 2011;96:137-40.
6. Watts R, Lane S, Hanslik T, et al. Development and validation of a consensus methodology for the classification of the ANCA-associated vasculitides and polyarteritis nodosa for epidemiological studies. Ann Rheum Dis. 2007;66:222-7.
7. Liu LJ, Chen M, Yu F, et al. Evaluation of a new algorithm in classification of systemic vasculitis. Rheumatology (Oxford). 2008;47:708-12.
8. Watts RA, Scott DG. ANCA vasculitis: to lump or split? Why we should study MPA and GPA separately. Rheumatology (Oxford). 2012;51:2115-7.
9. Mohammad AJ, Jacobsson LT, Mahr AD, et al. Prevalence of Wegener's granulomatosis, microscopic polyangiitis, polyarteritis nodosa and Churg–Strauss syndrome within a defined population in southern Sweden. Rheumatology (Oxford). 2007;46:1329-37.
10. Mahr A, Guillevin L, Poissonnet M, et al. Prevalences of polyarteritis nodosa, microscopic polyangiitis, Wegener's granulomatosis, and Churg–Strauss syndrome in a French urban multiethnic population in 2000: a capture–recapture estimate. Arthritis Rheum. 2004;51:92-9.
11. O'Donnell JL, Stevanovic VR, Frampton C, et al. Wegener's granulomatosis in New Zealand: evidence for a latitude-dependent incidence gradient. Intern Med J. 2007;37:242-6.
12. Lane SE, Watts RA, Bentham G, et al. Are environmental factors important in primary systemic vasculitis? A case–control study. Arthritis Rheum. 2003;48:814-23.
13. Watts RA, Gonzalez-Gay MA, Lane SE, et al. Geoepidemiology of systemic vasculitis: comparison of the incidence in two regions of Europe. Ann Rheum Dis. 2001;60:170-2.
14. Churg J, Strauss L. Allergic granulomatosis, allergic angiitis, and periarteritis nodosa. Am J Pathol. 1951;27:277-301.
15. Scott DG, Bacon PA, Tribe CR. Systemic rheumatoid vasculitis: a clinical and laboratory study of 50 cases. Medicine (Baltimore). 1981;60:288-97.
16. Bywaters EG, Scott JT. The natural history of vascular lesions in rheumatoid arthritis. J Chronic Dis. 1963;16:905-14.
17. Ball GV, Fessler BJ, Bridges SL Jr. Oxford Textbook of Vasculitis. Oxford University Press; 2014.

CHAPTER 2

Genetics of Vasculitis

John Mathew, Ramya J

INTRODUCTION

A common approach to establishing the genetic contribution to any disease is to conduct a stepwise family studies. General scheme involves the following:

- To establish familial aggregation of a phenotype in a family.
- Twin studies to look for a difference in concordance rates among mono- and dizygotic twins.
- Adoption studies to determine the degree of genetic contribution as compared to environmental influences.

Vasculitis being a group of rare heterogeneous disorders, it is difficult to carry out the above studies that require large sample sizes. Epidemiological studies have clearly pointed out the genetic predisposition in Behçet's disease[1] and Kawasaki disease (KD).[2-4] The differences in prevalence across geographic locations and ethnic background clearly point to the role of genetics in addition to environmental exposures in vasculitic disorders such as giant cell arteritis (GCA), Takayasu's arteritis (TA), and antineutrophil cytoplasmic antibodies (ANCA) associated vasculitis (AAV).

Candidate gene studies and genome-wide association studies (GWAS) are currently the methods by which diseases with complex genetics can be studied.[5]

Candidate genes are those with known functions implied in the expression of the investigated traits, which can be evaluated by an association analysis with the effects of the causative gene variants.[6] The genes in these studies are selected because of their possible etiological role for the disease, based on a biological pathway.[7] Association studies with candidate genes have been widely used for the study of complex diseases. It is limited by its inability to include all possible causative genes and polymorphisms. The pathogenesis of a disease needs to be at least partially understood to identify a candidate gene.

Genome-wide association studies can assess the genetic risk by assaying common variants across the genome, but to achieve statistical significance it requires a large sample size. This is difficult in rare diseases like vasculitis.

We shall proceed in order of the classification system of vasculitis.

LARGE-VESSEL VASCULITIS

Behçet's Disease (Variable-vessel Vasculitis)

The prevalence and severity of Behçet's disease is significantly higher in Middle East and Mediterranean.[8] Familial aggregation in various frequencies has been documented across the globe; highest being in Turkey (a country with highest prevalence) with a sibling recurrence risk of 18.2%.[1] Migrant Turks in West Berlin, Germany, have 40 times higher prevalence than their German peers.[9] Twin studies in Behçet's have found a concordance ratio of 2 in 6 for monozygotic twins and 1 in 8 for dizygotic twins[10] suggesting a significant genetic predisposition.[10] An earlier age at disease onset in children compared to their parents was present in 84% of the families studied suggesting genetic anticipation.[11]

Human Leukocyte Antigen Genes

Human leukocyte antigen (HLA)-B51 has been implicated as the strongest risk allele in several populations of diverse ethnicity.

Its contribution to genetic susceptibility is estimated to be 20%.[12] Although the prevalence of the HLA-B51 allele may vary in different population—its presence definitely confers increased risk when present. A meta-analysis quantifying the genetic effect of the HLA-B51/HLA-B5 allele on the risk of developing Behçet's showed a pooled odds ratio (OR) of 5.78 (CI 5–6.67) in carriers compared to noncarriers. Subgroup analysis of studies involving different ethnic populations showed similar odds ratios. Of the 89 subtypes of HLA-B51, HLA-B5101 is the commonest. Takemoto et al. have investigated the HLA-B5101 gene in Japanese, Turkish, Jordanian, and Iranian population and have found HLA-B510101 to be present in all patients.[13] The pathogenic role of HLA-B51 is not yet clear—it may be partly responsible for neutrophil hyperfunction.[14] 25% of patients are found to be HLA-B51 negative. Linkage studies have suggested HLA-A26:01, HLA-B15 and HLA-B57:01 as genetic risk factors independent of HLA-B51 in Japanese, Taiwanese, Greek and German populations.[12] This is supported by evidence from GWAS performed by Meguro et al.[12]

MHC-class I related gene A (MICA) although found to be associated in several studies appears to be in strong linkage dysequilibrium with HLA-B51.

Non-HLA Genes

The first GWAS study using pooled genetic data from Turkey identified five novel susceptibility loci—LOC100129342, KIAA1529, CPVL, UBASH3B, UBAC2 with an OR of 1.6–2.3.[15] These were new loci with no previously known associations. Further replication studies confirm the association of UBAC2 in four different replication cohorts.[12] UBASH 3B and UBAC2 code for ubiquitin and CPVL codes for carboxypeptidase.

GWAS by Remmers et al. established interleukin-10 (IL 10) variant (OR :1.45) and a variant located between IL 23 receptor and IL 12 receptor beta 2 gene (OR: 1.28) Mizuki et al replicated the same result in a GWAS performed in Japanese population.[12]

There have been several candidate gene studies on Behçet's disease. The most important of those are as follows: polymorphisms in E298D, which is a gene for endothelial nitric oxide synthase in cohorts in Turkey and Tunisia.[16] The other important studies involve mutations in (Mediterranean fever) gene that confers an increased risk with an OR of 2.96–4.55 in various studies involving middle-eastern population.[17,18] The role of MEFV explains the clinical observation that features of Behçet's and familial Mediterranean fever (FMF) are sometimes seen in the same patient. Carriage of MEFV mutation confers increased risk of developing vascular involvement and venous thrombosis in Behçet's disease.[19]

Takayasu's Arteritis

It is well known as a rare illness affecting young women of the south-eastern Asian origin. However, it is known to occur worldwide with varying demographics. Familial occurrence is considered rare in Takayasu—so far it has been reported in 32[61] families predominantly in Japan,[20,21] including two case reports of aortoarteritis in sisters in India.[22,23] Since familial occurrence is restricted to few case reports family/twin studies are rare. Fugito Numano et al. have done HLA A and B typing in 6 families with 2 more family members with Takayasu as early as 1972.[62] They found a common haplotype composed of A9, A10, B5 and BW 40 in Takayasu patients. Subsequently there has been several HLA associations in familial Takayasu cases but no further studies have been undertaken.

There are well-established association between HLA-B52 (HLA-B5201) in various population cohorts with high OR (3.7–10.2)—Indian, Mexican, Turkish and Japanese.[24] HLA-B51 bears strong homology to HLA-B52 differing by just two amino acids. HLA-B51, which has strong genetic association with Behçet's, is shown to have no association with TA.[25,26] Amino acid at 67th position in the HLA-B protein is particularly reported to be important.[27,28] Although previous studies have implicated HLA-B39 to be associated with severe disease, the results have not been replicated in the recent studies.[29]

Recent candidate gene studies from Japan have discovered the HLA-B67:01 allele as an independent association with TA.[30] However, this allele has not been reported in studies from Turkey/America—hence this may be an important association in patients of Asian origin. No difference has been found in clinical characteristics of patients who were positive/ negative for the above HLA alleles.

Two GWAS were published in 2013 simultaneously by Japanese and Turkish/US groups. The GWAS from the Japanese group identified two susceptibility loci: IL-12B region in chromosome 5 (OR = 1.75), MLX region (OR = 1.50), and HLA-B region.[31] The polymorphism in the IL-12B region was shown to have a synergistic effect on TA susceptibility in combination with HLA-B5201. The GWAS from Turkish/ US cohorts identified multiple susceptibility loci, including HLA-B/MICA (OR = 3.29) and HLA-DQB1/HLA-DRB1 (OR = 2.34/2.47).[24] The other susceptibility loci identified and confirmed were FCGR2A/FCGR3A locus on chromosome 1 (OR = 1.81) and IL-12B (OR = 1.54).[31] Future studies will make the understanding of TA better in the background of these susceptibility alleles detected in GWAS.

Giant Cell Arteritis

The well-known differences in the prevalence of GCA in western nordic population as compared to eastern countries may be related to lower frequency of the HLA-DRB1*0401 and HLA-DRB1*0404 alleles in Japanese healthy control population as compared to American control population.[32]

The prevalance of familial GCA is 1 in 83 (1 in 250 to 500 is expected by chance). 18 of the 32 (56%) familial patients assessed carried DR4 antigen.[33,63] The association with HLA-DRB1*04 has been consistently found in various North American and European cohorts. Initial studies showed weak association with major histocompatibility complex class I molecules. In the recent studies, notable association has been found between HLA-B*15 (OR = 2.7) and MICA A5 allele (OR = 2.2) (MHC class I polypeptide-related sequence A) gene in a Caucasian population in Spain.[34] The MICA gene encodes a stress-induced transmembrane molecule as an independent signal protein within MHC class I signaling. As we have discussed previously, it is found in association with Behçet's disease and TA as well.

A number of non-HLA polymorphisms have been associated with GCA. Most of these are in genes encoding inflammatory molecules (cytokines, cytokine receptors, molecules involved in endothelial function, genes of innate immunity) implicated in the pathogenesis of GCA. Most of these have not been replicated in other cohorts. A detailed discussion of these is beyond the scope of the current chapter.

MEDIUM-VESSEL VASCULITIS

Kawasaki Disease

There is ample proof for a genetic basis in KD. The incidence of KD in Japan is 10–20 times higher than Western countries.[4] The same level of incidence is maintained in Japanese ancestors living in Hawaii.[3] Kawasaki disease has significant familial aggregation—relative risk for siblings (λs) has been estimated to be 10.[2]

Candidate gene studies related to HLA molecules—initially identified HLA-Bw22 (currently Bw54) as a predominant susceptibility allele in Japanese.[35-38] Studies in Caucasians (English, Jewish) have identified association between HLA-Bw51 and KD.[39,40] During epidemics of KD in Japan and the United States in the past, several HLA class I molecules were identified, including HLA-B44, HLA-A2, Cw5. None of these were replicated in a study of HLA haplotypes in 23 affected sibs.[41] There is no significant association between KD and HLA class II antigens. Studies on non-HLA associations are too many and too complex for discussion here.[42]

Though linkage study using microsatellite markers—four genes were identified—most notable of these was polymorphism in the ITPKC-3 allele (kinase of inositol 1.4.5-triphosphate) with an OR of 1.74.[4] A polymorphism in ITPKC-3 leading to reduced mRNA expression was associated with susceptibility to KD and coronary abnormalities in Japanese population.

A GWAS study in Caucasian population identified eight susceptibility loci—all different than those reported in Japanese population.[43] Further studies are required to confirm association of these with KD susceptibility.

Polyarteritis Nodosa

In view of a definite etiological agent identified and rarity of familial aggregation, the possibility of genetic association is considered to be too poor. There have been only two previous case reports of polyarteritis nodosa (PAN) occurring in siblings, but in one of them both siblings were affected with hepatitis B infection.[44,45] MEFV mutations as a susceptibility factor were studied in 29 pediatric PAN patients—38% of the patients were found to have either of six mutation studies and three of them had homozygosity.[46] There was no control population studied and no further studies have been reported in the literature. A subset of multiply affected family members of childhood onset PAN is shown to be associated with mutation in CECR1 gene encoding adenosine deaminase-2 (autosomal recessive inheritance).[64]

SMALL-VESSEL VASCULITIS

ANCA Associated Vasculitis

The genetic predisposition of ANCA vasculitis is suggested by ethnic variation and familial aggregation. The overall prevalence of ANCA vasculitis is twice higher in subjects of European ancestry.[47] There is a significant difference in the prevalence of individual types of ANCA vasculitis in different ethnic groups—Granulomatosis with polyangiitis being more common in Norway and the UK, and microscopic polyangiitis (MPA) being more common in Spain and Japan.[48,49] A large registry-based epidemiological study has shown the relative risk of developing GPA in first degree relatives to be 1.54 (CI 0.35–6.9).[50] An earlier questionnaire-based study of 702 patients of GPA did not find a familial occurrence; 12 of the patients had an identical twin.[51] Overall these studies show that although there is a definite genetic association in AAV, association seems to be modest.

Among the candidate gene studies, the most reliable association so far has been with the rare Z null allele of the serpin A1 gene (SERPINA1) that encodes α-1 antitrypsin.[52] It occurs in 7–27% of Wegener's granulomatosis as compared to 1.5–4.7% of control populations (OR 3.01–9.36). However, this can only account for the risk in a subset of GPA. Of the several HLA genes implicated, strongest association is with HLA-DPB1*0401.[53]

The understanding of AAV has substantially changed after the publication of first GWAS in ANCA vasculitis. Genetically distinct MHC and non-MHC associations were found with AAV.[54] The strongest genetic association was found to be with antigenic specificity of ANCA and not with the clinical syndromes. Four single nucleotide polymorphisms (SNPs) acquired genome-wide significance. Three were in the MHC region—the most significant of which was gene encoding HLA-DP1. The other two SNPs in MHC region were in the COL11A2 gene—likely to be in linkage disequilibrium with HLA-DP. The only non-MHC SNP to acquire genome-wide significance was in the SERPINA1 locus at 14q32.

All three MHC-associated SNPs and SNP in the SERPINA1 locus were found in the cohort with granulomatosis with polyangiitis that were positive for PR 3 ANCA and not for myeloperoxidase (MPO) ANCA. They are also found in association with the PR 3 ANCA subgroup of microscopic polyangiitis. The PRTN3 gene, a major ANCA autoantigen, was found in association with granulomatosis with polyangiitis. A repeat GWAS in patient cohorts defined by ANCA specificity revealed a new SNP in HLA-DQ that reached genome-wide significance and was significantly associated with MPO ANCA.

It is clear from GWAS that HLA, SERPINA1, and PRTN3 are primarily aligned with ANCA specificity rather than clinically defined syndromes. It puts antiproteinase 3 autoreactivity at the center of the cause for AAV. It makes it imperative to consider including ANCA specificity in the classification criteria for ANCA-associated vasculitis in future.

Henoch-Schönlein Purpura

Henoch-Schönlein purpura (HSP) is proposed to have both infectious and genetic risk factors. Familial aggregation is limited. Three families in the Taiwanese study, two families in China, and eight cases in Japan have been reported as familial cases of HSP.[52-54] Interestingly, in middle-eastern countries there is high prevalence of vasculitis—mainly HSP (2.7%) and polyarteritis nodosa (0.9%)[54] among patients with FMF. Henoch-Schönlein purpura occurring in FMF patients was associated with homozygous M694V mutation.[55]

Based on the increased prevalence of HSP in FMF patients—several Israeli studies have looked into the association between FMF gene mutations in children with HSP. A total of 10% carried two mutated allele that is higher than that for general Israeli population (1–2%).[56] The presence

of the mutation does not found to have any effect on clinical presentation.[57]

Another Turkish study has found association between homozygous deletion of ACE I/D and HSP susceptibility (OR = 2.28/2.05).[58] Genetic association with HLA alleles has been found with HLA-DRB1*01 and *11 (OR 1.5–2.5), B35 and negative association with HLA-DRB1*07.[59] The presence of the C4 null allele (C4A or C4B) is associated with HSPs as seen in multiple cohorts of diverse ethnicity.[60]

KEY POINTS

- There have been significant advances in the way the genome is studied resulting in better understanding of the role of genetics in the etiopathogenesis of many diseases.
- This is true with possible polygenic diseases like vasculitis also.
- The currently available literature on the basis of candidate gene studies and GWAS gives further insight into the role of genetics in the etiopathogenesis of vasculitis.
- Multiple genetic predispositions have been identified for some of these diseases.

REFERENCES

1. Gul A, Inanc M, Ocal L, et al. Familial aggregation of Behçet's disease in Turkey. Ann Rheum Dis. 2000;59:622-5.
2. Fujita Y, Nakamura Y, Sakata K, et al. Kawasaki disease in families. Pediatrics. 1989;84:666-9.
3. Holman RC, Curns AT, Belay ED, et al. Kawasaki syndrome in Hawaii. Pediatr Infect Dis J. 2005;24:429-33.
4. Nakamura Y, Yashiro M, Uehara R, et al. Epidemiologic features of Kawasaki disease in Japan: results from the nationwide survey in 2005-2006. J Epidemiol. 2008;18:167-72.
5. Uehara R, Yashiro M, Nakamura Y, et al. Kawasaki disease in parents and children. Acta Paediatr. 2003;92:694-7.
6. Zhu M, Zhao S. Candidate gene identification approach: progress and challenges. Int J Biol Sci. 2007;3:420-7.
7. Collins FS, Guyer MS, Charkravarti A. Variations on a theme: cataloging human DNA sequence variation. Science. 1997;278:1580-1.
8. Dilsen N. History and development of Behçet's disease. Rev Rhum Engl Ed. 1996;63:512-9.
9. Zouboulis CC, Kotter I, Djawari D, et al. Epidemiological features of Adamantiades-Behçet's disease in Germany and in Europe. Yonsei Med J. 1997;38:411-22.
10. Masatlioglu S, Seyahi E, Tahir Turanli E, et al. A twin study in Behçet's syndrome. Clin Exp Rheumatol. 2010;28:S62-6.
11. Fresko I, Soy M, Hamuryudan V, et al. Genetic anticipation in Behçet's syndrome. Ann Rheum Dis. 1998;57:45-48.

12. Kaya TI. Genetics of Behçet's disease. Patholog Res Int. 2012;2012:912589.
13. Takemoto Y, Naruse T, Namba K, et al. Re-evaluation of heterogeneity in HLA-B*510101 associated with Behçet's disease. Tissue Antigens. 2008;72:347-53.
14. Fei Y, Webb R, Cobb BL, et al. Identification of novel genetic susceptibility loci for Behçet's disease using a genome-wide association study. Arthritis Res Ther. 2009;11:R66.
15. Sawalha AH, Hughes T, Nadig A, et al. A putative functional variant within the UBAC2 gene is associated with increased risk of Behçet's disease. Arthritis Rheum. 2011;63:3607-12.
16. Dursun A, Durakbasi-Dursun HG, Dursun R, et al. Angiotensin-converting enzyme gene and endothelial nitric oxide synthase gene polymorphisms in Behçet's disease with or without ocular involvement. Inflamm Res. 2009;58:401-5.
17. Ayesh S, Abu-Rmaileh H, Nassar S, et al. Molecular analysis of MEFV gene mutations among Palestinian patients with Behçet's disease. Scand J Rheumatol. 2008;37:370-4.
18. Imirzalioglu N, Dursun A, Tastan B, et al. MEFV gene is a probable susceptibility gene for Behçet's disease. Scand J Rheumatol. 2005;34:56-8.
19. Rabinovich E, Shinar Y, Leiba M, et al. Common FMF alleles may predispose to development of Behçet's disease with increased risk for venous thrombosis. Scand J Rheumatol. 2007;36:48-52.
20. Shima K, Yajima M, Numano F, et al. One family case of Takayasu disease. Nihon Naika Gakkai Zasshi. 1983;72:76-82.
21. Numano F, Isohisa I, Kishi U, et al. Takayasu's disease in twin sisters. Possible genetic factors. Circulation. 1978;58:173-7.
22. Tyagi S, Reddy NK, Khalilullah M. Familial occurrence of non-specific aortoarteritis in two sisters. Indian Heart J. 1991;43:193-4.
23. Naik N, Kothari SS, Sharma S. Familial Takayasu's aortoarteritis in two sisters. Indian Heart J. 1999;51:75-6.
24. Saruhan-Direskeneli G, Hughes T, Aksu K, et al. Identification of multiple genetic susceptibility loci in Takayasu arteritis. Am J Hum Genet. 2013;93:298-305.
25. Mehra NK, Jaini R, Balamurugan A, et al. Immunogenetic analysis of Takayasu arteritis in Indian patients. Int J Cardiol. 1998;66:S127-32; discussion S133.
26. Sahin Z, Bicakcigil M, Aksu K, et al. Takayasu's arteritis is associated with HLA-B*52, but not with HLA-B*51, in Turkey. Arthritis Res Ther. 2012;14:R27.
27. Terao C, Yoshifuji H, Mimori T. Recent advances in Takayasu arteritis. Int J Rheum Dis. 2014;17:238-47.
28. Vargas-Alarcon G, Flores-Dominguez C, Hernandez-Pacheco G, et al. Immunogenetics and clinical aspects of Takayasu's arteritis patients in a Mexican Mestizo population. Clin Exp Rheumatol. 2001;19:439-43.
29. Yoshida M, Kimura A, Katsuragi K, et al. DNA typing of HLA-B gene in Takayasu's arteritis. Tissue Antigens. 1993;42:87-90.
30. Terao C, Yoshifuji H, Ohmura K, et al. Association of Takayasu arteritis with HLA-B67:01 and two amino acids in HLA-B protein. Rheumatology (Oxford). 2013;52:1769-74.
31. Terao C, Yoshifuji H, Kimura A, et al. Two susceptibility loci to Takayasu arteritis reveal a synergistic role of the IL12B and HLA-B regions in a Japanese population. Am J Hum Genet. 2013;93:289-97.
32. Kobayashi S, Yano T, Matsumoto Y, et al. Clinical and epidemiologic analysis of giant cell (temporal) arteritis from a nationwide survey in 1998 in Japan: the first government-supported nationwide survey. Arthritis Rheum. 2003;49:594-8.
33. Carmona FD, Gonzalez-Gay MA, Martin J. Genetic component of giant cell arteritis. Rheumatology (Oxford). 2014;53:6-18.
34. Gonzalez-Gay MA, Rueda B, Vilchez JR, et al. Contribution of MHC class I region to genetic susceptibility for giant cell arteritis. Rheumatology (Oxford). 2007;46:431-4.
35. Kato S, Kimura M, Tsuji K, et al. HLA antigens in Kawasaki disease. Pediatrics. 1978;61:252-5.
36. Matsuda I, Hattori S, Nagata N, et al. HLA antigens in mucocutaneous lymph node syndrome. Am J Dis Child. 1977;131:1417-8.
37. Onouchi Y. Molecular genetics of Kawasaki disease. Pediatr Res. 2009;65:46R-54R.
38. Rowley AH. Kawasaki disease: novel insights into etiology and genetic susceptibility. Annu Rev Med. 2011;62:69-77.
39. Keren G, Danon YL, Orgad S, et al. HLA-Bw51 is increased in mucocutaneous lymph node syndrome in Israeli patients. Tissue Antigens. 1982;20:144-6.
40. Krensky AM, Berenberg W, Shanley K, et al. HLA antigens in mucocutaneous lymph node syndrome in New England. Pediatrics. 1981;67:741-3.
41. Harada F, Sada M, Kamiya T, et al. Genetic analysis of Kawasaki syndrome. Am J Hum Genet. 1986;39:537-9.
42. Onouchi Y, Tamari M, Takahashi A, et al. A genome-wide linkage analysis of Kawasaki disease: evidence for linkage to chromosome 12. J Hum Genet. 2007;52:179-90.
43. Burgner D, Davila S, Breunis WB, et al. A genome-wide association study identifies novel and functionally related susceptibility loci for Kawasaki disease. PLoS Genet. 2009;5:e1000319.
44. Mason JC, Cowie MR, Davies KA, et al. Familial polyarteritis nodosa. Arthritis Rheum. 1994;37:1249-53.
45. Reveille JD, Goodman RE, Barger BO, et al. Familial polyarteritis nodosa: a serologic and immunogenetic analysis. J Rheumatol. 1989;16:181-5.
46. Yalcinkaya F, Ozcakar ZB, Kasapcopur O, et al. Prevalence of the MEFV gene mutations in childhood polyarteritis nodosa. J Pediatr. 2007;151:675-8.
47. Mahr A, Guillevin L, Poissonnet M, et al. Prevalences of polyarteritis nodosa, microscopic polyangiitis, Wegener's granulomatosis, and Churg-Strauss syndrome in a French urban multiethnic population in 2000: a capture-recapture estimate. Arthritis Rheum. 2004;51:92-9.
48. Watts RA, Scott DG, Jayne DR, et al. Renal vasculitis in Japan and the UK—are there differences in epidemiology and clinical phenotype? Nephrol Dial Transplant. 2008;23:3928-31.
49. Willcocks LC, Lyons PA, Rees AJ, et al. The contribution of genetic variation and infection to the pathogenesis of ANCA-associated systemic vasculitis. Arthritis Res Ther. 2010;12:202.
50. Knight A, Sandin S, Askling J. Risks and relative risks of Wegener's granulomatosis among close relatives of patients with the disease. Arthritis Rheum. 2008;58:302-7.

51. Abdou NI, Kullman GJ, Hoffman GS, et al. Wegener's granulomatosis: survey of 701 patients in North America. Changes in outcome in the 1990s. J Rheumatol. 2002;29:309-16.

52. Mahr AD, Neogi T, Merkel PA. Epidemiology of Wegener's granulomatosis: lessons from descriptive studies and analyses of genetic and environmental risk determinants. Clin Exp Rheumatol. 2006;24:S82-91.

53. Heckmann M, Holle JU, Arning L, et al. The Wegener's granulomatosis quantitative trait locus on chromosome 6p21.3 as characterised by tagSNP genotyping. Ann Rheum Dis. 2007;67:972-9.

54. Lyons PA, Rayner TF, Trivedi S, et al. Genetically distinct subsets within ANCA-associated vasculitis. N Engl J Med. 2012;367:214-23.

55. Balbir-Gurman A, Nahir AM, Braun-Moscovici Y. Vasculitis in siblings with familial Mediterranean fever: a report of three cases and review of the literature. Clin Rheumatol. 2007;26:1183-5.

56. Gershoni-Baruch R, Broza Y, Brik R. Prevalence and significance of mutations in the familial Mediterranean fever gene in Henoch-Schonlein purpura. J Pediatr. 2003;143:658-61.

57. Dogan CS, Akman S, Koyun M, et al. Prevalence and significance of the MEFV gene mutations in childhood Henoch-Schonlein purpura without FMF symptoms. Rheumatol Int. 2013;33:377-80.

58. Nalbantoglu S, Tabel Y, Mir S, et al. Association between RAS gene polymorphisms (ACE I/D, AGT M235T) and Henoch-Schonlein purpura in a Turkish population. Dis Markers. 2013;34:23-32.

59. He X, Yu C, Zhao P, et al. The genetics of Henoch-Schonlein purpura: a systematic review and meta-analysis. Rheumatol Int. 2013;33:1387-95.

60. Stefansson Thors V, Kolka R, Sigurdardottir SL, et al. Increased frequency of C4B*Q0 alleles in patients with Henoch-Schonlein purpura. Scand J Immunol. 2005;61:274-8.

61. Kimberly A Morishita, et al. Familial Takayasu arteritis—a pediatric case and a review of the literature. Paediatric Rheumatology Online Journal. 2011;9:6.

62. Numano F, et al. Takayasu's disease in twin sisters. Possible genetic factors. Circulation, 1978.

63. Liozon E, et al. Familial aggregation in giant cell arteritis and polymyalgia rheumatica: a comprehensive literature review including 4 new families. Clin Exp Rheumatol. 2009: 27.

64. Navon Elkan P, et al. Mutant adenosine deaminase 2 in a polyarteritis nodosa vasculopathy. New Eng J Med. 214;370: 921-31.

CHAPTER 3

Classification of Vasculitis

Aman Sharma, Richard Watts

The systemic vasculitides are heterogeneous group medical disorders sharing a common feature in the form of vessel wall inflammation. Different disorders have predilection for different type and size of the blood vessels and thus are mostly classified according to this pattern. This distinction, however, is not exclusive, with various disorders having overlapping features. Various classification criteria have been proposed for these disorders from time to time, some based upon the size of the vessel and some on the presence/absence of granuloma formation on histopathological examination, and this highlights the lack of consensus for classification systems. Besides the classification criteria, a nomenclature system has also been proposed for having uniform definitions of some of these vasculitides. The Chapel Hill Consensus Conference Nomenclature System (CHCC) was proposed in 1993 and has been revised in 2012 (CHCC2012). While the classification systems are in place to have uniform criteria for research, they are not "diagnostic criteria". A diagnostic criterion is supposed to help in making a diagnosis in one patient and excluding other diagnosis. There are no validated diagnostic criteria as of now, though a study is presently underway to develop a diagnostic as well as classification criteria (DCVAS study).

The initial description of vasculitis in the 18th century by Heberden was in the form of case reports. The earliest description of a vasculitis that has been given a name was by Schönlein for a disorder characterized by joint pains, skin lesions, abdominal pains, and nephritis.[1,2] This was subsequently named as Henoch-Schönlein purpura. This name has now been revised to IgA vasculitis in CHCC2012. The first detailed pathological description of medium- and small-vessel vasculitis was given by Kussmaul and Maier in 1866.[3] As they observed that the inflammatory process also extended into the perivascular structures, they named it "periarteritis nodosa". This was subsequently named as polyarteritis nodosa (PAN), as it was understood that the vessel was the primary site of inflammation. The initial descriptions of PAN did not differentiate it from microscopic polyangiitis (MPA). Microscopic polyangiitis has a predominant small-vessel involvement, manifesting with lung hemorrhage and glomerulonephritis. These two features are not seen in PAN.

The understanding about the clinical manifestations and pathology increased significantly in the 20th century. Involvement of arterioles, capillaries, venules and granuloma formation were observed and recorded in some variants.[4-12] These observations also led to the naming of some of these disorders after the people who described them, e.g. Wegener's granulomatosis (WG) [now known as granulomatosis with polyangiitis (GPA)], Churg-Strauss syndrome [now known as eosinophilic granulomatosis with polyangiitis (EGPA)].[5,12] Kawasaki described a necrotizing arteritis with mucocutaneous lymph node syndrome, it was named after him.[13] One form of large-vessel vasculitis, identified in elderly, commonly involved the temporal arteries, and thus was initially called as temporal arteritis. Subsequently, it was shown that this can involve vessels without even involving temporal arteries in some patients, and as these also showed "giant cells", the term giant cell arteritis was used for this disorder.[14-16] A large-vessel vasculitis predominantly affecting young ladies presenting with pulseless disease was named Takayasu's arteritis (TAK).[17] Renaming of WG to GPA has been a major event in the history of nomenclature of these disorders.[18]

The first attempt to classify vasculitides was made by Zeek who described five distinct vasculitides from a review of literature. These were hypersensitivity angiitis, allergic granulomatous angiitis, rheumatic arteritis, periarteritis nodosa, and temporal arteritis. Her work is the basis of most of the modern classification systems.[7,8] Various other classification systems were proposed in the subsequent years.[19-22] Another attempt to classify these disorders was made by Lie who divided these into two broad categories of primary and secondary vasculitis.[23] Dependent upon the size of involved vessel, primary vasculitis had further subtypes. Vasculitis due to infection, drugs, essential mixed cryoglobulinemia, malignancy, hypocomplimentemia, and postorgan transplant was included in the secondary group.

AMERICAN COLLEGE OF RHEUMATOLOGY CRITERIA

The American college of rheumatology (ACR) proposed one of the most widely used and frequently cited classification criteria for seven types of vasculitides in 1990.[24-30] These included criteria for giant cell arteritis, TAK, GPA, EGPA, polyarteritis nodosa, Henoch-Schönlein purpura, and hypersensitivity vasculitis. The basis of these criteria was the pooled data from different centers. Data from 807 patients out of a cohort of 1,010 patients from 48 centers were analyzed. While evaluating the data of patients with suspected vasculitis, those with a diagnosis of Kawasaki disease (KD), insufficient evidence of vasculitis or secondary forms of vasculitis were excluded. The basis of diagnosis for these criteria was the expert opinion, which is often cited as a limitation of these criteria. Though these criteria were originally intended to be used only as classification criteria, and not diagnostic criteria, these have often been used to make a diagnosis. As classification criteria, they have a sensitivity and specificity between 71–95% and 78–99%, respectively. Some of the

other limitations of these criteria include the following: no description of MPA and no use of antineutrophil cytoplasmic antibodies (ANCA). The other concern has been the poor performance as diagnostic criteria with one patient fulfilling criteria of more than one disorder.[31,32]

CHAPEL HILL CONSENSUS CONFERENCE NOMENCLATURE SYSTEM

Chapel Hill Consensus Conference held in 1994 was a major milestone in the nomenclature of systemic vasculitides.[33] During this conference held in Chapel Hill, North Carolina, the names and definitions of common systemic vasculitides were given. It was also recognized here that MPA was a clinical entity distinct from PAN. The consideration was given that histology may not be always available and the concept of "surrogate markers of vasculitis" was introduced, though no list of such markers was provided. The main drawback of CHCC was that despite the recognition of ANCA at that time, role of ANCA was not appreciated. The other drawback was that vasculitis secondary to systemic disease or a known etiology was not included. The paper on CHCC was a landmark publication with more than 2,000 citations till now.[34] This CHCC nomenclature system was revised in a meeting held at Chapel Hill again in 2012 (CHCC2012) (Table 3.1).[35] In the revised CHCC2012, the small-vessel vasculitis group has been subdivided into immune complex and ANCA-associated vasculitis. There have been some changes in the names like change of WG to GPA, Churg-Strauss syndrome to EGPA,

Table 3.1 The names of vasculitides adopted by the 2012 International Chapel Hill Consensus Conference on the nomenclature of vasculitides

- **Large-vessel vasculitis (LVV)**
  - Takayasu arteritis (TAK)
  - Giant cell arteritis (GCA)
- **Medium-vessel vasculitis (MVV)**
  - Polyarteritis nodosa (PAN)
  - Kawasaki disease (KD)
- **Small-vessel vasculitis (SVV)**
  - ANCA-associated vasculitis
    - Microscopic polyangiitis (MPA)
    - Granulomatosis with polyangiitis (GPA)
    - Eosinophilic granulomatosis with polyangiitis (EGPA)
  - Immune complex SVV
    - Anti-GBM disease
    - Cryoglobulinemic vasculitis
    - IgA vasculitis (HSP)
    - Hypocomplementemic urticarial vasculitis
- **Variable-vessel vasculitis (VVV)**
  - Behçet's disease (BD)
  - Cogan's syndrome

- **Single-organ vasculitis (SOV)**
  - Cutaneous leukocytoclastic angiitis
  - Cutaneous arteritis
  - Primary angiitis of the CNS (PACNS)
  - Isolated aortitis
  - Others
- **Vasculitis associated with systemic disease**
  - Lupus vasculitis
  - Rheumatoid vasculitis
  - Sarcoid vasculitis
  - Others
- **Vasculitis with probable etiology**
  - HCV-associated cryoglobulinemic vasculitis
  - HBV-associated vasculitis
  - Syphilis-associated aortitis
  - Drug-associated immune complex vasculitis
  - Drug-associated ANCA-associated vasculitis
  - Cancer-associated vasculitis
  - Others

Source: Jennette et al. (2010).

and Henoch-Schönlein purpura to IgA vasculitis. Though the entity of anti-GBM disease as a true vasculitis has always been debated, it has been included in the new nomenclature system due to the similar clinical presentation. Categories of variable vessel vasculitis with Behçet's disease and Cogan's syndrome, single-organ vasculitis with cutaneous leukocytoclastic angiitis, cutaneous arteritis, primary angiitis of the CNS, isolated aortitis, vasculitis associated with systemic diseases and category of vasculitis with probable etiology of HCV-associated cryoglobulinemic vasculitis, HBV-associated vasculitis, syphilis-associated aortitis, drug-associated immune complex vasculitis, drug-associated ANCA-associated vasculitis, and cancer-associated vasculitis have been included.

EUROPEAN MEDICAL AGENCY ALGORITHM

In order to harmonize the ACR and CHCC definitions, a consensus methodology algorithm was proposed by Watts et al.[36] The initial development of this algorithm was based upon the analysis of data of 99 patients from a single center. A hierarchical approach is used in this algorithm. Increased sensitivity in classification of childhood GPA has been shown with this algorithm, and this algorithm has also been validated in various other populations including an Indian cohort.[37-40] The use of the new CHCC2012 nomenclature system in this algorithm has been published by the same group and has been shown to have good correlation with 2005 classification.[41]

As we can see that there is a lack of consensus for a true classification criteria, and these disorders can sometimes present with some very uncommon presenting manifestations, there is a need for a validated classification and a diagnostic criteria.[42] A very important step has been taken in the form of an ACR European League against Rheumatism (EULAR) study for the development of classification and diagnostic criteria of these vasculitides (DCVAS).[43] The patient recruitment is going on from centers all across the globe and the recruitment is likely to continue till 2015. It is hoped that this study will come up with a robust diagnostic and classification criteria. It is also possible that this study may come up with new disease entities like the genesis of MPA in CHCC.

CLASSIFICATION OF CHILDHOOD VASCULITIS

Childhood vasculitides were not considered as a separate entity in the initial classification systems like ACR classification

criteria. Thus, there was a need for a classification criteria derived from the cohort of childhood vasculitis. A working group of the Pediatric Rheumatology European Society (PRES) and EULAR met in Vienna in 2005 to study the adequacy of ACR criteria for childhood vasculitis and develop pediatric specific classification criteria (Table 3.2).[44] Consensus on the classification criteria of five diseases (HSP, KD, PAN, WG, and TA) was reached. There was a subdivision of small-vessel vasculitis group into granulomatous and nongranulomatous. Consensus on "Other Vasculitides" group comprising of Behçet's disease, vasculitis associated with infection, connective tissue disease, isolated angiitis of CNS, Cogan syndrome, and unclassified vasculitis was also reached. A definition of cutaneous PAN and MPA was also given with inclusion of myeloperoxidase (MPO) ANCA to the CHCC criteria of MPA. The fact that subglottic stenosis, tracheal stenosis, and endobronchial stenosis are common in children with GPA was included in the criteria along with ANCA (C ANCA or PR3). The angiographic definition was updated and hypertension was included as criteria for classification of TAK.

The initial proposal of these classification criteria were followed by a statistical validation process. There was also a large-scale web-based data collection. These activities were supported by PRES, EULAR, and Pediatric Rheumatology International Trials Organization (PRINTO).

Table 3.2 Classification of childhood vasculitis

- **Predominant larger vessel vasculitis**
  - Takayasu arteritis
- **Predominant medium-sized vessel vasculitis**
  - Cutaneous polyarteritis nodosa (c-PAN)
  - Cutaneous polyarteritis
  - Kawasaki disease
- **Predominant small vessel vasculitis**
  - Granulomatous
    - ◆ Wegener's granulomatosis
    - ◆ Churg-Strauss syndrome
  - Nongranulomatous
    - ◆ Henoch-Schönlein purpura
    - ◆ Microscopic polyangiitis
    - ◆ Hypocomplementemic urticarial vasculitis
- **Other vasculitides**
  - Behçet's disease
  - Vasculitis secondary to infection (including hepatitis B-associated PAN), malignancies, drugs, including hypersensitivity vasculitis
  - Vasculitis associated with connective tissue disease
  - Isolate angiitis of CNS
  - Cogan's syndrome
  - Unclassified

In order to validate these EULAR-endorsed classification criteria of childhood vasculitis, a consensus conference was held at Ankara in 2008.[45] Very minor changes were made to the 2005 criteria for GPA like any detected ANCA (immunofluorescence, MPO, and PR3). It was also proposed that the Richard Watt's European Medical Agency (EMEA) consensus methodology approach should be followed to differentiate GPA from MPA or EGPA. Since then, efforts are being made to have valid classification and diagnostic criteria and valid outcome measure in these disorders. It can be said that as far as classification criteria, diagnostic criteria, and nomenclature system of vasculitides are concerned, this is surely a "work in progress."[46,47]

KEY POINTS

- Various classification criteria have been proposed from time to time.
- Classification criteria play an important role in bringing uniformity to research.
- There are no validated diagnostic criteria.
- Ongoing DCVAS study is likely to come out with new diagnostic and classification criteria.

REFERENCES

1. Schönlein JL. Allegemeine und specielle Pathologie und Therapie, 3rd edition, vol. 2. Herisau, Germany: Literatur-Comptoir; 1837. p. 48.
2. Henoch E. Uber den zusammenhang von purpura und intestinal stoerungen. Berl Klin Wochenschur. 1868;5:517-9.
3. Kussmaul A, Maier R. Über eine bisher nicht beschreibene eigenthümliche Arterienerkrankung (Periarteriitis nodosa), die mit Morbus Brightii und rapid fortschreitender allgemeiner Muskellähmung einhergeht. Dtsch Arch Klin Med. 1866;1:484-518.
4. Wohlwill F. On the only microscopically recognizable form of periarteritis nodosa. Virchows Arch Pathol Anat Physiol Klin Med. 1923;246:377-411.
5. Arkin A. A clinical and pathological study of periarteritis nodosa. A report of five cases, one histologically healed. Am J Pathol. 1930;6:401-26.
6. Davson J, Ball J, Platt R. The kidney on periarteritis nodosa. Q J Med. 1948;17:175-202.
7. Zeek PM, Smith CC, Weeter JC. Studies on periarteritis nodosa: III. The differentiation between the vascular lesions of periarteritis nodosa and of hypersensitivity. Am J Pathol. 1948;24:889-917.
8. Zeek PM. Periarteritis nodosa: a critical review. Am J Clin Pathol. 1952;22:777-90.
9. Churg J, Strauss L. Allergic granulomatosis, allergic angiitis, and periarteritis nodosa. Am J Pathol. 1951;27:277-94.
10. Godman G, Churg J. Wegener's granulomatosis. Pathology and review of the literature. Arch Pathol Lab Med. 1954;58:533-53.
11. Klinger H. Grenzformen der Periarteriitis nodosa. Frankf Ztschr Pathol. 1931;42:455-80.
12. Wegener F. Über eine eigenartige rhinogene Granulomatose mit besonderer Beteiligung des Arteriensystems unter den Nieren. Beitr Pathol Anat. 1939;102:36-68.
13. Kawasaki T. MLNS showing particular skin desquamation from the finger and toe in infants. Allergy. 1967;16:178-89.
14. Hutchinson J. Diseases of the arteries. On a peculiar form of thrombotic arteritis of the aged which is sometimes productive of gangrene. Arch Surg (London). 1890;1:323-9.
15. Horton BT, Magath TB, Brown GE. Undescribed form of arteritis of temporal vessels. Proc Staff Meet Mayo Clin. 1932;7:700-1.
16. Gilmour JR. Giant-cell chronic arteritis. J Pathol. 1941;53:263-77.
17. Takayasu M. Case with unusual changes of the central vessels in the retina. Acta Soc Ophthalmol Jpn. 1908;12:554-5.
18. Falk RJ, Gross WL, Guillevin L, et al. "Granulomatosis with polyangiitis (Wegener's)": an alternative name for "Wegener's granulomatosis". A joint proposal of the American College of Rheumatology, the American Society of Nephrology, and the European League Against Rheumatism. Ann Rheum Dis. 2011;70:704.
19. Alargon-Segovia D, Brown AL. Classification and aetiological aspects of necrotising vasculitis. Mayo Clin Proc. 1964;39:205-22.
20. De Shazo RD. The spectrum of systemic vasculitis: a classification to aid diagnosis. Postgrad Med. 1975;58:78-82.
21. Gilliam JN, Smiley JD. Cutaneous necrotising vasculitis and related disorders. Ann Allergy. 1976;37:328-39.
22. Fauci AS, Haynes BF, Katz P. The spectrum of vasculitus: clinical, pathological, immunologic, and therapeutic considerations. Ann Intern Med. 1978;89:660-76.
23. Lie JT. Nomenclature and classification of vasculitis: plus ça change, plus c'est la même chose. Arthritis Rheum. 1994;37:181-6.
24. Hunder GG, Bloch DA, Michel BA, et al. The American College of Rheumatology 1990 criteria for the classification of giant cell arteritis. Arthritis Rheum. 1990;33:1122-8.
25. Arend WP, Michel BA, Bloch DA, et al. The American College of Rheumatology 1990 criteria for the classification of Takayasu arteritis. Arthritis Rheum. 1990;33:1129-34.
26. Leavitt RY, Fauci AS, Bloch DA, et al. The American College of Rheumatology 1990 criteria for the classification of Wegener's granulomatosis. Arthritis Rheum. 1990;33:1101-7.
27. Masi AT, Hunder GG, Lie JT, et al. The American College of Rheumatology 1990 criteria for the classification of Churg-Strauss syndrome (allergic granulomatosis and angiitis). Arthritis Rheum. 1990;33:1094-100.
28. Lightfoot RW Jr, Michel BA, Bloch DA, et al. The American College of Rheumatology 1990 criteria for the classification of polyarteritis nodosa. Arthritis Rheum. 1990;33:1088-93.
29. Mills JA, Michel BA, Bloch DA, et al. The American College of Rheumatology 1990 criteria for the classification of Henoch-Schönlein purpura. Arthritis Rheum. 1990;33:1114-21.

30. Calabrese LH, Michel BA, Bloch DA, et al. The American College of Rheumatology 1990 criteria for the classification of hypersensitivity vasculitis. Arthritis Rheum. 1990;33:1108-13.

31. Lane SE, Watts RA, Barker THW, et al. Evaluation of the Sørensen diagnostic criteria in the classification of systemic vasculitis. Rheumatology (Oxford). 2002;41:1138-41.

32. Lane SE, Watts RA, Shepstone L, et al. Primary systemic vasculitis: clinical features and mortality. QJM. 2005;98:97-111.

33. Jennette JC, Falk RJ, Andrassy K, et al. Nomenclature of systemic vasculitides. Proposal of an International Consensus Conference. Arthritis Rheum. 1994;37:187-92.

34. Jennette JC. What can we expect from a revised Chapel Hill Consensus Conference Nomenclature of Vasculitis? Presse Med. 2013;42:550-5.

35. Jennette JC, Falk RJ, Bacon PA, et al. 2012 revised international Chapel Hill Consensus Conference Nomenclature of Vasculitides. Arthritis Rheum. 2013;65:1-11.

36. Watts R, Lane S, Hanslik T, et al. Development and validation of a consensus methodology for the classification of the ANCA-associated vasculitides and polyarteritis nodosa for epidemiological studies. Ann Rheum Dis. 2007;66:222-7.

37. Uribe AG, Huber AM, Kim S, et al. Increased sensitivity of the European Medicines Agency algorithm for classification of childhood granulomatosis with polyangiitis. J Rheumatol. 2012;39:1687-97.

38. Liu L-J, Chen M, Yu F, et al. Evaluation of a new algorithm in classification of systemic vasculitis. Rheumatology. 2008;47:708-12.

39. Kamali S, Artim-Esen B, Erer B, et al. Re-evaluation of 129 patients with systemic necrotizing vasculitides by using classification algorithm according to consensus methodology. Clin Rheumatol. 2012;31:325-8.

40. Sharma A, Mittal T, Rajan R, et al. Validation of the consensus methodology algorithm for the classification of systemic necrotizing vasculitis in Indian patients. Int J Rheum Dis. 2014;17:408-11.

41. Abdulkader R, Lane S, Scott DGI, et al. Classification of vasculitis: EMA classification using CHCC2012 definitions. Ann Rheum Dis. 2013;72:1888.

42. Sharma A, Gopalakrishan D, Nada R, et al. Uncommon presentations of primary systemic necrotizing vasculitides: the Great Masquerades. Int J Rheum Dis. 2014;17:562-72.

43. Luqmani RA, Suppiah R, Grayson PC, et al. Nomenclature and classification of vasculitis—update on the ACR/EULAR diagnosis and classification of vasculitis study (DCVAS). Clin Exp Immunol. 2011;164:11-3.

44. Ozen S, Ruperto N, Dillon MJ, et al. EULAR/PRES endorsed consensus criteria for the classification of childhood vasculitides. Ann Rheum Dis. 2006;65:936-41.

45. Ozen S, Pistorio A, Iusan SM, et al. Paediatric rheumatology international trials organisation (PRINTO). ULAR/PRINTO/ PRES criteria for Henoch–Schönlein purpura, childhood polyarteritis nodosa, childhood Wegener granulomatosis and childhood Takayasu arteritis: Ankara 2008. Part II: final classification criteria. Ann Rheum Dis. 2010;69:798-806.

46. Sharma A. Outcome measures in primary systemic vasculitis— Indian perspective. Ind J Rheumatol. 2013;8:S68-69.

47. Sharma A. Nomenclature, classification and diagnostic criteria in systemic vasculitis—'a work in progress'. Ind J Rheumatol. 2013;8:99-101.

Basic Sciences

- Neutrophils in ANCA-associated Vasculitides
- Antineutrophil Cytoplasmic Antibodies
- Animal Models of ANCA Vasculitis
- Pathogenesis of Vasculitis
- Pathology of Cutaneous Vasculitis
- Pathology of Pulmonary Vasculitis
- Pathology of Renal Vasculitis
- Pathology of Central Nervous System and Peripheral Nerves

CHAPTER 4

Neutrophils in ANCA-associated Vasculitis

Véronique Witko-Sarsat, Arnaud Roccabianca, Luc Mouthon

INTRODUCTION

The pathogenesis of antineutrophil cytoplasmic antibodies (ANCA)-associated vasculitides (AAV) is poorly understood but consistent with a primary role of neutrophils in the acute injury. Neutrophils are key players in the pathophysiological process in AAV, since they are both targets of autoimmunity and effector cells responsible for endothelial damage. The two main target antigens of ANCA are the neutrophil granule proteins, proteinase 3 (PR3) and myeloperoxidase (MPO).[1] Anti-PR3 ANCAs are found in sera from patients with granulomatosis with polyangiitis (GPA) (Wegener), which is characterized by granulomatous inflammation of the upper and/or lower respiratory tract whereas anti-MPO ANCAs are present in sera from patients with microscopic polyangiitis (MPA), and less frequently in eosinophilic granulomatosis with polyangiitis (EGPA) (formerly Churg-Strauss syndrome), which associates late-onset asthma, hypereosinophilia, and small-vessel vasculitis. The selectivity of ANCA target antigens is surprising regarding the wide range of proteins stored within cytosolic granules of neutrophils (Fig. 4.1). It has recently been proposed that the formation of neutrophils extracellular traps (NETs) that are composed of DNA extruded from dying neutrophils, which bear all the cationic granule proteins including PR3 and MPO, could be involved in the pathophysiology of AAV.[2]

THE ANCA ANTIGENS PR3 AND MPO: KEYS IN THE PATHOPHYSIOLOGY OF ANCA-ASSOCIATED VASCULITIDES

PR3 and MPO are localized in the neutrophil azurophil granules and are both involved in the microbicidal activity of neutrophil. However, their structure and function differ dramatically. Thus, PR3 and MPO share proinflammatory

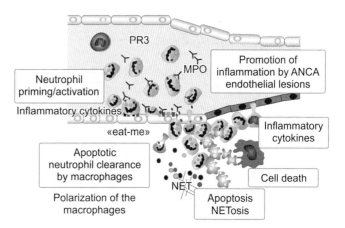

Fig. 4.1 Originally, an infection triggers on one hand, with priming of neutrophils, and on the other hand, an upregulation of endothelial adhesion molecules through proinflammatory cytokines occurs. This priming causes upregulation of neutrophil adhesion molecules and translocation of the ANCA antigens from granules to the cell surface. The interaction between the ANCAs and their antibodies on the cell surface activates the neutrophil, causing increased neutrophil–vessel wall adherence and transmigration. ANCA-mediated neutrophil activation also triggers reactive oxygen radical production and causes neutrophil degranulation leading to release proteolytic enzymes, injuring the vessel wall. Apoptotic neutrophils showing an "eat-me" signal, maintain an inflammatory polarization of macrophages after being cleared. During inflammation, neutrophils might be able to release NETs to fight against microorganisms, responsible for the release of PR3 and MPO

properties and are also able to modulate the inflammatory process during which they can have synergistic activities.[3] However, it is striking to note that, among the multiple proteins contained in neutrophils azurophil granules, these two biochemically very different proteins are preferred targets for the ANCA in AAV. Interestingly, the clinical presentation of patients with AAV differs, depending on the specificity of ANCA. Thus, in systemic GPA, characterized by glomerulonephritis and typically granulomatous involvement of lungs and upper airways, 85% of the patients have anti-PR3 ANCA and slightly less than 10% have anti-MPO ANCA. Interestingly, anti-MPO ANCAs are detected in 60–70% of patients with MPA, a systemic vasculitis typically characterized by pneumorenal syndrome, as well as in 30–38% of patients with EGPA. Importantly, these two types of antibodies are mutually exclusive and are very rarely detected in a same patient. It is of interest to mention that the distinct biochemical properties of MPO and PR3 were exploited empirically in the indirect immunofluorescence test of ANCA; thus, a perinuclear fluorescence is observed with anti-MPO ANCA, whereas a cytoplasmic fluorescence is noted with anti-PR3 ANCA.

Myeloperoxidase—An Oxidant-generating Protein

Myeloperoxidase is very abundant (up to 5% of dry weight) and is exclusively found in the azurophilic granules of neutrophils. It is a key element of the intracellular microbicide oxygen-dependent system,[4] synthesizing hypochlorous acid ($HOCl^-$) from superoxide anion that exerts its toxic effect not only on microorganisms (bacteria, fungi, and parasites) but also on the host cells by oxidizing a wide variety of molecules. In addition, hypochlorous acid can react with endogenous amines (R-NH2) to generate chloramines (SHR-Cl) that were baptized long-lived oxidants compared to free oxygen radicals whose life is extremely short, much less than 1 second. Hypochlorous acid can also oxidize plasma proteins and generate advanced oxidized protein products (AOPP) that have proinflammatory properties.[5] Finally, several teams focused their work on the characterization of the role of MPO in the mechanisms of inflammation in the absence of an infection. In this setting, the detection of MPO in atherosclerotic plaques unraveled the pathogenesis of atherosclerosis and marked the starting point of many efforts to demonstrate its involvement in atherogenesis, contributing to consider this condition at least in part as an inflammatory disease.[6] Indeed, MPO can oxidize low-density lipoproteins and proteins of the extracellular matrix in the blood vessel wall.[7]

Proteinase 3 Belongs to the Serprocidin: Neutrophil-derived Antibiotic Serine Proteinase

Proteinase 3 differs from MPO in many aspects. Thus, if biological activity of MPO is unique, since it is the only enzyme to generate chlorinated oxidants, PR3 has homologous proteins called serprocidins, which means antibiotic serine proteinases, namely elastase, azurocidin, and cathepsin G, which are also stored in azurophilic granules. Generally, the serine proteinases have a rather proinflammatory activity,[8,9] as demonstrated in several animal models using mice genetically deficient in elastase or cathepsin G or double deficient in elastase and PR3. Mice deficient in dipeptidyl peptidase enzyme required for cleavage of the prosequence of these serine proteases have been widely used to show the proinflammatory role of these enzymes. For example, it has been recently shown that neutrophil serine proteases have a deleterious role in a model of vasculitis associated with anti-MPO antibodies.[10]

Interestingly, elastase, which shares 56% of homology with PR3, is not a specific target of ANCA. Proteinase 3 was cloned, named myeloblastine, and described as a protein involved in the granulocytic differentiation. In fact, inhibition of its expression at the promyelocytic stage triggers the differentiation of these cells.[11] The PR3 has structural features that distinguish it from its counterparts, in particular its capacity to anchor to the plasmic membrane,[12,13] and therefore to be expressed at membrane of neutrophils in the absence of activation, which can have many implications on its biological functions. Furthermore, patients with a significant proportion of their neutrophils expressing membrane PR3 are at risk for developing vasculitis.[14] Proteinase 3 expression at the membrane of neutrophils is genetically determined. Thus, we had hypothesized studying two representative families that the percentage of neutrophils expressing PR3 could be a genetically transmitted character[14] and this hypothesis has not been refuted after a study of twins.[15] As it has been shown that ANCA can activate neutrophils, amplifying the inflammatory process, the accessibility of the autoantigen (PR3 and MPO) to the ANCA, is therefore a mechanistic prerequisite for cell activation by the ANCA. Moreover, the oxidative activity in response to ANCA is increased in neutrophils expressing membrane PR3 as compared to neutrophils not expressing PR3.[15] In addition, we have shown that PR3 was localized in the secretory vesicles, an easily mobilizable neutrophil compartment arising at the end of the differentiation of neutrophils, to increase the membrane receptors expression on the surface of the neutrophil, demonstrating that the PR3 did not follow the rules of compartmentalization "in use" in the neutrophil.[16] This observation opened new fields of investigation on membrane PR3, in particular its proteins partners and its functions.

Interestingly, the CD177, also called NB1,[17,18] is a membrane protein of neutrophils with a GPI anchorage that has a similar bimodal expression on human neutrophils and was involved in the migration process of neutrophils. NB1 was suggested to be a "receiver" of PR3 but the mechanisms by which the PR3 would be released, then caught by a neutrophil, in the absence of activation are not clear. Several groups demonstrated that PR3 can localize in the rafts or lipid rafts and join CD11b/CD18 and CD16,[19] contributing to explain its binding to the membrane. Interestingly and unlike its counterparts, PR3 is able to fit into lipid vesicles. Furthermore, molecular modeling studies using dynamics simulations allowed to demonstrate that, from the structural point of view, PR3 is able to bind to neutral or anionic membranes via a hydrophobic patch consisting of four hydrophobic amino acids,[12,13] which is not the case for the elastase. These four hydrophobic amino acids are crucial for the association of PR3 to the membrane[20] and might bind to CD177.[21] An association of PR3 and phospholipid scramblase I has also been identified. Phospholipid scramblase I is an enzyme responsible for the lipids scrambling during apoptosis.[22] The coexpression of PR3 and phospholipid scramblase was shown to be closely associated with the externalization of phosphatidylserine during apoptosis.[23] Thus, PR3 can be associated with various proteins, depending on the principle leading to its membrane expression: constitutive, initiated by degranulation or apoptosis.[24]

Importantly, membrane expression of PR3 increases during neutrophil apoptosis, thus interfering with phagocytosis by macrophages and inhibiting the resolution of inflammation. In this setting, an association between PR3 and calreticulin has been recently reported. Calreticulin, a chaperone protein described as an "eat-me" signal, promotes phagocytosis of apoptotic cell by macrophages.[25] Taken together, these mechanisms contribute to the persistence of apoptotic and/or necrotic neutrophils expressing PR3 at the inflammatory site, contributing to perturb the resolution of inflammation and promote autoimmune reaction.[25] Thus, a delay in the phagocytosis of apoptotic cells, in the setting of inflammation, might play a crucial role in the emergence of autoimmune manifestations, as observed in systemic lupus erythematosus. It was also suggested that the formation of NETs, composed of DNA expelled by dying neutrophils, which contain granules-derived cationic proteins including PR3 and MPO might be involved in the pathophysiology of AAV.[2] However, it is unclear how this mechanism might explain the selectivity of ANCA toward PR3 and MPO in AAV.

Neutrophils in ANCA-associated Vasculitides

Neutrophils play a major role in the pathophysiology of AAV, particularly in the mechanisms of endothelial injury and immune dysregulation associated with these conditions.

Thus, neutrophils are not simple terminal effector cells but are also capable of immunomodulation with the secretion of a variety of cytokines and chemokines[26] as a consequence of an active crosstalk with monocytes, dendritic cells, T lymphocytes, and B lymphocytes. For instance, neutrophils secrete high amounts of B-cell-activating factor (BAFF) and a proliferation-inducing ligand, which are both members of the TNF superfamily and involved in the B lymphocyte homeostasis.[27] In particular, serum BAFF levels are higher in patients with GPA as compared to controls.[28]

One of the possible mechanisms of presentation of target antigens, PR3 and MPO, are the formation of the formed DNA structures during a particular neutrophil death with a supposed antibacterial role: NETs.[29] Neutrophil extracellular traps exponents, PR3 and MPO, in ANCA vasculitides renal lesions have been reported.[2] The relevance of the antibacterial role of the NET has recently been called into doubt,[30] while the relevance of the formation of the NET is itself subject to interrogations. In addition, NET formation does not explain this selectivity of ANCA toward PR3 and MPO.

Enhanced Granular Protein Synthesis

Neutrophils from patients with AAV might have intrinsic defects that would contribute to amplify the pathogenetical process. Most of the studies performed in this setting focused on the interaction between neutrophils and ANCA, and relatively few studies were dedicated to the potential alteration of these cells during disease flare or in remission. Interestingly, at the time of disease flare, neutrophils of patients with GPA strongly re-express PR3 and MPO genes, while these genes are usually expressed only during the promyelocytic phase of the granulocytic differentiation, according to the "targeting by timing" theory.[31] Gene expression profiling studies on peripheral blood leukocytes identified more than 200 genes overexpressed in neutrophils of patients with ANCA-positive vasculitis.[32]

Increased Neutrophils Survival

Upon activation by ANCA, neutrophils from patients with AAV are characterized by increased apoptosis in vitro as compared to healthy controls.[33] On the other hand, it has been documented that the spontaneous apoptosis of neutrophils was delayed in patients with AAV.[34] Also, we recently reported that neutrophils from patients with GPA express increased expression of cytosolic proliferating cell nuclear antigen, a molecule known to be associated with increased neutrophil survival.[35] However, the potential consequences of these disturbances in the survival/apoptosis balance and the clearance of apoptotic neutrophils are not determined, which is the actual focus of ongoing research.

NEUTROPHIL ACTIVATION IN ANCA-ASSOCIATED VASCULITIDES: ROLE OF ANCA

During the pathological course of AAV, accumulation of neutrophils at the inflammatory site is initiated by the so-called "priming" of these cells. Priming of neutrophils can be induced by adhesion, bacterial products (lipopolysaccharide), inflammatory cytokines, or lipid mediators. Primed neutrophils are in a "ready to go" state, which results in a faster and amplified response upon exposure to a second stimulus. Priming is responsible for the induction of membrane expression of PR3 and MPO that can be targeted by ANCA, triggering neutrophil activation. When incubated in vitro with IgG purified from the serum of patients with anti-PR3 ANCA or anti-MPO ANCA, primed neutrophils produce superoxide anion and release lytic granular proteins.[36] Interestingly, to exert their biological effect, ANCAs must be intact since both antigen binding through the variable regions and Fcγ receptor (FcγRIIa or FcγRIIIb) binding through the Fc portion are required and β2-integrin must be engaged.[37] It has been suggested that ANCA-activated neutrophils release oxygen radicals, release destructive enzymes through degranulation and extrude NETs that have proinflammatory properties. Release of NETs (NETosis) by ANCA-activated neutrophils also contributes to endothelial injury and death. In parallel to studies performed in vitro in the human, animal models were developed, allowing to study in vivo the role of ANCA in AAV, providing evidence that anti-MPO ANCAs are pathogenic. However, whatever the presence or absence of ANCA, there is no doubt that activated neutrophils play a crucial role in endothelial cell damages. However, further investigations are needed to identify the molecular mechanisms regulating the interactions between ANCA, neutrophils, and endothelial cells, and their potential perturbations in AAV.

Although ANCA detection represents a valuable diagnostic tool, the use of ANCA as a biomarker to predict relapses is questionable. Thus, the detection of ANCA in the serum of patients reflects disease activity in some, but not all patients with AAV. In addition, a significant proportion of patients with biopsy-proven MPA or GPA have no detectable ANCA. Taken together, these observations raise again the question of the pathogenicity of anti-PR3 ANCA in vivo. A recent work has shown that there are more than 20 epitopes of MPO recognized by MPO ANCAs in patients with AAV. Interestingly, in this study, anti-MPO IgG ANCA from patients with active AAV recognized a large number of epitopes, including epitopes that were never recognized by anti-MPO IgG ANCA from patients with inactive disease and from healthy controls. Of note, low titers of anti-MPO IgG ANCA were detected, recognizing only a few MPO epitopes. Some patients with clinical and pathologic features of AAV who were negative for ANCAs using conventional clinical assays reacted with a specific MPO epitope. IgG ANCA binding to this MPO epitope was blocked by a fragment of ceruloplasmin, which is a natural inhibitor of MPO and binds to the portion of the MPO molecule that contains this epitope. This result suggests that the epitope specificity of ANCAs might influence their biological activity independently of the ANCA titers. In keeping with this concept, it has been shown that anti-PR3 antibodies can exert a dual biological effect according to their epitope specificity, thus raising the possibility of "good" and "bad" anti-PR3 ANCA, the first of which could contribute to limit, whereas other could potentiate inflammation. Interestingly, the occurrence of anti-PR3 antibodies in healthy individuals reinforces the need to clarify factors influencing the potential involvement of anti-PR3 ANCA in the pathogenesis of AAV.

Animal Models to Study the Pathogenicity of ANCA In Vivo

Twenty years after the description of the ANCA, the pathogenic role of anti-MPO in vivo has been demonstrated, which is not so obvious for the anti-PR3. In a mouse model invalidated for the MPO gene and immunized by murine MPO, an immune response against MPO was documented.[38] The transfer of purified serum IgG containing anti-MPO antibodies or spleen cells from these animals into *recombinase-associated gene* type-2 deficient mice that have no B-cell, T-cell, or antibodies, resulted in the occurrence of extracapillary glomerulonephritis,[38] thus demonstrating the pathogenic role of anti-MPO ANCA in vivo.[39] Interestingly, alternative complement pathway has also been shown to be involved in this model.[40] In human pathology, the occurrence of a pneumorenal syndrome in a newborn of a mother who had developed vasculitis with anti-MPO ANCA, confirming the in vivo pathogenetic role of these antibodies in humans.[41] Alternatively, a recent work points to the fact that there are dominant pathogenic epitopes for anti-MPO ANCA and that the absence of detection of ANCA in patients with MPA might result from the fact that anti-MPO ANCAs were associated with a fragment of ceruloplasmin and were eliminated during the purification of IgG from serum.[42] On the other hand, the demonstration of the pathogenicity of anti-PR3 ANCAs in vivo is still missing. The detection of circulating anti-PR3

ANCA reflects the activity of the disease among some patients suffering from vasculitides, but not all. In vivo, the immunization of mice invalidated for the HNE-PR3 gene with recombinant PR3 did not result in the appearance of vasculitis-compatible manifestations. Thus, the passive transfer of anti-PR3 ANCA in the presence of lipopolysaccharide gave similar result.[43] Another group used human PR3, murine recombinant PR3, and a chimeric human/mouse PR3, and demonstrated the presence of antibodies against these chimeric proteins in the absence of pathological manifestation, especially in the kidneys or lungs.[44] However, a recent model of a severe combined immunodeficiency (SCID) humanized mouse seems to reproduce pauci-immune glomerulonephritis induced by human anti-PR3 ANCA.[45] Chimeric mice were generated by the injection of human hematopoietic stem cells into irradiated NOD-SCID mice invalidated for the IL2 receptor encoding gene (NOD-SCID-IL2R). Paired chimeric mice were treated with serum IgG obtained from patients suffering from renal and pulmonary vasculitis with anti-PR3 antibodies, renal disease other than vasculitis or healthy controls. Mice receiving injections of anti-PR3 antibodies developed a moderate form of pauci-immune proliferative glomerulonephritis, with infiltration of human and murine leukocytes so that there were no glomerular changes in controls. No granuloma was observed in this model. Even if this result is a major step toward the demonstration of the pathogenetic role of anti-PR3 ANCA in vivo, it must be confirmed by other groups.

CONCLUSION

Pauci-immune necrotizing small-vessel vasculitides and extravascular granulomatosis are associated with ANCAs. The distinctive extremely destructive necrotizing vascular inflammation appears to be fueled by an amplification loop comprising ANCA-activated neutrophils that release factors that activate the alternative complement pathway that in turn attracts and activates more neutrophils. Promising therapies that can target multiple components of this vicious cycle (e.g. ANCAs, neutrophil activation, and complement activation) are under studies. The pathogenesis of these diseases is not known.

New perspectives in the research on neutrophils in AAV should include studies to determine whether some intrinsic dysregulation could favor a failure in the resolution of inflammation. A specific investigation of the functions and the immunomodulatory roles of the target antigens, either MPO or PR3, should be carried out in order to confirm their specific and presumably differential involvement in MPA and

GPA, respectively, as suggested by the recent genomic study comparing GPA and MPA.[46]

KEY POINTS

- The ANCA antigens PR3 and MPO are key elements in the pathophysiology of ANCA-associated vasculitides.
- Neutrophil activation by ANCA promotes inflammation.
- Neutrophils in AAV appear to have specific and probably intrinsic functional dysregulation.
- DNA released by neutrophils might be involved in the autoimmunity process.

REFERENCES

1. van der Woude FJ, Rasmussen N, Lobatto S, et al. Autoantibodies against neutrophils and monocytes: tool for diagnosis and marker of disease activity in Wegener's granulomatosis. Lancet. 1985;1:425-9.
2. Kessenbrock K, Krumbholz M, Schonermarck U, et al. Netting neutrophils in autoimmune small-vessel vasculitis. Nature Med. 2009;15:623-5.
3. Witko-Sarsat V, Rieu P, Descamps-Latscha B, et al. Neutrophils: molecules, functions and pathophysiological aspects. Lab Invest. 2000;80:617-53.
4. Klebanoff SJ, Kettle AJ, Rosen H, et al. Myeloperoxidase: a front-line defender against phagocytosed microorganisms. J Leukoc Biol. 2013;93:185-98.
5. Witko-Sarsat V, Gausson V, Nguyen AT, et al. AOPP-induced activation of human neutrophil and monocyte oxidative metabolism: a potential target for n-acetylcysteine treatment in dialysis patients. Kidney Int. 2003;64:82-91.
6. Witztum JL, Lichtman AH. The influence of innate and adaptive immune responses on atherosclerosis. Annu Rev Pathol. 2014;9:73-102.
7. Shao B, Oda MN, Oram JF, et al. Myeloperoxidase: an inflammatory enzyme for generating dysfunctional high density lipoprotein. Curr Opin Cardiol. 2006;21:322-8.
8. Korkmaz B, Horwitz MS, Jenne DE, et al. Neutrophil elastase, proteinase 3, and cathepsin G as therapeutic targets in human diseases. Pharmacol Rev. 2010;62:726-59.
9. Pham CT. Neutrophil serine proteases: specific regulators of inflammation. Nature Rev Immunol. 2006;6:541-50.
10. Schreiber A, Pham CT, Hu Y, et al. Neutrophil serine proteases promote IL-1 beta generation and injury in necrotizing crescentic glomerulonephritis. J Am Soc Nephrol. 2012;23:470-82.
11. Bories D, Raynal MC, Solomon DH, et al. Down-regulation of a serine protease, myeloblastin, causes growth arrest and differentiation of promyelocytic leukemia cells. Cell. 1989;59:959-68.
12. Hajjar E, Broemstrup T, Kantari C, et al. Structures of human proteinase 3 and neutrophil elastase—so similar yet so different. FEBS J. 2010;277:2238-54.

13. Hajjar E, Mihajlovic M, Witko-Sarsat V, et al. Computational prediction of the binding site of proteinase 3 to the plasma membrane. Proteins. 2008;71:1655-69.

14. Witko-Sarsat V, Lesavre P, Lopez S, et al. A large subset of neutrophils expressing membrane proteinase 3 is a risk factor for vasculitis and rheumatoid arthritis. J Am Soc Nephrol. 1999;10:1224-33.

15. Schreiber A, Busjahn A, Luft FC, et al. Membrane expression of proteinase 3 is genetically determined. J Am Soc Nephrol. 2003;14:68-75.

16. Witko-Sarsat V, Cramer EM, Hieblot C, et al. Presence of proteinase 3 in secretory vesicles: evidence of a novel, highly mobilizable intracellular pool distinct from azurophil granules. Blood. 1999;94:2487-96.

17. Bauer S, Abdgawad M, Gunnarsson L, et al. Proteinase 3 and CD177 are expressed on the plasma membrane of the same subset of neutrophils. J Leukoc Biol. 2007;81:458-64.

18. von Vietinghoff S, Tunnemann G, Eulenberg C, et al. NB1 mediates surface expression of the ANCA antigen proteinase 3 on human neutrophils. Blood. 2007;109:4487-93.

19. David A, Fridlich R, Aviram I. The presence of membrane proteinase 3 in neutrophil lipid rafts and its colocalization with FcgammaRIIIb and cytochrome b558. Exp Cell Res. 2005;308:156-65.

20. Kantari C, Millet A, Gabillet J, et al. Molecular analysis of the membrane insertion domain of proteinase 3, the Wegener's autoantigen, in RBL cells: implication for its pathogenic activity. J Leukoc Biol. 2011;90:941-50.

21. Korkmaz B, Kuhl A, Bayat B, et al. A hydrophobic patch on proteinase 3, the target of autoantibodies in Wegener granulomatosis, mediates membrane binding via NB1 receptors. J Biol Chem. 2008;283:35976-82.

22. Kantari C, Pederzoli-Ribeil M, Amir-Moazami O, et al. Proteinase 3, the Wegener autoantigen, is externalized during neutrophil apoptosis: evidence for a functional association with phospholipid scramblase 1 and interference with macrophage phagocytosis. Blood. 2007;110:4086-95.

23. Durant S, Pederzoli M, Lepelletier Y, et al. Apoptosis-induced proteinase 3 membrane expression is independent from degranulation. J Leukoc Biol. 2004;75:87-98.

24. Witko-Sarsat V, Reuter N, Mouthon L. Interaction of proteinase 3 with its associated partners: implications in the pathogenesis of Wegener's granulomatosis. Curr Opin Rheumatol. 2010;22:1-7.

25. Gabillet J, Millet A, Pederzoli-Ribeil M, et al. Proteinase 3, the autoantigen in granulomatosis with polyangiitis, associates with calreticulin on apoptotic neutrophils, impairs macrophage phagocytosis, and promotes inflammation. J Immunol. 2012;189:2574-83.

26. Mantovani A, Cassatella MA, Costantini C, et al. Neutrophils in the activation and regulation of innate and adaptive immunity. Nature Rev Immunol. 2011;11:519-31.

27. Scapini P, Nardelli B, Nadali G, et al. G-CSF-stimulated neutrophils are a prominent source of functional BLyS. J Exp Med. 2003;197:297-302.

28. Holden NJ, Williams JM, Morgan MD, et al. ANCA-stimulated neutrophils release BLyS and promote B cell survival: a clinically relevant cellular process. Ann Rheum Dis. 2011;70:2229-33.

29. Brinkmann V, Reichard U, Goosmann C, et al. Neutrophil extracellular traps kill bacteria. Science. 2004;303:1532-5.

30. Nauseef WM. Editorial: Nyet to nets? A pause for healthy skepticism. J Leukoc Biol. 2012;91:353-5.

31. Ciavatta DJ, Yang J, Preston GA, et al. Epigenetic basis for aberrant upregulation of autoantigen genes in humans with ANCA vasculitis. J Clin Invest. 2010;120:3209-19.

32. Alcorta DA, Barnes DA, Dooley MA, et al. Leukocyte gene expression signatures in antineutrophil cytoplasmic autoantibody and lupus glomerulonephritis. Kidney Int. 2007;72:853-64.

33. Harper L, Cockwell P, Adu D, et al. Neutrophil priming and apoptosis in anti-neutrophil cytoplasmic autoantibody-associated vasculitis. Kidney Int. 2001;59:1729-38.

34. Abdgawad M, Pettersson A, Gunnarsson L, et al. Decreased neutrophil apoptosis in quiescent ANCA-associated systemic vasculitis. PLoS One. 2012;7:e32439.

35. Witko-Sarsat V, Mocek J, Bouayad D, et al. Proliferating cell nuclear antigen acts as a cytoplasmic platform controlling human neutrophil survival. J Exp Med. 2010;207:2631-45.

36. Schreiber A, Kettritz R. The neutrophil in antineutrophil cytoplasmic autoantibody-associated vasculitis. J Leukoc Biol. 2013;94:623-31.

37. Hu N, Westra J, Kallenberg CG. Membrane-bound proteinase 3 and its receptors: relevance for the pathogenesis of Wegener's granulomatosis. Autoimmun Rev. 2009;8:510-4.

38. Xiao H, Heeringa P, Hu P, et al. Antineutrophil cytoplasmic autoantibodies specific for myeloperoxidase cause glomerulo-nephritis and vasculitis in mice. J Clin Invest. 2002;110:955-63.

39. Xiao H, Heeringa P, Liu Z, et al. The role of neutrophils in the induction of glomerulonephritis by anti-myeloperoxidase antibodies. Am J Pathol. 2005;167:39-45.

40. Xiao H, Schreiber A, Heeringa P, et al. Alternative complement pathway in the pathogenesis of disease mediated by anti-neutrophil cytoplasmic autoantibodies. Am J Pathol. 2007;170:52-64.

41. Bansal PJ, Tobin MC. Neonatal microscopic polyangiitis secondary to transfer of maternal myeloperoxidase-antineutrophil cytoplasmic antibody resulting in neonatal pulmonary hemorrhage and renal involvement. Ann Allergy Asthma Immunol. 2004;93:398-401.

42. Roth AJ, Ooi JD, Hess JJ, et al. Epitope specificity determines pathogenicity and detectability in ANCA-associated vasculitis. J Clin Invest. 2013;123:1773-83.

43. Pfister H, Ollert M, Frohlich LF, et al. Antineutrophil cytoplasmic autoantibodies against the murine homolog of proteinase 3 (Wegener autoantigen) are pathogenic in vivo. Blood. 2004;104:1411-8.

44. van der Geld YM, Hellmark T, Selga D, et al. Rats and mice immunised with chimeric human/mouse proteinase 3 produce autoantibodies to mouse PR3 and rat granulocytes. Ann Rheum Dis. 2007;66:1679-82.

45. Little MA, Al-Ani B, Ren S, et al. Anti-proteinase 3 anti-neutrophil cytoplasm autoantibodies recapitulate systemic vasculitis in mice with a humanized immune system. PLoS One. 2012;7:e28626.

46. Lyons PA, Rayner TF, Trivedi S, et al. Genetically distinct subsets within ANCA-associated vasculitis. N Engl J Med. 2012;367:214-23.

CHAPTER 5

Antineutrophil Cytoplasmic Antibodies

Ashish Aggarwal, Aman Sharma, Wolfgang L Gross

Systemic vasculitides are a heterogeneous group of disorders, characterized by blood vessel destruction, associated either with the ischemia of surrounding tissues or hemorrhage due to rupture of the weakened vessel wall. The diagnosis of vasculitis remains a challenge, even to the most experienced physician.[1] Discovery of antineutrophil cytoplasmic antibodies (ANCAs) has resulted in better understanding of pathogenesis and clinical manifestations of small vessel vasculitis. Chapel Hill Consensus Classification system 2012 has given a new nomenclature of ANCA-associated vasculitis (AAV) to a group of disorders comprising of granulomatosis with polyangiitis (GPA, previously Wegener's granulomatosis), microscopic polyangiitis (MPA), and eosinophilic GPA (EGPA).[2]

ANTINEUTROPHIL CYTOPLASMIC ANTIBODIES

In 1982, Davis and associates observed a diffuse cytoplasmic staining pattern (excluding nucleus) using indirect immunofluorescence (IIF) while studying antinuclear antibodies in serum samples from patients with segmental necrotizing glomerulonephritis.[3] This IIF pattern was because of ANCA, which first became widely recognized as a result of a publication in Lancet that described circulating autoantibodies that reacted with antigens in the cytoplasm of neutrophils and monocytes in patients with GPA.[4] Myeloperoxidase (MPO) and proteinase 3 (PR3) were recognized as the major autoantigens accounting for the cytoplasmic ANCA pattern of GPA.[5,6] Antineutrophil cytoplasmic antibodies are predominantly IgG autoantibodies directed against constituents of primary granules of neutrophils and monocytes' lysosomes. Clinically, ANCA directed to PR3 or MPO are studied extensively; however, the importance of other ANCA remains unknown. The vast majority of anti-PR3 antibodies yield a cytoplasmic ANCA pattern (c-PR3-ANCA), while most anti-MPO antibodies produce a perinuclear ANCA pattern (p-MPO-ANCA) on IIF.[7]

ANTINEUTROPHIL CYTOPLASMIC ANTIBODY-ASSOCIATED VASCULITIS

Antineutrophil cytoplasmic antibody-associated vasculitis is one of the most important subgroup of small vessel involvement associated with the presence of autoantibodies directed against cytoplasmic antigens in neutrophils with specificity against MPO or PR3.[8] GPA, MPA and EGPA are collectively referred to as AAV, as they share similar pathological features and positive correlation to ANCA. C-/PR3-ANCAs are mainly detected in patients with GPA, whereas p-/MPO-ANCAs are predominantly detected in patients with MPA and CSS.[4] Antineutrophil cytoplasmic antibody-associated vasculitis is associated with significant morbidity and mortality.

PRODUCTION OF ANCA

Natural autoantibodies are present in all healthy individuals. Autoimmune diseases are the result of deregulation of natural homeostatic autoimmunity.[9] Healthy individuals have low levels of circulating natural autoantibodies specific for MPO and PR3;[10] however, the epitope specificity of the repertoire of pathogenic MPO-ANCA differs from the repertoire of epitope specificity of natural MPO-ANCA. It may hence be stated as not all ANCAs are alike, healthy individuals have ANCA that react only with natural epitopes; patients in remission have ANCA reactive with natural and nonpathogenic epitopes while patients with active disease have ANCA reactive with any epitope, i.e. natural, nonpathogenic and pathogenic.[11,12] The transition from natural autoantibodies to pathogenic autoantibodies is associated with both quantitative and qualitative changes in immune regulatory mechanisms (mainly mediated by regulatory T cell and regulatory B cells).[13] The patients with active disease have defective Tregs[14] and Bregs.[15]

INTERACTION BETWEEN ANCAs AND THEIR TARGET ANTIGENS

The interaction between ANCAs and their target antigens has been suggested to play a multifactorial role in the pathogenesis of AAV. Guilpain et al. found that MPO-ANCA positive sera could activate MPO in vitro to generate hypochlorous acid, and the by-products of MPO activation exerted a strong cytolytic activity on endothelial cells in culture. This suggests that MPO-ANCA could play a pathogenic role in vivo by triggering an oxidative burst, leading to severe endothelial damage. Also, N-acetylcysteine, a potent antioxidant molecule abrogated HOCl production and endothelial lysis.[16]

PATHOPHYSIOLOGY OF AAV

As with many other autoimmune diseases, the etiology and pathogenesis of AAV appear to be multifactorial and involve the interplay of initiating and predisposing environmental and genetic factors, loss of immune tolerance and mediation of acute injury.[17] The exact mechanism of ANCA involvement in the pathogenesis of AAV is under investigations. It largely remained ambiguous whether ANCA is involved in the disease manifestation *per se* or is associated with the prognosis of the disease.

GENETIC ASSOCIATION OF AAV

Genetic predisposition influences the onset and mediation of AAV. The distribution of AAV is not uniform across geographical regions and ethnic and racial groups, suggesting that genetic and environmental factors affect the pathogenesis of these diseases.[18] Granulomatosis with polyangiitis has been associated with HLA-DP, SERPINA1 (encoding alpha1-antitrypsin), PRTN3 (encoding PR3, the main GPA-related autoantigen) and SEMA6A (semaphorin 6A), whereas MPA has been mainly associated with HLA-DQ.[19] Cao et al.[20] found that there is a 73.3-fold higher odds of having HLADRB1*15 alleles in African Americans. In AAV patients, DRB1*0405 might be an independent risk factor for the poor response to treatment and the deterioration of renal function, whereas

DPB1*0402 might be an independent risk factor for all-cause mortality.[21] The common allele associated with other autoimmune diseases, CTLA-4 (affecting T-cell activation) and PTPN22 (negative regulatory role in T-cell receptor signaling) have been implicated also in AAV.[22] Ciavatta et al. observed epigenetic modifications in ANCA autoantigen encoding genes that result in increased expression of PR3 and MPO in neutrophils of AAV patients.[23] This could predispose to both induction and mediation of ANCA disease by providing greater amounts of target autoantigens.

ENVIRONMENTAL FACTORS

Certain environmental factors including asbestos, silica,[24] high occupational solvent exposure, allergy in general,[25] pesticides,[26] infections (bacterial endocarditis, hepatitis C virus), and drugs (antithyroid medications) have been associated with AAV. Silica exposure alone may enhance the risk for ANCA positivity to sixfolds.[27] Because silica particles are powerful stimulators of T and B cells, their inhalation by susceptible individuals might trigger production of autoantibodies including ANCA. Moreover, release of PR3-ANCA or MPO-ANCA can be induced by activation of monocytes and macrophages by silica.[28] *Staphylococcus aureus* has long been known to be associated with GPA,[29,30] although the precise immunologic link has not been proven. Nasal *S. aureus* and bacterial endocarditis have been associated with the relapse of PR3-AAV. The infectious agent exposure may lead to the phenomenon of molecular mimicry, resulting in the generation of ANCA and its responses.[31] The mimicry may be indirect as postulated by the anticomplementary PR3 antibody theory or directed against neighboring molecules in the granules such as in the antilysosomal-associated membrane protein theory. Though sensitive and specific for certain forms of small-vessel primary vasculitides,[4] ANCAs have also been reported in other infectious diseases.[32,33] Prevalence of ANCA in tuberculosis (TB) is controversial in literature.[34,35] Antineutrophil cytoplasmic antibodies in TB patients are mainly directed against bactericidal/permeability increasing protein (BPI) and mostly appear after treatment.[36] The mechanism of production and effects of BPI-ANCA in the pathophysiology of disease is poorly understood.

PATHOGENIC B-CELL RESPONSE AND PRODUCTION OF ANCA

B-cell activation and downstream signaling are due to the interaction with specific B-cell receptors and coreceptor

CD19. CD19 expression has been shown to be 20% lower in naive B cells from patients with AAV.[37] In contrast, the memory B cells from some patients showed enhanced expression of CD19. Hence, it can be concluded that the mechanisms of self-tolerance may be lost in AAV, leading to production of autoreactive B cells. Preclinical studies in transgenic mice indicate that defective B-cell regulation during deletion of autoreactive B cells may also play a role in generating autoantibodies in AAV.[38] Also, B-cell activating factor of the TNF family (BAFF) expression had been shown to enhance in patients with GPA.[39] This BAFF may result in B-cell expansion resulting ANCA production.[40] Clinically, the relapse rates are positively correlated with the enhanced levels of B cells. Rituximab, a B-cell depletion therapy, also decreases ANCA levels in patients with AAV and induces disease remission.[41] The granulomatous lesions in GPA consist of clusters of PR3 surrounded by an infiltrate consisting of maturing B cells, antigen-presenting cells, and Th1-type CD4$^+$CD28$^-$ T cells. Hence, it may be concluded that endonasal B-cell maturation is antigen driven and that B cells generate ANCA via contact with PR3 or due to molecular mimicry.[42]

ABERRANT T-CELL RESPONSE AND GRANULOMA FORMATION

The efficacy of T-cell directed therapy in AAV underlines the involvement of autoreactive T cells in AAV pathogenesis. The active GPA patients had been reported to have not only the higher proportion of activated T cells but also the higher concentration of soluble T-cell activation markers, i.e. soluble IL-2 receptor (CD30).[43] Also, there is higher expression of effector memory T cells and decreased naive T cells in AAV patients.[13] A polarization toward a Th2-type response is predominant in patients with active generalized GPA or EGPA, while a Th1 response is dominant in patients with localized GPA or MPA, indicating that aberrant T-cell response plays a role in the disease process. Hence, conversion from Th1- to Th2-type response could underlie progression from localized to generalize GPA. Furthermore, Breg might regulate Th1 cells and are associated with Treg in quiescent AAV.[44] The effector CD4+CD28 cells migrate to the granulomas in AAV and are likely to play an important role in the granulomatous response in GPA and EGPA.[45] In ANCA-associated glomerulonephritis, effector T cells are the predominant T-cell subtype in the glomerular infiltrate. The Th17 cell type has also been expanded in in vitro stimulated peripheral blood cells from WG patients. The enhanced IL-17 secretion may release proinflammatory cytokines and also secrete neutrophil-attracting chemokines that together

are responsible for increasing expression of PR3 on the membrane of neutrophils.[46] It may be concluded that Th1, Th2, and Th17 responses may have a significant contribution in the pathogenesis of AAV by autoantibody and granulomas production.

MONOCYTE ACTIVATION AND AAV

The enhanced expression of PR3 on monocytes had not been correlated with the disease pathogenesis, though the ANCA-stimulated monocytes may release various cytokines and chemokines including IL-8, TNF-α, IL-1β, IL-6, monocyte chemotactic protein-1 (MCP-1), and thromboxane A. Pathological examination of renal tissue revealed the presence of monocytes in the glomerular crescents and granulomas from patients with AAV.[47]

ANCA-MEDIATED INTERACTION BETWEEN NEUTROPHILS AND ENDOTHELIAL CELLS

It is evident from the histopathological studies that endothelial damage, neutrophil invasion, and necrosis are the clinical features of AAV. In vitro studies have shown that in the presence of ANCA, there is an interaction between neutrophils and endothelial cells.[48] Antineutrophil cytoplasmic antibodies may also convert rolling neutrophils to stably adhered neutrophils to the endothelial layer. Interaction of neutrophils with endothelial cells activates PR3 receptors on the endothelial cells that further enhance the production of tissue factor (TF) by endothelial cells.[49] Anti-MPO antibodies could play a pathogenic role in vivo by triggering an oxidative burst, leading to severe endothelial damage.[16] Endothelial cell necrosis, and release of TF, may play a role in development of vasculitic lesions. Antineutrophil cytoplasmic antibodies may also bind to the endothelial cells directly and contribute to the pathogenesis of AAV.

ANCA IN THE DIAGNOSIS OF VASCULITIS

The association of ANCA with GPA started as soon as it was discovered.[4,50] Due to the relatively high incidence of disease and the evolution of AAV into a chronic relapsing disease with a 5-year 80% survival, ANCA serology is being increasingly used as a diagnostic marker of active disease.[51]

The international consensus statement on reporting of ANCA recommended both IIF and ELISA testing when seeking to identify ANCA, yet the gold standard remained the histological studies. They also recognized the association of other diseases with ANCAs that have atypical staining patterns on IIF or antigens other than the two described (PR3 and MPO). Furthermore, they recommend that negative results by IIF should also be tested by ELISA, as 5% of samples are only positive by ELISA.[52] Hence, it may conclude, as the ANCA detection by IIF is supplemented by the ANCA detection by ELISA.[51,53-55] Although neither included in the American College of Rheumatology (ACR 1990) nor in the Chapel Hill Consensus Conference (CHCC 1994) criteria for the classification of GPA or any systemic vasculitis, testing for c-ANCA is an important feature of the work-up for patients with suspected systemic vasculitis. Both the BSR[56] and EULAR[57] guidelines insist on the necessity of symptoms and signs of vasculitis in the presence of direct histological or serological evidence (positive ANCA) or specific indirect evidence such as imaging, mononeuritis multiplex or mononeuropathy on neurophysiological testing. According to the current recommendations, combining IIF and PR3 and MPO antigen-specific immunometric assays, in the proper clinical setting, assures the best diagnostic specificity.[58,59] The clinical value of serial ANCA testing in monitoring disease activity is still debated.

SHOULD ANCA TITERS MAY BE USED FOR THE MANAGEMENT OF ANCA-VASCULITIS?

It is advised that treatment should not be altered solely on the basis of a rise in ANCA titer, since only approximately half of such rises are followed by relapse, and around half of relapses occur in the absence of rises in ANCA titer.[60] Antineutrophil cytoplasmic antibody positivity (both at the onset as well as at the time of remission) increases the risk of recurrence four or more times. However, in AAV, a rise in or persistence of ANCA during remission is only modestly predictive of future disease relapse.[61] There is only 50% ANCA elevation that ended in relapses.[62,63] Controversy exists regarding the utility of serial measurements of ANCA in patients with AAV to predict disease relapse, though it can be used to assess prognosis in patients with AAV.[64] Birck et al. in their review article had concluded that the measurement of serial ANCA is not useful to monitor the disease activity.[65] A rise in ANCA during clinical remission is at best moderately predictive of relapse. Persistently positive ANCA during remission has a positive likelihood ratio of 1.97 and negative likelihood ratio of 0.73 for subsequent relapse of disease.[61] The available evidence suggests that treatment decisions should not be solely based upon ANCA titers.[66]

KEY POINTS

- The diagnosis of vasculitis remains a challenge, even to the most experienced physician.
- Antineutrophil cytoplasmic antibodies (ANCAs) have resulted in better understanding of pathogenesis and clinical manifestations of small-vessel vasculitis.
- The exact mechanism of ANCA involvement in the pathogenesis of AAV is under investigations.
- The distribution of AAV is not uniform across geographical regions, ethnic and racial groups.
- The international consensus statement on reporting of ANCA recommended both IIF and ELISA testing when seeking to identify ANCA.
- Controversy exists regarding the utility of serial measurements of ANCA in patients with AAV to predict disease relapse.
- The available evidence suggests that treatment decisions should not be solely based upon ANCA titers.

REFERENCES

1. Rich EN, Brown KK. Treatment of antineutrophil cytoplasmic antibody-associated vasculitis. Curr Opin Pulm Med. 2012;18:447-54.
2. Jennette JC, Falk RJ, Bacon PA, et al. 2012 revised International Chapel Hill Consensus Conference Nomenclature of Vasculitides. Arthritis Rheum. 2013;65:1-11.
3. Davies DJ, Moran JE, Niall JF, et al. Segmental necrotising glomerulonephritis with antineutrophil antibody: possible arbovirus aetiology? Br Med J (Clin Res Ed). 1982;285:606.
4. van der Woude FJ, Rasmussen N, Lobatto S, et al. Autoantibodies against neutrophils and monocytes: tool for diagnosis and marker of disease activity in Wegener's granulomatosis. Lancet. 1985;1:425-9.
5. Jenne DE, Tschopp J, Ludemann J, et al. Wegener's autoantigen decoded. Nature. 1990;346:520.
6. Jennette JC, Hoidal JR, Falk RJ. Specificity of anti-neutrophil cytoplasmic autoantibodies for proteinase 3. Blood. 1990;75:2263-4.
7. Drooger JC, Dees A, Swaak AJ. ANCA-positive patients: the influence of PR3 and MPO antibodies on survival rate and the association with clinical and laboratory characteristics. Open Rheumatol J. 2009;3:14-17.
8. Jennette JC, Falk RJ, Hu P, et al. Pathogenesis of antineutrophil cytoplasmic autoantibody-associated small-vessel vasculitis. Annu Rev Pathol. 2013;8:139-60.
9. Jennette JC, Falk RJ. The rise and fall of horror autotoxicus and forbidden clones. Kidney Int. 2010;78:533-5.

10. Cui Z, Zhao MH, Segelmark M, et al. Natural autoantibodies to myeloperoxidase, proteinase 3, and the glomerular basement membrane are present in normal individuals. Kidney Int. 2010;78:590-7.

11. Roth A, Ooi J, Hess J, et al. ANCA epitope specificity determines pathogenicity, detectability and clinical predictive value. Presse Med. 2013;42:664.

12. Roth AJ, Ooi JD, Hess JJ, et al. Epitope specificity determines pathogenicity and detectability in ANCA-associated vasculitis. J Clin Invest. 2013;123:1773-83.

13. Lepse N, Abdulahad WH, Kallenberg CG, et al. Immune regulatory mechanisms in ANCA-associated vasculitides. Autoimmun Rev. 2011;11:77-83.

14. Free ME, Bunch DO, McGregor JA, et al. Patients with antineutrophil cytoplasmic antibody-associated vasculitis have defective Treg cell function exacerbated by the presence of a suppression-resistant effector cell population. Arthritis Rheum. 2013;65:1922-33.

15. Bunch DO, McGregor JG, Khandoobhai NB, et al. Decreased CD5(+) B cells in active ANCA vasculitis and relapse after rituximab. Clin J Am Soc Nephrol. 2013;8:382-91.

16. Guilpain P, Servettaz A, Goulvestre C, et al. Pathogenic effects of antimyeloperoxidase antibodies in patients with microscopic polyangiitis. Arthritis Rheum. 2007;56:2455-63.

17. Charles Jennette J, Falk RJ. L1. Pathogenesis of ANCA-associated vasculitis: observations, theories and speculations. Presse Med. 2013;42:493-8.

18. Ugarte-Gil MF, Espinoza LR. Genetics of ANCA-associated vasculitides. Curr Rheumatol Rep. 2014;16:428.

19. Alberici F, Martorana D, Bonatti F, et al. Genetics of ANCA-associated vasculitides: HLA and beyond. Clin Exp Rheumatol. 2014;32:S90-97.

20. Cao Y, Schmitz JL, Yang J, et al. Drb1*15 allele is a risk factor for PR3-ANCA disease in African Americans. J Am Soc Nephrol. 2011;22:1161-7.

21. Chang DY, Luo H, Zhou XJ, et al. Association of HLA genes with clinical outcomes of ANCA-associated vasculitis. Clin J Am Soc Nephrol. 2012;7:1293-9.

22. Martorana D, Maritati F, Malerba G, et al. PTPN22 R620W polymorphism in the ANCA-associated vasculitides. Rheumatology (Oxford). 2012;51:805-12.

23. Ciavatta DJ, Yang J, Preston GA, et al. Epigenetic basis for aberrant upregulation of autoantigen genes in humans with ANCA vasculitis. J Clin Invest. 2010;120:3209-19.

24. Rihova Z, Maixnerova D, Jancova E, et al. Silica and asbestos exposure in ANCA-associated vasculitis with pulmonary involvement. Ren Fail. 2005;27:605-8.

25. Barragan-Martinez C, Speck-Hernandez CA, Montoya-Ortiz G, et al. Organic solvents as risk factor for autoimmune diseases: a systematic review and meta-analysis. PLoS One. 2012;7:e51506.

26. de Lind van Wijngaarden RA, van Rijn L, Hagen EC, et al. Hypotheses on the etiology of antineutrophil cytoplasmic autoantibody associated vasculitis: the cause is hidden, but the result is known. Clin J Am Soc Nephrol. 2008;3:237-52.

27. Hogan SL, Cooper GS, Savitz DA, et al. Association of silica exposure with anti-neutrophil cytoplasmic autoantibody small-vessel vasculitis: a population-based, case-control study. Clin J Am Soc Nephrol. 2007;2:290-9.

28. Gomez-Puerta JA, Gedmintas L, Costenbader KH. The association between silica exposure and development of ANCA-associated vasculitis: systematic review and meta-analysis. Autoimmun Rev. 2013;12:1129-35.

29. Tadema H, Heeringa P, Kallenberg CG. Bacterial infections in Wegener's granulomatosis: mechanisms potentially involved in autoimmune pathogenesis. Curr Opin Rheumatol. 2011;23:366-71.

30. Tadema H, Abdulahad WH, Lepse N, et al. Bacterial DNA motifs trigger ANCA production in ANCA-associated vasculitis in remission. Rheumatology (Oxford). 2011;50:689-96.

31. Pendergraft WF 3rd, Preston GA, Shah RR, et al. Autoimmunity is triggered by cPR-3(105-201), a protein complementary to human autoantigen proteinase-3. Nat Med. 2004;10:72-79.

32. Bosch X, Guilabert A, Font J. Antineutrophil cytoplasmic antibodies. Lancet. 2006;368:404-18.

33. Knight A, Ekbom A, Brandt L, et al. What is the significance in routine care of c-ANCA/PR3-ANCA in the absence of systemic vasculitis? A case series. Clin Exp Rheumatol. 2008;26:S53-56.

34. Flores-Suarez LF, Cabiedes J, Villa AR, et al. Prevalence of antineutrophil cytoplasmic autoantibodies in patients with tuberculosis. Rheumatology (Oxford). 2003;42:223-9.

35. Teixeira L, Mahr A, Jaureguy F, et al. Low seroprevalence and poor specificity of antineutrophil cytoplasmic antibodies in tuberculosis. Rheumatology (Oxford). 2005;44:247-50.

36. Esquivel-Valerio JA, Flores-Suarez LF, Rodriguez-Amado J, et al. Antineutrophil cytoplasm autoantibodies in patients with tuberculosis are directed against bactericidal/permeability increasing protein and are detected after treatment initiation. Clin Exp Rheumatol. 2010;28:35-39.

37. Culton DA, Nicholas MW, Bunch DO, et al. Similar CD19 dysregulation in two autoantibody-associated autoimmune diseases suggests a shared mechanism of B-cell tolerance loss. J Clin Immunol. 2007;27:53-68.

38. Bunch DO, Silver JS, Majure MC, et al. Maintenance of tolerance by regulation of anti-myeloperoxidase B cells. J Am Soc Nephrol. 2008;19:1763-73.

39. Krumbholz M, Specks U, Wick M, et al. BAFF is elevated in serum of patients with Wegener's granulomatosis. J Autoimmun. 2005;25:298-302.

40. Silva F, Cisternas M, Specks U. TNF-alpha blocker therapy and solid malignancy risk in ANCA-associated vasculitis. Curr Rheumatol Rep. 2012;14:501-8.

41. Zand L, Specks U, Sethi S, et al. Treatment of ANCA-associated vasculitis: new therapies and a look at old entities. Adv Chronic Kidney Dis. 2014;21:182-93.

42. Jennette JC, Falk RJ. B cell-mediated pathogenesis of ANCA-mediated vasculitis. Semin Immunopathol. 2014;36:327-38.

43. Sanders JS, Huitma MG, Kallenberg CG, et al. Plasma levels of soluble interleukin 2 receptor, soluble CD30, interleukin 10 and B cell activator of the tumour necrosis factor family during follow-up in vasculitis associated with proteinase 3-antineutrophil cytoplasmic antibodies: associations with disease activity and relapse. Ann Rheum Dis. 2006;65:1484-9.

44. Wilde B, Thewissen M, Damoiseaux J, et al. Regulatory B cells in ANCA-associated vasculitis. Ann Rheum Dis. 2013;72:1416-9.

45. Abdulahad WH, van der Geld YM, Stegeman CA, et al. Persistent expansion of CD4+ effector memory T cells in Wegener's granulomatosis. Kidney Int. 2006;70:938-47.

46. Velden J, Paust HJ, Hoxha E, et al. Renal IL-17 expression in human ANCA-associated glomerulonephritis. Am J Physiol Renal Physiol. 2012;302:F1663-73.

47. Wikman A, Lundahl J, Jacobson SH. Sustained monocyte activation in clinical remission of systemic vasculitis. Inflammation. 2008;31:384-90.

48. Halbwachs L, Lesavre P. Endothelium–neutrophil interactions in ANCA-associated diseases. J Am Soc Nephrol. 2012;23:1449-61.

49. Nolan SL, Kalia N, Nash GB, et al. Mechanisms of ANCA-mediated leukocyte–endothelial cell interactions in vivo. J Am Soc Nephrol. 2008;19:973-84.

50. Falk RJ, Jennette JC. Anti-neutrophil cytoplasmic autoantibodies with specificity for myeloperoxidase in patients with systemic vasculitis and idiopathic necrotizing and crescentic glomerulonephritis. N Engl J Med. 1988;318:1651-7.

51. Luxton G, Langham R. The CARI guidelines. ANCA serology in the diagnosis and management of ANCA-associated renal vasculitis. Nephrology (Carlton). 2008;13:S17-23.

52. Savige JA, Paspaliaris B, Silvestrini R, et al. A review of immunofluorescent patterns associated with antineutrophil cytoplasmic antibodies (ANCA) and their differentiation from other antibodies. J Clin Pathol. 1998;51:568-75.

53. Hagen EC, Daha MR, Hermans J, et al. Diagnostic value of standardized assays for anti-neutrophil cytoplasmic antibodies in idiopathic systemic vasculitis. EC/BCR project for ANCA assay standardization. Kidney Int. 1998;53:743-53.

54. Savige J, Neeson P, Trevisin M, et al. ELISA is the superior method for detecting antineutrophil cytoplasmic antibodies in the diagnosis of systemic necrotising vasculitis. J Clin Pathol. 2000;53:644-5.

55. Westman KW, Bygren PG, Olsson H, et al. Relapse rate, renal survival, and cancer morbidity in patients with Wegener's granulomatosis or microscopic polyangiitis with renal involvement. J Am Soc Nephrol. 1998;9:842-52.

56. Ntatsaki E, Carruthers D, Chakravarty K, et al. BSR AND BHPR guideline for the management of adults with ANCA-associated vasculitis. Rheumatology (Oxford). 2014. doi: 10.1093/rheumatology/keu009

57. Mukhtyar C, Guillevin L, Cid MC, et al. EULAR recommendations for the management of primary small and medium vessel vasculitis. Ann Rheum Dis. 2009;68:310-7.

58. Sinico RA, Radice A. Antineutrophil cytoplasmic antibodies (ANCA) testing: Detection methods and clinical application. Clin Exp Rheumatol. 2014;32:S112-7.

59. Csernok E, Moosig F. Current and emerging techniques for ANCA detection in vasculitis. Nature Rev Rheumatol. 2014;10: 494-501.

60. Carruthers D, Sherlock J. Evidence-based management of ANCA vasculitis. Best Pract Res Clin Rheumatol. 2009;23:367-78.

61. Tomasson G, Grayson PC, Mahr AD, et al. Value of ANCA measurements during remission to predict a relapse of ANCA-associated vasculitis—a meta-analysis. Rheumatology (Oxford). 2012;51:100-9.

62. Boomsma MM, Stegeman CA, van der Leij MJ, et al. Prediction of relapses in Wegener's granulomatosis by measurement of antineutrophil cytoplasmic antibody levels: a prospective study. Arthritis Rheum. 2000;43:2025-33.

63. Finkielman JD, Merkel PA, Schroeder D, et al. Antiproteinase 3 antineutrophil cytoplasmic antibodies and disease activity in Wegener granulomatosis. Ann Intern Med. 2007;147:611-9.

64. Specks U. Controversies in ANCA testing. Cleve Clin J Med. 2012;79:S7-11.

65. Birck R, Schmitt WH, Kaelsch IA, et al. Serial ANCA determinations for monitoring disease activity in patients with ANCA-associated vasculitis: systematic review. Am J Kidney Dis. 2006;47:15-23.

66. Rua-Figueroa Fernandez de Larrinoa I, Erausquin Arruabarrena C. Treatment of ANCA-associated systemic vasculitis. Rheumatol Clin. 2010;6:161-72.

CHAPTER 6

Animal Models of ANCA Vasculitis

Mark Little, Alice Coughlan

INTRODUCTION

Easily manipulated small animal models of disease provide the opportunity to examine complex disease processes *in vivo*, as well as providing a method of testing new therapies and biomarkers, and are therefore essential tools in biomedical research. In order to study ANCA-associated vasculitis (AAV) *in vivo*, considerable effort has been made

to develop rodent models of the disease, resulting in the emergence of four accepted models: the passive transfer model, the bone marrow transplant model, the experimental autoimmune vasculitis (EAV) mouse model, and EAV rat model (Figs 6.1A to D).

Of these, three are based on mice that reflect the relatively large number of knockout and genetically manipulated mouse strains available. Importantly, each model has

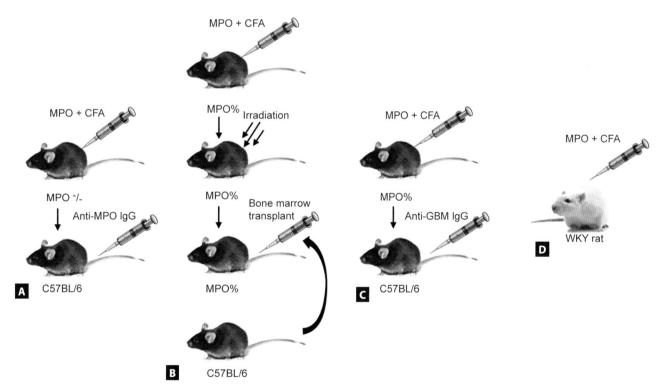

Figs 6.1A to D Overview of disease induction in the four most commonly used rodent models of ANCA vasculitis. (A) The passive transfer model; (B) The bone marrow transplant model; (C) The EAV mouse model; (D) The EAV rat model. C57BL/6 mice are a strain of wild-type, that is genetically unmodified, mice.
Abbreviations: MPO, myeloperoxidase; CFA, complete Freund's adjuvant; GBM, glomerular basement membrane; WKY, Wistar-Kyoto rats

its own strengths and weakness, with the most suitable model depending heavily on the experimental question being asked.

PASSIVE TRANSFER MODEL

The first breakthrough in the development of *in vivo* models of AAV came when Xiao et al. discovered that transfer of anti-MPO antibodies into mice induces a pauci-immune, crescentic glomerulonephritis (GN) that closely resembles human AAV.[1] In this model, anti-myeloperoxidase (anti-MPO) antibodies are raised through immunization of MPO-deficient mice with murine MPO. These antibodies are then transferred into wild type mice (i.e. mice with native MPO), which go on to develop disease (Fig. 6.1A). This is commonly known as *the passive transfer model* and remains the most widely used model of MPO-ANCA vasculitis.

While the passive transfer model provided the first evidence that ANCA are, in and of themselves, pathogenic, there remains several limitations associated with the model. Firstly, it should be noted that disease is mild, with, on average, 5–10% of glomeruli affected. With a slight modification to the model, in the form of systemic administration of the proinflammatory stimulus lipopolysaccharide (LPS), a more severe phenotype can be induced.[2] However, despite this, the GN seen in mice remains relatively mild when compared to human disease. The reason for this may be due to the fact that the model engages only the innate immune response, with passively transferred antibody interacting with neutrophils to induce disease. However, while neutrophils are the key effector cell in early AAV, it is highly likely that other cell types, for example effector T cells, also play a significant role in human disease pathogenesis. Finally, the passive transfer model is not in the strictest sense an autoimmune model, as antibodies are raised against a foreign antigen. Thus, it is possible, and perhaps likely, that the response we see does not fully reflect what is happening in humans.

BONE MARROW TRANSPLANT MODEL

The *bone marrow transplant model* is a variation of the passive transfer model in which MPO-deficient mice immunized with MPO are irradiated, following the development of anti-MPO antibodies, and then immediately transplanted with bone marrow from MPO-sufficient mice (Fig. 6.1B).[3] As the antibody-producing plasma cells are relatively resistant to irradiation, they remain in the mouse, resulting in the continued production of anti-MPO antibodies. This then allows investigation of the chronic phase of disease. In addition, it allows one to separate out the impact of bone marrow-derived cells on the pathogenesis, and to use genetically manipulated mice as bone marrow donors.

Although arguably an improvement on the passive transfer model, the bone marrow transplant model has many of the same limitations. The bone marrow transplant model is a relatively mild model of a severe human disease, which depends on the effect of an antibody raised against a foreign antigen with no break in tolerance. The disease in the bone marrow transplant model also takes considerably longer to develop than in the passive transfer model: up to 8 weeks for the bone marrow transplant model compared to 1 week for the passive transfer model.

MOUSE MODEL OF AUTOIMMUNE VASCULITIS

Using a different approach to disease induction, Ruth et al. immunized wild-type C57BL/6 mice with MPO, leading to a break in tolerance and the development of both humoral and cellular immune responses against MPO.[4] Unfortunately, this was not sufficient to induce renal damage, possibly due to the relatively low levels of antibody produced. However, a local renal immune response in the glomeruli, resulting in pauci-immune crescentic GN, can be induced by administration of subnephritogenic levels of sheep-derived anti-glomerular basement membrane (anti-GBM) antibodies (Fig. 6.1C). The anti-GBM antibody in this model probably serves to attract neutrophils to the glomeruli and induce degranulation, leading to the deposition of MPO. This MPO then acts as a planted autoantigen for MPO-specific antibodies and CD4[+] T cells, leading to glomerular damage and thus a disease phenotype similar to that seen in humans.

In contrast to the passive transfer and bone marrow transplant models, and as the title suggests, this model involves a break in tolerance and is thus a model of autoimmunity. However, the fact that the disease is triggered by administration of anti-GBM antibody, of which there is no direct equivalent in human disease, complicates the model and represents a limitation to this approach.

RAT MODEL OF EXPERIMENTAL AUTOIMMUNE VASCULITIS

Shortly before the development of the autoimmune vasculitis mouse model, an analogous model was established in rats. Using a similar approach to Ruth et al. Little et al. immunized Wistar-Kyoto (WKY) rats with human MPO (Fig. 6.1D).[5] This resulted in the generation of MPO-ANCA and MPO-reactive T cells, ultimately leading to the development of a mild crescentic, pauci-immune GN in approximately 60% of the animals treated. Interestingly, pulmonary capillaritis was also observed in a proportion (approximately 40%) of treated animals. Although disease was not induced in all animals in this study, a subsequent study went on to show that more severe disease could be induced in all animals treated through the addition of pertussis toxin to the complete Freund's adjuvant (CFA) used during the immunization stage.[6]

As with the mouse model of autoimmune vasculitis, this model involves a break in tolerance. Indeed, although the initial antibodies and T cells produced are anti-human, they are cross reactive with rat MPO, which displays significant homology to the human molecule, and thus the immune response leading to disease is to an autoantigen. There are, however, disadvantages associated with this model. Firstly, genetically modified strains of rats, used to examine particular aspects of disease pathogenesis, are not nearly as readily available as genetically modified mouse strains. In addition, disease can only be induced in a particular strain of rats, the WKY rats, which are already predisposed to the development of GN.[6] Thus, although genetically modified rat strains are slowly becoming more readily available, it remains difficult to acquire genetically modified rats that would be susceptible to disease induction. Finally, disease induction can take up to 8 weeks, and the disease phenotype is relatively mild.

RODENT MODELS OF PR3-ANCA DISEASE

To date, there is no widely accepted model of PR3-ANCA-induced disease. This is despite numerous attempts at generating a model, many using approaches that proved successful for MPO-ANCA-induced disease. Briefly, disease induction strategies that have been tried include the following:

- *Immunization of rats and mice with combinations of human or murine PR3 or chimeric molecules:* Although anti-PR3 antibodies could be generated in this manner, disease was not observed.[7]
- *The passive transfer of anti-PR3 antibodies into LPS-primed mice:* In this model, anti-PR3 antibodies were generated by immunization of PR3- and elastase-deficient mice with murine PR3. While no renal or pulmonary disease was found, transferred anti-PR3 antibodies did exacerbate inflammation in tumor necrosis factor (TNF)-α-primed skin.[8]
- *The transfer of PR3-ANCA-producing splenocytes, isolated from recombinant murine PR3 immunized nonobese diabetic (NOD) mice, into naive NOD-severe combined immunodeficiency (SCID) recipients (which lack T and B cells):* Although mice developed vasculitis and necrotizing crescentic GN, there is evidence to suggest that it was

not pauci immune. Additionally, transfer of PR3-ANCA-producing splenocytes did not induce disease in C57BL/6 mice, making the use of genetically modified mouse strains difficult.[9]

- *The passive transfer of patient-derived human anti-PR3 antibodies into humanized mice:* In this context, humanized mice refer to highly immunodeficient NOD-SCID interleukin-2 (IL-2) receptor gamma knockout mice transplanted with human stem cells and thus possessing human immune cells. Humanized mice that received human PR3-ANCA developed mild GN and lung hemorrhage. Although the results from this study are promising, further work is required if this model is to become widely applied.[10]

The failure of these various strategies to provide a robust model of PR3-ANCA-associated disease is likely to be related to the differences between human and rodent PR3, in particular with regards their cellular expression.[11] Thus, and taking into account promising preliminary data with regards the humanized mouse model, future attempts to develop a PR3-ANCA model will likely rely on the use of humanized or transgenic *in vivo* systems.

INSIGHTS FROM ANIMAL MODELS

Despite their limitations, the various animal models of AAV remain useful tools to study disease pathogenesis and to test potential therapies in vivo, with several major discoveries in the field of AAV having been made through their use.

Using the passive transfer model, it has been shown that neutrophils are the key effector cells in AAV, with their depletion completely preventing disease.[12] Furthermore, it has been shown that the co-administration of LPS with anti-MPO antibody exacerbates disease in a toll-like receptor (TLR)-4 dependent manner.[2] When taken together, these findings support the theory that, following infection, pro-inflammatory stimuli act synergistically with MPO-ANCA to induce disease. While this was an important finding, defining how we think about disease pathogenesis, it was not unexpected. In contrast, the finding that the complement system plays a substantial role in AAV, a pauci-immune disease with little or no complement deposition, came as a surprise. However, using both the passive transfer and bone marrow transplant models, several studies have shown that mice deficient in C5a, its receptor and alternative complement factor B, are completely protected from GN.[13-15] Importantly, it was also shown that use of a C5a-depleting antibody attenuated kidney disease even when treatment was started post disease induction.[13] Thus, these in vivo studies highlighted a potential, and unexpected, therapeutic target. In addition to the role of complement, studies carried out in these two models have identified several signaling pathways important in AAV pathogenesis including the phosphoinositide 3-kinase (PI3K) pathway[16] (the bone marrow transplant model), the p38 mitogen-activated protein kinase (MAPK) pathway[17] (the passive transfer model), and the Fc receptor signaling pathway[18,19] (the passive transfer model).

One of the most significant findings to emerge from the use of animal models is that MPO-specific CD4[+] T cells potentially play an important role in AAV pathogenesis, outside of their helper cell capacity.[4] Indeed, the mouse model, which depends on CD4[+] T cells to induce GN, has been used to show that Th17 cells, a proinflammatory CD4[+] T cell subset, are likely play a key role in GN.[20] Furthermore, this model has been used to show that TLR2, through its ability to enhance Th17 responses, and TLR9, through its ability to enhance Th1 responses, are also likely to have roles in disease pathogenesis.[20] Importantly, and as mentioned earlier, pertussis toxin has the ability to exacerbate GN in the rat model of disease. Thus, as pertussis toxin activates both naive CD4[+] T cells and TLR2/4, which skews T cells toward Th1 and Th17 phenotypes, this further supports a role for these cells in AAV.[21] In addition to highlighting the role of CD4[+] T cells in disease, the rat model has also been used to examine leukocyte–endothelial cell interactions, with anti-MPO IgG being shown to increase leukocyte adhesion and migation to venules,[5] and to test anti-TNF-α as a potential therapeutic target.[22] In the case of the former study, anti-TNF-α antibodies attenuated MPO-ANCA-induced GN, illuminating a potential therapeutic target.

CONCLUSION

Several groups have successfully generated pathology in mice and rats that closely resembles human MPO-ANCA-associated vasculitis and thus have provided the opportunity for researchers to examine, and ultimately manipulate, the complex interactions involved in disease pathogenesis in an in vivo setting. Indeed, the passive transfer and bone marrow transplant models have been used to better understand the interplay of neutrophils, ANCA and endothelial cells in vivo, in addition to providing evidence that the complement system plays a fundamental role in AAV pathogenesis. Concurrently, active immunization of mice and rats with MPO has allowed the study of both the cellular and humeral immune response, highlighting the importance of effector T cells in disease pathogenesis and providing models suited to long-term trials of novel therapeutics. Importantly, while there is currently no model that reflects all aspects of human disease, if interpreted

with caution, and combined with appropriate in vitro data collected using patient samples, as well as cell-based assays, data obtained from animal studies can yield exciting and important results that may provide the basis for future therapeutic interventions.

KEY POINTS

- MPO-ANCA vasculitis has been modeled using:
  - Passive transfer of high titer anti-mouse MPO antibody into an array of genetically modified naive murine recipients.
  - Transfer of mouse MPO-replete bone marrow into MPO-immunized MPO-deficient recipients.
  - Breaking tolerance to MPO in the mouse by immunization with human MPO, with focusing of the consequent immune response in the kidney by administration of antiglomerular basement antibody.
  - Breaking tolerance to MPO in the Wistar-Kyoto rat by immunization with human MPO; cross reactivity of the consequent adaptive immune response with rat MPO results in the pathological features of ANCA vasculitis.
- PR3-ANCA vasculitis has proved difficult to model, with approaches similar to those used to model MPO-ANCA vasculitis failing to induce disease, probably because of differences in structure and cellular location between the mouse and human PR3 molecule. Transgenic approaches to introduce the human counterpart into the mouse, or use of hematopoietic stem cells to induce a human immune system in immunodeficient mouse strains, hold promise for the future.

REFERENCES

1. Xiao H, Heeringa P, Hu P, et al. Antineutrophil cytoplasmic autoantibodies specific for myeloperoxidase cause glomerulo-nephritis and vasculitis in mice. J Clin Invest. 2002;110:955-63.
2. Huugen D, Xiao H, van Esch A, et al. Aggravation of anti-myeloperoxidase antibody-induced glomerulonephritis by bacterial lipopolysaccharide: role of tumor necrosis factor-alpha. Am J Pathol. 2005;167:47-58.
3. Schreiber A, Xiao H, Falk RJ, et al. Bone marrow-derived cells are sufficient and necessary targets to mediate glomerulonephritis and vasculitis induced by anti-myeloperoxidase antibodies. J Am Soc Nephrol. 2006;17:3355-64.
4. Ruth AJ, Kitching AR, Kwan RY, et al. Anti-neutrophil cytoplasmic antibodies and effector CD4[+] cells play nonredundant roles in anti-myeloperoxidase crescentic glomerulonephritis. J Am Soc Nephrol. 2006;17:1940-9.

5. Little MA, Smyth CL, Yadav R, et al. Antineutrophil cytoplasm antibodies directed against myeloperoxidase augment leukocyte-microvascular interactions in vivo. Blood. 2005;106:2050-8.

6. Little MA, Smyth L, Salama AD, et al. Experimental autoimmune vasculitis: an animal model of anti-neutrophil cytoplasmic autoantibody-associated systemic vasculitis. Am J Pathol. 2009;174:1212-20.

7. van der Geld YM, Hellmark T, Selga D, et al. Rats and mice immunised with chimeric human/mouse proteinase 3 produce autoantibodies to mouse pr3 and rat granulocytes. Ann Rheum Dis. 2007;66:1679-82.

8. Pfister H, Ollert M, Frohlich LF, et al. Antineutrophil cytoplasmic autoantibodies against the murine homolog of proteinase 3 (Wegener autoantigen) are pathogenic in vivo. Blood. 2004;104:1411-8.

9. Primo VC, Marusic S, Franklin CC, et al. Anti-PR3 immune responses induce segmental and necrotizing glomerulonephritis. Clin Exp Immunol. 2010;159:327-37.

10. Little MA, Al-Ani B, Ren S, et al. Anti-proteinase 3 antineutrophil cytoplasm autoantibodies recapitulate systemic vasculitis in mice with a humanized immune system. PLoS One. 2012;7:e28626.

11. Wiesner O, Litwiller RD, Hummel AM, et al. Differences between human proteinase 3 and neutrophil elastase and their murine homologues are relevant for murine model experiments. FEBS Lett. 2005;579:5305-12.

12. Xiao H, Heeringa P, Liu Z, et al. The role of neutrophils in the induction of glomerulonephritis by anti-myeloperoxidase antibodies. Am J Pathol. 2005;167:39-45.

13. Huugen D, van Esch A, Xiao H, et al. Inhibition of complement factor C5 protects against anti-myeloperoxidase antibody-mediated glomerulonephritis in mice. Kidney Int. 2007;71:646-54.

14. Schreiber A, Xiao H, Jennette JC, et al. C5a receptor mediates neutrophil activation and ANCA-induced glomerulonephritis. J Am Soc Nephrol. 2009;20:289-98.

15. Xiao H, Schreiber A, Heeringa P, et al. Alternative complement pathway in the pathogenesis of disease mediated by antineutrophil cytoplasmic autoantibodies. Am J Pathol. 2007;170:52-64.

16. Schreiber A, Rolle S, Peripelittchenko L, et al. Phosphoinositol 3-kinase-gamma mediates antineutrophil cytoplasmic autoantibody-induced glomerulonephritis. Kidney Int. 2010;77:118-28.

17. van der Veen BS, Chen M, Muller R, et al. Effects of p38 mitogen-activated protein kinase inhibition on anti-neutrophil cytoplasmic autoantibody pathogenicity in vitro and in vivo. Ann Rheum Dis. 2011;70:356-65.

18. Nolan SL, Kalia N, Nash GB, et al. Mechanisms of ANCA-mediated leukocyte–endothelial cell interactions in vivo. J Am Soc Nephrol. 2008;19:973-84.

19. van Timmeren MM, van der Veen BS, Stegeman CA, et al. IgG glycan hydrolysis attenuates ANCA-mediated glomerulonephritis. J Am Soc Nephrol. 2010;21:1103-14.

20. Summers SA, Steinmetz OM, Gan PY, et al. Toll-like receptor 2 induces Th17 myeloperoxidase autoimmunity while toll-like receptor 9 drives Th1 autoimmunity in murine vasculitis. Arthritis Rheum. 2011;63:1124-35.

21. Nasso M, Fedele G, Spensieri F, et al. Genetically detoxified pertussis toxin induces Th1/Th17 immune response through MAPKs and IL-10-dependent mechanisms. J Immunol. 2009;183:1892-9.

22. Little MA, Bhangal G, Smyth CL, et al. Therapeutic effect of anti-TNF-alpha antibodies in an experimental model of anti-neutrophil cytoplasm antibody-associated systemic vasculitis. J Am Soc Nephrol. 2006;17:160-9.

CHAPTER 7

Pathogenesis of Vasculitis

Durga Prasanna Misra, Anupam Wakhlu, Vikas Agarwal

INTRODUCTION

The term "vasculitis" refers to inflammation of the vessel wall that may result in dysfunction in the organ/s supplied by the involved blood vessel. Blood vessel of all sizes—small, medium, and large—may be affected; however, each vasculitis differs in pathogenetic mechanisms.

CLASSIFICATION AND NOMENCLATURE

The vasculitides are a group of multisystem disorders tied together by a common thread of vessel wall inflammation. They are classified depending on the predominant type of blood vessel affected (large—aorta and its major branches; medium—visceral arteries and their branches, and small—intraparenchymal arteries, arterioles, capillaries, and venules). Of note, such a classification refers to the dominantly affected vessel type and does not imply that in a particular type of vasculitis, other types of vessels cannot be affected. The nomenclature of vasculitis as suggested by the Chapel Hill Consensus Conference 2012 is already mentioned in the previous chapter. The clinical features consequent to the different types of vasculitis vary accordingly. Large-vessel vasculitides cause pulse loss, asymmetry of blood pressure, limb claudication, bruits in the stenosed vessels, renovascular hypertension, and vessel dilatation secondary to scarring. Medium-vessel vasculitis manifests as cutaneous involvement in the form of ulcers, livedo reticularis, nodules and digital gangrene, renovascular hypertension, mononeuritis multiplex resulting from vasa nervorum involvement, and microaneurysms demonstrable on visceral vessel imaging. Small-vessel vasculitis can affect the kidneys (glomerulonephritis), upper respiratory tract (sinusitis, collapse of nasal bridge, ear discharge, and hearing loss), lower respiratory tract (subglottic stenosis, pulmonary

alveolar capillaritis causing pulmonary hemorrhage, and respiratory failure), peripheral nerves (mono or polyneuropathy), eyes (scleritis, episcleritis, uveitis, and orbital granulomas), and skin (leukocytoclastic vasculitis, purpura, vesiculobullous lesions, urticaria, and cutaneous granulomata).[1] We shall consider separately pathogenesis of vasculitis predominantly involving large, medium, and small (immune-complex-mediated and ANCA-associated) vessels, taking into account animal models, genetic predisposition, environmental influences, and immune aberrations.

PATHOGENESIS OF LARGE-VESSEL VASCULITIS

Giant Cell Arteritis

Pathology

Temporal artery biopsy usually shows transmural inflammation encompassing all the layers of the artery with infiltration with lymphocytes and macrophages in the form of granulomas, usually near the disrupted internal elastic lamina. Intimal hyperplasia is seen leading to vessel occlusion.[2]

Pathogenesis

Genetics: The increased frequency of HLA alleles DRB1*0401 and B1*0404/08 has been demonstrated in patients with giant cell arteritis (GCA).

Innate immunity: Each vessel in the vascular tree exhibits a distinct toll-like receptor (TLR) profile and supports selective T-cell responses, accounting for the differences in vessel involvement in GCA and Takayasu's arteritis (TA).[3] Activated dendritic cells (DCs) produce CCL18, CCL19, and CCL21 and bind chemokine receptor CCR7 expressed on their cell surface, with resultant trapping in the aortic wall. Activated DCs colocalize with T cells in the inflamed aortic wall and express costimulatory CD86, driving T-cell-mediated inflammation (in contrast to immature DCs that are tolerogenic to nearby T cells). It is hypothesized that DCs provide antigenic stimulation to CD4+ cells in GCA and link innate and adaptive immune responses in this disease.[2]

Adaptive immunity: Giant cell arteritis is predominantly a T-cell-driven disease. It results in recruitment and activation of Th1 cells, which secrete IFN-γ leading to granulomatous inflammation and macrophage activation with smooth muscle migration and intimal proliferation due to PDGF and VEGF.[2] An important role of Th17 cells in large-vessel vasculitis pathogenesis has been demonstrated, with suppression of Th17 response by corticosteroids (as opposed to lack of suppression of Th1 response).[4] A strong expression of the NOTCH receptor and its ligands Jagged1 and Delta1 has been demonstrated in temporal arteries of GCA patients, with pharmacological disruption of NOTCH pathway in a murine model causing inhibition of T-cell activation both in early and late phases of vascular inflammation (offering a potential therapeutic target down-regulating both Th1 and Th17 responses).[5]

Takayasu's Arteritis

Pathology

Biopsies are unusual from patients with TA; whenever biopsies have been obtained at time of angioplasties, an inflammatory cell infiltrate comprising helper and cytotoxic T cells, macrophages, neutrophils, gamma delta T cells (γδ T cells), and natural killer cells, with noncaseating granulomas in the wall of large vessels have been demonstrated.[6]

Pathogenesis

Genes and environment: It was thought previously that environmental factors like mycobacterial infection have a role in pathogenesis of TA. This is supported by increased humoral immune response to the mycobacterial HSP (mHSP65) in TA patients and correlation between reactive T cells to mHSP65 with its human homologue mHSP60 as well as between titers of anti-mHSP65 and anti-mHSP60 antibody in sera of TA patients.[7,8] 65kD HSP is markedly induced in media and vasa vasorum of TA patients and serves as a target for γδ T

cells. Later, this theory was not given much importance due to an inability to demonstrate mycobacteria or *M. tuberculosis* genome in histopathological tissues from aorta of TA patients.[8] An increased frequency of HLA B52 and HLA DR4 alleles in TA patients suggest a genetic basis to this disease.[9]

Innate immunity: Seko et al. described infiltration of γδ T lymphocytes, natural killer cells, macrophages, cytotoxic T lymphocytes, and T helper cells in aortic tissue samples from seven patients with TA.[10] This suggests that both the innate and adaptive immune systems are involved in the pathogenesis of large-vessel vasculitis. Each vessel in the vascular tree exhibits a distinct TLR profile and supports selective T-cell responses, accounting for the differences in vessel involvement in the two large-vessel vasculitides, TA (aorta and its branches), and GCA (extracranial branches of aorta).[3] Involvement of apoptotic pathways in TA pathogenesis is evidenced by expression of 4-1BBL, Fas and MICA (MHC Class 1 Chain-related A) on aortic tissue, and 4-1BB, FasL and NKG2D on infiltrating cells (natural killer cells and γδ T cells).[11]

Adaptive immunity: Recruitment of adaptive immune cells results from elevated sVCAM1, endothelin-1 and VEGF in blood, and ICAM-1, and HLA Class I and II in aortic tissues. Activated Th1 cells secrete IFN-γ leading to granulomatous inflammation and macrophage activation releasing both VEGF (causing increased neovascularization) and PDGF (and consequent smooth muscle migration and intimal proliferation). These lymphocytes are sensitized to aortal antigen, demonstrating *in vitro* increased cytotoxicity to cultured human umbilical cord endothelial cells and increased proliferation to purified human aortal antigen extract.[6] Recently, our group has demonstrated the expansion of Th17 cells in peripheral blood of patients with TA.[12] Patients with TA show increased mRNA expression on TNF-α, IFN-γ, IL-2, IL-3, IL-4, IL-12 (after LPS stimulation) and decreased IL-10 mRNA expression, suggesting a pathogenic role of these cytokines.[13] MMP-2, -3, and -9 levels are elevated in TA patients with correlation of MMP3 and 9 levels with disease activity, which could be due to IL-6 and RANTES induction of MMP production.[14] Furthermore, anti-TNF-α therapy[15] and anti-IL-6 therapy (tocilizumab)[16,17] have shown efficacy in treatment of difficult-to-treat TA, even over long-term follow-up. Serum levels of soluble receptor for advanced glycation end products are found to be elevated in TA.[18] A role of B cells in TA has recently found credence with demonstration of the increased frequency of peripheral blood antibody secreting cells in active TA versus controls, with B-cell depletion therapy (Rituximab) showing therapeutic efficacy in active refractory TA.[19] Elevated anti-endothelial cell antibodies and anti-cardiolipin antibodies have also been reported in patients with TA.[20,21]

PATHOGENESIS OF MEDIUM-VESSEL VASCULITIS

Polyarteritis Nodosa

Pathology

Biopsy samples from affected tissues, commonly from muscle and kidney, show focal and segmental transmural necrotizing inflammation affecting medium-sized vessels. There is a variable infiltration with lymphocytes and neutrophils in acute vascular lesions with scarring and fibrosis seen in chronic lesions. Immune complexes are usually not demonstrable on immunofluorescence.

Pathogenesis

Genes and environment: Although no well-characterized animal models exist, *Cynomolgus macaques* monkeys are known to spontaneously develop a disease closely mimicking human polyarteritis nodosa (PAN).[22] The relatively lesser prevalence of PAN and the reduction in incidence following universal Hepatitis B vaccination makes large-scale genetic studies like GWAS impractical. Single gene mutations are rarely known to cause PAN—a recent paper described mutations in CECR1, a gene encoding ADA2 causing a familial PAN in Jewish and German families.[23] Although no specific antigenic trigger has been identified, the close association with Hepatitis B infection (HBV) suggests a significant role of environment. Polyarteritis nodosa may be the first manifestation of HBV infection and usually occurs early in the course of infection (within six months). It is associated with higher HBeAg titers and is responsive to treatment for HBV—this suggests the role of direct viral replication in the affected vessels. However, precore mutants that do not express HBeAg still can develop PAN.[24]

Immune response: Also, it is proposed that either circulating immune complexes are deposited in affected vessels, or there is in situ immune complex formation—this is further evidenced by decreased titers of complements during active PAN. Complement activation at sites of vessel inflammation cause endothelial damage and secretion of IL-2, IL-8, and IFN-γ from the endothelium; TNF-α and IL1-β are also elevated. This further promotes upregulation of ICAM, VCAM, and HLA Class I molecules on the endothelium causing CD8+

T lymphocyte and monocyte recruitment to sites of damage. Presentation of the putative antigen to T cells by HLA Class I molecules perpetuates the vessel inflammation. Therapy of PAN is dependent on whether it is associated with HBV or not. HBV-associated PAN requires removal of culprit circulating immune complexes by plasmapheresis along with short course of potent corticosteroid therapy to rapidly control vessel inflammation; this must be accompanied by antiviral therapy to suppress HBV replication—seroconversion of HBeAg has been noted to go hand in hand with remission of PAN. In contrast, non-HBV-associated PAN requires more prolonged conventional immunosuppression akin to the anti-neutrophil cytoplasmic antibody (ANCA)-associated small-vessel vasculitides.[22,25,26]

Kawasaki Disease

Pathology

Pathological changes in the coronary arteries are seen at the end of the first week, when there is a dissociation in the tunica media. By the 10th day, there appears intense inflammatory infiltrate with lymphocytes, macrophages, and neutrophils occurring from both the lumen and the adventitia, gradually engulfing the whole vessel wall. There is granulomatous inflammation of the arterial wall. Stasis of blood occurring in the vessel wall and the lumen can predispose to in situ thrombosis, manifesting as acute coronary syndrome. By the 25th day, the inflammatory infiltrate begins to subside and almost completely disappears; by day 40 scarring is usually the only sequel leading on to coronary arterial aneurysms.[27]

Pathogenesis

Genes and environment: There are no established animal models for KD. A role of genetics is suggested by increased prevalence in Japanese compared to the West. Differing genetic polymorphisms have also been described—FCGR2A, CASP3, ITPKC, HLA, and CD40 have been described in Asian populations; FCGR2A and ABCC4 in Caucasians. The role of environmental factors is suggested by an increased incidence in winter months as well as well-defined epidemics of the disease in Japan. Although no causality with an inciting microbe has been demonstrated, low adenoviral titers have been demonstrated in these patients. Also, many of the symptoms such as fever, perioral erythema, conjunctival inflection, and desquamation of palms are similar to those of staphylococcal toxic shock syndrome; hence, the role of superantigens released by bacteria like TSST may have some pathogenic significance.

Immune response: At the sites of coronary arterial lesions, the predominant cause of morbidity and mortality, oligoclonal IgA secreting plasma cells have been demonstrated along with macrophages, monocytes, and lymphocytes by the 10th day of symptoms. This suggests the possible generation of these plasma cells following a respiratory infection. Inflammatory cells secrete a variety of mediators such as TNF-α, IFN-γ, IL1-β, IL-6, and MCP-1—these cause increased expression of E-selectin and ICAM-1 on vascular endothelium, resulting in increased adhesion of circulating leucocytes and subsequent recruitment to sites of coronary arteritis. Aneurysms have been shown to develop by the 12th day; inflammation usually subsides by the 25th day and is self-limited by the end of the sixth week. This emphasizes the need for early diagnosis and treatment of these children, with intravenous immunoglobulin therapy before the 10th day having demonstrated efficacy in markedly reducing sequelae of coronary aneurysms.[27,28]

PATHOGENESIS OF IMMUNE-COMPLEX-MEDIATED SMALL-VESSEL VASCULITIS

Pathology

Biopsies from affected tissues are characterized by immune complex deposits, containing immunoglobulins and complement fragments. Skin biopsies show inflammation in capillaries and venules, with variable infiltration with lymphocytes and neutrophils, endothelial swelling and proliferation, leukocytoclasia, and fibrinoid vessel wall necrosis.

Pathogenesis

Cryoglobulinemic Vasculitis

It is usually associated with HCV infection; 86% patients in a series of patients were reported to have HCV positivity.[29] Patients with HCV-related cryoglobulinemia are usually older, have longer duration of HCV infection, have type II cryoglobulins, higher titers of cryoglobulins, and clonal B-cell expansion.[30] The pathogenesis possibly represents unregulated clonal B lymphocyte expansion in response to chronic antigenic stimulation by HCV. A population of B lymphocytes bearing the translocation t(14;18) (causing Bcl2 activation and hence enhanced B-cell survival) has been described in these patients.[31] Also hypothesized is molecular mimicry to NS5A and HCV core proteins.[32,33] The ability of HCV E2 protein to bind to CD81 on B cells is also proposed to reduce the threshold for activation of these cells.[34] In contrast, the pathogenetic mechanisms for other etiologies of cryoglobulinemic vasculitis, namely malignancy or connective tissue disease associated, are less clearly defined. Deposition of immune complexes bearing cryoglobulins on the vessel wall induces complement activation and vessel wall inflammation leading on to tissue injury.

Henoch-Schönlein Purpura Vasculitis

Elevated serum IgA levels (specifically IgA1) are seen in patients with Henoch-Schönlein Purpura (HSP); these correlate with active nephritis. In addition, the circulating IgA1 is galactose deficient, rendering it less susceptible to uptake and clearance by asialoglycoprotein in liver and hence more likely to get deposited in kidneys and other tissues.[35] Once deposited, complement activation through both alternate and MBL pathways has been proposed to play a role in ensuing tissue damage.[36] Also implicated has been a role for eosinophils—elevated IgE levels have been seen in patients with HSP.[37] Circulating IgA anticardiolipin antibodies are also elevated and correlate with the degree of nephritis.[38] Also, increased expression of α-smooth muscle actin has been demonstrated in renal biopsies of HSP patients and correlates with increased severity of nephritis.[39]

Hypocomplementemic Urticarial Vasculitis

Complexes containing C1q/anti-C1q antibodies are almost universally demonstrable in patients with hypocomplementemic urticarial vasculitis. Deposition of these complexes on the vessel wall causes localized complement activation by the classical pathway; this results in degranulation of mast cells causing localized inflammatory cytokine release, increase in vascular permeability, and further recruitment of inflammatory cells to the site of insult. Additionally, C1q has a role in apoptotic cell clearance; this is impaired in the presence of antibodies to C1q and can lead on to further autoantibody formation. Also immune complexes bearing C1q antibodies are known to cause T-cell stimulation.[40]

Other Immune-complex-mediated Vasculitis (Associated with Systemic Lupus Erythematosus, Sjögrens Syndrome, and Rheumatoid Arthritis)

The pathogenesis basically involves immune complex formation, which is deposited on vessel walls; as discussed above, it causes localized complement activation leading on to tissue damage, inflammatory cell recruitment, and cell death at the site of insult. In the presence of abnormal apoptotic cell clearance in the milieu of lupus and Sjögren's, the process of autoantibody synthesis is further perpetuated by the necrotic cell debris, causing more immune complex formation and accentuating the vascular damage.[41]

ANCA-ASSOCIATED SMALL VESSEL VASCULITIS

Pathology

There is a pauci-immune vasculitis in all forms of ANCA-associated small-vessel vasculitis (AAV); little or no complement deposits are seen on immunofluorescence. Characteristically, there is involvement of small vessels (capillaries and venules) irrespective of organ involved. Acute vascular lesions have a dense neutrophilic infiltrate, with fibrinoid necrosis of the vessel wall and leukocytoclasia. Within a week, the inflammatory infiltrate changes to one comprising monocytes, macrophages, and lymphocytes; varying degrees of sclerosis appear from the end of the first week. Skin biopsy shows dermal capillaritis and venulitis; renal biopsies reveal evidence of segmental fibrinoid necrosis in glomerular capillary tufts that can progress to sclerosis (usually segmental). Lung biopsies are consistent with hemorrhagic alveolar capillaritis. In GPA and EGPA, characteristic extravascular granulomas are seen (comprising palisading macrophages and multinucleate giant cells surrounding a central area of necrosis) in biopsies from upper or lower respiratory tract, but not usually from other sites. Additionally, EGPA has a dense eosinophilic infiltrate in affected tissues.[42]

Pathogenesis

Genes and Environment

Varying rates of incidence and prevalence depending on populations and a prevalent North-South gradient demonstrable in the Northern Hemisphere[43] suggest significant contribution of environmental factors to the development of AAV. A case-control study from the UK described farming, silica exposure, and history of allergy to be significant risk factors for AAV.[44] Hydrocarbon exposure has been linked to ANCA vasculitis, with a propensity for pulmonary hemorrhage in those exposed.[45] The association of drugs and ANCA positivity as well as ANCA vasculitis is well described.[46] Usually MPO-ANCA results from drug exposure. Varying mechanisms have been described—sulfasalazine induces neutrophil apoptosis; DNA released during acetaminophen-induced liver injury stimulates TLR 9 and causes NALP3 inflammasome activation; metabolites of PTU are cytotoxic in the presence of activated neutrophils

and also cause abnormal neutrophil extracellular traps (NETs)[47] causing presentation of neutrophil cytoplasmic antigens against that an immune response can be mounted. The association of leukotriene receptor antagonists and omalizumab with EGPA seems independent of a decreased steroid requirement causing unmasking of AAV.[48,49] Infections have often been noted to precede onset or precipitate flares of AAV. A study showed decreased relapse rates in patients with GPA on cotrimoxazole.[50] Increased risk of relapse of GPA with *Staphylococcus aureus* nasal carriage has been linked to toxic shock syndrome toxin-1 produced by the microorganism, which putatively acts as a superantigen and causes neutrophil activation.[51] The link between infection and AAV has been more clearly defined after discovery of anti-lysosomal-associated membrane protein2 (LAMP2) antibodies in sera of patients with focal necrotizing glomerulonephritis, which correlated with active disease. Similar disease could be induced in animal models after immunizing with LAMP2.[52]

Single-gene defects have rarely been described to cause a phenotype similar to ANCA vasculitis. Defective transporter-associated protein-1 expression resulting in HLAClass I deficiency causes a phenotype similar to GPA with necrotizing granulomatous lesions of upper respiratory tract and skin associated with recurrent bacterial respiratory infections and skin vasculitis. Anti-PR3 positivity is seen; however, increased NK and γδ T cells are detected, unlike classical GPA. *In vitro* correction of the defect restored normal HLA-Class I expression and prevented self-reactivity of patients' cells.[53]

The genetic associations for AAV have been widely studied across populations; various associations (HLA and non-HLA—involved in various stages of lymphocyte activation) have been described and are summarized in Table 7.1.[54-62] A recent GWAS study from the UK showed distinct genetic associations with respect to either anti-PR3 (HLA-DP, SERPINA1, PRTN3) or anti-MPO ANCA (HLA-DQ) positivity but not with the clinical phenotype,[63] suggesting

Table 7.1 Genetic associations of AAV[54-62]

Gene	Disease	Population
HLA-DRB1*0901	MPA	Asians
HLA-DRB1*04, DPB1*0401	GPA	German
HLA-DRB4	EGPA	Italian
HLA-DRB1*15	PR-3 ANCA vasculitis	African Americans
CTLA 4, PTPN22	AAV	United Kingdom
PRTN3 (A546G poly)	GPA	German
AAT polymorphisms (SERPINA1)	GPA GPA and MPA	American European

Unconfirmed/conflicting associations—IL2RA, IL10, LILRA2, CD226, FCRIIIb that future classification of ANCA vasculitis may be based on the specificity of ANCA rather than the clinical phenotype as is the norm today. Another recent paper emphasized the same when it was discovered that TLR 9 polymorphisms are associated with PR3-ANCA vasculitis as opposed to MPO-ANCA vasculitis.[64] Not only genetics, epigenetic influences also have a role, with decreased histone demethylation at PR3 and MPO loci described in AAV patients, resulting from increased JMJD3 and decreased RUNX3, enzymes involved in histone methylation.[65]

Innate immunity: The role of alternate complement pathway in promoting disease is evidenced by C5 or factor B knockout mice failing to produce clinical disease in animal models.[66] Similar findings could be demonstrated on blocking C5a receptor with decreased neutrophil activation and decreased severity of renal disease after MPO transfer.[67]

Neutrophils are indispensable for the genesis of ANCA vasculitis; clinical disease could be ameliorated in mouse models of MPO transfer if neutrophils were depleted prior to antibody transfer.[42] Abnormal NETs have been demonstrated on activating neutrophils with ANCA derived from human sera; these abnormal NETs also contain PR3 and MPO and may have a role in aberrant antigen presentation. Neutrophil extracellular traps have also been demonstrated in glomerular lesions on kidney biopsy specimens. Also the number of circulating immune complexes resulting from aberrant NETs was demonstrated to be greater in patients with active ANCA vasculitis compared to those in remissions or with healthy controls.[68] One of the proposed mechanisms of propylthiouracil-induced ANCA vasculitis is aberrant NET formation; this has been demonstrated in murine experiments.[13]

Neutrophils are required to be in an activated state for ANCA vasculitis to occur; blocking neutrophil activation by knocking out or inhibiting PI3Kγ[69] or inhibiting p38 MAP kinase in mice[70] significantly reduced severity of ANCA-mediated glomerular injury. Also decreased macrophage recruitment to sites of glomerular lesions were seen a week after the initial insult on blocking p38 MAP kinase, suggesting macrophages also have a role in the perpetuation of ANCA-mediated vasculitis.[39] Neutrophils on activation express MPO and PR3 on their surface enabling further activation by antibodies to these normally cryptic cellular constituents.

Eosinophils are the predominant effector cells implicated in EGPA; although eosinophils do not contain PR3 or MPO, it has been proposed that activated neutrophils recruit and activate eosinophils—these eosinophils further secrete IL-1, IL-3, IL-5, TGF-α, and TGF-β, which recruit T helper 2 cells, perpetuate granuloma formation and fibrosis.[42]

Endothelial progenitor cells (EPCs) are involved in endothelial repair, and they have recently gained attention as potential mechanisms of aberrant endothelial repair and accelerated atherosclerosis in rheumatic diseases.[71] Reduced circulating EPCs have been found to predict relapse in ANCA vasculitis.[72] Also, elevated circulating angiopoietin-2 levels (a regulator of endothelial detachment) have been found in active renal AAV (as compared to inactive renal disease and limited GPA) and correlate with disease activity.[73]

Adaptive immunity: How do antibodies form against PR3 and MPO found inside neutrophil granules? Are these antibodies pathogenic? Robust animal models have been described for MPO-ANCA vasculitis. It has been observed that MPO knockout mice immunized with MPO developed robust immune response with high titer anti-MPO antibodies but do not develop clinical disease like MPO vasculitis. However, when these anti-MPO antibodies were transferred to other strains of mice, heterogeneous disease ranging from limited to systemic vasculitis of varying severity was seen depending on the strain of mice. This suggests that autoantibody (ANCA) is pathogenic, and akin to humans, disease severity varied depending on the genetic vulnerability of the strain of mice used.[74] Necrotizing crescentic glomerulonephritis (NCGN) and systemic vasculitis were also induced on anti-MPO transfer to Rag2 knockout mice (which intrinsically lack T and B lymphocytes), suggesting that T lymphocytes are not indispensable for the genesis of AAV. However, more severe disease was seen in the presence of T lymphocytes. Such well-established animal models have yet to be described for anti-PR3-mediated vasculitis. In NOD mice (a strain predisposed to autoimmunity), anti-PR3 antibodies were produced on immunizing with recombinant PR3 but failed to produce clinical disease; however, when these antibodies were transferred onto a background of NOD-SCID mice, a phenotype resembling human disease with segmental NCGN and systemic vasculitis and early death was seen.[75,76]

The role of B cells is demonstrable by the pathogenicity of ANCA and the established efficacy of B-cell depletion therapy in AAV. Also patients with ANCA vasculitis have elevated circulating levels of B-lymphocyte stimulator that is one of the proposed mechanisms of breakage of tolerance as it promotes survival of autoreactive B cells in germinal centers.[77] Immunoglobulins isolated from B lymphocytes from granulomas in GPA showed specificity toward lysosomal transmembrane protein 9B (TMEM9B—which colocalizes inside lysosomes with LAMP-1 and is involved in the proinflammatory response resulting from the TNF signaling cascade) and tetraspanin 7 (which interacts with integrins thereby regulating neutrophil activation and adhesion).[78]

As we have seen, T cells are not essential for AAV to occur, but disease is more severe in their presence. Myriad abnormalities have been described with respect to T helper cell populations in ANCA vasculitis—Th1 skewing has been shown in localized GPA; Th2 skewing and Th17 expansion have been demonstrated in systemic GPA and EGPA.[79] Although defective T regulatory cells (Tregs) had been previously described in AAV,[42] a clearer role has emerged recently. Not only were Tregs in AAV patients defective in their ability to suppress T effector cells (an altered splice variant of FoxP3 was demonstrated to be responsible), but also the T effector cells were abnormal—a CD25 intermediate population could be demonstrated in peripheral blood resistant to suppression by Tregs from healthy volunteers.[80] The role of T lymphocytes is emphasized by a recent trial demonstrating efficacy of open-label abatacept (which blocks T lymphocyte activation through CTLA4) in nonsevere GPA, with 18/20 patients attaining disease control and 16/20 attaining remission.[81] A recent publication from the UK highlighted increased circulating follicular B-helper T cells (TFH—involved in immune regulation at germinal centers) along with decreased Tregs in patients with GPA; interestingly rituximab therapy caused depletion of these TFH as disease went into remission, but the same was not demonstrated with the use of other immunosuppressants (cyclophosphamide, mycophenolate mofetil, methotrexate, or azathioprine).[82]

To summarize, on a favorable genetic background, environmental influences (including drugs and infections) lead on to genesis of ANCA. Formation of ANCA is mediated by complex interactions between B and T cells resulting from loss of immune tolerance. These autoantibodies activate neutrophils through alternative complement pathway, and cause more exposure on ANCA outside neutrophils leading to accelerated antibody production against the same. Also these activated neutrophils cause endothelial damage and migrate to affected tissues, later on being replaced by macrophages at sites of granuloma formation.[42,83] The acute vascular lesion shows localized neutrophil influx, with leucocytoclasia, vessel wall necrosis, and fibrin accumulation. Over time (within a week), these lesions predominantly contain monocytes, macrophages, and T lymphocytes and progress early to sclerotic lesions.[48]

KEY POINTS

- Vasculitis is a rare disease; pathogenesis of various subtypes is heterogeneous.
- Broadly, there is abnormal immune activation (both innate and acquired) likely due to environmental influences on a susceptible genetic background.
- The pathogenic processes sometimes precede the onset of disease by a significant duration.
- Understanding pathogenesis enable exploring newer directed therapies acting on these mechanistic pathways involved in genesis and perpetuation of vasculitis.

REFERENCES

1. Jennette JC, Falk RJ, Bacon PA, et al. 2012 revised international Chapel Hill consensus conference nomenclature of vasculitides. Arthritis Rheum. 2013;65:1-11.
2. Weyand CM, Goronzy JJ. Medium- and large-vessel vasculitis. N Engl J Med. 2003;349:160-9.
3. Pryshchep O, Ma-Krupa W, Younge BR, et al. Vessel-specific toll-like receptor profiles in human medium and large arteries. Circulation. 2008;118:1276-84.
4. Deng J, Younge BR, Olshen RA, et al. Th17 and Th1 T-cell responses in giant cell arteritis. Circulation. 2010;121:906-15.
5. Piggott K, Deng J, Warrington K, et al. Blocking the notch pathway inhibits vascular inflammation in large-vessel vasculitis. Circulation. 2011;123:309-18.
6. Arnaud L, Haroche J, Mathian A, et al. Pathogenesis of Takayasu's arteritis: a 2011 update. Autoimmun Rev. 2011;11:61-7.
7. Aggarwal A, Chag M, Sinha N, et al. Takayasu's arteritis: role of mycobacterium tuberculosis and its 65 kda heat shock protein. Int J Cardiol. 1996;55:49-55.
8. Kumar Chauhan S, Kumar Tripathy N, Sinha N, et al. Cellular and humoral immune responses to mycobacterial heat shock protein-65 and its human homologue in Takayasu's arteritis. Clin Exp Immunol. 2004;138:547-53.
9. Flores-Dominguez C, Hernandez-Pacheco G, Zuniga J, et al. [alleles of the major histocompatibility system associated with susceptibility to the development of Takayasu's arteritis]. Gac Med Mex. 2002;138:177-83.
10. Seko Y, Minota S, Kawasaki A, et al. Perforin-secreting killer cell infiltration and expression of a 65-kd heat-shock protein in aortic tissue of patients with Takayasu's arteritis. J Clin Invest. 1994;93:750-8.
11. Seko Y, Sugishita K, Sato O, et al. Expression of costimulatory molecules (4-1bbl and fas) and major histocompatibility class I chain-related a (mica) in aortic tissue with Takayasu's arteritis. J Vasc Res. 2004;41:84-90.
12. Misra DP, Chaurasia S, Misra R. 332. Increased circulating TH17 and natural killer T cells in Takayasu's arteritis. Rheumatology. 2014;53:i184.

13. Tripathy NK, Chauhan SK, Nityanand S. Cytokine mRNA repertoire of peripheral blood mononuclear cells in Takayasu's arteritis. Clin Exp Immunol. 2004;138:369-74.

14. Matsuyama A, Sakai N, Ishigami M, et al. Matrix metallo-proteinases as novel disease markers in Takayasu arteritis. Circulation. 2003;108:1469-73.

15. Hoffman GS, Merkel PA, Brasington RD, et al. Anti-tumor necrosis factor therapy in patients with difficult to treat Takayasu arteritis. Arthritis Rheum. 2004;50:2296-304.

16. Nishimoto N, Nakahara H, Yoshio-Hoshino N, et al. Successful treatment of a patient with Takayasu arteritis using a humanized anti-interleukin-6 receptor antibody. Arthritis Rheum. 2008;58:1197-200.

17. Youngstein T, Peters JE, Hamdulay SS, et al. Serial analysis of clinical and imaging indices reveals prolonged efficacy of TNF-alpha and IL-6 receptor targeted therapies in refractory Takayasu arteritis. Clin Exp Rheumatol. 2014;32:S11-8.

18. Mahajan N, Dhawan V, Malik S, et al. Serum levels of soluble receptor for advanced glycation end products (srage) in Takayasu's arteritis. Int J Cardiol. 2010;145:589-91.

19. Hoyer BF, Mumtaz IM, Loddenkemper K, et al. Takayasu arteritis is characterised by disturbances of B cell homeostasis and responds to B cell depletion therapy with rituximab. Ann Rheum Dis. 2012;71:75-9.

20. Eichhorn J, Sima D, Thiele B, et al. Anti-endothelial cell antibodies in Takayasu arteritis. Circulation. 1996;94:2396-401.

21. Misra R, Aggarwal A, Chag M, et al. Raised anticardiolipin antibodies in Takayasu's arteritis. Lancet. 1994;343:1644-5.

22. Colmegna I, Maldonado-Cocco JA. Polyarteritis nodosa revisited. Curr Rheumatol Rep. 2005;7:288-96.

23. Navon Elkan P, Pierce SB, Segel R, et al. Mutant adenosine deaminase 2 in a polyarteritis nodosa vasculopathy. N Engl J Med. 2014;370:921-31.

24. Cacoub P, Terrier B. Hepatitis B-related autoimmune manifestations. Rheum Dis Clin North Am. 2009;35:125-37.

25. Lhote F, Cohen P, Guillevin L. Polyarteritis nodosa, microscopic polyangiitis and Churg-Strauss syndrome. Lupus. 1998;7:238-58.

26. Trepo C, Guillevin L. Polyarteritis nodosa and extrahepatic manifestations of HBV infection: the case against autoimmune intervention in pathogenesis. J Autoimmun. 2001;16:269-74.

27. Takahashi K, Oharaseki T, Yokouchi Y. Pathogenesis of kawasaki disease. Clin Exp Immunol. 2011;164:20-2.

28. Dimitriades VR, Brown AG, Gedalia A. Kawasaki disease: pathophysiology, clinical manifestations, and management. Curr Rheumatol Rep. 2014;16:423.

29. Ferri C, La Civita L, Longombardo G, et al. Hepatitis C virus and mixed cryoglobulinaemia. Eur J Clin Invest. 1993;23:399-405.

30. Ferri C, Mascia MT. Cryoglobulinemic vasculitis. Curr Opin Rheumatol. 2006;18:54-63.

31. Machida K, Cheng KT, Sung VM, et al. Hepatitis C virus induces a mutator phenotype: enhanced mutations of immunoglobulin and proto-oncogenes. Proc Natl Acad Sci USA. 2004;101:4262-7.

32. Hosui A, Ohkawa K, Ishida H, et al. Hepatitis C virus core protein differently regulates the jak-stat signaling pathway under interleukin-6 and interferon-gamma stimuli. J Biol Chem. 2003;278:28562-71.

33. Park KJ, Choi SH, Choi DH, et al. 1Hepatitis C virus NS5A protein modulates c-jun N-terminal kinase through interaction with tumor necrosis factor receptor-associated factor 2. J Biol Chem. 2003;278:30711-8.

34. Pileri P, Uematsu Y, Campagnoli S, et al. Binding of hepatitis C virus to cd81. Science. 1998;282:938-41.

35. Mestecky J, Tomana M, Crowley-Nowick PA, et al. Defective galactosylation and clearance of IgA1 molecules as a possible etiopathogenic factor in IgA nephropathy. Contrib Nephrol. 1993;104:172-82.

36. Lau KK, Suzuki H, Novak J, et al. Pathogenesis of Henoch-Schonlein purpura nephritis. Pediatr Nephrol. 2010;25:19-26.

37. Kawasaki Y, Hosoya M, Suzuki H. Possible pathogenic role of interleukin-5 and eosino cationic protein in Henoch-Schönlein purpura nephritis. Pediatr Int. 2005;47:512-7.

38. Kawakami T, Yamazaki M, Mizoguchi M, et al. High titer of serum antiphospholipid antibody levels in adult Henoch—Schönlein purpura and cutaneous leukocytoclastic angiitis. Arthritis Rheum. 2008;59:561-7.

39. Silva GE, Costa RS, Ravinal RC, et al. Mast cells, TGF-beta1 and alpha-SMA expression in IgA nephropathy. Dis Markers. 2008;24:181-90.

40. Jara LJ, Navarro C, Medina G, et al. Hypocomplementemic urticarial vasculitis syndrome. Curr Rheumatol Rep. 2009;11:410-5.

41. Munoz LE, Lauber K, Schiller M, et al. The role of defective clearance of apoptotic cells in systemic autoimmunity. Nat Rev Rheumatol. 2010;6:280-9.

42. Jennette JC, Falk RJ, Hu P, et al. Pathogenesis of antineutrophil cytoplasmic autoantibody-associated small-vessel vasculitis. Annu Rev Pathol. 2013;8:139-60.

43. Mahr AD, Neogi T, Merkel PA. Epidemiology of Wegener's granulomatosis: lessons from descriptive studies and analyses of genetic and environmental risk determinants. Clin Exp Rheumatol. 2006;24:S82-91.

44. Lane SE, Watts RA, Bentham G, et al. Are environmental factors important in primary systemic vasculitis? A case-control study. Arthritis Rheum. 2003;48:814-23.

45. Pai P, Bone JM, Bell GM. Hydrocarbon exposure and glomerulonephritis due to systemic vasculitis. Nephrol Dial Transplant. 1998;13:1321-3.

46. Csernok E, Lamprecht P, Gross WL. Clinical and immunological features of drug-induced and infection-induced proteinase 3-antineutrophil cytoplasmic antibodies and myeloperoxidase-antineutrophil cytoplasmic antibodies and vasculitis. Curr Opin Rheumatol. 2010;22:43-8.

47. Nakazawa D, Tomaru U, Suzuki A, et al. Abnormal conformation and impaired degradation of propylthiouracil-induced neutrophil extracellular traps: implications of disordered neutrophil extracellular traps in a rat model of myeloperoxidase antineutrophil cytoplasmic antibody-associated vasculitis. Arthritis Rheum. 2012;64:3779-87.

48. Bibby S, Healy B, Steele R, et al. Association between leukotriene receptor antagonist therapy and Churg-Strauss syndrome: an analysis of the FDA AERS database. Thorax. 2010;65:132-8.

49. Wechsler ME, Wong DA, Miller MK, et al. Churg-Strauss syndrome in patients treated with omalizumab. Chest. 2009;136:507-18.

50. Stegeman CA, Tervaert JW, de Jong PE, et al. Trimethoprim-sulfamethoxazole (co-trimoxazole) for the prevention of relapses of Wegener's granulomatosis. Dutch co-trimoxazole Wegener study group. N Engl J Med. 1996;335:16-20.

51. Popa ER, Stegeman CA, Abdulahad WH, et al. Staphylococcal toxic-shock-syndrome-toxin-1 as a risk factor for disease relapse in Wegener's granulomatosis. Rheumatology (Oxford). 2007;46:1029-33.

52. Kain R, Exner M, Brandes R, et al. Molecular mimicry in pauci-immune focal necrotizing glomerulonephritis. Nat Med. 2008;14:1088-96.

53. Villa-Forte A, de la Salle H, Fricker D, et al. HLA class I deficiency syndrome mimicking Wegener's granulomatosis. Arthritis Rheum. 2008;58:2579-82.

54. Gencik M, Borgmann S, Zahn R, et al. Immunogenetic risk factors for anti-neutrophil cytoplasmic antibody (ANCA)-associated systemic vasculitis. Clin Exp Immunol. 1999;117:412-7.

55. Morris H, Morgan MD, Wood AM, et al. ANCA-associated vasculitis is linked to carriage of the Z allele of alpha(1) antitrypsin and its polymers. Ann Rheum Dis. 2011;70:1851-6.

56. Tsuchiya N, Kobayashi S, Hashimoto H, et al. Association of HLA–DRB1*0901-DQB1*0303 haplotype with microscopic polyangiitis in Japanese. Genes Immun. 2006;7:81-4.

57. Tsuchiya N, Kobayashi S, Kawasaki A, et al. Genetic background of Japanese patients with antineutrophil cytoplasmic antibody-associated vasculitis: association of HLA–DRB1*0901 with microscopic polyangiitis. J Rheumatol. 2003;30:1534-40.

58. Vaglio A, Martorana D, Maggiore U, et al. HLA-DRB4 as a genetic risk factor for Churg–Strauss syndrome. Arthritis Rheum. 2007;56:3159-66.

59. Cao Y, Schmitz JL, Yang J, et al. DRB1*15 allele is a risk factor for PR3–ANCA disease in African Americans. J Am Soc Nephrol. 2011;22:1161-7.

60. Carr EJ, Niederer HA, Williams J, et al. Confirmation of the genetic association of CTLA 4 and PTPN22 with anca-associated vasculitis. BMC Med Genet. 2009;10:121.

61. Gencik M, Meller S, Borgmann S, et al. Proteinase 3 gene polymorphisms and Wegener's granulomatosis. Kidney Int. 2000;58:2473-7.

62. Mahr AD, Edberg JC, Stone JH, et al. Alpha(1)-antitrypsin deficiency-related alleles Z and S and the risk of Wegener's granulomatosis. Arthritis Rheum. 2010;62:3760-7.

63. Lyons PA, Rayner TF, Trivedi S, et al. Genetically distinct subsets within ANCA-associated vasculitis. N Engl J Med. 2012;367:214-23.

64. Husmann CA, Holle JU, Moosig F, et al. Genetics of toll like receptor 9 in ANCA-associated vasculitides. Ann Rheum Dis. 2014;73:890-6.

65. Ciavatta DJ, Yang J, Preston GA, et al. Epigenetic basis for aberrant upregulation of autoantigen genes in humans with ANCA vasculitis. J Clin Invest. 2010;120:3209-19.

66. Xiao H, Schreiber A, Heeringa P, et al. Alternative complement pathway in the pathogenesis of disease mediated by anti-neutrophil cytoplasmic autoantibodies. Am J Pathol. 2007;170:52-64.

67. Schreiber A, Xiao H, Jennette JC, et al. C5a receptor mediates neutrophil activation and ANCA-induced glomerulonephritis. J Am Soc Nephrol. 2009;20:289-98.

68. Kessenbrock K, Krumbholz M, Schonermarck U, et al. Netting neutrophils in autoimmune small-vessel vasculitis. Nat Med. 2009;15:623-5.

69. Schreiber A, Rolle S, Peripelittchenko L, et al. Phosphoinositol 3-kinase-gamma mediates antineutrophil cytoplasmic autoantibody-induced glomerulonephritis. Kidney Int. 2010;77:118-28.

70. van der Veen BS, Chen M, Muller R, et al. Effects of p38 mitogen-activated protein kinase inhibition on anti-neutrophil cytoplasmic autoantibody pathogenicity in vitro and in vivo. Ann Rheum Dis. 2011;70:356-65.

71. Castejon R, Jimenez-Ortiz C, Valero-Gonzalez S, et al. Decreased circulating endothelial progenitor cells as an early risk factor of subclinical atherosclerosis in systemic lupus erythematosus. Rheumatology (Oxford). 2014;53:631-8.

72. Zavada J, Kideryova L, Pytlik R, et al. Reduced number of endothelial progenitor cells is predictive of early relapse in anti-neutrophil cytoplasmic antibody-associated vasculitis. Rheumatology (Oxford). 2009;48:1197-201.

73. Kumpers P, Hellpap J, David S, et al. Circulating angiopoietin-2 is a marker and potential mediator of endothelial cell detachment in ANCA-associated vasculitis with renal involvement. Nephrol Dial Transplant. 2009;24:1845-50.

74. Xiao H, Heeringa P, Hu P, et al. Antineutrophil cytoplasmic autoantibodies specific for myeloperoxidase cause glomerulonephritis and vasculitis in mice. J Clin Invest. 2002;110:955-63.

75. Coughlan AM, Freeley SJ, Robson MG. Animal models of anti-neutrophil cytoplasmic antibody-associated vasculitis. Clin Exp Immunol. 2012;169:229-37.

76. Salama AD, Little MA. Animal models of antineutrophil cytoplasm antibody-associated vasculitis. Curr Opin Rheumatol. 2012;24:1-7.

77. Schneeweis C, Rafalowicz M, Feist E, et al. Increased levels of BLyS and sVCAM-1 in anti-neutrophil cytoplasmatic antibody (ANCA)-associated vasculitides (AAV). Clin Exp Rheumatol. 2010;28:62-6.

78. Thurner L, Muller A, Cerutti M, et al. Wegener's granuloma harbors B lymphocytes with specificities against a pro-inflammatory transmembrane protein and a tetraspanin. J Autoimmun. 2011;36:87-90.

79. Wilde B, Thewissen M, Damoiseaux J, et al. T cells in ANCA-associated vasculitis: what can we learn from lesional versus circulating T cells? Arthritis Res Ther. 2010;12:204.

80. Free ME, Bunch DO, McGregor JA, et al. Patients with antineutrophil cytoplasmic antibody-associated vasculitis have defective Treg cell function exacerbated by the presence of a suppression-resistant effector cell population. Arthritis Rheum. 2013;65:1922-33.

81. Langford CA, Monach PA, Specks U, et al. An open-label trial of abatacept (ctla4-ig) in nonsevere relapsing granulomatosis with polyangiitis (Wegener's). Ann Rheum Dis. 2014;73:1376-9.

82. Zhao Y, Lutalo PM, Thomas JE, et al. Circulating T follicular helper cell and regulatory T cell frequencies are influenced by B cell depletion in patients with granulomatosis with polyangiitis. Rheumatology (Oxford). 2014;53:621-30.

83. Chen M, Kallenberg CG. ANCA-associated vasculitides—advances in pathogenesis and treatment. Nat Rev Rheumatol. 2010;6:653-64.

CHAPTER 8

Pathology of Cutaneous Vasculitis

BD Radotra

INTRODUCTION

Cutaneous vasculitis is a commonly encountered condition in clinical practice. It is not a disease per se; rather it is a manifestation of a diverse group of diseases. As skin is commonly affected in vasculitic disorders, it offers an accessible tissue for a confirmatory diagnosis. Vasculitis is defined as inflammation of the blood vessel with evidence of vascular damage. The damage may be occlusive or nonocclusive, causing necrosis and hemorrhagic manifestations, respectively. Small hemorrhagic lesions are termed petechiae (<3 mm) and larger lesions are called ecchymosis (>3 mm).

There is considerable controversy regarding the diagnostic criteria of vasculitis. However, most pathologists consider that there should be two components on microscopic examination for diagnosis of skin vasculitis: (1) inflammation of vascular wall and (2) evidence of vessel wall injury.[1] The inflammation in the vessel wall may be composed of neutrophils (which is the commonest), eosinophils, lymphocytes, granulomatous, or mixed in nature. Perivascular lymphocytic infiltrate without evidence of vessel wall damage should not be considered as vasculitis since it is observed in many of the dermatopathological conditions. The extent of inflammation may vary, ranging from mild to severe and depends on the age of the lesion. In long-standing cases or during healing stage, the inflammation may be very minimal. Vascular injury is characterized by endothelial swelling, leukocytoclasis, fibrinoid necrosis, and extravasations of RBCs. Fibrinoid necrosis is considered as one of the most specific pieces of evidence of vascular injury. The presence of fibrin thrombi is also considered as vascular injury but it is not specific, as it can be seen in prethrombotic conditions as well.

Skin vasculitis may be a primary or secondary to other diseases. Secondary vascular injury such as inflammation, necrosis, or fibrin thrombi may also occur in blood vessels due to some adjacent inflammatory pathology like infection or ulceration. Therefore, one has to keep these facts in mind before evaluating a skin biopsy and decide whether it is a cause or effect. Histological examination alone is not sufficient to classify a vasculitic disease process. A diagnosis of underlying cause of vasculitis requires additional investigations like direct immunofluorescence (DIF), demonstration of serum antibodies like antinuclear antibody (ANA), and antineutrophilic cytoplasmic antibody (ANCA).

The vasculitic process is classified according to the size of the blood vessel. There is lot of confusion regarding the classification and nomenclature of vasculitis. In recent 2012 revised International Chapel Hill Consensus Conference nomenclature of vasculitides (CHCC2012), it has been classified according to the size, etiology, pathology, pathtogenesis, demographics, clinical manifestations, and organ involvement and divided into many classes.[2] In cutaneous vascular pathology, large- or medium-vessel vasculitides are rarely encountered; mostly they are small-vessel vasculitis. A new category has been recognized in this recent nomenclature system, i.e. single-organ vasculitis that includes cutaneous leukocytoclastic angiitis and cutaneous arteritis among others.

LARGE-VESSEL VASCULITIS

Cutaneous vasculitis is rare in large-vessel vasculitis (LVV). The examples of LVV are Takayasu arteritis (TA) and giant cell arteritis (GCA). Takayasu arteritis affects aorta and its major branches, whereas the GCA affects temporal artery. However,

LVV may involve smaller vessels as well. Both these diseases are more common in females; TA is seen more in younger individuals (<50 years) whereas GCA more in elderly patients. Pathologically both may show granulomatous inflammation of the vessel wall with disruption of elastic fibers.

MEDIUM-VESSEL VASCULITIS

Medium-vessel vasculitis (MVV) predominantly involves medium arteries that include the main visceral arteries and their branches. Major variants of MVV are polyarteritis nodosa (PAN) and Kawasaki disease. Polyarteritis nodosa shows multisystem involvement. Characteristic lesion in PAN is a panarteritis in different stages of development involving medium- and small-sized arteries. Cutaneous manifestations of PAN include subcutaneous nodules, ecchymosis, and digital gangrene. Affected skin often shows only small-vessel disease. The skin biopsy shows that arterial involvement is typically focal and predominantly shows necrotizing nongranulomatous small- and medium-sized vasculitis.[3] Tests for ANCA are usually absent. In the early stage, the infiltrate in predominantly neutrophilic coupled with fibrinoid necrosis of the vessel wall and disruption of elastic lamina. In the late or healing stage there is vascular occlusion due to intimal proliferation and thrombosis (Fig. 8.1). The inflammatory infiltrate in the late stage may be minimal. The small vessels in the superficial dermis show nonspecific perivascular lymphocytic infiltration.

SMALL-VESSEL VASCULITIS

Small-vessel vasculitis (SVV) is most commonly found in skin and usually presents as palpable purpura. Small vessels are arteries, arterioles, capillaries, venules, and veins. According to CHCC2012, small-vessel vasculitis is of two major types: ANCA-associated vasculitis (AAV) and immune-complex SVV. The exact etiology of SVV can be determined only by additional investigations rather than the skin biopsy as will be discussed subsequently. Morphologically, the two commonest patterns of SVV are leukocytoclastic vasculitis and granulomatous vasculitis. Although not specific, usually AAV produces granulomatous vasculitis and immune-complex SVV produces a leukocytoclastic vasculitic pattern.

Leukocytoclastic Vasculitis

Leukocytoclastic vasculitis (LCV) is the commonest form of small-vessel vasculitis of skin. A large number of conditions including infectious and noninfectious diseases can produce LCV. Apart from palpable purpura it also presents with extracutaneous manifestations. The disease is most often induced by immune-complex deposition and subsequent complement activation. It may be idiopathic or may be caused by an underlying disease or drugs.[4] Leukocytoclastic vasculitis predominantly involves postcapillary venules. The vascular involvement may be restricted in the upper dermis (Fig. 8.2) or there may be florid involvement with

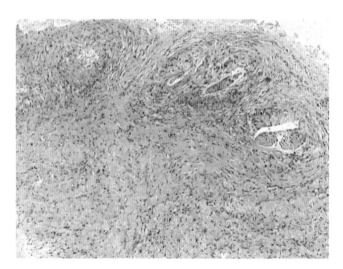

Fig. 8.1 The deep-dermal medium-sized artery shows panarteritis with occlusion of lumen in a case of PAN

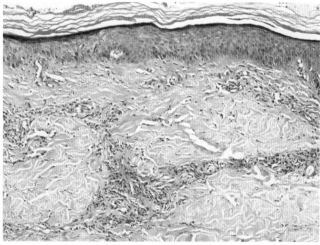

Fig. 8.2 The small blood vessels in the upper dermis are involved by inflammation that obscures their outlines

dermal necrosis. The inflammatory infiltrate in the vessel wall predominantly consists of neutrophils, and often there is fragmentation of their nuclei (leukocytoclasis) (Fig. 8.3). There is also evidence of vascular injury. In early, mild cases there may be only endothelial swelling accompanied by extravasation of RBCs and edema, whereas fibrinoid necrosis of the vessel wall is seen in florid cases (Fig. 8.4). Dermal edema, if extensive, may produce subepidermal blister. Many diseases may produce this common pattern of vascular injury; the major causes remain infection and immune-mediated inflammation. Thus, the histology must be interpreted in the context of clinical information and additional investigation findings. An infectious etiology must be ruled out as the treatment of infectious vasculitis is drastically different

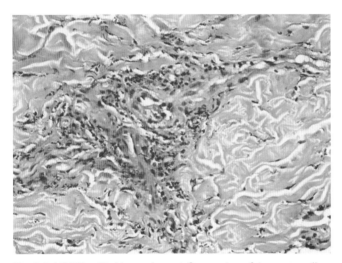

Fig. 8.3 LCV: The skin biopsy shows inflammation of the postcapillary dermal venules consisting of neutrophils with fragmentation of their nuclei (leukocytoclasis)

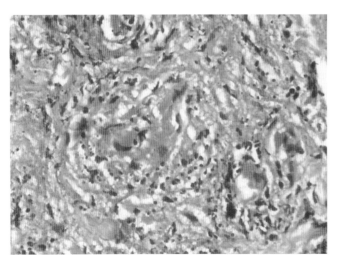

Fig. 8.4 Small-vessel vasculitis: The neutrophilic infiltrate is accompanied by fibrin deposition in the vessel wall

from immune-mediated vasculitis. The skin biopsy shows deposition of immunoglobulins and complement fractions around the blood vessels.

Henoch-Schönlein Purpura

Henoch-Schönlein purpura (HSP) is a subset of small-vessel vasculitis that predominantly affects children. The hallmark of the disease is palpable purpura of buttock and lower extremities, hematuria, and abdominal pain. It usually follows streptococcal upper respiratory tract infection and shows a self-limiting course with resolution expected within 6–16 weeks. Histologically, HSP cannot be differentiated from other causes of LCV (Figs 8.5A and B). Direct immunofluorescence shows deposition of IgA along capillary walls. Vascular deposition of IgA immune complexes is responsible for this multisystem disorder. A number of underlying factors such as drugs, infections, vaccinations, and various malignancies has been associated with HSP.[5]

Urticarial Vasculitis

The urticarial vasculitis is characterized by persistent wheals (lasting more than 24 hours) with faint purpura. The course is usually self-limiting. Some patients present with the low level of complement and presence of anti-C1q antibody (hypocomplementic urticarial vasculitis or anti-C1q vasculitis). These patients have likelihood of more severe and recurrent disease. Histological examination reveals leukocytoclastic vasculitis with variable degree of perivascular and interstitial neutrophilic infiltrate.

Cryoglobulinemic Vasculitis and Small-Vessel Vasculitis Associated with Paraproteins

Small-vessel vasculitis (SVV) may be associated with paraproteins including cryoglobulins, cryofibrinogens, macroglobulins, and heavy chains in the serum. Cryoglobulins may be monoclonal or polyclonal in nature. Monoclonal cryoglobulinemia type I is usually associated with lymphoproliferative disorders or plasma cell dyscrasias. Polyclonal cryoglobulinemia types II and III are frequently associated with hepatitis C infection and connective tissue disorders; idiopathic forms are termed as essential mixed cryoglobulinemia. Morphology of the blood vessels reveals deposition of pale, eosinophilic, amorphous material along the wall of blood vessels as well as within the lumen, giving rise to thrombus-like appearance.[6] This deposit is brightly PAS positive. Accompanying inflammation may be minimal and extravasation of RBCs is a dominant finding. Apart from

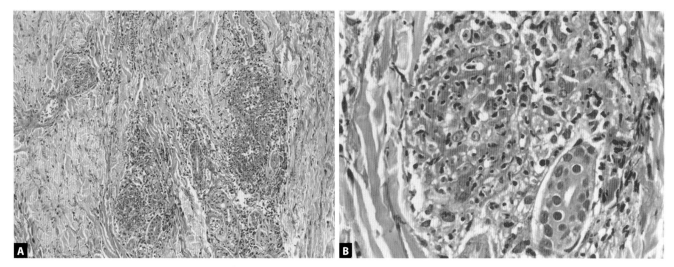

Figs 8.5A and B HSP: The dermal vessels show leukocytoclastic vasculitis. There is fibrinoid necrosis of the vessel wall with extravasation of RBCs

skin, glomeruli and peripheral nerves are also commonly involved. Direct immunofluorescence shows deposition of monoclonal or polyclonal immunoglobulins (usually IgG and IgM) in the vessel wall.

Others

Other conditions like serum sickness, connective tissue disorders like SLE, rheumatoid arthritis, autoimmune diseases, and drugs may also produce leukocytoclastic vasculitis.

Granulomatous Vasculitis

A number of conditions may produce granulomatous small-vessel vasculitis, among which AAV and infection top the list. In these conditions granuloma formation occurs with no or minimal vessel wall damage. However, it should be kept in mind that these conditions produce predominantly LCV and granulomatous response may be seen only focally, so the absence of granulomatous vasculitis does not exclude a diagnosis of AAV.

ANCA-Associated Vasculitis

ANCA-associated vasculitis (AAV) includes granulomatosis with polyangiitis (GPA, Wegener's granulomatosis), eosinophilic granulomatosis with polyangiitis (EGPA, Churg-Strauss), and microscopic polyangiitis (MPA). All these conditions in common produce necrotizing vasculitis

and granulomatous inflammation. Microscopic polyangiitis is a systemic disease typically affecting arterioles and capillaries of kidney, lung, skin, and less commonly other organs. Skin involvement in MPA is seen in 30–40% of cases. It predominantly shows leukocytoclastic vasculitis affecting arterioles, capillaries, and venules. Rarely cutaneous palisading granuloma may be seen.[7] Wegener's granulomatosis is a systemic disease involving predominantly the upper and lower respiratory tracts and kidney. Skin involvement may range from 10% to 50% cases. It shows necrotizing small-vessel vasculitis and variable granulomatous inflammation (Figs 8.6A and B). Small foci of necrosis with palisaded histiocytes may also be seen.[8] The presence of multinucleated giant cells is a helpful histological finding (Figs 8.7A and B). EGPA also shows multisystem involvement and classical triad of asthma, hypereosinophilia, and systemic vasculitis may be seen. The predominantly involved organs are lung, gastrointestinal tract, nerves, and heart. Skin involvement is variable and clinically manifest as cutaneous hemorrhage or subcutaneous nodules. Histologically, it shows mainly leukocytoclastic vasculitis with an excess of eosinophilic infiltrate.[9] Dermis in addition shows palisading necrotizing granulomas. The central portion of these granulomas contains degenerated collagen that appears bright red, surrounded by palisading histiocytes and multinucleated giant cells. However, this change is not specific for EGPA. Although AAV show characteristic morphology, there is considerable overlap. So a proper clinical background and ANCA positivity are required for the establishment of their diagnosis.

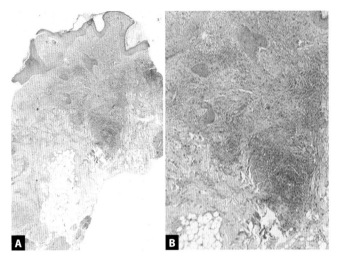

Figs 8.6A and B Skin biopsy from a case of Wegener's granulomatosis shows granulomatous vasculitis involving deep dermal blood vessels

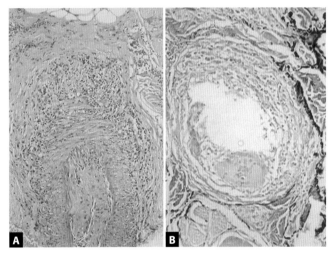

Figs 8.7A and B Wegener's granulomatosis: The muscular artery shows chronic granulomatous inflammation with multinucleate giant cells. (A) H & E; (B) EVG stain

Others

Other conditions such as PAN, cutaneous Crohn's disease, drug reaction, connective tissue disease, and granuloma annulare can also rarely produce granulomatous cutaneous vasculitis.

KEY POINTS

- Cutaneous vasculitis is a manifestation of a diverse group of diseases.
- Cutaneous vasculitis consists of medium-vessel vasculitis and small-vessel vasculitis; the former is rarely encountered but typically shows focal and

predominantly necrotizing nongranulomatous arteritis affecting small- as well as medium-sized vessels of skin.

- Small-vessel vasculitis is common and consists of two major types: ANCA-associated vasculitis (AAV) and immune-complex SVV. Although not specific, usually AAV produces granulomatous vasculitis and immune-complex SVV produces a leukocytoclastic vasculitic pattern.
- The term lymphocytic vasculitis should be avoided since commonly encountered perivascular lymphocytic infiltrate seen in a variety of dermatopathologic disorders can be easily mistaken for it.
- A skin biopsy is considered to be a gold standard for diagnosis; however, a diagnosis of the underlying cause of vasculitis requires additional investigations like direct immunofluorescence (DIF), demonstration of serum antibodies like antinuclear antibody (ANA), and antineutrophilic cytoplasmic antibody (ANCA).
- A deep skin biopsy, extending to subcutis and taken from the earliest, most symptomatic, reddish, or purpuric lesion is ideal for obtaining a high-yielding diagnostic sample.

REFERENCES

1. Carlson JA. The histological assessment of cutaneous vasculitis. Histopathology. 2010;56:3-23.
2. Jennette JC, Falk RJ, Bacon PA, et al. 2012 revised International Chapel Hill Consensus Conference Nomenclature of Vasculitides. Arthritis Rheum. 2013;65:1-11.
3. Díaz-Pérez JL, De Lagrán ZM, Díaz-Ramón JL, et al. Cutaneous polyarteritis nodosa. Semin Cutan Med Surg. 2007;26:77-86.
4. Tai YJ, Chong AH, Williams RA, et al. Retrospective analysis of adult patients with cutaneous leukocytoclastic vasculitis. Australas J Dermatol. 2006;47:92-6.
5. Magro CM, Crowson AN. A clinical and histologic study of 37 cases of immunoglobulin A-associated vasculitis. Am J Dermatopathol. 1999;21:234-40.
6. Cohen SJ, Pittelkow MR, Su WP. Cutaneous manifestations of cryoglobulinemia: clinical and histopathologic study of seventy-two patients. J Am Acad Dermatol. 1991;25:21-7.
7. Seishima M, Oyama Z, Oda M. Skin eruptions associated with microscopic polyangiitis. Eur J Dermatol. 2004;14:255-8.
8. Barksdale SK, Hallahan CW, Kerr GS, et al. Cutaneous pathology in Wegener's granulomatosis. A clinicopathologic study of 75 biopsies in 46 patients. Am J Surg Pathol. 1995;19:161-72.
9. Davis MD, Daoud MS, McEvoy MT, et al. Cutaneous manifestations of Churg-Strauss syndrome: a clinicopathologic correlation. J Am Acad Dermatol. 1997;37:199-203.

CHAPTER **9**

Pathology of Pulmonary Vasculitis

Amanjit Bal, Ashim Das

INTRODUCTION

Pulmonary vasculitis is a heterogeneous disease affecting arteries, veins, and capillaries. The common vasculitic syndromes affecting the lungs include granulomatosis with polyangiitis (GPA), eosinophilic granulomatosis with polyangiitis (EGPA), microscopic polyangiitis (MPA), and antiglomerular basement membrane (anti-GBM) disease.[1-3] Pulmonary involvement is rare in polyarteritis nodosa, Kawasaki disease, Henoch-Schönlein purpura, and cryoglobulinemic vasculitis. The pathology of primary pulmonary vasculitis is often complicated by several forms of secondary vasculitis especially infection-associated vasculitis and vasculitis associated with connective tissue diseases. This is common in developing countries where infection-associated vasculitis due to tuberculosis and fungal infection are more frequently encountered by surgical pathologists. Thus, the diagnosis of pulmonary vasculitides requires clinical, radiological, laboratory, and pathological correlation. Table 9.1 enlists the vasculitides involving the lungs.

PRIMARY VASCULITIDES

Granulomatosis with Polyangiitis

Granulomatosis with polyangiitis (GPA) is a systemic disease characterized clinically by the involvement of the upper and lower respiratory tracts with involvement of kidney. Localized GPA involving the lungs is also known to occur. It is characterized by the presence of diffuse anti-neutrophilic cytoplasmic antibody (c-ANCA) positivity with specificity for PR3.[4] Pathologically, it is characterized by granulomatous inflammation involving upper and lower respiratory tracts and segmental necrotizing glomerulonephritis and extra-glomerular granulomatous inflammation of the kidneys.

Table 9.1 Vasculitides involving the lungs

Primary ANCA (pauci-immune)-associated small-vessel vasculitis

Granulomatosis with polyangiitis (Wegener's) (GPA)

Microscopic polyangiitis (MPA)

Eosinophilic granulomatosis with polyangiitis (Churg-Strauss) (EGPA)

Primary immune complex-mediated small-vessel vasculitis

Antiglomerular basement membrane (anti-GBM) disease

IgA vasculitis (Henoch-Schönlein) (IgAV)

Cryoglobulinemic vasculitis (CV)

Secondary vasculitis

Infection-associated vasculitis

Systemic lupus erythematosus and other connective tissue diseases

Lymphoproliferative lesions

Sarcoid vasculitis

Drugs

Although, it is categorized as small vessel vasculitis but any caliber vessels can be affected in this process.

Pathology Findings (Figs 9.1 to 9.3)

The pathological findings in the lungs are also variable and range from exudative lesions to healed lesions depending on the clinical stage of the disease.

The gross pathology at autopsy in GPA shows multiple nodular and hemorrhagic lesions. These firm nodules may cavitate and are often associated with overlying fibrinous pleuritis. These nodular lesions are usually related to the vascular involvement.

Microscopically, the features include combinations of geographic necrosis and vasculitis of either granulomatous

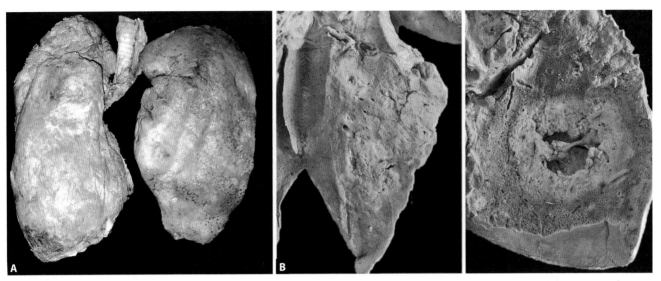

Figs 9.1A and B Granulomatosis with polyangiitis. (A) Consolidation of the right lung with nodular lesion in the left lung as seen from pleural surface with pleuritis; (B) Cut surface showing nodular lesions with the central cavitation

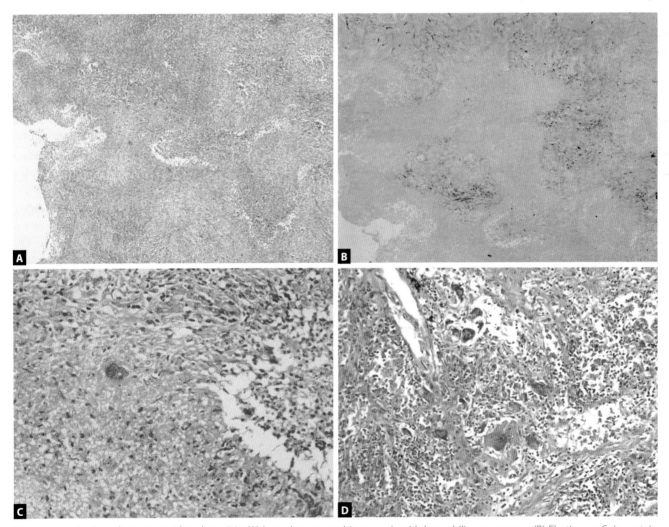

Figs 9.2A to D Granulomatosis with polyangiitis: (A) Irregular geographic necrosis with basophilic appearance; (B) Elastic von Geison stain highlighting destruction of underlying lung parenchyma in necrotic areas; (C) and (D) Granulomatous vasculitis with necrosis of the vessel wall and loose collections of epithelioid and giant cells in extravascular locations

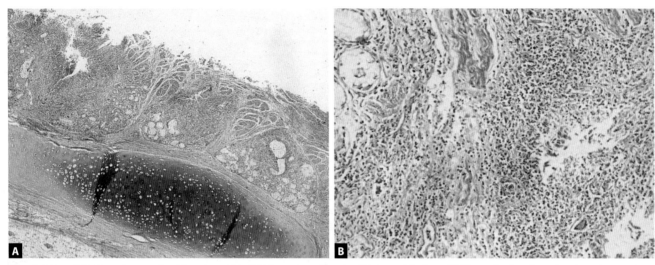

Figs 9.3A and B Granulomatosis with polyangiitis. (A) Ulceration of tracheal lining epithelium; (B) The wall of trachea showing characteristic loose collections of epithelioid cells with giant cells

or non-granulomatous nature.[5] Many non-specific histopathologic features are also seen.

Necrosis: The necrosis may be classic geographic with palisading histiocytes but small areas of necrosis with neutrophilic abscess formation are also seen. Surrounding these necrotic areas, isolated epithelioid cells with or without giant cells or sometimes only scattered giant cells can be seen along with neutrophils and eosinophils.

Vasculitis: The vasculitis may be classical granulomatous vasculitis or may be necrotizing; depending on the age of the lesions. Any size of vessels may be affected; arteries, capillaries, and venules. The granulomas are never well formed as seen in tuberculosis but are loose collections of epithelioid histiocytes with a few giant cells. The granulomatous inflammation may be missing in the early phase of the disease and can be mistaken as microscopic polyangiitis.

Other changes: There are many other pathological changes described in GPA such as diffuse pulmonary hemorrhage, tissue eosinophilia, intra-alveolar organization, and lipoid pneumonia. Diffuse pulmonary hemorrhage may be a rare serious complication of GPA. Brochiolocentric granulomatosis has also been described in this condition.

The changes in the upper airways including paranasal sinuses may be nonspecific inflammation or necrotizing inflammation with or without granulomatous reaction. The above-mentioned changes are more classically seen in autopsy material but open lung surgical biopsy can

show classical changes of GPA like geographic necrosis and granulomatous vasculitis but the diagnostic yield of endobronchial or transbronchial biopsies is extremely low.

Differential Diagnosis

The findings of necrosis with ill-defined granulomatous inflammation in GPA will also bring the differential diagnosis of tuberculosis and fungal infections in the developing country. The ill-defined granulomas with some giant cell in the presence of vasculitis may help to negate a diagnosis of tuberculosis. Many lymphomas like angiocentric lymphoma can simulate the histologic features of vasculitis. The involvement of upper respiratory tracts particularly sinuses and the subglottis are usually involved in GPA, which helps in differentiating from other primary vasculitides where biopsy does not reveal classical granulomatous vasculitis.

Microscopic Polyangiitis

Microscopic polyangiitis as the name suggests is a systemic vasculitis affecting small vessels, however, medium sized vessels can also be affected. It is associated with perinuclear antineutrophil cytoplasmic antibodies (pANCA) with specificity for myeloperoxidase that is considered pathogenic. In Chapel Hill classification, it is categorized under pauci-immune small-vessel vasculitis, thus associated with a few or no immune deposits.[6] Clinically, it can present as isolated renal involvement or as pulmonary-renal syndrome with rapidly progressive glomerulonephritis and alveolar hemorrhage. Pulmonary involvement in MPA most often presents as alveolar hemorrhage, with a chest radiograph characteristically showing patchy air space shadows. Rarely patients can have associated pleurisy and pleural effusions.

Pathology Findings (Figs 9.4A to D)

The pathological hallmarks of MPA include neutrophilic capillaritis leading to disruption of alveolar capillary basement membrane and resulting in diffuse pulmonary hemorrhage. Diffuse pulmonary hemorrhage is reflected in the gross as hemorrhagic appearance of the lungs and presence of intra-alveolar hemorrhage on microscopy. Chronic hemorrhage can be present as collection of hemosiderin-laden macrophages in the air spaces. The neutrophilic capillaritis is characterized by neutophilic infiltrate in the interalveolar septa along with nuclear debris of neutrophils undergoing apoptosis. The mere presence of neutrophils in the interstitium, which is also a common finding in active infections, does not qualify for capillaritis. The presence of nuclear debris, which is also termed as leukocytoclasia, represents true capillaritis and differentiates it from neutrophilic stasis seen in interstitial vessels.[7] Sometimes there is spilling over of neutrophils into the air spaces and resemble acute pneumonia. In such cases, identification of capillaritis in adjacent lesser involved lung parenchyma helps in distinguishing vasculitic process from infection. With recurrent episodes of diffuse alveolar hemorrhage (DAH), both obstructive lung disease and pulmonary fibrosis have been described as chronic complications.

Differential Diagnosis

Microscopic polyangiitis needs to be differentiated from GPA especially in small biopsies that may not demonstrate granulomatous vasculitis. In such cases, clinical picture of the patient and ANCA status helps in differentiating these two entities.[8] The presence of destructive inflammatory disease of the upper respiratory tract points toward a diagnosis of GPA. The presence of granulomatous either vascular or extravascular locations should points toward a diagnosis of GPA. Microscopic polyangiitis should also be differentiated from other small-vessel vasculitic syndromes such as Henoch-Schönlein purpura, cryoglobulinemic vasculitis, and lupus vasculitis. However, MPA has no immune deposits in contrast to other small-vessel vasculitis that have known immune complex deposits.

Eosinophilic Granulomatosis with Polyangiitis (Churg-Strauss)

Eosinophilic granulomatosis with polyangiitis, previously known as Churg-Strauss syndrome, was first described by Churg and Strauss in 1951 as "allergic granulomatosis, allergic angiitis, and periarteritis nodosa". It was characterized as a systemic disease that in addition to pulmonary vasculitis is associated with the presence of asthma, peripheral eosinophilia, and systemic vasculitis. The involvement of upper respiratory tract is less severe with no significant destruction and the renal involvement is usually milder than GPA.

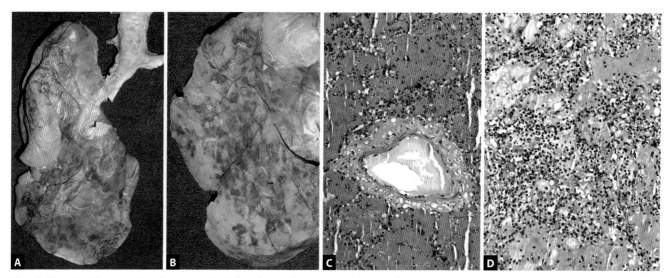

Figs 9.4A to D Microscopic polyangiitis. (A) Diffuse hemorrhagic consolidation of the lung as viewed from pleural surface; (B) Cut surface showing extensive areas of parenchymal hemorrhages; (C) Fresh intra-alveolar hemorrhages; (D) Neutrophilic infiltrate in the alveolar walls with nuclear debris in the background of alveolar hemorrhage

Pathology Findings (Figs 9.5A to C)

The characteristic histologic features include combination of necrotizing vasculitis, extensive eosinophilic infiltrate, and the presence of extravascular granulomas. However, recent data indicate that this definition is too narrow as EGPA is characterized by sequence of events, and the prevasculitic phase of the disease is not recognized leading to cases of EGPA being missed. Before vasculitis appears, there is often extravascular infiltration of tissues by eosinophils, and this is the diagnostic hallmark of early-stage EGPA. Thus, the American College of Rheumatology (ACR) criteria now allow tissue eosinophilia in the absence of pathologic vasculitis to serve as one criterion for the diagnosis of EGPA.[9]

Prevasculitic phase of EGPA, in the lung, takes the form of the dense peripheral radiographic airspace infiltrates of chronic eosinophilic pneumonia (CEP). This early stage of EGPA histologically mimics CEP in which foci of eosinophil necrosis and scattered giant cells may be observed.

The vasculitic phase of EGPA is characterized by an eosinophil-rich necrotizing vasculitis involving small arteries, arterioles, venules, and veins; and necrotizing granulomas centered on necrotic eosinophils. In many instances, the vasculitis of EGPA consists of infiltration of the vessel wall by inflammatory cells without any obvious tissue necrosis and is termed non-necrotizing vasculitis. The granulomas in EGPA consist of necrotic eosinophils and surrounding palisade epithelioid histiocytes with or without giant cells. However, the presence of granulomas is not mandatory for the diagnosis of EGPA; thus, their absence should not influence against a diagnosis of EGPA.

The postvasculitic phase of EPGA is characterized by healed vasculitis, organized thrombi in vessels, and lack of significant eosinophilic infiltrate.

Differential Diagnosis

The eosinophilic infiltrate of prevasculitic phase of EGPA has to be distinguished from conditions, such as eosinophilic pneumonia, allergic bronchopulmonary aspergillosis (ABPA), and parasitic infections.[10] Of these, the major differential is ABPA. These patients also have asthma and eosinophilia, along with serum precipitins against *Aspergillus*. The pulmonary changes of ABPA include bronchiectasis, allergic mucin impaction, eosinophilic pneumonia, and bronchocentric granulomatosis along with presence of hyphae of *Aspergillus* fungi in mucin. Pulmonary eosinophilic infiltrates may also be seen in tropical eosinophilia, in drug reactions, hypereosinophilic syndrome. However, these patients do not have underlying asthma.

Antiglomerular Basement Membrane Disease/Goodpasture's Syndrome

Antiglomerular basement membrane (anti-GBM) antibody disease is a rare cause of pulmonary-renal syndrome and is defined by the presence of serum anti-GBM antibody. The clinical presentation is of acute rapidly progressive glomerulonephritis with biopsy findings of severe crescentic glomerulonephritis and a linear deposition of IgG along the GBM as evidenced by immunofluorescence (IF). When accompanied by pulmonary involvement, it is referred to as anti-GBM disease or "Goodpasture syndrome". Lung involvement occurs in patients who smoke, presumably because of lung injury and the exposure of new epitopes to the immune system. Other exposures have also been implicated as causal factors, including hydrocarbons, cocaine use, hard metal dust, and *D*-penicillamine. Recently, several studies have been published suggesting the role of silica as one of etiological factors in ANCA associated vasculitis and glomerulonephritis. Silicosis and mineral

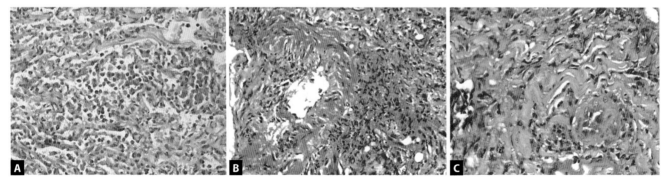

Figs 9.5A to C Eosinophilic granulomatosis with polyangiitis. (A) Tissue infiltration by eosinophils in air spaces simulating eosinophilic pneumonia; (B) Eosinophilic vasculitis without the vessel wall necrosis; (C) Eosinophilic infiltrate is extending into the surrounding tissue

dust pneumoconiosis have been linked to an increase in autoantibodies, immune complexes, and excess production of immunoglobulins, even in the absence of a specific autoimmune disease.

The hallmark of anti-GBM disease is circulating autoantibodies, which are principally directed against the glomerular/alveolar basement membrane. The antibodies are targeted against the type IV collagen, and the specific epitope is the NC1 domain of the alpha 3 chain. However, binding antibodies against the alpha 5 (IV) and alpha 4 (IV) chains of type IV collagen have also been detected.[11] These anti-GBM antibodies are usually IgG class, in the patient's serum or tissue, however rarely; the circulating autoantibodies can belong to IgA class rather than IgG.

Pathology Findings (Figs 9.6A to F)

Pulmonary lesions present histologically as alveolar hemorrhages, with numerous hemosiderin-containing macrophages, and prominence of type II pneumocytes. Necrosis of alveolar walls with polymorphonuclear cell infiltration can also be detected however no capillaritis is seen. This is in contrast to MPA where capillaritis is pathognomonic pathology finding for diagnosis. Although the pulmonary lesions lack overt leukocyte infiltration, anti-GBM disease is classified as vasculitis because cellular and humoral inflammatory mechanisms are responsible for the injury. On IF examination, linear binding of IgG is usually detected along the alveolar basement membrane. However, on ultrastructural examination no electron dense deposits are seen along alveolar capillaries possibly due to uniform binding of circulating autoantibodies to GBM epitopes rather than the formation of clumps of deposits (Figs 9.6A to F).

Approximately 10–38% of patients with anti-GBM antibody disease also have ANCA positivity (pANCA) and may have signs of systemic vasculitis.[12] Patients with dual antibodies are considered to be a vasculitis variant of anti-GBM antibody disease. Such patients may not have a typical presentation of pulmonary–renal syndrome, resulting in delay of the correct diagnosis and initiation of treatment. The prognosis of dual-positive patients is comparable to patients with isolated anti-GBM disease. However, similar to isolated ANCA disease patients, these dual-positive cases have higher frequency of active relapses.

Table 9.2 highlights the differentiating points of primary vasculitides involving the lungs.

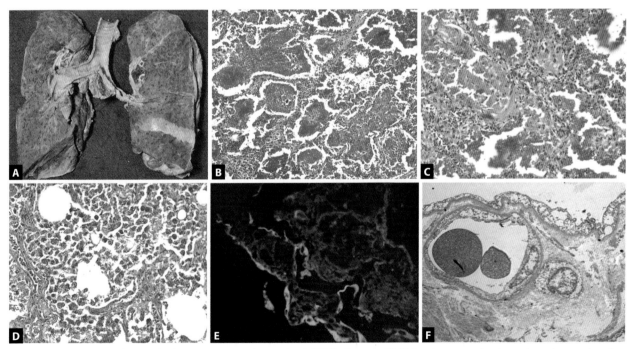

Figs 9.6A to F Anti-glomerular basement membrane (anti-GBM) disease. (A) Voluminous, and subcrepitant lungs showing hemorrhagic consolidation; (B) Dominantly fresh alveolar hemorrhages; (C) Neutrophilic stasis in alveolar septa, however, no capillaritis seen; (D) Collection of hemosiderin laden macrophages in the alveolar spaces indicative of old hemorrhages; (E) Linear IgG deposits on alveolar lining and capillary basement membrane by immunofluorescence; (F) Ultrastructural examination does not show any electron dense deposits in alveolar capillaries

Table 9.2 Distinguishing features of primary pulmonary vasculitides.

	GPA	MPA	EGPA	Anti-GBM
Dominant organ involvement	• Upper and lower respiratory tract • Kidneys • Pulmonary or renal limited GPA is known	• Lower respiratory tract • Kidneys	• Lungs (with history of asthma) • No significant involvement of sinuses or upper respiratory tract • No significant renal involvement	• Kidneys • Lungs
Vessel involvement	• Mainly small-vessel vasculitis but any sized vessel can be involved	• Mainly small-vessel involvement	• Small-vessel involvement but medium-sized vessel involvement may be seen	• Exclusively capillaries, venules, and arterioles
ANCA	cANCA associated dominantly	pANCA associated dominantly	pANCA or cANCA	No, serum anti-GBM autoantibodies
Gross findings	Nodules and cavities	Hemorrhagic consolidation	Nodules or consolidation	Hemorrhagic consolidation
Histological hallmarks	• Geographic necrosis • Granulomatous or nongranulomatous vasculitis • Poorly formed extra vascular granulomatous reactions	• Capillaritis • Alveolar hemorrhage • No granulomatous reactions	• Tissue eosinophilic infiltrate • Eosinophilic vasculitis • Extra vascular granulomas	• Alveolar hemorrhage • No capillaritis
Immune complexes	No immune complexes	No immune complexes	No immune complexes	Linear IgG deposits

Abbreviations: GPA: Granulomatosis with polyangiitis; MPA: Microscopic polyangiitis; EGPA: Eosinophilic granulomatosis with polyangiitis; anti-GBM: Antiglomerular basement membrane disease.

SECONDARY VASCULITIDES

Infection Associated Vasculitis

The findings of granulomatous inflammation in granulomatosis with polyangiitis also bring the differential diagnosis of tuberculosis and fungal infections in the developing country. Also antineutrophilic cytoplasmic antibody may not be diagnostic of pulmonary vasculitis, as this has been found to be positive in other situations also. Moreover, the biopsy findings vary in the different time frame of the disease. Thus, the immunosuppressive treatment in a wrongly diagnosed case of GPA may prove fatal for tuberculosis and fungal infections as all three diseases are characterized by granulomatous inflammation.

The vasculitic process is well known in various infections. Infectious vasculitis is caused by direct invasion of the pathogen in vessel walls that causes inflammation. Tuberculosis can result in granulomatous arteritis leading to vessel wall thickening, aneurysm formation, and stenoses mimicking primary vasculitis (Figs 9.7A and B). Also ANCA levels may be raised in *Mycobacterial tuberculosis* and *nontubercular Mycobacteria* infections.

When considering a diagnosis of pulmonary vasculitis, it is prudent to exclude tuberculous infections by tissue diagnosis and stains and cultures for *mycobacteria* should be performed. Similarly, fungal infections also cause secondary vasculitis by direct infiltration into the vessel wall especially the *Aspergillus* and Mucor (Figs 9.8A to D). Special stains such as Periodic acid Schiff and Grocott's stain aid in identification of fungi.

Systemic Lupus Erythematosus (SLE) and Other Collagen Vascular Disorders

Respiratory complications are frequent in collagen vascular or connective tissue disorders and these are frequent in SLE. Previously, the lung histology of bland DAH has been reported in association with SLE. However, more recent studies indicate the frequent presence of small-vessel vasculitis in the form of arteriolitis, venulitis, and capillaritis in association with DAH in SLE (Figs 9.9A to D). Immune complex deposition is often found in the lungs of patients with SLE vasculitis and DAH. The presence of granular immune deposits distinguishes the DAH of SLE from that of Wegener's granulomatosis, microscopic polyangiitis that has no immune deposits (pauci-immune), and from Goodpasture's syndrome that has linear immune deposits. Small-vessel pulmonary vasculitis has also been recently reported in polymyositis, rheumatoid arthritis, and scleroderma causing alveolar hemorrhage. Thus, serologic testing for evaluation of DAH should be done to identify the underlying disease entities.

Sarcoid Vasculitis

Sarcoidosis is a multisystem disease of unknown etiology and the lungs are affected in more than 90% of patients. The

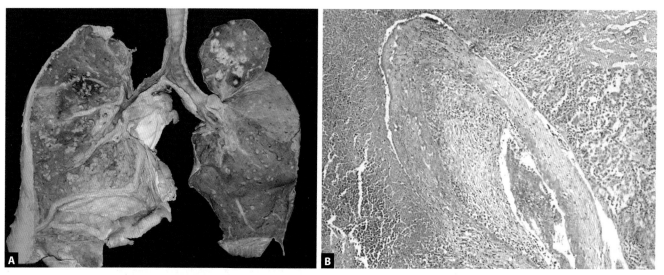

Figs 9.7A and B Tuberculosis vasculitis. (A) Gross photograph of the lungs showing numerous nodular caseating areas; (B) Evidence of vasculitis (inset: Acid-fast bacilli on Ziehl Neelsen stain).

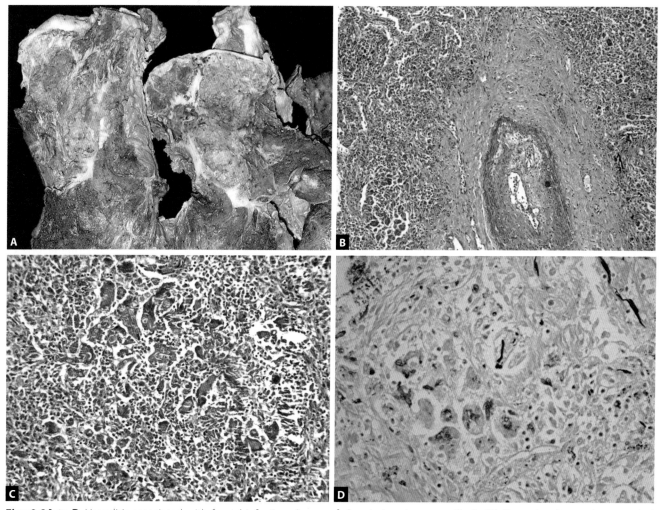

Figs 9.8A to D Vasculitis associated with fungal infection. A case of chronic invasive aspergillosis. (A) Gross showing cavitatory apical lesion; (B) The vessel wall shows infiltration by giant cells; (C) Giant cells show presence of fungal hyphae; (D) Fungal hyphae highlighted by Grocott's stain

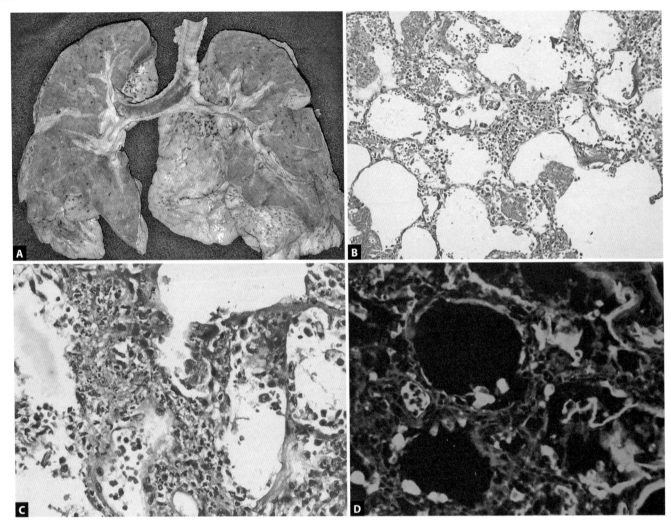

Figs 9.9A to D Lupus associated vasculitis. (A) Grossly showing hemorrhagic consolidation; (B) and (C) Presence of small-vessel vasculitis in the form of capillaritis involving interalveolar capillaries with nuclear debris, mimicking MPA; (D) However, immunofluorescence showing granular IgG deposits along capillary walls

etiological factors implicated in its pathogenesis include chronic immunologic response produced by a genetic susceptibility and exposure to specific environmental factors, and association with HLA-DRB1 and infectious agents such as *Mycobacteria*, Herpes virus, and *Helicobacter pylori*.

The morphologic diagnosis of sarcoidosis depends upon location and appearance of granulomas and exclusion of an alternative causes. The sarcoid granulomas follow the lymphangitic pattern, i.e. are present along subpleura, interlobular septa, around bronchovascular regions, and interalveolar interstitium. The granulomas are compact, circumscribed, non-necrotizing composed of epithelioid cells surrounded by rim of fibroblasts, and can have multinucleated giant cell. In early stages of the disease, granulomas are cellular and discrete, but they become more fibrotic and hyalinized as the disease advances.

Necrotizing sarcoid granulomatosis (NSG) is a rare variant of sarcoidosis and mimics pulmonary vasculitis. The diagnostic feature of NSG is the presence of sarcoid-like granulomas in the walls of blood vessels; the small arteries, veins, and venules. This results in irregular areas of necrosis of parenchyma and the vessel walls. Necrotizing sarcoid granulomatosis principally affects the lungs and the differential diagnosis includes EGPA, GPA, and lymphomatoid granulomatosis. However, in both GPA and EGPA, the hilar lymph node enlargement is uncommon.

Vasculitis in Lymphoproliferative Lesions

Many lymphomas such as angiocentric lymphoma and lymphomatoid granulomatosis can simulate the histologic features of vasculitis. Lymphomatoid granulomatosis,

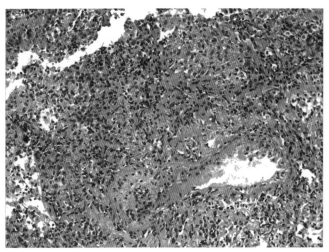

Fig. 9.10 Lymphomatoid granulomatosis: polymorphous population of lymphoid cells infiltrating the vessel wall mimicking vasculitis

which shows angiodestructive polymorphous inflammatory infiltrate with scattered large atypical cells, was described previously as pulmonary angiitis just like GPA (Fig. 9.10). Initially, it was thought to be T-cell lymphoproliferative process, but now it is considered as Epstein-Barr Virus (EBV) associated B-cell lymphoma. Grade I lesions that have very few atypical lymphoma cells can pose diagnostic challenge and histologically mimics GPA (Fig. 9.10). However, grade II and III lesions, which have many atypical cells, are diagnostic of this being a lymphomatous process than primary vasculitis.

KEY POINTS

- Pulmonary involvement by vasculitis is mainly limited to small-vessel vasculitis.
- Granulomatosis with polyangiitis as compared to other vasculitis involves both upper and lower respiratory tract.
- Granulomatosis with polyangiitis and eosinophilic granulomatosis with polyangiitis usually presents with nodules and cavities and show granulomatous vasculitis on morphology similar to infection-associated vasculitis.

- Microscopic polyangiitis and anti-GBM disease present as hemorrhagic consolidation and show DAH with and without capillaritis, respectively.
- In the differential diagnosis between GPA and MPA, the presence of either vascular or extravascular granulomatous lesions should points toward the diagnosis of GPA.
- For definite diagnosis, clinical picture and laboratory findings along with pathology findings should be taken into consideration.

REFERENCES

1. Brown KK. Pulmonary vasculitis. Proc Am Thorac Soc. 2006;3:48-57.
2. Jennette CJ, Falk RJ, Bacon PA, et al. 2012 revised International Chapel Hill Consensus Conference nomenclature of vasculitides. Arthritis Rheum. 2013;65:1-11.
3. Peachell MB, Müller NL. Pulmonary vasculitis. Semin Respir Crit Care Med. 2004;25:483-9.
4. Savage COS, Harper L, Adu D. Primary systemic vasculitis. Lancet. 1997;349:553-8.
5. Yoshikawa Y, Watanabe T. Pulmonary lesions in Wegener's granulomatosis: a clinicopathologic study of 22 autopsy cases. Hum Pathol. 1986;17:401-10.
6. Jennette JC, Falk RJ. Small vessel vasculitis. N Engl J Med. 1997;337:1512-23.
7. Smyth L, Gaskin G, Pusey CD. Microscopic polyangiitis. Semin Respir Crit Care Med. 2004;25:523-32.
8. Schwarz MI, Brown KK. Small-vessel vasculitis of the lung. Thorax. 2000;55:502-10.
9. Churg A. Recent advances in the diagnosis of Churg–Strauss syndrome. Mod Pathol. 2001;14:1284-93.
10. Travis WD. Pathology of pulmonary vasculitis. Semin Respir Crit Care Med. 2004;25:475-82.
11. Lahmer T, Heemann U. Anti-glomerular basement membrane antibody disease: a rare autoimmune disorder affecting the kidney and the lung. Autoimmun Rev. 2012;12:169-73.
12. DE Zoysa J, Taylor D, Thein H, et al. Incidence and features of dual anti-GBM-positive and ANCA-positive patients. Nephrology. 2011;16:725-9.

CHAPTER 10

Pathology of Renal Vasculitis

Ritambhra Nada, Manish Rathi, Aman Sharma, J Charles Jennette

Vasculitides are categorized into infectious vasculitis, caused by direct invasion and proliferation of pathogens in vessel walls with resultant inflammation (*Aspergillus or Mucomycosis* arteritis, rickettsial vasculitis, and syphilitic aortitis), or noninfectious vasculitis. The recent revision of the Chapel Hill Consensus Conference Nomenclature of Vasculitis (CHCC 2012)[1,2] addresses only noninfectious vasculitis; though indirectly etiopathogenetic associations with infections are known, e.g. cryoglubulinemic vasculitis (CV) associated with hepatitis C virus infection.

Renal parenchymal injury is seen in most systemic vasculitis, most prominently in SVV. It is very important to realize that medium-vessel vasculitis (MVV) and even large vessel vasculitis (LVV) can also affect small arteries.

In CHCC 2012, the first categorization level is again based on the predominant type and size of vessels involved, i.e. large, medium, and small vessel vasculitis. These vessels differ not only in size but also in structural and functional attributes, hence different predilections of involvement in different type of vasculitis. Please note that though LVV affects large arteries more often than medium or small vessel vasculitis, MVV affects predominantly medium arteries, and SVV affects predominantly small arteries and other small vessels, but, importantly, all three major categories can affect any size artery. This can have bearing on renal parenchymal involvement in any of these vasculitides.

Another point to remember is that dominant types of inflammation occur in specific forms of vasculitis but this may be seen only during active disease. Most medium and small vessel vasculitides have necrotizing arteritis with extensive vascular necrosis during the acute phase, a finding that differs from the more chronic and granulomatous inflammation of the large vessel vasculitides. In this context, the early phase of granulomas in SVV, granulomatosis with polyangiitis (GPA), and eosinophilic granulomatosis with polyangiitis (EGPA) have acute-suppurative features, whereas the granulomatous inflammation of LVV has more conventional features with a predominance of macrophages. Unlike the large vessel vasculitides, which rarely affect intraparenchymal vessels, the medium vessel vasculitides and especially the small vessel vasculitides often involve renal parenchyma, which manifests as significant renal dysfunction. The necrotizing vascular inflammation is characterized by segmental fibrinoid necrosis with neutrophilic infiltration and leukocytoclasia of arteries, arterioles, capillaries, venules, veins, and glomeruli in SVV, and only arteries in medium-vessel vasculitides.

SMALL-VESSEL VASCULITIS

- Small-vessel vasculitis is a vasculitis predominantly affecting small vessels, defined as small intraparenchymal arteries, arterioles, capillaries, and venules.
- Medium arteries and veins may be affected.

In essence, all intraparenchymal vessels are small vessels, with the exception of the initial penetrating branches of medium arteries. Small biopsy specimens usually contain only small vessels; therefore, the largest arteries in such biopsies are small arteries. The two major categories of SVV are following:

1. *Antineutrophil cytoplasmic antibody (ANCA)-associated vasculitis (AAV):* It is characterized by a paucity of deposition of immunoglobulins in the vessel wall and includes:
   - *Microscopic polyangiitis (MPA)*
   - *Granulomatosis with polyangiitis (Wegener's) (GPA)*
   - *Eosinophilic granulomatosis with polyangiitis (Churg-Strauss) (EGPA)*
   - *Renal-limited AAV.*

2. *Immune complex SVV:* It is characterized by prominence of deposition of immunoglobulins in the vessel wall. It includes:
   – Antiglomerular basement membrane (anti-GBM) disease
   – Cryoglobulinemic vasculitis (CV)
   – IgA vasculitis (Henoch-Schönlein) (IgAV)
   – Hypocomplementemic urticarial vasculitis (anti-C1q vasculitis).

ANCA-associated Vasculitis

ANCA-associated vasculitis is necrotizing vasculitis, with few or no immune deposits, predominantly affecting small vessels (i.e., capillaries, venules, arterioles, and small arteries), associated with ANCA specific for myeloperoxidase (MPO-ANCA) or proteinase 3 (PR3-ANCA). A prefix should be added to the name to indicate ANCA reactivity, i.e.
- MPO-ANCA
- PR3-ANCA
- ANCA-negative
  Patients with ANCA-negative AAV may have ANCA that cannot be detected with currently available methods or may have ANCA of unknown specificity, or truly not associated with ANCA.

  The small amount or lack of immune deposits in vessel walls that is a characteristic of AAV differs from the moderate to marked vessel wall immune deposition that is characteristic of immune complex SVV. However, the cut-off for the presence of fewer deposits in AAV versus more immune deposits in immune complex SVV is subjective and not based on any precise quantitative measures.

Microscopic Polyangiitis

- Microscopic polyangiitis (MPA) is necrotizing vasculitis, with few or no immune deposits, predominantly affecting small vessels (i.e. capillaries, venules, or arterioles).
- Necrotizing arteritis involving small and medium arteries may be present.
- Necrotizing glomerulonephritis is very common.
- Pulmonary capillaritis often occurs.
- Inflammation that is *not centered on vessels*, including *granulomatous inflammation, is absent.*

Granulomatosis with Polyangiitis (Wegener's)

- Granulomatosis with polyangiitis (GPA) is necrotizing granulomatous inflammation, usually involving the upper and lower respiratory tract.

- Necrotizing vasculitis affecting predominantly small-to-medium vessels (e.g., capillaries, venules, arterioles, arteries, and veins).
- Necrotizing glomerulonephritis is common.
- Ocular vasculitis and pulmonary capillaritis with hemorrhage are frequent.
- Granulomatous and nongranulomatous extravascular inflammations are common.
- Limited expressions of GPA occur, especially disease confined to the upper or lower respiratory tract or the eye. These patients may have no identifiable evidence of systemic vasculitis; however, they should be kept under close follow-up. Whenever, they exhibit clinical and pathological changes identical to those seen in GPA, especially if they are ANCA positive, they should be included in the GPA category.

Eosinophilic Granulomatosis with Polyangiitis (Churg-Strauss)

- Eosinophilic granulomatosis with polyangiitis (EGPA) is eosinophil-rich and necrotizing granulomatous inflammation that often involves the respiratory tract.
- There is necrotizing vasculitis, predominantly affecting small-to-medium vessels.
- It is invariably associated with asthma and eosinophilia.
- Nasal polyps are common.
- Antineutrophil cytoplasmic antibody is more frequent when glomerulonephritis is present. Only 25% of patients with EGPA who have no renal disease are ANCA positive, whereas 75% with any renal disease and 100% with documented necrotizing glomerulonephritis have ANCA.
- The prominence of eosinophils in the blood and tissue is an essential feature of EGPA, and hence the name.
- Limited expressions of EGPA confined to the upper or lower respiratory tract may occur.
- Granulomatous and nongranulomatous extravascular inflammations, such as nongranulomatous eosinophil-rich inflammation of lungs, myocardium, and gastrointestinal tract are common.

Gross Pathology of AAV[3] (Figs 10.1 and 10.2)

- In severe disease, the kidneys show flea-bitten appearance due to presence of blood in Bowman's spaces and tubules.
- There can be areas of small hemorrhagic or pale infarcts.
- Rarely, papillary necrosis can be seen when there is medullary angiitis.

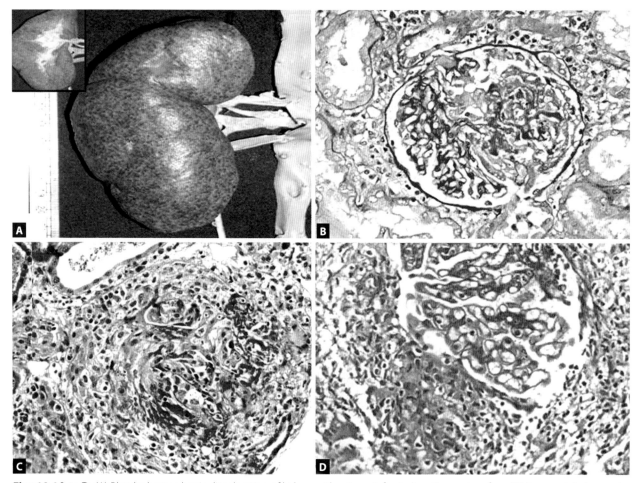

Figs 10.1A to D (A) Blotchy hemorrhagic discoloration of kidney without any infarcts (inset) on cut surface; (B) Segmental glomerular tuft necrosis with segmental cellular crescent. Adjacent normal capillaries suggest pauci-immune or antiglomerular basement membrane (GBM) glomerulonephritis; (C) Global circumferential crescents with red fibrin in tuft necrosis and crescent; (D) Segmental tuft necrosis with granulomatous glomerulonephritis with occasional giant cells (B and D PAS, C Masson's Trichrome, ×40 original magnification). (B to D) Pauci-immune glomerulonephritis and anti-GBM glomerulonephritis cannot be distinguished based on light microscopic features. Both can have granulomatous glomerulonephritis and thus this feature is not specific for granulomatosis with polyangiitis

- Gross lesions as aneurysm or thrombosis can be seen when medium-sized arteries or its branches such as arcuate or interlobar arteries with SVV. Such lesions are rare in AAV when compared with MVV.

Light Microscopy[3]

Glomeruli

- Characteristic acute histological lesions of acute pauci-immune ANCA glomerulonephritis are fibrinoid necrosis of glomerular tuft with the presence of crescents.

  The fibrinoid necrosis usually is accompanied by crescent formation. Foci of fibrinoid necrosis in pauci-immune crescentic glomerulonephritis often contain neutrophil granule constituents. Presence of relatively normal glomerular segments adjacent to severe fibrinoid necrosis in same glomerulus or other glomeruli is seen in pauci-immune AAV and acute anti-GBM glomerulonephritis.

  Whereas presence of varying degree of glomerular endocapillary hypercellularity, less glomerular necrosis in adjacent segments, or other glomeruli is indicative of immune complex crescentic glomerulonephritis. Similarly, there is little or no disruption of Bowman's capsule, and less periglomerular inflammation in immune complex crescentic glomerulonephritis.

- Crescent formation occurs at the point of basement membrane rupture but can be circumferential.

  Range of severity varies from focal segmental fibrinoid necrosis and crescent formation in < 10% of glomeruli to severe diffuse global necrotizing and crescentic glomerulonephritis.

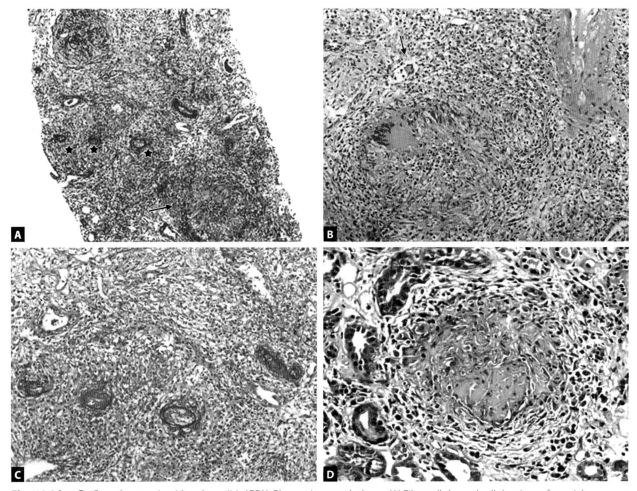

Figs 10.2A to D Granulomatosis with polyangiitis (GPA). Photomicrograph shows (A) Fibrocellular and cellular circumferential crescents with glomerulonephritis and granulomatous inflammation around small artery (asterisks) showing fibrinoid necrosis. (B) Granulomatous glomerulonephritis with giant cell and scattered giant cells in interstitium favoring diagnosis of GPA. (C) Granulomatous inflammation around small artery with fibrinoid necrosis. (D) Fibrous crescent with globally sclerosed glomerulus merging with interstitium (PAS—A, B, H&E—B, Masson's trichrome—D, ×10–A, ×20–C, ×40–B, D—magnification). Presence of granulomatous inflammation in relation to artery in the interstitium and scattered interstitial giant cell exclude microscopic polyangiitis and are clues for GPA.

On an average in a given renal biopsy specimen, 45–55% of glomeruli have crescents and 20–25% of glomeruli have fibrinoid necrosis.

Comparatively mild, possibly early, acute disease with focal necrosis but no crescents was observed in only 3% of specimens.

Similarly, extensive crescent formation involving >50% of glomeruli in the absence of active necrosis was seen in 4%.

Either focal (4%) or diffuse (12%) sclerosing glomerulonephritis with no necrosis and no cellular crescents can be seen in 16% of specimens, presumably, representing a chronic phase of disease.

Rare biopsy specimens from patients with clinical evidence for ANCA glomerulonephritis may have no lesions identified by light microscopy (LM) (1%) or only tubulointerstitial inflammation (1%). These patients may have focal ANCA glomerulonephritis that is not sampled in the renal biopsy. However, serial sections should be done to look for small segmental lesions.

- The histological features of renal-limited pauci-immune crescentic glomerulonephritis are indistinguishable from those of pauci-immune crescentic glomerulonephritis that occurs as a component of systemic vasculitis (i.e. MPA, GPA, and EGPA).

- There is no difference in glomerular crescents, necrosis, and sclerosis in patients with ANCA-negative pauci-immune glomerulonephritis and patients with ANCA-positive pauci-immune glomerulonephritis.

- The extent of crescent formation is not different between patients with PR3-ANCA versus MPO-ANCA.

- Breaks in Bowman's capsule are common in pauci-immune crescentic glomerulonephritis. There can be granulomatous glomerulitis and severe inflammatory periglomerulitis that resemble inflammation seen in extraglomerular vessels in the interstitium in GPA. Although interstitial granulomatous inflammation is not a feature of MPA, granulomatous glomerulonephritis is a nonspecific finding that can be seen in MPA, GPA, and anti-GBM disease. It may be more frequent in MPO-ANCA disease than in PR3-ANCA disease. Occasional multinucleated giant cells in the glomerular or periglomerular infiltrates can be seen without granuloma, possibly at point of fragmentation of Bowman's capsule.

- With time, the necrotic glomerular lesions of pauci-immune crescentic glomerulonephritis lead to segmental or global sclerosis. Presence of focal chronic sclerotic lesions and focal acute necrotizing lesions, suggest episodic nature of lesions where lesions with sclerosis represent previous episode that have caused scarring and necrotizing lesions represent acute exacerbations of disease.

Dual Lesions

- The possibility of concurrent immune complex and ANCA disease must be considered when there is endocapillary hypercellularity or thick capillary walls, in ANCA-positive patient with glomerular fibrinoid necrosis or crescent formation that will be corroborated by immunofluorescence and electron microscopy.
- Similarly, in the presence of more extensive necrosis or crescent formation with confirmed immune complex disease such as membranous glomerulopathy with exclusively subepithelial deposits or IgA nephropathy with exclusively mesangial deposits, coexisting ANCA disease must be considered.

Blood Vessels

Arteries, arterioles, and medullary vasa recta should be examined for the possibility of accompanying necrotizing SVV, i.e. renal arteritis, arteriolitis, and medullary angiitis in pauci-immune crescentic glomerulonephritis. The interlobular arteries are the most commonly affected arteries, but any artery may be involved. Hilar arteriolar necrosis is often continuous with glomerular necrosis.

Presence of vasculitis in biopsy or presence of pauci-immune crescentic glomerulonephritis should prompt a search for clinical, serological, and other pathological tests for systemic vasculitis.

- Histological features of acute arterial and arteriolar lesions in the kidney and elsewhere in pauci-immune

SVV is segmental fibrinoid necrosis with associated mural and perivascular infiltration of neutrophils or mononuclear leukocytes or both. This necrotizing arteritis of pauci-immune SVV is histologically indistinguishable from the necrotizing arteritis of polyarteritis nodosa (PAN). *Presence of glomerulonephritis* indicates that this necrotizing arteritis is a component of a SVV rather than medium-sized vasculitis, such as PAN.

- Arteritis in not seen frequently in biopsies, e.g. only 13% of renal biopsies with ANCA glomerulonephritis have vasculitis. Vasculitis has been documented in 19–23% of MPA, and 23% of with PR3-ANCA glomerulonephritis.
- Acute arteritis has intramural and perivascular infiltrates containing many neutrophils, often with leukocytoclasia. If biopsied later, it will have predominantly mononuclear leukocytes. Numerous eosinophils are not specific but should raise suspicion for EGPA (Churg–Strauss syndrome).
- Thrombosis may be present at sites of vascular inflammation and necrosis.
- Perivascular inflammatory infiltrates that occur adjacent to necrotic segments of arteries may have a granulomatous appearance with palisading macrophages and may be multinucleated giant cells. This perivascular inflammatory response is similar to the periglomerular granulomatous inflammatory response that occurs around severely injured glomeruli in pauci-immune crescentic glomerulonephritis. Perivascular granulomatous inflammation is most frequent in patients with GPA but also may occur in patients with EGPA. It is not seen in MPA.
- Acute necrotizing arterial lesions result in progressive sclerosis that evolves into segmental vascular scarring with or without associated mononuclear leukocytes and macrophages. Necrotic areas are replaced by distorted vessel wall usually with thickened intima and fibrotic muscularis and breaks in elastic lamina.
- Occasionally necrotizing, leukocytoclastic angiitis affecting the medullary vasa recta results in medullary angiitis resulting in ischemia and coagulative necrosis that may lead to sloughing of the necrotic papillary tip (papillary necrosis). Focal interstitial hemorrhage may also be present.

Tubules and Interstitium

- Interstitial edema and focal tubular epithelial flattening are common with severe acute pauci-immune crescentic glomerulonephritis. Tubular lumens may contain numerous red blood cells, which in absence of glomerular lesions in ANCA-positive patient should prompt multiple serial sections to find focal necrotizing glomerular lesions. Interstitial infiltration by leukocytes is common and is most pronounced adjacent to severely inflamed glomeruli or vessels. Tubulitis may be seen. Interstitial eosinophils often occur in EGPA (Churg-Strauss syndrome), but these are not specific as they can occur in any AAV and in PAN.

- Focal zones of tubular coagulative necrosis should raise the possibility of an accompanying vasculitis that has caused infarction.
- Pauci-immune crescentic glomerulonephritis, especially as it progresses, is accompanied by interstitial leukocyte infiltration that has two patterns that usually coexist: tubulointerstitial and periglomerular. Interstitial

leukocyte infiltration and interstitial fibrosis tend to be more pronounced with MPO-ANCA glomerulonephritis than with PR3-ANCA glomerulonephritis.

- There may be plasma cell-rich infiltrate in about one-third cases that can have moderate amount of IgG4 positive cells.[4]

Granulomas in AAV[5] (Figs 10.3A to D)

The acute lesions of GPA (WG) are not granulomatous. It is rather purulent, more like an abscess that may have occasionally giant cells (a component associated with granulomas) and progressively attracts more and more macrophages that form a zone of granulomatous inflammation around the central zone of neutrophil-rich

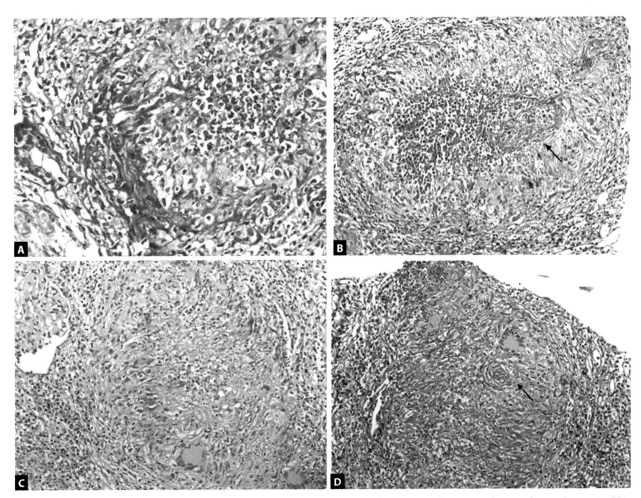

Figs 10.3A to D Granulomatosis with polyangiitis (GPA). Photomicrographs show evolutionary phases of granulomas in GPA. (A) Suppurative granuloma with neutrophils. (B) Granuloma in relation to artery (arrow) show bluish debri with degenerating neutrophils in the center and palisading macrophages at the periphery. (C) Eosinophilic necrosis in center of granuloma in interstitium with two giant cells. (D) Periarterial (arrow) granuloma and giant cells (PAS—A, B, D, H&E—C ×40 original magnification). Early stages of granulomatosis have a central zone rich in neutrophils resembling a microabscess with a marginal zone of palisading macrophages. Granulomas do not classically look like caseating/noncaseating granulomas of tuberculosis/sarcoidosis

necrosis. This purulent neutrophil-rich infiltrate later convert to areas of necrosis with slightly basophilic hue as it evolves from extensive karyorrhectic (leukocytoclastic) debris. These ages into amorphous acidophilic material with a peripheral zone of palisading macrophages and scattered multinucleated giant cells. This stage has a granulomatous appearance. These multinucleated cells generally have engulfed apoptotic and necrotic neutrophil debris. The typical well-defined granulomatous inflammation composed of epithelioid cells and giant cells as seen in sarcoidosis or tuberculosis are not a feature of GPA. However, stain for acid-fast bacilli should be done in all cases with granulomas, even suppurative ones as in places where tuberculosis is prevalent, any morphological pattern described above can be seen.

- Periglomerular granulomatous inflammation secondary to severe necrotizing glomerular injury should not be confused with the rare occurrence in patients with GPA of interstitial necrotizing granulomatous inflammation. Interstitial granulomas have irregular, jagged outline with central zone of necrosis surrounded by a loose infiltrate of mononuclear leukocytes, neutrophils, and scattered multinucleated giant cells. Glomerulocentric granulomas are rounded in contours and contain fragments of Bowman's capsule and GBM. Interstitial granulomas are component of the systemic necrotizing granulomatosis of GPA or EGPA. Perivascular interstitial inflammation occurs adjacent to the sites of segmental necrotizing inflammation in cortical arteries and arterioles and in the medullary vasa recta. Any type of inflammatory cells may be seen. Many eosinophils in the vasculitic and perivasculitic infiltrates can occur in MPA and GPA as well as in EGPA. Therefore, a diagnosis of EGPA cannot be made on the basis of numerous eosinophils in the vasculitic infiltrate. History of asthma and blood eosinophilia should be present.
- As disease progresses, interstitial fibrosis and tubular atrophy with tubulitis can be seen.

Extrarenal Pathology

- Based on a biopsy alone, a pathologist can only give a descriptive diagnosis (such as necrotizing arteritis or leukocytoclastic angiitis) along with a differential diagnosis of categories of vasculitis that could be causing the lesions.

  For example, histologically indistinguishable necrotizing arteritis in a biopsy specimen from intestines, skeletal muscle, peripheral nerve, or skin can be caused by PAN, MPA, GPA, and EGPA. Similarly, leukocytoclastic angiitis in the dermis can be caused not only by the ANCA

small-vessel vasculitides, but also by immune-mediated SVV such as IgAV (Henoch-Schönlein purpura), CV, and rheumatoid vasculitis.

- Antineutrophil cytoplasmic antibody small-vessel vasculitides, especially MPA and GPA, are the common causes of pulmonary-renal vasculitic syndrome that is also a feature of anti-GBM disease. However, there are differences in histology. Hemorrhagic necrotizing pulmonary alveolar capillaritis is frequent. The acute alveolar capillaritis with marked neutrophil infiltration in alveolar septa, often with leukocytoclasia is seen in AAV, whereas less conspicuous neutrophils and destruction of alveolar capillary basement membranes are seen in anti-GBM disease (Goodpasture's syndrome).

Immunofluorescence Microscopy

- By definition, pauci-immune crescentic glomerulo-nephritis does not have immunofluorescence microscopy findings that would be diagnostic for anti-GBM disease or immune complex disease. However, the term pauci-immune rather than nonimmune staining is used because many patients have a low level of staining for immunoglobulin (i.e. <2+ on a scale of 0–4+).
- The paucity of staining for immunoglobulin is seen in renal-limited ANCA associated necrotizing and crescentic glomerulonephritis as well as ANCA-associated systemic SVV.
- When staining for immunoglobulins is present, it may be for any combination of IgG, IgM, or IgA. The staining usually is confined to or predominantly in the mesangium; however, the distribution is extremely variable. Segmental trapping in sclerosed or necrotic areas should be carefully interpreted.
- When IgA staining is dominant or codominant, the possibility of concurrent ANCA disease and IgA nephropathy is a consideration.
  - Diagnosis of pauci-immune crescentic glomerulo-nephritis, if there is IgA-dominant staining that is less than 2+ intensity in the setting of glomerular necrosis and crescents.
  - Diagnosis of concurrent ANCA glomerulonephritis and IgA nephropathy, if there is 2+ or greater IgA-dominant staining in a patient with necrosis, crescents, and ANCA, especially if there also is well-defined endocapillary hypercellularity in nonnecrotic glomeruli.
- Pauci-immune crescentic glomerulonephritis with minor granular subepithelial staining for IgG versus

ANCA glomerulonephritis with concurrent membranous glomerulopathy
- ANCA glomerulonephritis concurrent with membranous glomerulopathy should only be considered, if 50% of glomeruli have over 50% of the tufts involved with 2+ or greater granular staining for IgG in a patient with necrosis, crescents, and ANCA.
- The presence of intense linear staining of glomeruli in an ANCA-positive patient with crescentic glomerulonephritis raises the possibility of concurrent anti-GBM disease. The presence of ANCA alters the phenotype of disease, likely to have systemic SVV that is not expected with anti-GBM disease alone. Thus, testing for ANCA may provide useful information not only in patients with pauci-immune glomerulonephritis and vasculitis but also in patients with anti-GBM glomerulonephritis or crescentic immune complex glomerulonephritis.

Electron Microscopy

- Most patients with pauci-immune crescentic glomerulonephritis, MPA, GPA, and EGPA have no or scanty glomerular or vascular immune complex type electron-dense deposits.
- Pauci-immune crescentic glomerulonephritis with no electron-dense deposits cannot be distinguished from anti-GBM glomerulonephritis, which also lacks electron-dense deposits.
- Presence of extensive immune complex type electron-dense deposits is not consistent with a diagnosis of pauci-immune glomerulonephritis; however, this does not rule out an ANCA-positive glomerulonephritis because ANCA positivity, with associated glomerular necrosis and crescent formation, can be superimposed on immune complex glomerulonephritis.
- The ultra-structural features of pauci-immune crescentic glomerulonephritis are the same in patients with renal-limited disease as those in patients with systemic vasculitis.

Classification of ANCA-associated Glomerulonephritis[6]

A classification of ANCA-associated glomerulonephritis has been proposed. The phenotypical order of the classes corresponds to the order of severity of renal function impairment during follow-up.
- Patients with focal ANCA-associated glomerulonephritis present with relatively preserved renal function and have a relatively favorable renal outcome.

- Patients with crescentic ANCA-associated glomerulonephritis present with highly active renal disease and severely reduced renal function but stand a good chance for renal function recovery.
- Patients with a mixed phenotype have an intermediate outcome profile.
- Patients with sclerotic ANCA-associated glomerulonephritis at the time of biopsy run the highest risk for not recovering renal function and also have a higher risk for death within the first year after diagnosis.

Following criteria and algorithm have been proposed that has been validated in terms of prediction of renal outcome.

Class	Inclusion criteria
Focal	>50% normal glomeruli
Crescentic	>50% glomeruli with cellular crescents
Sclerotic	>50% sclerosed glomeruli
Mixed	< 50% normal glomeruli, glomeruli with cellular crescents, and sclerosed glomeruli

Inclusion Criteria

Pauci-immune staining pattern on immunofluorescence microscopy and ≥ 1 glomerulus with necrotizing or crescentic glomerulonephritis on LM are required for inclusion in all four classes.

Exclusion Criteria

- A coarse granular staining with positivity for mesangial IgA has been described in a small number of patients with ANCA-associated glomerulonephritis. This staining pattern was not an exclusion criterion for the current classification.
- This classification does not take into account patients with comorbid diseases or overlap syndromes, such as ANCA-associated glomerulonephritis in combination with anti-glomerular basement membrane (GBM) nephritis. Patients who are double-positive serologically for anti-GBM antibodies and ANCA (usually MPO-ANCA) and whose biopsies show distinct, intense linear staining for IgG are known to have a worse renal outcome that is defined by the anti-GBM nephritis component. Biopsies of these patients should not be classified according to this system.
- This exclusion criterion of comorbid disease also applies for all other renal diseases. ANCA-associated glomerulonephritis have also been described in combination with:
- Diabetic nephropathy

- Lupus nephritis
- Membranous glomerulonephritis.

Following algorithm to be followed:

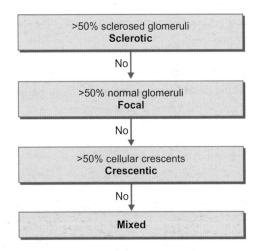

These glomeruli need to be defined by following definitions.

Normal Glomeruli

- A normal glomerulus should not show vasculitic lesions or global glomerulosclerosis. It also should not show endocapillary proliferation, extensive endothelial swelling, or proliferation in more than one capillary loop or more than four intracapillary inflammatory cells (neutrophils, lymphocytes, or monocytes) in all of the glomerular capillary bed.
- Normal glomeruli should not have synechiae or local/segmental sclerosis.
- Subtle signs of ischemia such as slight collapse of tuft, focal Bowman's capsule splitting, or focal wrinkling of the GBM or prominent parietal epithelium of Bowman's capsule may be seen in normal glomerulus.

Crescents

- Crescent with cellular components ≥10% is considered cellular crescent, irrespective of amount of fibrous component, segmental or circumferential involvement, presence of fibrin, periglomerular granulomatous reaction, breaks in Bowman's capsule. Presence of glomerular fibrinoid necrosis is not important for this classification.
- Segmental and circumferential crescents show extracapillary proliferation in ≤50% and ≥50% of the circumference of Bowman's space respectively.
- Fibrous crescents have >90% extracellular matrix.

Global Glomerulosclerosis

Global glomerulosclerosis is considered when sclerosis is in ≥ 80% of the tuft irrespective of etiopathogenesis of sclerosis.

This classification takes into account only the glomerular lesions. Tubulointerstitial changes may also be of prognostic value in ANCA-associated vasculitis. They should be mentioned when they are unusual such as:

- Dominance of any cell type in the infiltrate (plasma cells or eosinophils)
- A high number of interstitial granulomas
- Extensive arteriosclerosis.

These findings may have clinical importance or be clue to differential diagnosis of other diseases, such as drug hypersensitivity, infection, or cardiovascular disease.

Immune Complex Small Vessel Vasculitis (Figs 10.4 and 10.5)

Immune complex SVV is vasculitis with moderate-to-marked deposition of immunoglobulins and/or complement in the vessel wall, predominantly, affecting small vessels (i.e. capillaries, venules, arterioles, and small arteries).

- Glomerulonephritis is frequent.
- Arterial involvement is much less common in immune complex SVV compared to ANCA SVV.

It can be categorized as a vasculitis associated with probable etiologies depending on clinical and other relevant diagnostic tests, e.g.

- Anti-glomerular basement membrane (anti-GBM) disease
- Hepatitis C virus-associated cryoglobulinemic vasculitis
- Vasculitis-associated with systemic disease
- Lupus vasculitis
- Rheumatoid vasculitis.

Anti-glomerular Basement Membrane Disease

Anti-glomerular basement membrane disease (Anti-GBM) disease is a SVV-restricted to glomerular capillaries, pulmonary capillaries, or both that manifests as glomerulonephritis with fibrinoid necrosis with or without crescents and pulmonary hemorrhages with basement membrane deposition of antibasement membrane autoantibodies.

This immune-mediated glomerulonephritis is different as here there is *in situ* formation of immune complexes composed of autoantibodies bound to basement membrane

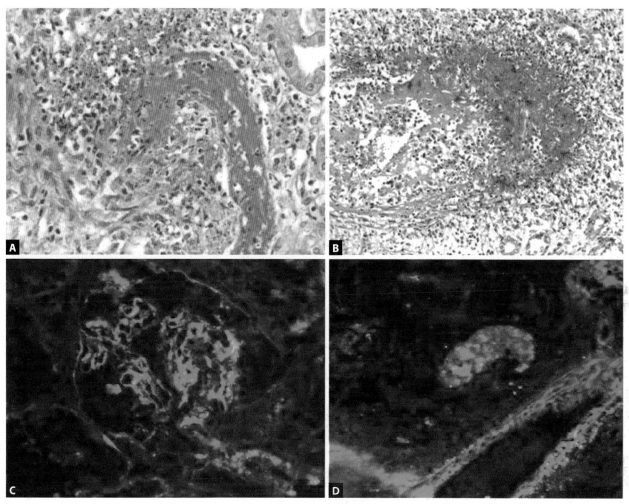

Figs 10.4A to D Noninflammatory immune-mediated necrotizing vasculitis. Photomicrographs show (A) fibrinoid necrosis of a small artery that was confirmed by (B) red-stained fibrin deposition in arterial wall, (C) IgG, and (D) fibrin was co-deposited in these areas of necrosis in arterioles and arteries in addition to full-house mesangial deposits of immunoglobulins and compliments (H&E—A, MSB—B, immunofluorescence IgG–C, fibrin—D, ×40—A–D original magnification). Noninflammatory immune-mediated necrotizing vasculitis in lupus nephritis class II

in glomerular and pulmonary alveolar capillaries. The pulmonary hemorrhages often lack overt leukocyte infiltration.

Pathology of Anti-GBM Disease[7]

Gross

Kidneys in case with severe disease are enlarged with flea-bitten appearance. No infracts are likely to be there.

Light Microscopy

Glomeruli

Histopathological examination shows segmental glomerular fibrinoid necrosis and crescent formation:

- Glomeruli with crescents can show little or no change to extensive necrotizing destruction of the tuft.
- Unlike other forms of immune complex crescentic glomerulonephritis, the intact capillary walls in anti-GBM glomerulonephritis have normal thickness. Normal glomeruli or glomerular segments indicate presence of anti-GBM or ANCA-related glomerulonephritis, whereas in immune complex crescentic glomerulonephritis there is marked hypercellularity and thickening of capillary walls in the intact tufts.
- More than 90% of anti-GBM disease has some degree of crescent formation. About three quarter of glomeruli have crescents, which is in general more than that seen in AAV.
- Biopsy without crescents has mild focal segmental fibrinoid necrosis.

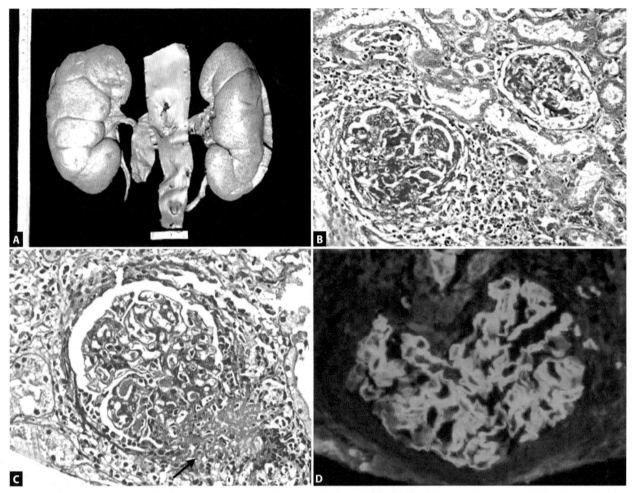

Figs 10.5A to D Antiglomerular basement membrane (anti-GBM) glomerulonephritis. Photographs show (A) Flea-bitten kidney and no infarcts. (B) Focal and global fibrinoid necrosis of glomerular tuft with circumferential crescent in one with granulomatous glomerulitis. (C) Segmental fibrinoid necrosis of glomerular tuft that extends to hilar afferent arteriole that can be seen in anti-GBM glomerulonephritis. (D) Linear staining of glomerular basement membrane with breaks and crescent (H&E, PAS, Masson's trichrome, EVG, immunofluorescence, ×40 original magnification). Absence of endocapillary hypercellularity or capillary wall thickening in adjacent tuft makes immune complex-mediated glomerulonephritis less likely. Presence of vasculitis at glomerular hilum is permissible in anti-GBM, but presence of non-hilar vasculitis should raise suspicion of coexisting antineutrophil cytoplasmic antibody-associated vasculitis

- Normal glomerulus but linear staining on IF can be seen with dominant pulmonary symptoms.
- Crescents can have multinucleated giant cells and a granulomatous appearance.
- Extensive fibrinoid necrosis, focal destruction of Bowman's capsule, and disordered crescents are features common to both anti-GBM glomerulonephritis and ANCA glomerulonephritis. Immune complex crescentic glomerulonephritis usually has minimal or no fibrinoid necrosis, more orderly crescents, and intact Bowman's capsules.
- Periglomerular interstitial inflammation includes multinucleated giant cells may accompany severe glomerular injury, with disruption of Bowman's capsule.

- Acute lesions progress to sclerosis. Sclerotic lesions and necrotizing lesions may be present in same biopsy although anti-GBM glomerulonephritis more often has synchronous lesions that are predominantly acute or predominantly chronic compared to ANCA glomerulonephritis that more often has a mixture of acute and chronic lesions. This is in accord with the natural history of anti-GBM disease that is characterized as one episode that rarely recurs versus the remitting and relapsing course of ANCA disease.

Tubules

Tubules are normal or show features of mild acute kidney injury in the form of flattening. There is accompanying edema in severe cases. Interstitial fibrosis replaces the edema in later stages.

Interstitium

- Variable tubulointerstitial inflammation composed of mixed inflammatory cells (neutrophils, eosinophils, lymphocytes, monocytes, and macrophages) can be seen depending upon severity, activity, and chronicity of the glomerular disease.
- Occasional interstitial multinucleated giant cells may be seen.
- Extensive disruption of Bowman's capsule with accentuated periglomerular inflammation may be seen. It may be granulomatous inflammation.

Blood Vessels

Glomerular fibrinoid necrosis and inflammation can extend into proximal part of contiguous hilar arterioles. Presence of necrotizing arteriolitis, necrotizing arteritis, and leukocytoclastic medullary angiitis in biopsy in areas other than glomerular hilum should raise suspicion of existence of ANCA-associated vasculitis, which may be present in about one-third of cases.

Immunofluorescence

Global and diffuse linear staining of glomerular basement membranes in all cases irrespective of degree of fibrinoid glomerular necrosis or crescents. IgG is almost always the dominant immunoglobulin although there may be staining for IgA and IgM. There are very rare cases with IgA-dominant anti-GBM antibodies. Granular or discontinuous linear staining for C3 is common.

Some cases do have similar linear staining around distal tubular basement membranes.

Electron Microscopy

No changes in GBM or mesangium are seen in anti-GBM disease other than focal breaks in the GBM.

IgA Vasculitis (Henoch-Schönlein) (Figs 10.6A to D)

IgA vasculitis (IgAV) is vasculitis with IgA1-dominant immune deposits, affecting small vessels (predominantly capillaries, venules, or arterioles).

- IgA vasculitis often involves the skin and gastrointestinal tract, and frequently causes arthritis.
- Small bowel is most commonly involved, though any part of gastrointestinal tract may be involved.
- Glomerulonephritis indistinguishable from IgA nephropathy may occur.
- There can be single-organ IgAV such as renal-limited IgAN or cutaneous IgAV. They may subsequently develop systemic IgAV.
- Onset of symptomatic IgAV is often associated with episodes of an upper respiratory tract or gastrointestinal infection.
- IgA vasculitis can be seen with other diseases, such as liver disease, inflammatory bowel disease, and ankylosing spondylitis.

Cryoglobulinemic Vasculitis

Cryoglobulinemic vasculitis (CV) is a vasculitis characterized by deposition of cryoglobulin immune deposits in small vessels (predominantly capillaries, venules, or arterioles) and is associated with serum cryoglobulins.

It has predilection for:
- Skin
- Glomeruli
- Peripheral nerves

It should be further classified with prefix as:
- Idiopathic or essential to indicate unknown etiology
- Hepatitis C-associated CV—according to known etiology

MEDIUM-VESSEL VASCULITIS

Vasculitis predominantly affecting medium arteries, i.e., the main visceral arteries and their branches is MVV. However, arteries of any size may be affected.

It has two main variants:
1. Polyarteritis nodosa
2. Kawasaki disease (KD)

At the onset, MVV has more acute and necrotizing inflammation compared to rather chronic and granulomatous inflammation in LVV.

Polyarteritis Nodosa (Figs 10.7A to D)

Polyarteritis nodosa is a necrotizing arteritis of medium or small arteries.

- Glomerulonephritis or vasculitis in arterioles, capillaries, or venules is absent by definition.

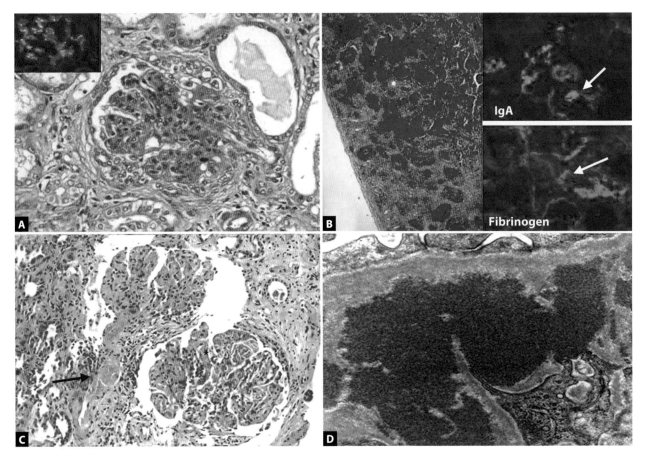

Figs 10.6A to D Immune complex glomerulonephritis and vasculitis. Photomicrographs show (A) Proliferative glomerulonephritis with crescent and IgA-dominant deposits (inset)—IgA nephropathy. (B) This patient had massive pulmonary hemorrhages with IgA-dominant immune complex vasculitis with fibrin in alveolar capillaries —IgA vasculitis. (C) Membranoproliferative glomerulonephritis (MPGN) with hyaline thrombi (asterisks) and fibrinoid necrosis of arterioles in patient with cryoglobulinemia. (D) Immune complex deposits showed short microtubular structures confirming cryoglobulins (H&E—A–C, immunofluorescence—A, B, uranyl acetate—D, ×40A–C—original magnification, d—80,000). IgA nephritis with crescents and IgA vasculitis in lungs resulted in massive pulmonary hemorrhage, which is very rare in IgA vasculitis. Vasculitis and hyaline thrombi in MPGN should raise suspicion of cryoglobulemic MPGN and vasculitis. Serology and EM can confirm the diagnosis

- It is not associated with ANCA.
- PAN and ANCA-associated vasculitis can exhibit clinically and pathologically indistinguishable necrotizing arteritis of medium and small arteries. Antineutrophil cytoplasmic antibodies status and absence of glomerulonephritis is an important discriminating feature in such scenario.

Gross Pathology[3]

The most common organs showing gross lesions are:
- Kidneys
- Gastrointestinal tract
- Heart

Arterial pseudoaneurysms with complicating thrombosis or rupture and resultant parenchymal infarction are common gross findings.

Lesions of different age are known to exist in the same organ.

Arteries of any caliber in the kidney can be affected and gross findings depend upon size of artery involved:
- Main renal artery is rarely involved.
- Interlobar and arcuate arteries are involved most often.
- Large and medium artery inflammation result in nodular inflammatory lesions and pseudoaneurysms those are grossly visible.
- Inflammation of small arteries (i.e. interlobular arteries) results in microscopic lesions.

Nodules are palpable grossly and longitudinal or oblique sections bring out the relationship with arteries better than cross-sections through the pseudoaneurysm.
- Nodular lesions have predilection for points of arterial bifurcation. Hence, observed most often at the

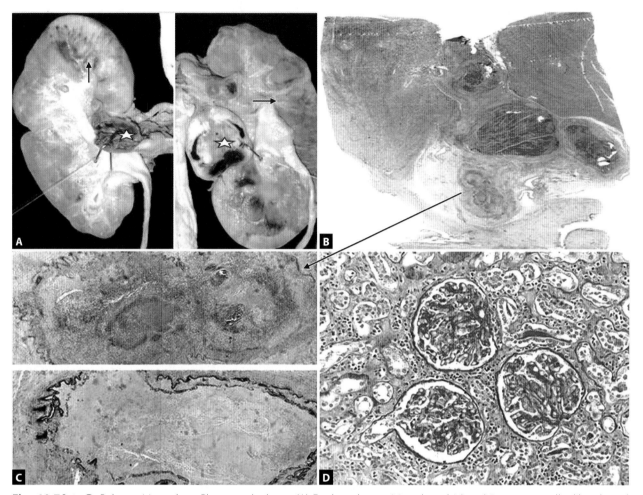

Figs 10.7A to D Polyarteritis nodosa. Photograph shows (A) Fresh and organizing thrombi (stars) in aneurysmally dilated renal arteries at hilum resulting in renal infarcts (arrows). (B) Renal arteries (interlobar and arcuate) with segmental fibrinoid necrosis and inflammatory arteritis with superimposed fresh PAS positive thrombi and sclerosing arteritis with organizing thrombi. (C) Broken elastic lamina and inflammation are evidence of past vasculitis with fibrinoid necrosis. (D) Absence of glomerulonephritis favors diagnosis of PAN (PAS—B–D, EVG—C, scanner view—B, ×20—D, C ×40 original magnification). Segmental arteritis with acute and sclerosing arteritis with thrombi of different ages and absence of glomerulonephritis favor diagnosis of PAN. Arteritis of this caliber artery and aneurysm could be seen in antineutrophil cytoplasmic antibody (ANCA)-associated vasculitis (AAV) also, although AAV preferentially affects interlobular arteries. Absence of glomerulonephritis and negative ANCA serology favors former

corticomedullary junction and in the renal sinus adjacent to the columns of Bertin (i.e. arcuate and interlobar arteries).

- Infarcts are wedge-shaped; color of infarct and border depends upon the age of infarct.
- Color of lesion is determined by nature of inflammation.
- Fibrinoid necrosis and leukocyte infiltration are pale.
- Aneurysms, especially when they contain thrombi, are dark red.
- Thrombosed arteries without pseudoaneurysm are better palpated.
- Rupture of a renal aneurysms results in retroperitoneal hematoma or hemorrhagic ascitis.

Light Microscopy

Microscopic findings follow two dictums:
1. Segmental arterial involvement.
2. Inflammation and necrosis of different ages coexist, i.e.
   - An acute necrotizing phase,
   - A chronic sclerotic phase.

Lesions of different ages may be observed simultaneously in the same artery and different arteries. Acute lesions have fibrinoid necrosis and acute inflammations in sclerotic phase replaced by chronic inflammation and fibroplasia, and organize as varying degrees of vascular sclerosis and ectasia.

There is fibrinoid necrosis and infiltration of predominantly neutrophils with varying numbers of eosinophils initially confined to the inner parts of the arterial wall, which later become transmural with perivascular extension. This centrifugal spread from within to perivascular adventia is classic.

Destruction of internal elastic lamina results in ectasia and pseudoaneurysm formation. Break in internal elastic lamina indicates the presence vascuilitis in the past.

Thrombi can get recanalized, because lesions are segmental careful grossing and sections at multiple levels are important.

Renal parenchymal injury is in the form of wedge-shaped infarcts with coagulative necrosis replacing renal parenchyma. Infarcts are bordered by neutrophils during initial stages. They result in depressed fibrous scars. Glomeruli at periphery of infracts can have collapse-like morphology with crown of podocytes that should not be considered crescent formation.

Adjacent parenchyma shows evidence of acute kidney injury with simplified tubular epithelium that later can be seen as ischemic wrinkled areas of tubular atrophy and fibrosis.

Presence of Glomerulonephritis Excludes Diagnosis of PAN

Immunofluorescence and Electron Microscopy

Immunofluorescence microscopy and electron microscopy typically do not reveal evidence of vascular immune complex deposition.

Differential Diagnosis

A major clinical differential diagnostic consideration is between PAN and MPA.
- Overt clinical evidence for glomerulonephritis or a positive ANCA, either of that essentially rules out PAN.
- Extensive pulmonary hemorrhage caused by capillaritis rules out PAN.
- Polyarteritis nodosa typically has extensive fibrinoid material, whereas the acute lesions of kawasaki disease (KD) have lesser amounts of fibrinoid material and more edema.

Kawasaki Disease

- Kawasaki disease presents as mucocutaneous lymph node syndrome usually in infants and young children.
- Associated with arteritis predominantly affecting medium and small arteries.

- Coronary arteries are often involved.
- Aorta and large arteries may be involved.

Clinically, significant renal disease in KD is rare. Postmortem studies have shown that inflammatory lesions in renal arteries are seen in one-fourth to three-fourths of patients. The difference in frequency of renal involvement pathologically may be a result of different sampling times because the frequency of the acute visceral vasculitis lesions of KD peaks during the first week of the illness and is markedly reduced after one month. Glomerulonephritis and hemolytic-uremic syndrome have been reported in KD, but are rare. Renovascular hypertension caused by postvasculitic stenosis of the renal artery is a rare renal complication.

Pathology of Kawasaki Disease[3] (Figs 10.8 and 10.9)

Gross

- The arteritis of KD affects small- and medium-sized arteries and it has a predilection for the coronary arteries followed by renal arteries.
- Pseudoaneurysms and thrombosis may occur. Thrombosis of inflamed coronary arteries in patients with KD is the most common cause of childhood myocardial infarction.
- Frequencies of renal artery involvement are as follows:
  - Interlobar arteries
  - Occasionally affect main renal and arcuate arteries
  - Only rarely involve interlobular arteries
- Sections of renal sinus are very important.

Light Microscopy

- Acute arteritis of KD is a necrotizing process, but it typically has less conspicuous fibrinoid change and more edema than PAN.
- Inflammatory changes are most pronounced in the intima and media to begin with resulting in thickened intima by infiltrating leukocytes.
- Media shows edema, vacuolization of myocytes, disassociation of myocytes, and focal rupture of the internal elastic lamina.
- Even in acute phase has mixture of neutrophils, monocytes, and macrophages.
- Arteritis spreads centrifugally into media to become transmural in some segments with necrosis and extensive disruption of elastic laminae in the most severely inflamed areas. Pseudoaneurysm formation ensues.
- Thrombosis may occur at sites of arteritis, resulting in distal ischemia.

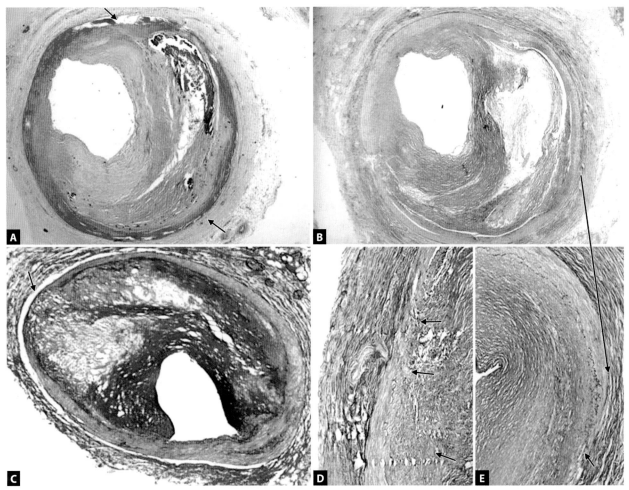

Figs 10.8A to E Chronic Kawasaki disease in coronary arteries. Photomicrographs show coronary arteries of young female (21 years old) with hypertension and breathlessness since age of 12. (A) Intimal thickening with calcification and segmental thinning of media with ectasia (arrows), (B and C) vascular ectasia at the point of thinning of media, and (D and E) Broken internal lamina (arrows) indicating past vasculitis (H&E–A, EVG—B–E, A–C×20, D–E×40 original magnification). Medium-vessel vasculitis in coronary arteries (medium size arteries) in chronic phase in young patient with hypertension and no atherosclerotic disease is consistent with Kawasaki disease and her renal arteries at hilum were examined (see Fig. 10.9)

Renal parenchymal injury as renal infarct is rare; myocardial infarction is a common complication of KD coronary arteritis.

Secondary ischemic and hypertensive changes in renal parenchyma may be seen.

LARGE-VESSEL VASCULITIS

Large-vessel vasculitis affects large arteries more often than do other vasculitides. Two major variants are:
1. Takayasu arteritis (TAK)
2. Giant cell arteritis (GCA)

No large vessels are inside organs including muscles, nerves, kidney, and skin. Large-vessel vasculitis affects large arteries much more often than does vasculitis of any other category, but LVV also involves medium and small vessels, and thus can affect arteries within the viscera, including arteries in the kidney.

Involvement of smaller branches of arteries (especially, medium arteries) may be the cause of most symptoms in patients with LVV. For example, large artery injury may not be the cause of lower backache that causes significant morbidity, but rather injury to smaller branches of the spinal arteries causes this problem.

The histopathological features of TAK and GCA are indistinguishable. Primarily because there are no specific biomarkers for TAK and GCA, it is not possible to know if any or all examples of single-organ LVV (e.g. aortitis) are limited expressions of TAK or GCA. Isolated aortitis can also be

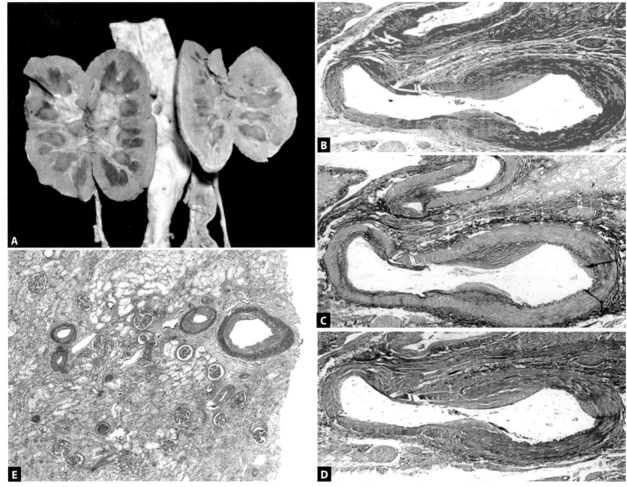

Figs 10.9A to E Chronic Kawasaki disease in renal arteries. Photographs of renal arteries at hilum of suspected Kawasaki disease because of coronary artery arteritis with ectasia (see Fig.10.8) shows (A) normal cortex and congested medulla and absence of atherosclerotic changes in aorta. (B to D) Ectatic renal artery at renal hilum with segmental intimal fibrous thickening with loss of underlying elastic lamina and adjacent media with mild segmental fibrosis. (E) Smaller intraparenchymal arteries showed only hypertensive changes with severe concentric intimal fibrosis (H&E—B, EVG—C, Masson's trichrome—D, PAS—E, ×40—B–D, ×10—E original magnification). Young female (21 years old) with hypertension and breathlessness since age of 12 was worked up extensively during life for causes of secondary hypertension and all caused were negative. Autopsy confirmed presence of chronic vasculitis with ectasia in medium-sized arteries, i.e. coronaries and extra parenchymal renal arteries consistent with the sclerotic phase of Kawasaki disease. Coronary and renal angiograms should be performed in young patients with clinical suspicion of Kawasaki disease

associated with an infection (e.g. syphilis) or systemic disease. For example, some patients with IgG4-related systemic disease develop aortitis as the only vasculitic manifestation.

Takayasu Arteritis (Figs 10.10 to 10.14)

Gross Pathology [3]

Aortic segments can show any of these lesions:
- Segmental stenosis (80% of patients),
- Dilatation without overt aneurysm (60%),
- Aneurysm (20%),
- Dissection (10%).

The abdominal aorta is the most common segment of the aorta involved especially in Indian series. Arteries affected by TAK typically have segments with thickened, firm walls, and narrowed lumen. Occasionally, the lumen may be completely obliterated, usually by firm pale fibrous material rather than acute thrombus.

Renal artery ostia may be obliterated resulting hypertensive arterionephrosclerotic changes.

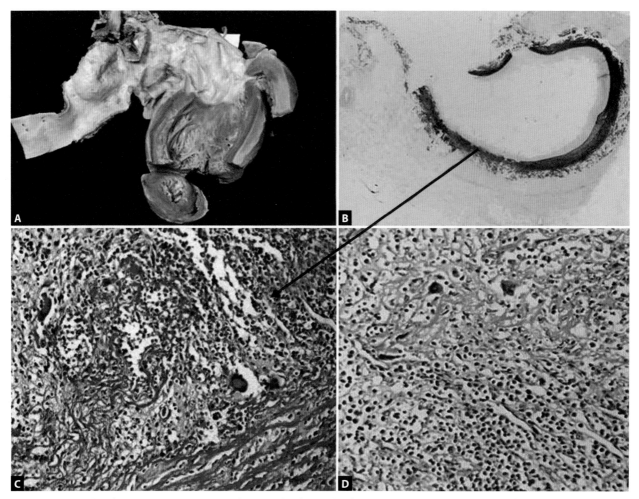

Figs 10.10A to D Takayasu arteritis (aortitis). Photographs show (A) Takayasu arteritis with aneurysmal dilatation of arch of aorta. (B) Moth eaten appearance of medial-adventitial junction (which is main site of inflammation) and adventitial widening and secondary intimal thickening. (C) Granulomatous inflammation with giant cells in relation to broken elastic fibers. (D) Giant cells adjacent to fragmented elastic fibers along with mononuclear leukocytes response (EVG—B, H&E—C, D, ×40—C, ×20—D original magnification). Takayasu arteritis shows granulomatous reaction that may be initiated by degenerating elastic tissue engulfed by giant cells predominantly at the junction of media-adventitia resulting in loss of medial elastic tissue and medial and adventitial fibrosis. Secondary involvement of intimal is common.

Light Microscopy

- Takayasu arteritis is a panarteritis.
- There is granulomatous inflammation in relation to adventitia and media with giant cells having phagocytozed elastic tissue. In acute phase, collections of neutrophils are also seen that are replaced by mononuclear cells over the time.

There is chronic inflammation around vasa vasorum with resultant destruction of elastic tissue in media resulting in moth-eaten appearance.

Renal parenchyma shows evidence of nephrosclerosis or, rarely, malignant hypertensive nephropathy.

Takayasu arteritis has caused persistent renal artery stenosis resulting in ischemic atrophy characterized by:
- Crowding of normal glomeruli
- Endocrinization of tubules
- No/minimal interstitial inflammation/fibrosis.

Giant Cell Arteritis

Giant cell arteritis is the arteritis, often granulomatous and usually affecting the aorta and/or its major branches, with a predilection for the branches of the carotid and vertebral arteries.

Giant cells are frequently but not always observed in biopsy specimens from patients with active GCA.

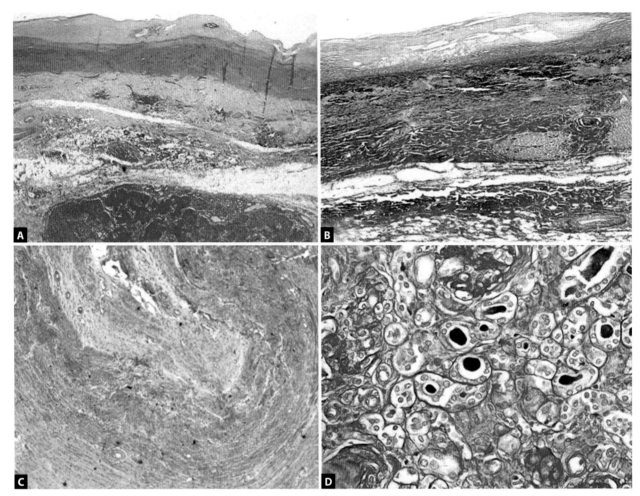

Figs 10.11A to D Takayasu arteritis. Photomicrographs show (A) Adventitial inflammation and fibrosis that extends to media and intima with secondary intimal fibrosis with calcification, (B) Moth-eaten appearance of media due to loss of elastic fibers and adventitial thickening, (C) Renal artery in this case showed renal artery stenosis with similar fibrosis in adventitia and intima resulting in (D) Endocrinization of tubules in renal cortex (H&E—A, EVG—B, Masson's trichrome—C, PAS—D, 10—A, ×20—B, ×40—C–D original magnification). In Takayasu arteritis, adventitial inflammation and fibrosis are seen in all cases. Intimal fibrosis thickening and fibrosis are common. Renal artery stenosis causes chronic ischemia with endocrinization of cortical tubules, which reduces the distance between glomeruli

Involvement of intrarenal arteries by GCA has been documented in autopsies. None of them had glomerulonephritis. None had clinical manifestations of renal dysfunction.

Microscopic hematuria with dysmorphic red blood cells in 48% of 42 patients with GCA has been documented. None of the patients with hematuria had hypertension, renal insufficiency, or significant proteinuria, and only one had red blood cell casts. The lack of accompanying proteinuria and red blood cell casts indicates that the hematuria is caused directly by the arteritis rather than by glomerulonephritis.

KEY POINTS

- Renal biopsy helps in diagnosis of renal limited and systemic vasculitis.
- Glomerular morphology gives vital clues for diagnosing small-vessel vasculitis (SVV).
- Immunofluorescence findings in the glomeruli and arteries have an important role to play in interpretation of morphological changes. Renal pathology also has an important role in predicting the prognosis.

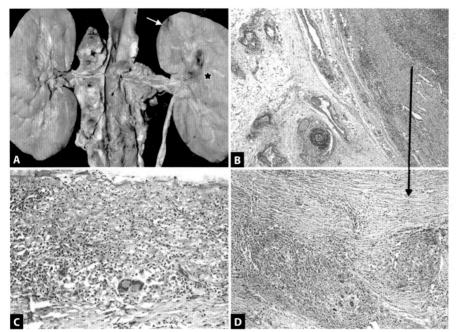

Figs 10.12A to D Takayasu arteritis with renal arteritis and thrombosis resulting in renal infarct. Photographs of case of Takayasu arteritis show (A) Infrarenal aortic aneurysmal dilatation with thrombosed renal artery (asterisk) at hilum with renal infarct (arrow), (B) Adventitia shows hyperplastic vasa vasorum and periadventitial inflammation, (C) Lymphomononuclear inflammation with giant cells in the media, and (D) Granulomatous response with giant cells in the adventitia (H&E—B–D, ×10—B, ×40—C, ×20—D original magnification). In Takayasu arteritis, vasa vasorum is hyperplastic with occlusion resulting in medial fibrosis. Granulomatous inflammation can be present all the layers of artery. Renal artery is shown in Figure 10.13

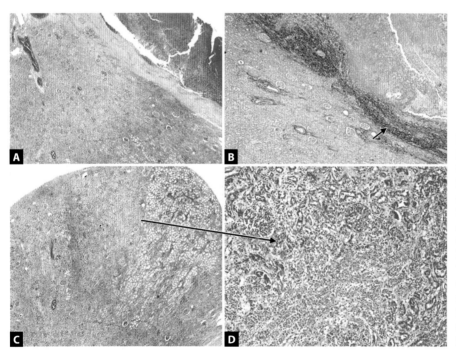

Figs 10.13A to D Takayasu aortitis with healed arteritis of renal artery with ostial thrombotic occlusion resulting in renal infarct. Photomicrographs show (A) Renal artery with thrombus, (B) Loss of elastic tissue indicating healed vasculitis, (C and D) Arterial occlusion resulting in renal infarct (H&E—A, C, D, EVG—B, ×10—A, D, × 20—B–D original magnification). In this case of Takayasu arteritis, changes of inflammation extended to medium-sized artery with overlying thrombosis resulting in renal infarct. In large-vessel vasculitis, changes in any caliber arteries may be seen and result in dominant presenting feature

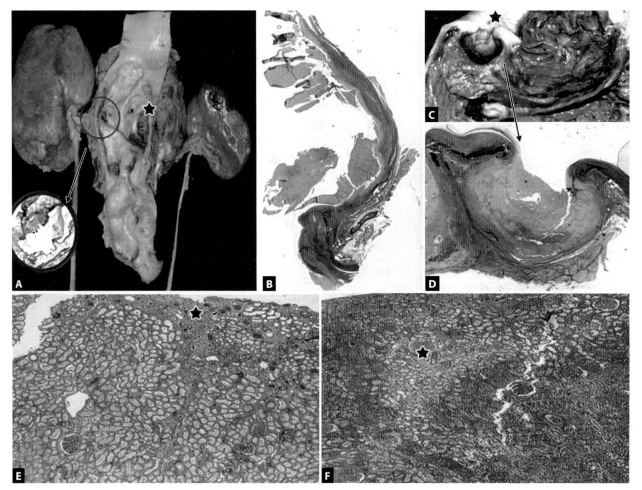

Figs 10.14A to F Takayasu aortitis without renal arteritis can produce embolic renal infarcts. Photographs show (A) complicated abdominal Takayasu aortitis with diffuse aneurysmal dilatation having occluded lumina and normal left kidney (confirmed organized thrombus—inset) with arterionephrosclerotic subcapsular scars (asterisk). (E) Fresh thrombotic occlusion of right aneurysmally dilated renal artery ostia. (C, D, F) Embolic infarct (asterisk) in smaller right kidney. (B) Pseudoaneurysm with overlying thrombus in Takayasu arteritis (H&E—F, PAS—E, EVG—B–D, ×10—B, E, F, x20—D original magnification). In Takayasu arteritis, renal infarct can be embolic. Arterionephrosclerosis can be seen due to arteriosclerosis

REFERENCES

1. Jennette JC, Falk RJ, Bacon PA, et al. Revised International Chapel Hill Consensus (2012) Conference Nomenclature of vasculitides. Arthritis Rheum. 2013;65:1-11.
2. Jennette JC. Overview of the 2012 revised International Chapel Hill Consensus Conference nomenclature of vasculitides. Clin Exp Nephrol. 2013;17:603-6.
3. Jennette JC, Thomas DB. Pauci-immune and antineutrophil cytoplasmic autoantibody mediated crescentic glomerulonephritis and vasculitis. In: Jennette JC, Olson JL, Schwartz M (Eds). Hepinstall's Pathology of the Kidney, 6th edition. Lippincott Williams & Wilkins, Philadelphia. 2007. pp. 644-73.
4. Raissian Y, Nasr SH, Larsen CP, et al. Diagnosis of IgG4-related tubulointerstitial nephritis. J Am Soc Nephrol. 2011;22:1343-52.
5. Jennette JC. Nomenclature and classification of vasculitis: lessons learned from granulomatosis with polyangiitis (Wegener's granulomatosis). Clin Exp Immunol. 2011; 164:7-10.
6. Berden AE, Ferrario F, Hagen EC, et al. Histopathologic classification of ANCA-associated glomerulonephritis. J Am Soc Nephrol. 2010;21:1628-36.
7. Jennette JC, Nickeleit V. Anti-glomerular basement membrane glomerulonephritis and Goodpasture's syndrome. In: Jennette JC, Olson JL, Schwartz M (Eds). Hepinstall's Pathology of the Kidney, 6th edition. Lippincott Williams & Wilkins, Philadelphia. 2007. pp. 615-41.

CHAPTER 11

Pathology of Central Nervous System and Peripheral Nerves

BD Radotra, RK Vasishta

Central nervous system vasculitis is a heterogeneous group of disorders with varying and multiple etiologies, which may develop either as a primary condition or secondary to an underlying disease such as infection, collagen vascular disease, and malignancy.[1] It manifests as inflammation and/or necrosis involving blood vessels. The diverse and varying symptoms of CNS vasculitis are the cause for difficulty in making a correct clinical diagnosis. The pathologist also faces the same dilemma because the histology may be also quite variable and nonspecific. The important diagnostic modalities include imaging techniques such as conventional angiography or MR angiography. Brain biopsy may be required to confirm diagnosis in some cases.[2] Depending upon the disease suspected, it is important to sample a precise and accurate brain area for biopsy (usually tip of nondominant temporal lobe) for a definite diagnosis. Meningeal and superficial blood vessels should be included in biopsy particularly in collagen vascular disorders and primary angiitis of CNS.

Central nervous system vasculitis may also be classified on the basis of pathogenetic mechanisms such as cell-mediated, immune-complex-mediated, and ANCA-mediated inflammations, but basically the diseases covered in this classification are the same as given in Table 11.1.

NONINFECTIOUS CENTRAL NERVOUS SYSTEM VASCULITIDES

Takayasu's Arteritis

Also known as pulseless disease, Takayasu's arteritis (TA) generally affects aorta and its major branches in young Asian women of less than 50 years of age. The involvement of carotid and subclavian arteries is important from a neurologist or neuropathologist's point of view. A specific etiology is not known for TA. In India, an association of tuberculosis

Table 11.1 Classification of CNS vasculitis

Noninfectious type	Infectious type
Primary CNS involvement: • Takayasu's arteritis • Giant cell arteritis • PACNS • Kawasaki disease	Bacterial Viral Fungal
Manifestation of systemic disorder: • PAN • SLE • Wegener's granulomatosis • Behçet's syndrome	HIV-related
• Drug-related • Malignancy-related	

and granulomatous lesions in the vessel walls pointed to tuberculosis as an etiological factor. However, in our experience on our autopsy material we have not found any direct evidence.[3] The involved carotid arteries or subclavian artery appear rigid due to concentric thickening of the wall that results in severe luminal occlusion with sometimes superimposed thrombosis (Fig. 11.1). The reduced blood flow leads to ischemia and cerebral infarction (Figs 11.2A and B). Generally, intracranial arteries such as internal carotid artery and vertebral arteries do not reveal significant involvement. Histologically, TA shows inflammation of media with disruption of elastic tissue accompanied by secondary fibrosis (Fig. 11.3). Granulomatous inflammation with giant cells may be seen. In long-standing cases, there is splaying of the elastic tissue that extends into thickened adventitia. It should be remembered that histological changes are concentric and affect media and adventitia more than intima (Figs 11.4A and B). This is in contrast to atherosclerosis where eccentric plaques are located mainly in the intima. However, accelerated atherosclerosis may be seen in blood vessels affected by Takayasu's arteritis. In active lesions, lymphocytic

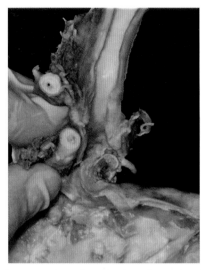

Fig. 11.1 Takayasu arteritis. The major branches arising from the arch of aorta show complete occlusion due to concentric fibrosis of the wall (arrow). The aorta shows severe atherosclerosis

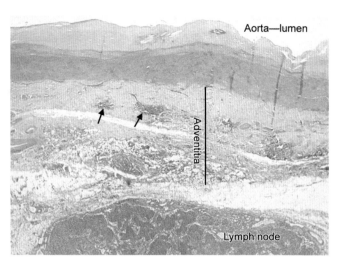

Fig. 11.3 Takayasu arteritis. Histology of the aorta shows intimal proliferation, medial, and adventitial fibrosis with perivascular lymphocytic infiltration of vasa vasorum (arrows). Periaortic lymph node with reactive hyperplasia is also seen

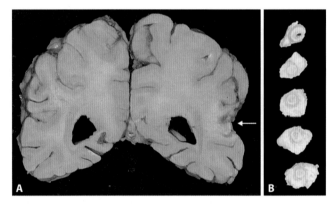

Figs 11.2A and B Takayasu arteritis. (A) This coronal slice of the brain shows an old healed infarct affecting the right parietal lobe with shrunken cerebral cortex (arrow) and collapsed meninges. The corresponding area on the left side reveals normal appearance of gray and white matter. The transverse cuts of neck arteries in the same case showed the complete narrowing of lumen (B)

infiltrate around vasa vasorum is common (Figs 11.4A and B). In chronic cases, fibrosis and thickening persists and the arteries may show dilatation.

Giant Cell Arteritis

Temporal arteritis is perhaps a common form of vasculitis in neurological practice but pathologists in India do not see it quite often. Perhaps it is a systemic vasculitis but the disease mainly affects large- and medium-size extracranial arteries of head and neck. The intracranial arteries are most often spared. Involvement of superficial temporal and ophthalmic arteries is well known. Since the intracranial arteries are not affected, the stroke or transient ischemic attack is rare manifestation. The characteristic clinical features are localized, sharp aching, and throbbing headache, thickened temporal artery with tenderness and claudication of muscles of mastication. Visual symptoms may be seen. The morbidity is mostly associated with involvement of the ophthalmic artery with ischemic retinal injury and blindness.

Histology: The temporal artery is most often biopsied since it is easy to obtain it. Grossly, temporal artery becomes thick, tortuous, and tender with reduced pulsations. The chosen abnormal segments provide the best diagnostic yield. The lesions are focal and segmental [like polyarteritis nodosa (PAN) and hence need for serial sections] and hence it is advised that a long segment should be sampled. A negative biopsy does not exclude the disease. The classic histology is a mixed infiltrate of neutrophils and lymphocytes in the intima and muscularis. Characteristically, the internal elastic lamina is fragmented and frayed (on elastic Van Gieson stain) that never returns to its normal architecture (Figs 11.5A and B). Multinucleated giant cells are often seen but are not essential. Older lesions show intimal thickening and fibrosis of the wall indicating an episode of previous injury [thus, Masson trichrome stain or immunohistochemistry for antismooth muscle (SMA) is useful]. In later stages due to fibrosis, there is blurring of distinction between media and adventitia. Rarely, fibrotic vessels may show aneurysmal dilatation. Sometimes thrombosis may be seen due to local injury. Giant cell arteritis may involve aorta and its major branches with a predilection of extracranial branches of carotid artery and it may be indistinguishable from Takayasu's arteritis, except for age (>50 years).

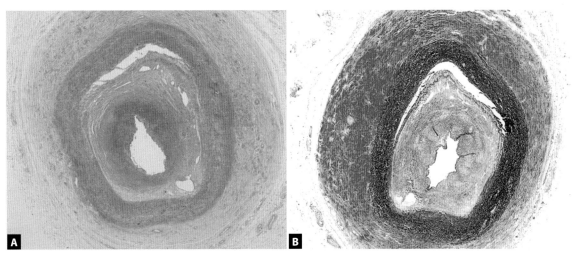

Figs 11.4A and B Takayasu arteritis. Marked fibrosis of the arterial wall and narrowing of lumen of a neck artery is seen. Note that the adventitial fibrosis is predominant

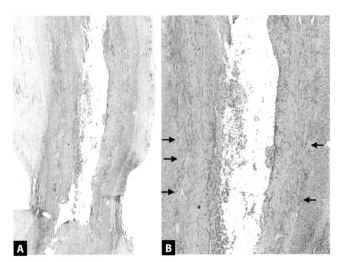

Figs 11.5A and B The longitudinal section of a temporal artery that shows fibrosis of the wall and fragmentation of internal elastic lamina (arrows)

PRIMARY ANGIITIS OF CENTRAL NERVOUS SYSTEM (PACNS)

This was also known as granulomatous angiitis of nervous system. It usually affects adults and presents with recurring headaches, multifocal neurological deficits, diffuse encephalopathy, and intracranial hemorrhage. Although angiographic findings in PACNS are nonspecific and mimic many other vasculitis, yet the affected vessels show narrowed segments of cerebral arteries. The diagnosis is usually confirmed on brain biopsy that should contain leptomeninges and superficial cortical tissue to provide enough number of blood vessels for histological examination. Many times such cases are picked up at autopsy after a massive ischemic or hemorrhagic cerebral event.[4,5] Since the disease is segmental, a negative biopsy does not exclude the diagnosis. Cerebral veins may also be affected in this disease. Usually, nondominant temporal lobe tip biopsy is advised. The blood vessels may show granulomatous or nongranulomatous inflammation affecting the walls. Multinucleate giant cells may be seen.

Polyarteritis Nodosa

It is a multisystem disease in which the classic presentation is vasculitic skin lesions, mononeuritis, and renal disease. The cranial involvement is not common; however, peripheral nervous system is commonly affected (50% patients) that manifests as mononeuritis multiplex. Therefore, sural nerve biopsies are commonly performed to diagnose PAN. Classically, PAN presents as necrotizing vasculitis of small- and medium-sized muscular arteries. An association with HBsAg is noted in 10–50% of cases. Polyarteritis nodosa shows segmental and multifocal lesions along the length of an affected artery.[6] Therefore, acutely inflamed necrotic segments may be seen adjacent to relatively normal segment of an artery. The lesions in PAN are of varying age. Early lesions show fibrinoid necrosis (Figs 11.6A and B) of the vessel wall with a mixed cellular infiltrate including neutrophils. Presence of neutrophils should be considered as a good indicator of the vasculitis being PAN. The older lesions show resolution of the inflammation with fibrosis (Figs 11.7A to D). Some pathologists prefer to do an immunostain using SMA antibody to demonstrate the loss of muscle fibers in tunica media of healed lesions. The nerve biopsy mostly demonstrates loss of myelinated nerve fibers by luxol fast blue/PAS stain as well as axonal loss on immunohistochemistry using antineurofilament protein antibody (Figs 11.8A to C). Because of segmental and multifocal involvement serial sections should always be done in a nerve biopsy sent for a diagnosis of PAN.

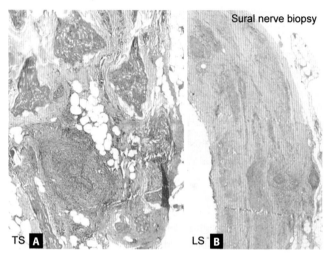

Figs 11.6A and B Sural nerve biopsy: Transverse cut (TS) of the nerve reveals a medium-sized artery affected by fibrinoid necrosis and mixed inflammation. Longitudinal section (LS) shows perineural fibrosis and multiple small arteries are inflamed

Cerebral involvement is rare in PAN whereas systemic involvement includes the vessel of the kidney, viscera, joints, and skin; and there is relative sparing of the lungs [contrary to common lung involvement in granulomatosis with polyangiitis (GPA) and eosinophilic GPA]. The cerebral involvement is characterized by ischemic events as well as intracranial hemorrhage secondary to cerebral aneurysms.[7] The cerebral arterial aneurysms are formed because the segmental arterial lesions heal by fibrosis and result into weakening of the vessel wall and such arteries show beaded appearance on angiography.

Eosinophilic Granulomatosis with Polyangiitis (Churg-Strauss Syndrome)

It is a syndrome of asthma, peripheral eosinophilia, and multiorgan vasculitis. It characteristically affects the lungs (like GPA, but unlike classic PAN) and CNS is rarely affected. Fibrinoid necrosis, eosinophil-rich granulomatous inflammation with multinucleated giant cells affects small- and medium-sized arteries, capillaries, and venules.

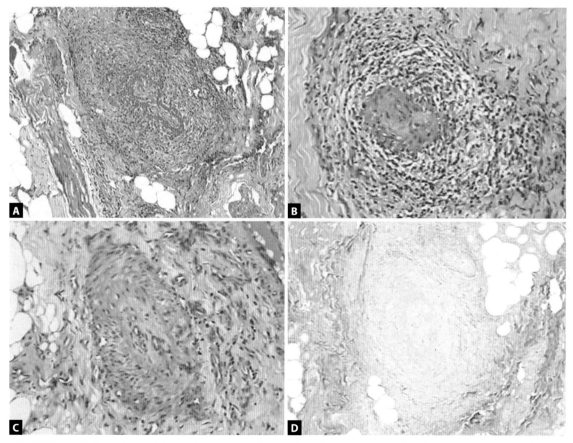

Figs 11.7A to D A sural nerve biopsy shows acute inflammation of entire arterial wall with fibrin deposition resulting in the loss of arterial wall architecture

that can mimic tuberculosis in any organ such as necrosis, granulomas, fibrosis, vasculitis, and infarction. Special stains are necessary to exclude one or the other.

Lymphomatoid Granulomatosis

Lymphomatoid granulomatosis typically affects lungs but it can involve CNS in 10–15% of patients. It is perhaps a controversial entity and some people consider it to be a variant of primary CNS (angiotropic) lymphoma. The brain shows small foci of necrosis that contain small blood vessels with transmural inflammation. Histology reveals angiocentric and angiodestructive polymorphous cellular infiltrate containing atypical lymphocytes. Sometimes patchy fibrinoid necrosis may be seen.

Vasculitis Associated with Collagen Vascular Disease

SLE Vasculitis

Vasculitis associated with systemic lupus erythematosus (SLE) can affect brain and cause acute neurological manifestations such as seizures, cerebrovascular accidents and delirium. Neuropsychiatric manifestations are known to occur in about 30–40% patients of SLE.[9] Being an autoimmune disease, it is characterized by hyperactivation of B- and T-lymphocytes resulting in the overproduction of autoantibodies, tissue deposition of immune complexes, and high levels of inflammatory cytokines, cumulatively resulting in a systemic proinflammatory state.[10,11] Sometimes, there may be no gross pathology, but small infarcts and hemorrhages can be identified (Figs 11.9A and B). Microinfarcts are commonly

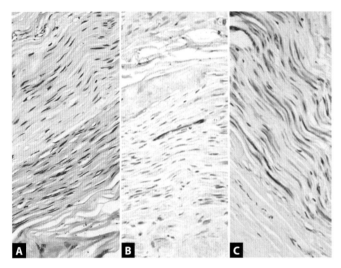

Figs 11.8A to C (A) The nerve biopsy shows loss of myelin; (B) immunostain for neurofilament protein shows loss of axons; and (C) shows a nerve containing normal axons in a sural nerve for comparison to (B)

Granulomatosis with Polyangiitis (Wegener Granulomatosis)

Granulomatosis with polyangiitis is known to affect CNS in 7–11% patients[8] and is associated with presence of c-ANCA in the serum. It is characterized by a necrotizing and granulomatous vasculitis that affects small arteries, veins, and capillaries. A distinctive triad of organ involvement: (1) ear, nose, and/or throat; (2) lung; and (3) kidney are characteristic. While the triad defines GPA, the disease is still a systemic necrotizing vasculitis involving many other organs. In Indian context, the disease produces lesions

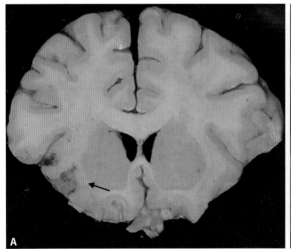
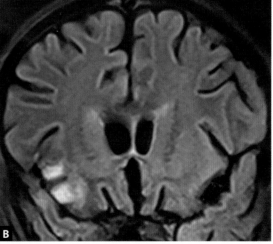

Figs 11.9A and B (A) A case of SLE shows small infarct with a hemorrhagic component in the left insular cortex; (B) The corresponding areas on neuroimaging show edema and hyperintensity

seen that result from vascular thrombi and small-vessel vasculitis (Figs 11.10A and B). In some cases, meningeal as well as parenchymal vessels may show organized thrombi with recanalization as a consequence of the organization (Figs 11.11A to D).

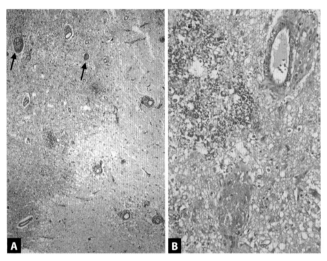

Figs 11.10A and B Histology of the brain (Fig. 11.9) shows vascular thrombi (arrow), pale infarct, and hemorrhages

CENTRAL NERVOUS SYSTEM VASCULITIS DUE TO INFECTIONS

Central nervous system angiitis may be a complication of many infections such as bacterial, viral, fungal, or rickettsial infection. Among viral infections, HIV-1, cytomegalovirus, and varicella zoster virus infections can be seen in AIDS patients. Bacterial infections such as syphilis and *Borrelia burgdorferi* are rarely seen. Among bacterial infections that complicates as CNS vasculitis tubercular meningitis (TBM) is the most important. This is followed by fungal vasculitis in our set-up. The infectious pathology can directly involve the vessels or it may be immunologically mediated.

- Vascular involvement in TBM is a well-known serious complication that results in significant morbidity and mortality. It may manifest as panarteritis, periarteritits, endothelitis, and/or necrosis.[12] These lesions may occur either in isolation or in different combinations. Necrotizing lesions may occur either as fibrinoid necrosis alone or in combination with spectrum of inflammatory infiltrate (Figs 11.12A to D). Proliferative lesions can be endarteritis obliterans due to fibrointimal proliferation with or without inflammatory infiltrate. In our experience, on autopsy

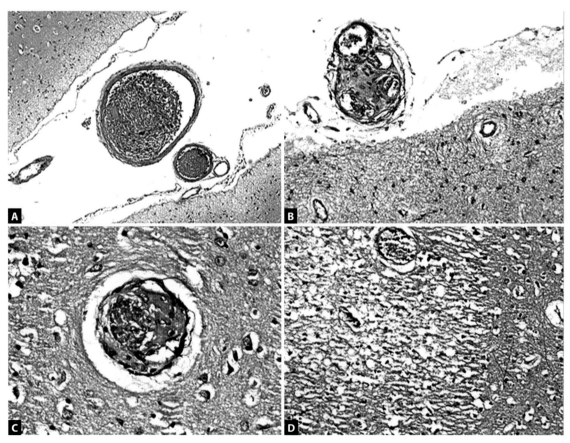

Figs 11.11A to D These photographs show fresh (A) and organized (B) thrombi in meningeal arteries. The parenchymal small blood vessel shows fibrin thrombus (C) and microinfarct (D)

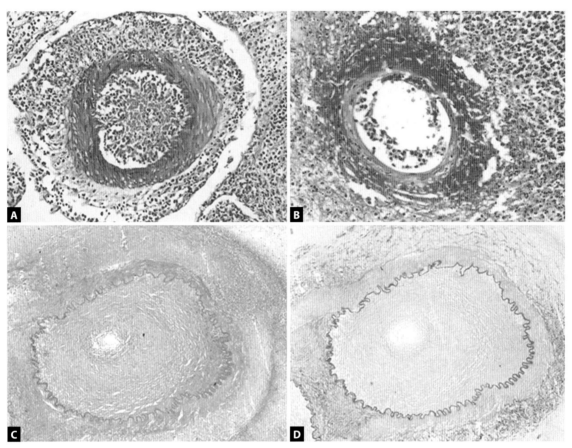

Figs 11.12A to D Tuberculous meningitis. (A) Panarteritis with inflammation involving all layers of the arterial wall; (B) Extensive fibrinoid necrosis of the vessel wall; (C) Severe occlusion of lumen of an artery due to fibrointimal proliferation; (D) Elastic Van Geison stain of (C)

cases, proliferative changes are more common in larger arteries whereas necrotizing lesions were predominant in arterioles and smaller arteries. Additionally, necrotizing lesions are more common in patients with acute, fulminant course whereas proliferative lesions were common in subacute cases. These vascular changes reduce cerebral perfusion and result in cerebral infarction, which may be large arterial infarcts or microscopic infarcts. Microscopic infarcts are commonly seen in brainstem in autopsy cases of TBM and these are not detected by imaging studies. Such changes may be a cause of significant mortality in many cases. The pathogenesis of vascular pathology in TBM is not clearly understood. It is speculated that the arterial inflammation starts from periarterial location because of direct effect of proinflammatory cytokines such as tumor necrosis factor-alpha and interleukins secreted by lymphocytes and macrophages. Tumor necrosis factor-alpha demonstrated in cerebrospinal fluid of TBM patients may induce vasculotoxicity due to its prothrombotic activity. Because of thick exudates in basal meninges and sylvian fissure, the small vessels that arise from middle cerebral artery and supply lentiform nuclei get encased in thick inflammation that explains why basal ganglia infarction is commonly in TBM.

- The angioinvasive fungi such as *aspergillus* and zygomecetes (mucor) commonly affect cerebral blood vessels in acute disseminated invasive fungal infections. We have experienced it commonly in our autopsy material. These fungi directly invade blood vessels of all sizes both in the meninges and parenchyma, and produce necrotizing vasculitis, thrombosis, and sometimes aneurysm formation (Figs 11.13A and B). Usually, there are no multinucleate giant cells or granulomatous reaction in such cases compared to chronic fungal granuloma that present as space occupying lesion of brain. The spectrum of histopatholocal changes includes infarcts, hemorrhage, necrosis, and a combination of all three. It is very easy-to-demonstrate presence of fungi in such lesions even without special stains as the number of fungi is numerous in the invaded vessel wall.

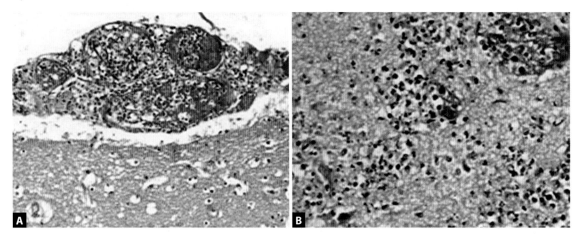

Figs 11.13A and B (A) The meningeal blood vessels show acute vasculitis, thrombosis, and numerous fungal profiles; (B) Acute necrotizing inflammation of the parenchyma with fibrin exudation

KEY POINTS

- CNS vasculitis constitutes a wide range of conditions characterized by inflammation of walls of vessels of the CNS.
- In isolated angiitis of the CNS, only vessels of the CNS are involved.
- Brain tissue biopsy helps in confirmation of the diagnosis and is considered to be the gold standard for diagnosis of isolated angiitis of CNS.

REFERENCES

1. West SG. Central nervous system vasculitis. Curr Rheumatol Rep. 2003;5:116-27.
2. Salvarani C, Brown RD Jr, Hunder GG. Adult primary central nervous system vasculitis. Lancet. 2012;380:767-77.
3. Sharma BK, Jain S, Radotra BD. An autopsy study of Takayasu arteritis in India. Int J Cardiol. 1998;66:S85-90.
4. Radotra BD, Chopra JS. Non-infectious granulomatous angiitis of central nervous system: an autopsy report. Indian J Pathol Microbiol. 1992;35:365-9.
5. Panda KM, Santosh V, Yasha TC, et al. Primary angiitis of CNS: neuropathological study of three autopsied cases with brief review of literature. Neurol India. 2000;48:149-54.
6. Vankalakunti M, Joshi K, Jain S, et al. Polyarteritis nodosa in hairy cell leukaemia: an autopsy report. J Clin Pathol. 2007;60:1181-2.
7. Sharma S, Kumar S, Mishra NK, et al. Cerebral miliary micro-aneurysms in polyarteritis nodosa: report of two cases. Neurol India. 2010;58:457-9.
8. Seror R, Mahr A, Ramanoelina J, et al. Central nervous system involvement in Wegener granulomatosis. Medicine (Baltimore). 2006;85:54-65.
9. Stock AD, Wen J, Putterman C. Neuropsychiatric lupus, the blood brain barrier, and the TWEAK/Fn14 Pathway. Front Immunol. 2013;4:484.
10. Ludovico Iannetti, Roberta Zito, Simone Bruschi, et al. Recent understanding on diagnosis and management of central nervous system vasculitis in children. Clin Dev Immunol. Hindawi Publishing Corporation; 2012;2012:1-9.
11. Fanouriakis A, Boumpas DT, Bertsias GK. Pathogenesis and treatment of CNS lupus. Curr Opin Rheumatol. 2013; 25:577-83.
12. Lammie GA, Hewlett RH, Schoeman JF, et al. Tuberculous cerebrovascular disease: a review. J Infect. 2009;59:156-66.

CHAPTER 12

Imaging in Vasculitis

Chirag Ahuja, NK Khandelwal

INTRODUCTION

Vasculitis, as the name suggests, is inflammation of the vessels. It is a relatively rare group of pathologies characterized by inflammation of the walls of the vessels. Vascular inflammation may lead to changes in the vascular morphology in the form of wall thickening, luminal narrowing, complete occlusion, and formation of aneurysms and pseudoaneurysms. Alternatively, it may lead to anatomical and physiological changes in the organ that are perfused by the diseased vessels. A yet another manifestation may be secondary to involvement of organs in nonperfused territory of the diseased vessel as a possible concomitant involvement of the organ system. The vasculitides are classified into the following categories (discussed elsewhere in the book) based on vessel involvement:[1] (a) large vessel, (b) medium vessel, (c) small vessel, (d) variable vessel, (e) vessels of single organ, and (f) vasculitis with systemic involvement.

Catheter angiography and currently digital subtraction angiography (DSA) form the gold-standard imaging technique for the diagnosis of vasculitis. Magnetic resonance imaging (MRI) and MR angiography (MRA) play a substantial role in the diagnostic algorithm of many vasculitides due to the noninvasive nature of the investigation and excellent soft tissue resolution capabilities. However, many a times, imaging only behaves as an adjunct, and the diagnosis requires a detailed clinical work-up including laboratory results in conjunction with appropriate angiographic data. With significant progress in medical technology over the last few decades, imaging has transformed the approach to medical disorders, so also vasculitis and has led to marked improvement in the detection, diagnosis, and management of diseases. The various imaging modalities currently in the diagnostic armamentarium of radiologists are ultrasonography (US), computed tomography (CT), MRI, and DSA. The former three, in addition to vascular imaging, have cross-sectional capability and are helpful for demonstrating end-organ effects and complications of the vasculitic process. Each modality is discussed in detail in the following section.

ULTRASONOGRAPHY

Ultrasonography employs high-frequency sound waves that are directed to the area of interest in human body. The image generation occurs from the echoes reflected by the tissues and their interfaces.[2] Image depiction occurs on a gray-scale with reasonably good anatomical details, especially in superficially located vessels. Vessel wall thickness and echogenicity of the diseased vessel can be evaluated. Intraluminal details regarding thrombosis, stenosis, and occlusion can be assessed. Dynamic evaluation of blood flow is also possible by duplex mode and color Doppler in form of quantitative assessment of blood velocities and flow waveforms including direction of flow. The advantages of US include easy and widespread availability, quick results, and low cost. However, there are some limitations of the technique such as operator dependency, dependence on a good acoustic window (which is absent in some obese patients and certain locations such as mediastinum), and relatively compromised reproducibility.

COMPUTED TOMOGRAPHY

Computed tomography employs the principle of image formation by X-ray attenuation during transmission through a slab of human body. The current generation CT scanners have evolved phenomenally leading to rapid data acquisition with greater scan coverage.[3] Its advantages include quick acquisition, widespread availability, multiplanar reconstructing capabilities with fine spatial resolution, and good parenchymal and intraluminal vascular details. The depiction of vessel wall calcifications and easy reproducibility of results are added advantages. Disadvantages include the risk of ionizing radiation, requirement of intravascular iodinated contrast (which may lead to allergic reactions in certain individuals and be harmful for already compromised kidneys). Nevertheless, CT gives precise details of the vessel lumen as well as end-organs that are being perfused by diseased arteries. Multiphasic acquisition may need to be performed, i.e. precontrast phase, arterial phase, parenchymal phase, and delayed phase depending on the information required. Currently, CT is the most common modality being used for vascular and parenchymal evaluations in suspected vasculitis.

MAGNETIC RESONANCE IMAGING

Magnetic resonance imaging employs magnetic properties of protons in the body tissues to create images. By using variable gradient field strength and direction, the protons are allowed to resonate at a frequency and direction that is dependent on applied field and its immediate environment. The basic MR sequences that were commonly used are T1- and T2-weighted sequences that though time consuming gave good tissue contrast. With significant advances in this field, faster and better quality images can be produced. Gadolinium-enhanced MR provides the enhancement pattern of pathologies, thus classifying them better. The evaluation of vasculitis by MR usually includes angiography, vessel wall imaging, and occasionally myocardial assessment. Magnetic resonance angiography can depict the intraluminal details exquisitely.[4] Advantages of MRI include excellent contrast resolution, multiplanar capabilities, and no use of ionizing radiation. Some disadvantages are limited availability, long examination time, contraindication in patients with pacemakers and other such implantable devices, and tubular examination chamber that may lead to claustrophobia in certain patients.

DIGITAL SUBTRACTION ANGIOGRAPHY

The principle of DSA involves attenuation of the X-ray beams by iodinated contrast that leads to formation of images. It involves selective contrast injection into the vessel of interest and its dynamic visualization as it passes across the desired territory that is captured by continuous sequential X-ray beams in the form of fluoroscopy.[5] Modern techniques use powerful image intensifiers with precise subtraction technology that depict exquisite details of the vessel of interest. Thus, DSA is the gold-standard technique for the evaluation

of vascular details, especially the intraluminal aspect. Its advantages include rapid image acquisition, excellent spatial resolution, dynamic evaluation of flowing blood and capability of interventional management, and treatment of diseases. Its disadvantages are radiation exposure, drawbacks of nephrotoxic iodinated contrast, and invasive nature of the investigation.

IMAGING: WHAT TO LOOK FOR?

Vasculitis primarily involves the blood vessels including the arteries and veins. Secondary involvement of the organ system can occur in the perfusion zones of these diseased vessels. There may sometimes be remote changes occurring elsewhere, distant to the territory of the involved vessel but falling into the continuum of the disease process. Thus, imaging requires demonstration of changes occurring at both vascular and parenchymal levels for optimal diagnosis. A detailed evaluation of the following aspects should be done.
- Clinical presentation including onset and progress
- Appropriate past and ancillary history
- Details of vessel involvement like the vessel order, pattern of involvement, mural and intraluminal changes
- Details of organ involvement including distribution of involvement and nature of changes.

Vessel involvement: Vascular assessment involves a number of aspects of which recognizing the order and pattern of vessels involved is an important one, which can narrow down the diagnostic possibilities based on revised Chapel Hill classification of vasculitides. Large-vessel involvement is seen in Takayasu's arteritis (TA) and giant cell arteritis (GCA), medium vessel in polyarteritis nodosa (PAN) and Kawasaki disease (KD), while small-vessel involvement is seen in antineutrophil cytoplasmic antibody (ANCA)-associated vasculitis (AAV) such as Wegener's granulomatosis and Churg–Strauss vasculitis, and immune complex small-vessel vasculitis (SVV) such as anti-glomerular basement membrane (anti-GBM) disease, cryoglobulinemic vasculitis, and IgA vasculitis (Henoch-Schönlein). Variable vessels are involved in Behçet's disease (BD) and Cogan's syndrome (CS). Intraluminal vascular evaluation can be done by angiographic methods such as DSA, CT, or MR angiography of which the former is the best, as discussed previously. Ultrasonography can be used in superficial vessels. The changes include luminal irregularity, stenosis (partial or complete), thrombotic occlusion, ectasia, dissection, and formation of aneurysms and pseudoaneurysms. Mural changes that can be seen are wall thickening, calcifications, wall thrombi, or hematomas. Apart from helping in reaching at a conclusive diagnosis, these changes also help in the follow-up of diseases in the form of judging treatment response and disease progression.

Parenchymal involvement: Secondary organ involvement can occur as a result of perfusion deficit or direct involvement when small vessels of the organ are affected. Many a times, parenchymal involvement gives an indirect indication toward small-vessel vasculitides, as direct visualization of small arteries is often beyond the scope of available imaging modalities. The various effects of small artery stenosis or occlusion are development of ischemic zones or infarcts. Mural changes of wall weakening can lead to localized or dissipated hemorrhage secondary to aneurysm rupture. Venous side occlusions may lead to congestive parenchymal changes with resultant venous ischemia. Indirect features may be in the form of parenchymal nodules and masses (lungs, liver), interstitial thickening (lungs), mesenteric ischemia (abdomen), etc., most of which occur secondary to perivascular inflammation. The concerned organs can be evaluated by cross-sectional imaging techniques, i.e., US, CT, or MRI. As a general rule, CT is good for evaluation of lungs and mediastinum as well as neck and abdomen. Ultrasonography can be employed in superficial structures such as neck including thyroid gland, extremities, scrotum, and abdomen. Magnetic resonance is useful in brain and certain abdominal organs. It is, however, prudent to consult a radiologist who can guide regarding what to choose from for best possible results.

LARGE-VESSEL VASCULITIS

Large-vessel vasculitis (LVV) predominantly affects large arteries, though medium-sized arteries can be involved too, e.g., predominant involvement of temporal and ophthalmic arteries is seen in GCA; however, there also occurs involvement of retinal and ciliary arteries. Two major types include TA and GCA.

Takayasu's Arteritis

Takayasu's arteritis is a LVV of unknown etiology that primarily affects the aorta and its branches. Pulmonary arteries may occasionally be involved. Though the precise etiology is still unknown, genetic predisposition is being increasingly recognized in many patients[6] and so are links with tuberculosis. The disease pathogenesis includes progressive inflammation of the outer media and adventitia of large-sized arteries. There is an initial acute or "active" phase of the illness with an inflammation and mural thickening of the vessels, which in due course leads to a stenotic phase (Figs 12.1A

to D) with progressive fibrosis, firm thickened arterial wall, consequent narrowing, pseudoaneurysm formation, and opening of collateral channels. The early symptoms or signs are the result of local and systemic inflammation that may be absent at times leading to delayed diagnosis. Late effects (pulseless disease) are secondary to tissue ischemia from progressive arterial narrowing.

The angiographic classification is based on the pattern of vessel involvement and categorizes the disease into six types:[7]
1. Type I involves only the branches of the aortic arch.
2. Type IIa involves ascending aorta, aortic arch and its branches.
3. Type IIb affects ascending aorta, aortic arch and its branches, and thoracic descending aorta.
4. Type III involves the descending thoracic aorta, the abdominal aorta, and/or the renal arteries.
   The ascending aorta, the aortic arch and its branches are not affected.
5. Type IV involves only the abdominal aorta and/or renal arteries.
6. Type V has combined features of Type IIb and IV.

US, CT, and MRI are useful modalities and are more helpful in TA than in any other vasculitides due to the large size of vessels involved that can be imaged with either of these modalities. Digital subtraction angiography also plays a role, but more so for the depiction of intraluminal changes than vessel wall changes.

Demonstration of mural thickening with luminal narrowing forms the mainstay of diagnosis in the early phase. Ultrasonography of carotid and subclavian arteries depicts the typical signs of an inflamed vessel (smooth, homogeneous, hypoechoic, and concentric wall thickening) sometimes termed the "macaroni sign."[8] The thickening is relatively more echogenic than in GCA due to less wall edema and more chronic course of TA.[9] It tends to be relatively homogeneous, circumferential, and most commonly involves the proximal 50–75% segment of the common carotid artery. Progressive narrowing of the vessel can be seen as the disease progresses. Thus, US can be a noninvasive guide to monitor disease progression and assess the effect of therapy. CT and MRI also help in detecting mural thickening with reasonable accuracy especially in the aorta that cannot be visualized by US due to poor acoustic window. Normally, the aortic wall is less than 1 mm in thickness, and its outer wall is well circumscribed. Mural inflammation leads to ill-defined outer margin in addition to wall thickening. Increased wall attenuation has been noted that is attributed to fibrous and connective tissue proliferation and calcium deposition in the adventitia and media on noncontrast CT.[10] Contrast-enhanced computed tomography may show

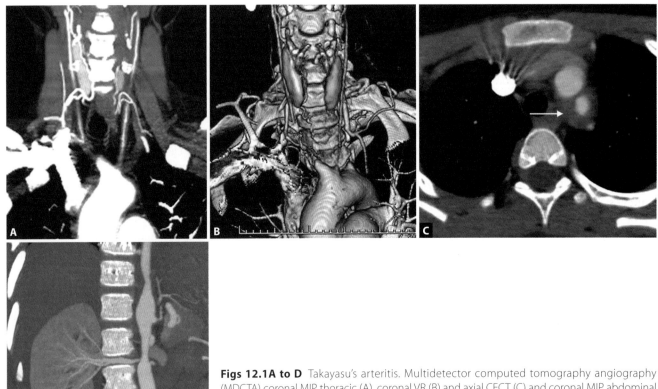

Figs 12.1A to D Takayasu's arteritis. Multidetector computed tomography angiography (MDCTA) coronal MIP thoracic (A), coronal VR (B) and axial CECT (C) and coronal MIP abdominal images show segmental stenosis of supra-aortic arteries with variable distal formation. Concentric mural thickening of proximal left subclavian artery can be appreciated (arrow). Segmental stenosis of the abdominal aorta leads to right renal artery stenosis at origin (D)

a double ring pattern of wall thickening, best seen in the arterial phase acquisition.[11] One school of thought attributes the inner, poorly enhancing ring to mucoid or gelatinous swelling of the intima and the outer enhancing ring to active medial and adventitial inflammation due to enlarged vasa vasorum. According to others, the intima represents the hypoenhancing rim-sandwiched between luminal contrast and outer enhancing rim of medial and adventitial inflammation.[10] Same changes can be appreciated on a well-performed MRI that does not require contrast administration to visualize the wall. However, the pattern of enhancement of the wall can be assessed only after administering intravenous gadolinium.

During the late stage of the disease, intimal and adventitial thickening leads to arterial occlusion (pulseless stage). This can be demonstrated by angiography or less invasive techniques like the CTA and MRA. Computed tomography has proven to be convenient and efficacious with > 93% sensitivity and specificity for luminal changes in the thoracic aorta and its major branches. Progressive disease leads to long and diffuse or short segmental irregular narrowing of involved arteries.[12] Skip areas are common in form of

stenosis while mural thickening is appreciated on cross-sectional imaging in the intervening angiographically normal areas (Figs 12.1A to D). Aneurysmal dilatation (saccular and fusiform) of the aorta and its branches can be seen. Magnetic resonance imaging may be helpful in functional assessment of flow across the stenotic sites and also to assess regurgitation across the aortic valve when involved. Similar assessment can also be performed with duplex ultrasound especially in arteries that are more superficial and accessible to the probe.

Pulmonary arteries can be involved with predilection for upper lobar branches and their segmental divisions. Progressive mural thickening may lead to stenosis and distal vascular "pruning." Consequent central arterial dilatation occurs leading to pulmonary arterial hypertension, which needs differentiation from pulmonary artery thromboembolism. Secondary parenchymal changes subsequently ensue and can be seen in form of mosaic attenuation in lungs, centrilobular nodules, subpleural reticulonodular changes, and pleural thickening. Chronic arterial inflammation leads to mural calcifications, apart from stenosis, which can be imaged by CT scan.

Giant Cell Arteritis

The typical symptoms and findings of GCA can many a times be misinterpreted that may lead to a delay in the otherwise urgently needed treatment. This entity was first described clinically in late 19th century and referred to as "arteritis of the aged."[13] It manifests in patients over the age of 50 years and has significant association with polymyalgia rheumatic. In the 2012 revised version of the International Chapel Hill Consensus Conference (CHCC) nomenclature, GCA is defined as a LVV, affecting the aorta and its large arterial branches. The characteristic vessels involved in GCA are the branches of the carotid and vertebral arteries that are preferentially affected by the inflammatory process.[14]

Histologically, GCA is characterized by granulomatous inflammation with lymphocytes, macrophages, and giant cells in the vascular wall. The inflammatory edema and the vascular wall thickening can be picked up with medical imaging techniques and can point toward the diagnosis. Progressive inflammation may lead to stenosis or vascular occlusion. Bitemporal headaches refractory to analgesia occurs in a majority of patients.[15] Other symptoms considered specific are activity-related accentuated pain on chewing (jaw claudication) and swallowing occurring as a result of ischemia of the masticatory muscles.

Imaging modalities used for evaluating the disease are US, MRA, and CTA, which form the noninvasive method to visualize the luminal and mural details. Typical findings include hypoattenuating mural thickening, stenosis, occlusions, and skip lesions. The vascular segments more commonly involved are distal subclavian artery, carotid arteries, and branches of the external carotid arteries, especially the temporal artery. Aortic aneurysms are common than in the general population.[16] Aortic dissection may occur, following weakening of the wall that may also lead to aortic insufficiency. Giant cell arteritis is diagnosed on the basis of the combination of symptoms, clinical findings, laboratory results, and diagnostic imaging.[16-18] Ultrasound plays a major role in evaluating the superficial arteries, most commonly the superficial temporal artery (STA). An intermediate frequency transducer (at least 9 MHz) is essential. Inflammatory edema of the vascular wall is seen as hypoechoic wall thickening ("halo sign"). Volpe et al.[19] reported that the "halo sign" is well visualized by color Doppler and gray-scale US (Figs 12.2A to C). The dimensions of the halo sign seem to be very important with maximum widths ≥ 1 mm being correlated with high specificity (93%).[20]

Vascular stenoses and occlusions of the affected vessels are seen in the later disease course. Duplex sonography also helps in hemodynamic flow assessment of the stenosed segments and can reveal any reversal of flow with inverse

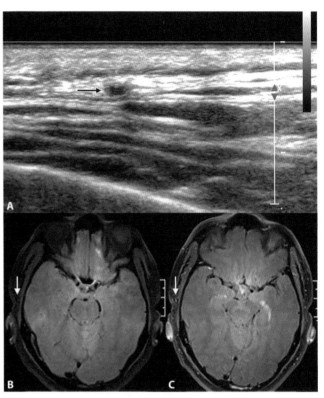

Figs 12.2A to C Giant cell arteritis. Ultrasound examination of the right temporal region (A) shows thickened hypoechoic temporal artery wall-"halo sign" (arrow). Axial pregadolinium (B) and post-gadolinium (C) Images confirm the wall thickening and abnormal enhancement (arrows)

cerebral supply via the temporal artery, in which case biopsy is contraindicated. Color-coded duplex ultrasound has been reported to have 90% sensitivity and 98% specificity for detecting lesions. Magnetic resonance imaging also allows detailed imaging of the walls and lumina of the superficial cranial arteries.[21,22] The inflamed vessels show enhancement following gadolinium administration. This is particularly helpful when planning a temporal biopsy, as a directed biopsy leads to optimal results. Magnetic resonance also shows involvement of the aorta, the supra-aortic arteries (Figs 12.2A to C), and the great arteries of the viscera that cannot be imaged with duplex ultrasound. In one of the studies, the authors reported sensitivity of MRI for detecting temporal artery inflammation as 100% with specificity of the same magnitude.[22] Magnetic resonance imaging can also be useful for follow-up of patients for assessing treatment response following steroid therapy.

MEDIUM-VESSEL VASCULITIS

Medium-vessel vasculitis (MVV) predominantly affects medium arteries, defined as the main visceral arteries and their branches of any size. Polyarteritis nodosa and KD are the major variants. The onset of inflammation in MVV is more acute and necrotizing than the onset of inflammation in LVV.

Polyarteritis Nodosa

Polyarteritis nodosa is necrotizing arteritis of medium or small arteries classically involving renal and visceral arteries without glomerulonephritis or vasculitis in arterioles, capillaries, or venules, and not associated with ANCAs. The kidneys are involved in 70–80% of cases, while gastrointestinal tract, coronary arteries, peripheral nerves, and skin are affected in approximately 50% of patients.[23]

Cross-sectional imaging plays a relatively limited role because of subnominal resolution in the detection of changes of stenosis, ectasias, and occlusions that are better picked by catheter angiography. Multiple microaneurysms (< 5 mm) form the hallmark of PAN. This however cannot be taken as diagnostic of the disease, as it may not be seen at times. CTA/MRA may not detect microaneurysms but may depict the stenosis, occlusions, and pseudoaneurysms of the main renal artery and beyond, till its segmental divisions. Microaneurysms (Figs 12.3A and B) are exquisitely demonstrated by catheter angiography that forms the gold standard to diagnose PAN, with sensitivity and specificity of 89 and 90%, respectively.[24] They arise secondary to weakening of the vessel wall secondary to destruction of the elastic lamina with the media undergoing fibrinoid necrosis. All the stages of vessel wall destruction namely acute necrosis, thrombosis, occlusion, and stenosis can all exist at a given time in an individual. The consequent parenchymal changes

occur in the form of ischemia/infarction of the organ being supplied (classically seen as peripherally located wedge-shaped infarcts in kidneys and liver and mesenteric ischemia in the bowel). Rupture of aneurysms may lead to subcapsular/perirenal hematoma formation and hemoperitoneum (rupture of mesenteric aneurysms) that can be seen with ultrasound. The microaneurysms respond to glucocorticoid treatment.

Imaging findings in chest include round-shaped or wedge-shaped ischemic areas with infiltrates seen in the lungs that are a depiction of ensuing ischemia. Some of this nodular/patchy consolidation may undergo cavitation. Mediastinal changes may be seen in the form of cardiomegaly with pericarditis, pericardial thickening, and/or pericardial effusion. Cardiac failure in late stages may lead to pulmonary edema with or without pleural effusion. These changes can be assessed with the help of CT scan and echocardiography. Coronary artery involvement is seen in 40–60% of patients having a clinical cardiac disease[25] in form of thrombosis, irregularity, ectasia, and aneurysm formation.

Apart from demonstrating the manifestations of PAN, imaging helps to exclude other diagnosis, especially tuberculosis and malignancy that can lead to similar clinical manifestations and may mimic vasculitis. Angiography, though an invasive modality for diagnosis of vasculitis, is very helpful in tackling of ruptured aneurysms through embolization of the involved vessel that immediately leads to cessation of bleeding. Revascularization/thrombolysis can be attempted in acutely thrombosed vessels as well.

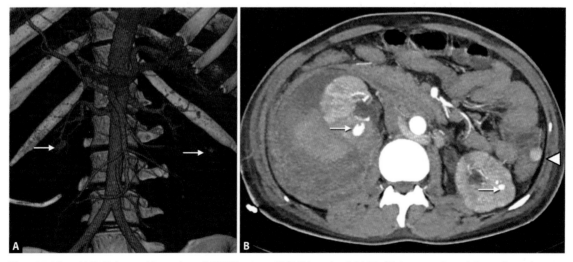

Figs 12.3A and B Polyarteritis nodosa. MDCTA coronal VR (A) and axial MIP (B) images show bilateral renal artery aneurysms (arrows) and left splenic artery aneurysm (arrowhead). Note the right-sided large subcapsular hematoma due to rupture of an aneurysm causing parenchymal compression

KAWASAKI DISEASE

Kawasaki disease is an acute arteritis causing systemic vasculitis associated with mucocutaneous lymph node syndrome and predominantly affecting medium and small arteries. It primarily affects infants and young children. Coronary arteries are often involved with aneurysms occurring in 15–20% of cases; aorta and other medium-to-large-size arteries may be involved, e.g., axillary, renal, or iliac arteries.

Echocardiography is an excellent noninvasive modality to detect coronary artery abnormalities and aneurysms. Catheter angiography, however, still forms the gold standard for diagnosis. Of late, advancement in technology has led to the development of cardiac-gated MRI as an excellent tool to evaluate the coronary arterial and cardiac functional abnormalities. Echocardiography identifies coronary aneurysms accurately with sensitivity and specificity of 95 and 99%, respectively.[26]

The American Heart Association recommends that KD patients should be evaluated by echocardiography at presentation, at 2 weeks and after 6–8 weeks. Echo has also been used to follow treatment response and also assesses regional wall motion. It has a limitation in detecting stenosis, partial thrombosis, especially in distal arteries. In patients with large body habitus, in whom the visualization of coronary arteries by echocardiography is more difficult, other imaging modalities such as angiography or MRA should be used.[27] Magnetic resonance imaging has an excellent capability to visualize mural as well as luminal details along with blood flow measurements. Magnetic resonance imaging's lack of ionizing radiation and noninvasive nature makes it preferable in children and young adults with KD over other modalities such as CT and invasive catheter angiography. It can accurately detect the aneurysm size, its extent, presence of thrombus, and stenosis length, and can be helpful in the assessing treatment response and follow-up of such patients. Using bright- and dark-blood imaging, Suzuki et al.[28] replicated the equivalence of MRI with conventional angiography and superiority over echocardiography in detecting aneurysms and stenosis in patients ranging from 4 months to 37 years. Other sites where aneurysms develop in KD patients are aorta, iliac arteries, and axillary and renal arteries. Computed tomography currently forms a noninvasive modality for the evaluation of the aneurysm and follow-up for change in size, thrombus extent, and calcifications, etc.

SMALL-VESSEL VASCULITIS

Small-vessel vasculitis predominantly affects small vessels, defined as small intraparenchymal arteries, arterioles, capillaries, and venules. Medium arteries and veins may also be affected rarely. Small vessels are actually the intraparenchymal vessels. The two categories of SVV are characterized by a paucity of vessel wall immunoglobulin in one and a prominence of vessel wall immunoglobulin in the other. Antineutrophil cytoplasmic antibody-associated vasculitis is one of the major vasculitis having paucity of vessel of wall immunoglobulin. The major clinicopathological variants of AAV are microscopic polyangiitis, granulomatosis with polyangiitis (Wegener's), eosinophilic granulomatosis with polyangiitis (Churg–Strauss), and single-organ AAV (for example, renal-limited AAV). Immune complex SVV has moderate-to-marked vessel wall deposits of immunoglobulin and/or complement, predominantly affecting small vessels. Glomerulonephritis is frequent. Arterial involvement is much less common in immune complex SVV compared to ANCA SVV. Immune complex vasculitis can be categorized as a vasculitis associated with probable etiologies (e.g. hepatitis C virus-associated cryoglobulinemic vasculitis) or as a vasculitis associated with systemic disease (e.g. systemic lupus vasculitis or rheumatoid vasculitis). The imaging findings in most of these disorders are a manifestation of end-organ injury, as the order of vascular involvement is very distal, with ramifications being within the parenchyma of the organ affected. Renal manifestations may be in the form of raised cortical echogenicity with accentuated or ill-defined corticomedullary differentiation with renomegaly in the acute phase and shrunken kidney in the chronic phase. Similarly, pulmonary parenchymal changes may be in the form of cavitating nodules, interstitial thickening, and serositis in the form of pleural and/or pericardial effusion. On the same analogy, liver and bowel may be affected with areas of differential enhancement/ischemia with peritoneal inflammation and ascites. None of these changes are diagnostic of any particular pathology but serve as valuable corroborative information in diagnosing these vasculitides. Systemic lupus and rheumatoid vasculitis warrant special mention, as certain imaging features in these along with the background disease activity may lead us to a conclusive diagnosis or stage of the pathology.

Rheumatoid Vasculitis

It is basically a complication of the underlying process of rheumatoid arthritis. Vascular inflammation (ascending aortitis), aneurysms, stenosis, and vessel occlusions may occur with eventual end-organ damage in form of infarctions and hemorrhages in the abdomen. Many of the features resemble those of PAN. Depending on the location and type of pathology, the evaluation may be done by US, CT, or MRI.

Systemic Lupus Vasculitis

Systemic lupus erythematosus leads to thrombus formation in the vessels, especially the veins. Extremity thrombosis may be evaluated by ultrasound Doppler while the central (renal, superior and inferior vena cava, cerebral venous sinuses, etc.) thrombosis requires cross-sectional modality such as the CT or MRI with angiography (venography). Contraindication to contrast in case of allergies or renal dysfunction prompts a noncontrast MRA that gives reasonably good results. Lupus arteritis has been reported in form of aortitis.[29] There occurs diffuse concentric mural thickening that may appear as hyperattenuating on CT with patchy contrast enhancement. Conventional angiography can, at times, miss this especially in the early stages when there is no significant luminal compromise. Computed tomography or magnetic resonance imaging is also useful in evaluating the response to treatment. Other manifestations may be in the form of lupus nephritis (manifests as renal parenchymal disease on imaging), renal vein thrombosis, renal subcapsular hematomas, and lupus mesenteric vasculitis that may lead to ischemia and even perforation. The latter usually involves the superior mesenteric artery territory with presence of "Comb sign" (increased thickened nontapering vessels giving the appearance of a comb). The corresponding bowel loop usually shows thickening (> 3 mm) and may show a "double halo sign" (central hypodensity with hyperattenuating inner and outer layers). Pneumatosis intestinalis and portal venous gas indicate ischemia with extraluminal contrast/fluid signifying perforation of the involved bowel. Central nervous system (CNS) manifestations are in the form of white matter changes with infarcts (Figs 12.4A to C) and associated sinovenous thrombosis.

VARIABLE-VESSEL VASCULITIS

Variable-vessel vasculitis can affect vessels of any size (small, medium, and large) and type (arteries, veins, and capillaries). Behçet's disease and CS are included in this class.

Behçet's Disease Vasculitis

It is a multisystem disorder and can affect any artery, vein, or organ of the body. It is characterized by recurrent oral and/or genital aphthous ulcers accompanied by cutaneous, ocular, articular, gastrointestinal, and/or CNS inflammatory lesions. Small-vessel vasculitis, arteritis, arterial aneurysms and, venous and arterial thromboangiitis, and thrombosis may occur. Venous inflammation and consequent thrombosis are more common than arterial inflammation. Arterial manifestation is seen in less than 3% of cases. It can be divided into three categories: arterial occlusions, arterial aneurysms, and pulmonary artery aneurysms.[30] It is thus one of the very rare causes of pulmonary artery aneurysms that are usually multiple, are prone to rupture, and respond to steroids. They can be exquisitely demonstrated by pulmonary CTA or MRA. Nonresponding pulmonary artery aneurysms can be treated by endovascular embolization with coils or vascular plugs. However, extra caution should be taken, as these patients are prone to develop aneurysms and thrombus at the sites of vascular punctures. There are reports of successful treatment of arterial aneurysm by the endovascular route.[31]

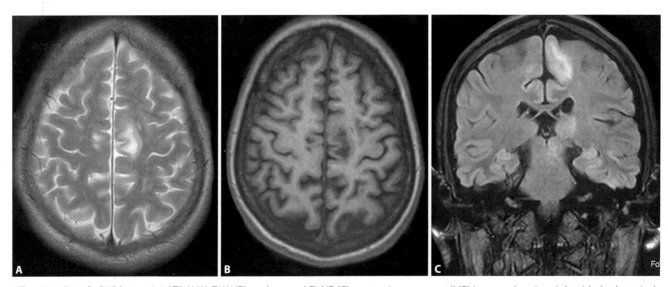

Figs 12.4A to C CNS lupus. Axial T2W (A), T1W (B), and coronal FLAIR (C) magnetic resonance (MR) images showing right-sided subcortical white matter T2 hyperintensities and left-sided infarct secondary to vasculitis involving the intracranial arteries

The typical sites of venous involvement are inferior vena cava, superior vena cava, and common iliac veins.[32] Superficial thrombophlebitis of the lower extremity and cerebral sinus venous thrombosis are few examples that can be imaged by Doppler ultrasound and MRI with MR venography, respectively. Arterial aneurysms and pseudoaneurysms can be evaluated by noncontrast MRA (time of flight MRA), gadolinium-enhanced MRA in conjunction with T1/T2/gradient-based sequences. Common arterial sites are femoropopliteal, pulmonary, subclavian, carotid arteries, and aorta.[33] Other lesions that have been reported are mesenteric vasculitis,[34] renal artery aneurysm,[35] and internal carotid artery dissection.[36]

Cogan's Syndrome Vasculitis

It is characterized by ocular inflammatory lesions, including interstitial keratitis, uveitis, and episcleritis, and inner ear disease,[37] including sensorineural hearing loss and vestibular dysfunction. Vasculitic manifestations may include arteritis (affecting small, medium, or large arteries),[38] aortitis,[39] aortic aneurysms, and aortic and mitral valvulitis.

The small vessels in the vascularized layers of the anterior globe are the ones most commonly involved in CS vasculitis.[40] Inflamed small blood vessels invade the adjacent normally avascular corneal stroma and cause the very distinctive interstitial keratitis of CS.

SINGLE-ORGAN VASCULITIS

Single-organ vasculitis is vasculitis in arteries or veins of any size in a single organ, with no features that indicate that it is a limited expression of a systemic vasculitis. The involved organ and vessel type should be included in the name [e.g. cutaneous SVV, testicular vasculitis, and CNS vasculitis (Figs 12.5A to C)]. Vasculitis distribution may be unifocal or multifocal (diffuse) within an organ or organ system.

VASCULITIS ASSOCIATED WITH SYSTEMIC DISEASE

Vasculitis can be associated with and may be caused by a systemic disease. The name (diagnosis) should have a prefix term specifying the systemic disease (e.g. rheumatoid vasculitis, lupus vasculitis, sarcoidosis vasculitis, and relapsing polychondritis vasculitis). This category of vasculitis associated with systemic diseases and the following category associated with probable etiologies often are considered to be secondary vasculitides.

INFECTION-RELATED VASCULITIS

Another category that has distinctly been classified as a separate class is the secondary vasculitis following infectious agents (e.g. *Treponema*, *Salmonella*, *Staphylococci*, *Streptococci*, and *Myobacteria*). Most of these organisms involve the aorta resulting in aortitis. Apart from the imaging manifestations of mural thickening, aneurysm formation, valvular incompetence, stenosis, etc., systemic manifestations occur depending upon the microbe. Cross-sectional imaging, especially CT scan, plays a major role in the detection of lesions and deciphering their precise details for planning future treatment. Aggressive antibiotics often have to be combined with major surgical resections, anastomoses, and

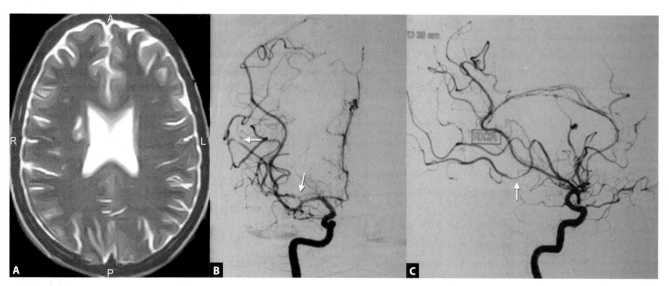

Figs 12.5A to C CNS vasculitis. Axial T2W MRI (A) demonstrating the right periventricular white matter infarct. Right internal carotid artery (ICA) DSA-frontal (B) and lateral (C) projections showing segmental stenosis of ICA branches (arrows)

bypassing for optimal results. Surgical morbidity is high in these patients.

Vasculitides are a vast group of disorders characterized by a common denominator of inflammation of the vessels. Some vasculitides have specific imaging features that are diagnostic for that particular entity while most of the others have a combination of stenosis, aneurysms, occlusions, and end-organ changes. Significant advances have been made in the diagnosis and treatment of these lesions over the last few decades that has led on to a better understanding of the disease entities of this group of disorders. Molecular imaging has been an exciting recent advancement in this group of disorders.[41] With dedicated research being performed in the field of vasculitis, one hopes to have better clarity and understanding of vasculitides in times to come.

KEY POINTS

- The main aim of imaging in vasculitis is to identify inflammation in the vessel wall, the extent of vascular involvement, and consequences of hypoperfusion to the distal-fed organ.
- Mural changes of vasculitis are in the form of thickened, hypoechoic wall forming the "halo" sign on US and "double ring" sign on CT secondary to inflammation of the vessel wall.
- Luminal changes of vasculitis may be in the form of thrombosis, stenosis, ectasia, aneurysm or pseudoaneurysm formation of the vessel involved, and are best shown by DSA.
- Large- and medium-vessel vasculitides are easier to diagnose than SVV due to the larger size of vessels involved and their relatively accessible location.
- Takayasu's arteritis or pulseless disease shows extensive aortic involvement including its major branches. Depending on the vessels involved, it is classified into six types.
- Giant cell arteritis (GCA) involves superficial temporal artery (STA) that, being superficial, can be easily accessed and biopsied. Typical "halo sign" due to concentric mural hypoechogenicity of the STA wall is characteristic.
- Polyarteritis nodosa (PAN) characteristically shows multiple microaneurysms (< 5 mm) in the renal and mesenteric arteries.
- Coronary artery aneurysms along with aortic involvement strongly indicate toward KD.
- Small-vessel vasculitis usually leads to ischemic changes in the organs secondary to small-vessel inflammation and thrombosis.

REFERENCES

1. Jennette JC, Falk RJ, Bacon PA, et al. 2012 revised International Chapel Hill Consensus Conference Nomenclature of Vasculitides. Arthritis Rheum. 2013;65:1-11.
2. Shriki J. Ultrasound physics. Crit Care Clin. 2014;30:1-24.
3. Horton KM, Sheth S, Corl F, et al. Multidetector row CT: principles and clinical applications. Crit Rev Comput Tomogr. 2002;43:143-81.
4. Wheaton AJ, Miyazaki M. Non-contrast enhanced MR angiography: physical principles. J Magn Reson Imaging. 2012;36:286-304.
5. Foley WD, Milde MW. Intra-arterial digital subtraction angiography. Radiol Clin North Am. 1985;23:293-319.
6. Schmidt J, Kermani TA, Bacani AK, et al. Diagnostic features, treatment, and outcomes of Takayasu arteritis in a US cohort of 126 patients. Mayo Clin Proc. 2013;88:822-30.
7. Zhu F, Luo S, Wang ZJ, et al. Takayasu arteritis: imaging spectrum at multidetector CT angiography. Br J Radiol. 2012;85:e1282-92.
8. Nicoletti G, Mannarella C, Nigro A, et al. The "Macaroni Sign" of Takayasu's arteritis. J Rheumatol. 2009;36:2042-3.
9. Vaideeswar P, Deshpande JR. Pathology of Takayasu arteritis: a brief review. Ann Pediatr Cardiol. 2013;6:52-8.
10. Sharma S, Sharma S, Taneja K, et al. Morphologic mural changes in the aorta revealed by CT in patients with nonspecific aortoarteritis (Takayasu's arteritis). Am J Roentgenol. 1996;167:1321-5.
11. Park JH. Conventional and CT angiographic diagnosis of Takayasu arteritis. Int J Cardiol. 1996;54:S165-71.
12. Khandelwal N, Kalra N, Garg MK, et al. Multidetector CT angiography in Takayasu arteritis. Eur J Radiol. 2011;77(2):369-74.
13. Horton BT, Magath TB, Brown GE. An undescribed form of arteritis of the temporal vessels. Proc Mayo Clin. 1932;7:700-1.
14. Jennette JC, Falk RJ, Andrassy K, et al. Nomenclature of systemic vasculitides. Proposal of an international consensus conference. Arthritis Rheum. 1994;37:187-92.
15. Vaith P, Warnatz K. Clinical and serological findings of giant-cell arteritis. Z Rheumatol. 2009;68:124-31.
16. Evans JM, O'Fallon WM, Hunder GG. Increased incidence of aortic aneurysm and dissection in giant cell (temporal) arteritis. A population-based study. Ann Intern Med. 1995;122:502-7.
17. Ness T, Auw-Hadrich C, Schmidt D. Temporal arteritis (giant cell arteritis). Clinical picture, histology, and treatment. Ophthalmologe. 2006;103:296-301.
18. Kale N, Eggenberger E. Diagnosis and management of giant cell arteritis: a review. Curr Opin Ophthalmol. 2010;21:417-22.
19. Volpe A, Caramaschi P, Marchetta A, et al. B-flow ultrasound in a case of giant cell arteritis. Clin Rheumatol. 2007;26:1955-7.
20. Salvarani C, Silingardi M, Ghirarduzzi A, et al. Is duplex ultrasonography useful for the diagnosis of giant-cell arteritis? Ann Intern Med. 2002;137:232-8.
21. Bley TA, Uhl M, Carew J, et al. Diagnostic value of high-resolution MR imaging in giant cell arteritis. Am J Neuroradiol. 2007;28:1722-7.

22. Bley TA, Wieben O, Uhl M, et al. High-resolution MRI in giant cell arteritis: imaging of the wall of the superficial temporal artery. Am J Roentgenol. 2005;184:283-7.

23. Colmegna I, Maldonado-Cocco JA. Polyarteritis nodosa revisited. Curr Rheumatol Rep. 2005;7:288-96.

24. Hekali P, Kajander H, Pajari R, et al. Diagnostic significance of angiographically observed visceral aneurysms with regard to polyarteritis nodosa. Acta Radiol. 1991;32:143-8.

25. Chandrakantan A, Kaufman J. Renal hemorrhage in polyarteritis nodosa: diagnosis and management. Am J Kidney Dis. 1999;33:e8.

26. Hiraishi S, Misawa H, Takeda N, et al. Transthoracic ultrasonic visualisation of coronary aneurysm, stenosis, and occlusion in Kawasaki disease. Heart. 2000;83:400-5.

27. Newburger JW, Takahashi M, Gerber MA, et al. Diagnosis, treatment, and long-term management of Kawasaki disease: a statement for health professionals from the Committee on Rheumatic Fever, Endocarditis and Kawasaki Disease, Council on Cardiovascular Disease in the Young, American Heart Association. Circulation. 2004;110:2747-71.

28. Suzuki A, Takemura A, Inaba R, et al. Magnetic resonance coronary angiography to evaluate coronary arterial lesions in patients with Kawasaki disease. Cardiol Young. 2006;16:563-71.

29. Brinster DR, Grizzard JD, Dash A. Lupus aortitis leading to aneurysmal dilatation in the aortic root and ascending aorta. Heart Surg Forum. 2009;12(2):E105-8.

30. Park JH, Han MC, Bettmann MA. Arterial manifestations of Behçet disease. Am J Roentgenol. 1984;143:821-5.

31. Kim SW, Lee do Y, Kim MD, et al. Outcomes of endovascular treatment for aortic pseudoaneurysm in Behçet's disease. J Vasc Surg. 2014;59:608-14.

32. Terzioglu E, Kirmaz C, Uslu R, et al. Superior vena cava syndrome together with multiple venous thrombosis in Behçet's disease. Clin Rheumatol. 1998;17:176-7.

33. Berkmen T. MR angiography of aneurysms in Behçet disease: a report of four cases. J Comput Assist Tomogr. 1998;22:202-6.

34. Yokota K, Akiyama Y, Sato K, et al. Vasculo-Behçet's disease with non-traumatic subcapsular hematoma of the kidney and aneurysmal dilatations of the celiac and superior mesenteric arteries. Mod Rheumatol. 2008;18:615-8.

35. Ozkurt H, Oztora F, Tunc S, et al. Pseudoaneurysm of the renal interlobar artery in Behçet's disease. Acta Radiol. 2006;47:1000-2.

36. Pannone A, Lucchetti G, Stazi G, et al. Internal carotid artery dissection in a patient with Behçet's syndrome. Ann Vasc Surg. 1998;12:463-7.

37. Greco A, Gallo A, Fusconi M, et al. Cogan's syndrome: an autoimmune inner ear disease. Autoimmun Rev. 2013;12:396-400.

38. Lydon EJ, Barisoni L, Belmont HM. Cogan's syndrome and development of ANCA-associated renal vasculitis after lengthy disease remission. Clin Exp Rheumatol. 2009;27:S144.

39. Gasparovic H, Djuric Z, Bosnic D, et al. Aortic root vasculitis associated with Cogan's syndrome. Ann Thorac Surg. 2011;92:340-1.

40. Yaginuma A, Sakai T, Kohno H, et al. A case of atypical Cogan's syndrome with posterior scleritis and uveitis. Jpn J Ophthalmol. 2009;53:659-61.

41. Su HS, Nahrendorf M, Panizzi P, et al. Vasculitis: molecular imaging by targeting the inflammatory enzyme myeloperoxidase. Radiology. 2012;262:181-90.

CHAPTER 13

Positron Emission Tomography and Vasculitides

Enrico Tombetti, Justin C Mason

PRINCIPLES OF PET IMAGING

Positron emission tomography (PET) is a technology that uses β^+ decay of positron-emitting radioisotopes for image formation.[1,2] As in other nuclear medicine techniques, radioisotopes are included in radiotracers that act as molecular probes reporting specific biochemical processes *in vivo*. During β^+ decay, a proton in the nucleus of an unstable atom (the radioisotope) is converted into a neutron while releasing a positron (β^+) and an *electron neutrino* (ν_e, an electrically neutral subatomic particle with very low mass and interacting power with matter). β^+ decay is an isobaric nuclear decay process (i.e. without change in the mass number of the nucleus):

$$_m^n X \rightarrow _{m-1}^n Y + \beta^+ + \nu_e$$

Energy decay is converted into the generation of β^+ and ν_e particles and kinetic energy, which is variable according to the parent and daughter nuclei.

Positrons are the antimatter counterparts of electrons. According to the mass–energy equivalence, the resting energy of both positrons and electrons is 511 keV. Upon collision, positrons and electrons annihilate each other producing a pair of 511 keV *annihilation photons* (γ rays). The PET detectors are arranged in a ring to allow different detectors to register the coincident arrival of the annihilation photons. Only photons registered within a narrow *time-window of coincidence* (typically between 3 and 15 ns) are registered as an event of annihilation, which is assumed to have occurred somewhere on the straight line between the two detectors, known as the *coincidence line*. Numerous recorded annihilations in intersecting coincidence lines provide information concerning the distribution of positron-emitting radiotracers in the body. The positron kinetic energy influences the mean distance traveled (known as *range*) before annihilation and contributes to limiting the spatial resolution of PET imaging.

This distance is also influenced by the density of the matter crossed by the proton, being lower in the bone than in the lungs. Annihilation respects the laws of conservation of energy and linear momentum. As such, the two g-photons are emitted in opposite directions, at approximately 180° from each other. The nonabsolute colinearity of annihilation photons is another factor limiting the spatial resolution of PET, in a way dependent upon detector ring diameter. Intrinsic detector spatial resolution, mainly influenced by detector size, is the other main factor influencing the spatial resolution of PET. The detector characteristics also influence the dose of radiotracers required and the time needed for the scan.

The distribution of radiotracers in the body reports selective biochemical processes and not the composition of anatomical structures. As such, PET scans provide mainly functional information with little anatomical detail, making it difficult to define the structural significance of the radiotracer uptake. The choice of β^+-emitting radioisotope depends on: (i) the radiotracer used, which has to be labeled through a feasible chemical reaction; (ii) the ability to generate the radiotracer using a cyclotron; (iii) the half-life of its β^+ decay; (iv) the likelihood of other (non-β^+) decays, and (v) the stability of the product(s) of decay. For these reasons, ^{18}F is favored as it has a half-life of 109 minutes. Radiotracers report selective biological processes. [18]Fluorodeoxyglucose (^{18}F-FDG) is the radiotracer most widely used clinically and will be the main focus of this chapter. It competes with glucose for entry into the cell via glucose transporters. Once inside the cell, ^{18}F-FDG is phosphorylated to ^{18}F-FDG-6-phosphate without undergoing further metabolism, thereby becoming trapped in the cells. The possibility of dephosphorylation by glucose-6-phospatase, highly expressed in the liver and moderately in mononuclear cells, is an important exception. Thus, ^{18}F-FDG targets cells with an active glucose metabolism, including numerous malignant tumors, inflamed or infected tissues, active muscles, and the central nervous system.[2,3]

Radiotracer uptake into tissues is influenced by other variables, such as the injected dose, blood glucose level, volume of distribution of the radiotracer, *uptake time* (i.e. the timeframe between radiotracer infusion and scanning), acquisition time, the scanner, settings, and reconstruction technique utilized.[3] Thus, evaluation of tissue uptake is not straightforward. Absolute quantitation is not feasible in clinical practice and several other modalities have been proposed for the purpose. Qualitative assessment is the most straightforward and has been shown on many occasions to be as accurate as are semiquantitative methods. Assessment relies on visual comparison of uptake with the reference uptake of normal tissues, usually liver, blood pool, or lung, creating a four-point scale. *Standardized uptake value* (SUV) represents the mainstay of semiquantitative assessments. Of the several methods of calculating SUV, the simplest and most widely used is based on weight as measurement of body size:

$$SUV = \frac{\text{Activity concentration in tissue}}{\left(\dfrac{\text{Injected activity}}{\text{Body size}} \right)}$$

Guidelines are available for reducing variability of SUV measurements and allowing comparison between different examinations.[4,5] SUV_{mean} and SUV_{max}, respectively, represent the mean or maximum SUV of all voxels within a volume of interest, while SUV_{peak} represents the average SUV in a small group of voxels surrounding the voxel with highest activity.[3] Major limitations of SUV_{mean}, SUV_{max}, and SUV_{peak} are, respectively, the interobserver variability in the definition of the volume of interest, the sensitivity to noise, and the underestimation of SUV for small lesions.[3] Other diffuse and promising semiquantitative methods require standardization of the activity of the region of interest with a reference such as liver, blood pool, or lung.

The possibility of dephosphorylation and late washout of ^{18}F-FDG-6-phosphate in mononuclear cells has led to dual time point or delayed scanning for distinguishing malignant from inflammatory tissues being recommended.[2] Current PET scans with ^{18}F-FDG have a maximum spatial resolution for soft tissues of approximately 3–4 mm. The typical uptake period is 60 minutes, with a subsequent scanning time of 20–45 minutes. The mean effective dose per scan varies between scanners and is continuing to fall. A recent study in patients suffering from lymphoma revealed a mean effective dose of 39.3 mSv (range 7.1–100).[6] Patients are required to fast for approximately 4–6 hours and blood glucose should be less than 150 mg/dL to enhance ^{18}F-FDG uptake. Patients should

avoid physical exercise before the procedure and absolute rest is required during the uptake phase of ^{18}F-FDG before scanning.[1,2]

In the last decade, combined scanners allowing coregistration of PET and CT have become available. The main advantages of PET/CT are: (i) combination of functional data from PET with anatomical details from CT, allowing coupling of a hypermetabolic focus with its anatomical counterpart; (ii) better correction for attenuation of annihilation photons traveling through tissues with the transmission data obtained from CT, improving the quality of PET images.[1,2] Two general approaches are used for transmission CT scans: (a) a low-dose CT to provide attenuation correction and anatomical detail; (b) a standard CT with diagnostic quality. As yet, no consensus has been agreed regarding the optimal approach.

^{18}F-FDG PET/CT IN VASCULITIDES

The functional data conveyed by ^{18}F-FDG PET/CT have been proposed as a method for assessing inflammatory activity in the vasculitides. Positron emission tomography can localize inflammation in large arteries and on occasion in medium-sized vessels. Inflammation of organs as a consequence of small-vessel vasculitis can also be detected. However, the majority of data concerning ^{18}F-FDG PET use in this field refer to the LVVs.

^{18}F-FDG/CT PET in Large-Vessel Vasculitides

Coregistration of PET and CT has proved to be a pivotal advance in this field, enabling LVV to be distinguished from perivascular uptake due to brown fat metabolic activity or periadventitial diseases including chronic periaortitis and retroperitoneal fibrosis. Vascular complications of LVVs, specifically aneurysms and ischemia following arterial stenosis or occlusion, are the events that most clearly affect prognosis. Morphological imaging based on ultrasonography (US), magnetic resonance (MR), and CT can identify anatomical derangements in large vessels but not in smaller vessels such as the posterior ciliary or the ophthalmic arteries in giant cell arteritis (GCA). Functional imaging, additionally allows evaluation of the characteristics of the wall of large arteries secondary to disease involvement. The pathogenesis of either aneurysmal or steno-occlusive vascular progression in LVVs is poorly understood. This process is probably related to both vascular flogosis and an excessive remodeling response, to both the inflammation and mechanical strain related to distorted anatomy and changes in blood flow. Although it has been proposed that ^{18}F-FDG uptake identifies active vascular wall inflammation, the role of active arterial remodeling in uptake has yet to be determined. Thus, ^{18}F-FDG PET/CT has been studied as a promising tool for the diagnosis of the active phases of LVVs, as well as in the assessment of disease activity and response to therapies.

Diagnosis

Giant cell arteritis: In up to 20% of patients, the diagnosis of GCA is not straightforward. The clinical picture of GCA can be atypical or paucisymptomatic, with nonspecific features of malaise, weight loss, and fever of unknown origin. The temporal arteries may be normal on clinical examination and the patients lack the typical symptoms of headache, scalp tenderness, and jaw claudication. Definitive diagnosis requires histological evidence of GCA in a temporal artery biopsy (TAB) or in other arterial specimens. Unfortunately, TAB sensitivity is low and other arterial specimens are rarely available, except following surgery in cases of ascending aortic aneurysm. Ultrasound studies may identify edema in the temporary artery wall as the halo sign, which correlates well with positive histology.[7] However, diagnostic insensitivity remains to some extent as US may not recognize subtle histological involvement, such as inflammation of vasa vasorum or of periadventitial small vessels.[8] Furthermore, in some patients the disease is confined to large arteries and temporal arteries may not be involved. Other morphological imaging modalities predominantly detect large-vessel involvement, MR detects arterial wall thickening, as well as luminal changes due to stenosis or ectasia/aneurysms. It can also demonstrate inflammation of the arterial wall as evidenced by contrast-medium enhancement.[9] Similarly, ^{18}F-FDG PET/CT scanning has been investigated for its utility in the evaluation of inflammation in extracranial large arteries, for both diagnosis and assessment of disease extent.

Individual GCA studies and meta-analyses report FDG-PET/CT sensitivity of ~80% and specificity ~90%.[10-13] Positron emission tomography appears particularly useful for atypical cases, influencing both the diagnosis and therapeutic choices,[10] and in elderly patients with fever of unknown origin, also helping to exclude infection and underlying malignancy. Positron emission tomography appears to have a similar diagnostic performance to MRI in untreated GCA patients.[14-16] A typical FDG-PET/CT scan in a patient with GCA is shown in Figures 13.1A to C. Arterial involvement is usually symmetric, including most frequently the subclavian arteries, followed by the thoracic and abdominal aorta and the axillary arteries.[17] Patients may also have PET findings suggestive of concurrent polymyalgia rheumatica (PMR).

Intense aortic FDG uptake at diagnosis appears to have an important prognostic significance, correlating with the

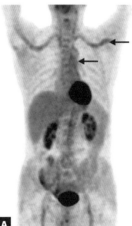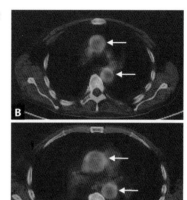

Figs 13.1A to C [18]FDG-PET-CT scanning in giant cell arteritis. The patient presented with fever, malaise, lethargy, weight loss, and a raised acute-phase response, without the classical signs of headache, scalp tenderness, and jaw claudication. The temporal arteries were normal on clinical examination and the diagnosis was revealed by the PET-CT scan. (A) Increased FDG uptake is apparent in the subclavian and axillary arteries and the thoracic aorta (arrows). (B and C) show the coregistered CT and PET images with intense FDG uptake in the thoracic aorta (arrows)

future development of aortic aneurysms,[18] which is the major cause of disease-related death in GCA. Of note, arterial FDG uptake rises with advancing age.[19,20] Importantly, active atherosclerosis can also result in arterial FDG uptake.[19] Distinction between active atherosclerosis and active GCA is usually based on the arterial sites involved, the presence of arterial wall calcification, the pattern of uptake ("patchy or focal" in atherosclerosis and "smooth linear or long segmental" in GCA),[12] and the intensity of uptake (higher in GCA).

In patients with ascending aortic aneurysm and histological evidence of granulomatous giant cell inflammation, FDG-PET/CT can reveal involvement of other arterial sites including the descending aorta and subclavian–axillary trunks, allowing the differentiation between GCA and isolated giant cell aortitis, a recently described condition for which prognosis and need for systemic therapies are still to be defined.[21-23]

Current potential pitfalls in the use of FDG-PET/CT for diagnosis of GCA are: (i) Positron emission tomography cannot evaluate involvement in the cervical branches of carotid arteries. They are too small or too near to the intense constitutive uptake in the brain. Large artery inflammation has been shown to occur in about 30% of patients with other diagnostic modalities,[24,25] and PET may not recognize patients with purely cephalic involvement. However, the latter are usually easier to diagnose, on account of a higher frequency of typical cranial symptoms and positive temporal artery biopsies.[24,26] Moreover, PET can identify subclinical large artery involvement in GCA with high frequency. Increased arterial FDG uptake was observed in 80% of 32 biopsy proven GCA patients.[13] (ii) FDG-PET for the diagnosis of GCA has not been standardized and there is no concordance with respect to quantification of the signal.[12,27] Qualitative assessment may allow the pattern and intensity of arterial uptake to be distinguished from atherosclerosis and may have higher specificity but lower sensitivity.[11] Recent studies have proposed that the arterial-to-blood pool ratio might be the parameter with the highest accuracy.[28] Similarly, it has been proposed that longer uptake times might improve FDG-PET performance,[29] and that combined assessment of supra-aortic branches might yield a higher diagnostic value.[13] The identification of cutoff values for semiquantitative uptake indices may be hampered by control populations with different age and prevalence of atherosclerosis.[11] (iii) Diagnostic sensitivity of PET is reduced by concurrent corticosteroid or immunosuppressive regimens, and in these situations the clinical utility of PET is less clear.[10,12,30]

Takayasu arteritis: The means to achieve earlier diagnosis of Takayasu arteritis (TA) represents an unresolved medical issue: it is a rare disease and a high level of suspicion is required for its identification. Moreover, the presentation of TA is typically nonspecific with constitutional symptoms. The

acute-phase response is frequently less intense than in GCA, and clinical or laboratory evidence of systemic inflammation may be absent at disease onset in up to 20% of subjects.[31,32] Histology is considered the gold standard for diagnosis, but arterial specimens in TA are limited to cases in which surgery has to be performed. Thus, diagnosis is often delayed until the clinical manifestations of large arteries stenoses, occlusions, or development of aneurysms.[33] Imaging can uncover TA before these significant luminal alterations take place (i.e. in the so-called prestenotic phase): indeed morphological analysis may reveal typical arterial wall thickening, which is highly specific for LVV. Arterial uptake at FDG-PET/CT has also been proposed for the early diagnosis of TA and the evaluation of disease extent.[34] However, disease rarity has prevented a definitive definition of the role of PET for the diagnosis and management of TA.

Individual FDG-PET studies on small groups of patients during the active phase of TA, suggest a good diagnostic sensitivity between 80 and 100%.[35-39] The majority of these studies evaluating FDG-PET for the diagnosis of TA are based on a qualitative assessment of arterial wall uptake. Coregistration of PET and CT increases sensitivity for arterial uptake.[40] Diagnostic specificity of FDG-PET seems to be very high, since arterial uptake in young patients is seldom related to causes other than arteritis. A typical FDG-PET/CT scan in a patient with TA is shown in Figures 13.2A and B. In the early phases of disease, FDG pattern of uptake is typically

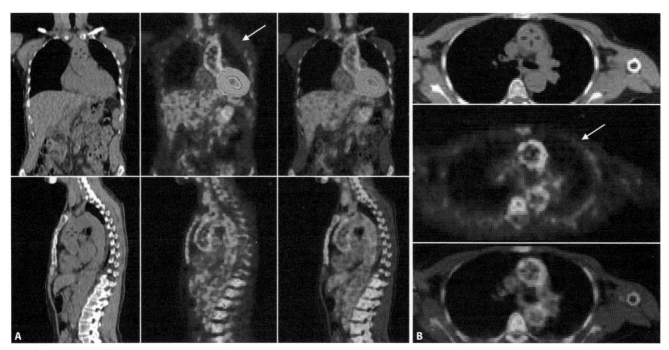

Figs 13.2A and B [18]FDG-PET-CT scanning in Takayasu arteritis. A 54-year-old female patient affected by Takayasu arteritis. (A and B) Coronal, sagittal and axial CT, PET, and fused PET/CT images show intense uptake in the aortic arch and descending thoracic aorta (SUVmax 9.8) (arrows)

continuous or segmental, outlining the arteries as tubular structures. After therapy initiation or spontaneous remission of disease, the pattern of uptake, if still present, may become patchier but still in a linear distribution.[41]

When TA is suspected, FDG-PET/CT may not only be useful for early diagnosis, but will also help to evaluate the disease extent. It has been reported that FDG-PET identifies more involved arterial regions than MR[35] and can detect arterial uptake even in absence of wall thickening.[40]

Potential pitfalls in the use of FDG-PET for TA at diagnosis are: (i) lack of sensitivity in the case of late diagnoses, after spontaneous remission or therapy initiation. (ii) Radiation exposure associated with repeat PET/CT scans in young patients. (iii) Absence of data suggesting a higher sensitivity of FDG-PET/CT for the diagnosis of TA in the prestenotic phase, in comparison to other established imaging modalities such as MR, although FDG-PET may have higher sensitivity than MR in detecting single arterial lesions in the prestenotic phase, and is potentially better for defining disease extent.[35] (iv) No data are available concerning the prognostic significance of the intensity or the extent of arterial FDG uptake in TA.

Other diseases with large-vessel vasculitis: Beside GCA and TA, LVV can occur in isolated idiopathic aortitis, as well as in other rheumatic conditions. Although data regarding the role of FDG-PET/CT scanning in these conditions are embryonic, it may be useful for evaluating vascular as well as extravascular involvement. Aortitis in the setting of spondyloarthropathies, rheumatoid arthritis, and systemic lupus erythematous will not be discussed further in this chapter.

Relapsing polychondritis (RP) is a rare disease with recurrent episodes of inflammation demonstrating preferential tropism to cartilage, especially hyaline cartilage. Airway involvement is present in up to 50% of patients and represents a major cause of morbidity and mortality.[42,43] Large artery involvement is well described in RP and it is more often confined to the aorta. Diagnosis of RP is often delayed until the cartilage destruction becomes clinically evident. Computed tomography can identify cartilaginous destruction and fibrotic replacement, but it is inaccurate for evaluation of early inflammatory involvement. Preliminary data suggest that FDG-PET/CT may be a sensitive means for the diagnosis of RP and in the assessment of disease extent, including airways and large arterial involvement.[44-46] Moreover, FDG-PET/CT may help to guide biopsies for diagnostic confirmation of RP and may detect inflammation before irreversible cartilaginous destruction. Lastly, FDG-PET/CT is a promising technique for disease activity assessment.[44-46]

Behçet disease (BD) is a multisystem, chronic relapsing vasculitis characterized by mucocutaneous, ocular, articular, neurological, gastrointestinal, and cardiovascular manifestations. Vasculitis primarily affects the small-blood vessels and veins, but medium and large arteries may be involved, with aneurysms, pesudoaneurysms, and arterial occlusions. Although arterial involvement is seen in only 14% of BD patients, it represents one of the leading causes of death.[47] Single case reports and a small series of eight patients have described the utility of FDG-PET for the identification of active arterial involvement in patients with known BD.[48-50] Similarly, single case reports have suggested that FDG-PET in BD may help to identify other sites of disease.

Cogan's syndrome, a very rare vasculitis that primarily affects the ocular and audiovestibulary systems, may exhibit widespread involvement of small, medium, or large blood vessels in more than 10% of cases.[51] Case reports have described the use of FDG-PET/CT for studying extraocular and extra-audiovestibular disease, such as arthritis or aortitis.[52-54]

Differential Diagnosis

Polymyalgia rheumatica: In the absence of specific features, the diagnosis of PMR requires exclusion of mimics, including GCA, elderly-onset rheumatoid arthritis, and malignancies. FDG-PET may help to discriminate. Typical PMR FDG-PET/CT scans show symmetric uptake at sites of bursitis and large-joint synovitis (Fig. 13.3).[55-57] Hip and shoulder involvement

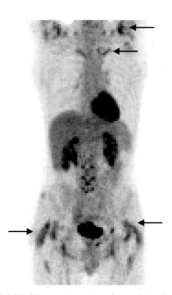

Fig. 13.3 [18]FDG-PET-CT scanning in polymyalgia rheumatica (PMR). The scan shows the characteristic uptake seen in a patient with untreated PMR. Increased uptake is seen at the shoulders suggestive of subacromial bursitis and there is evidence of symmetrical ischial bursitis (arrows). There is also increased uptake at the site of the posterior longitudinal ligament of the cervical spine and interspinous bursitis in the lumbar region (arrows) (maximum SUV 5.05).

are common, but increased uptake in the ischial tuberosities, greater trochanters, and spinous processes is more specific: the presence of at least two of the latter has 86% sensitivity for PMR and 88% specificity when compared to a control group of active rheumatic disease or polyarthritis.[56]

Although PMR and GCA are associated and proposed to be part of the same spectrum of disease, identification of isolated PMR has important prognostic and therapeutic implications. Distinction on the basis of absence of symptoms of cranial or large-vessel involvement may not always be accurate, as GCA may manifest after PMR or can purely involve large arteries. FDG-PET/CT shows large-vessel inflammation in approximately 30% of isolated PMR patients. These patients present a similar distribution of arterial uptake to GCA patients, although usually with lower intensity.[55] Thus, should PET be performed in PMR looking for smoldering arteritis? Scarce evidence suggests that asymptomatic vasculitis neither shares the same risk of complications as GCA,[58] nor represents a subset of PMR with more refractory disease.[55] We believe that PET may be useful in the identification of PMR and its mimics, but should not be performed on a regular basis until further data clarify this.

Infectious aortitis: It may mimic the arterial involvement of LVVs, since constitutional signs and symptoms raised inflammatory markers and some imaging aspects may be shared between the two groups. Infectious aortitis may be due to pyogenic bacteria including *Salmonella* species, *Staphylococcus aureus*, *Enterococcus* species, *Streptococcus pneumonia*, and *Clostridium* species, *Mycobacterium* species, *Treponema pallidum* and viruses such as HIV-related aortitis. Clinical history as well as radiological variables may help to distinguish infectious and noninfectious aortitis.[59] FDG-PET may be useful in subacute and chronic infectious aortitis, e.g. syphilitic aortitis, where it can detect aortitis before possible life-threatening complications occur.[60] However, although FDG-PET/CT can identify infectious aortitis, it cannot *per se* differentiate between infectious and noninfectious causes: only matching PET results with clinical, laboratory, and morphological imaging data allows differentiation between these conditions.

Chronic Periaortitis, IgG4-Related Disease, and Other Periaortic Fibrotic Disorders

Chronic periaortitis (CP) encompasses a specific range of rare diseases characterized by the presence of fibroinflammatory tissue around the abdominal aorta and/or the iliac arteries. These include idiopathic retroperitoneal fibrosis, inflammatory abdominal aortic aneurysm, and

perianeurysmal retroperitoneal fibrosis.[61] Other causes of retroperitoneal fibrosis and/or periaortitis include IgG4-related disease (IgG4-RD), Erdheim-Chester disease, chemicals, infections, surgery, radiation therapy, and malignancies. Periaortic inflammation is amongst the differential diagnoses of the LVVs, since both conditions can have nonspecific inflammatory symptoms and arterial involvement. Fibrous encasement of retroperitoneal structures and absence of aortic stenosis may allow clinical distinction from aortitis. Morphological imaging with MRI or CT usually clearly identifies the periarterial nature of these diseases, typically, showing a soft-tissue mass surrounding the aorta and/or iliac arteries. The presence of intimal or medial calcification at the internal border of a thickened arterial wall helps to identify the adventitial and periadventitial nature of the tissue.

Typical FDG-PET/CT findings in CP are shown in Figures 13.4A to C. The periaortic tissue usually demonstrates avid FDG uptake in the active inflammatory phase, and this associates with the presence of contrast enhancement on the CT scan.[62] In up to 40% of patients with CP, FDG-PET/CT shows vascular uptake in the thoracic aorta and/or its branches, suggesting that CP may represent a systemic LVV, where adventitial and periadventitial tissue are primarily involved.[63] Involvement of other retroperitoneal structures, such as the ureters or the inferior vena cava, may be seen as well (Figs 13.4A to C). Small heterogeneous studies have reported that FDG-PET/CT has good diagnostic sensitivity for CP. These studies have proposed FDG-PET/CT for evaluating disease activity and extent as well as for guiding medical and operative decisions including ureteral stent removal.[64-68] A single prospective study reported a sensitivity of FDG-PET of 77% for diagnosis of CP.[68] Patients without FDG-avid periaortic tissue may still respond to tamoxifen, and FDG-PET/CT performed after 3 months of therapy was inaccurate in the identification of response to tamoxifen.[68] Other studies report a better performance of FDG-PET/CT, with a sensitivity of 95% and a specificity of 90% in identifying active CP.[62] Beam-hardening artifact due to aortic calcification or ureteral stents may cause overcorrection for transmission and a falsely elevated SUV value in inactive CP. In conclusion, PET may be a useful tool for assessing the activity of CP. This is of particular importance, since acute-phase reactants are often inaccurate and iodinated contrast medium may be contraindicated in patients with renal insufficiency.

IgG4-related disease demonstrates protean manifestations and diverse organ involvement, characterized by lesions exhibiting storiform fibrosis, obliterative phlebitis, and a lymphoplasmacytic infiltrate enriched with IgG4-positive

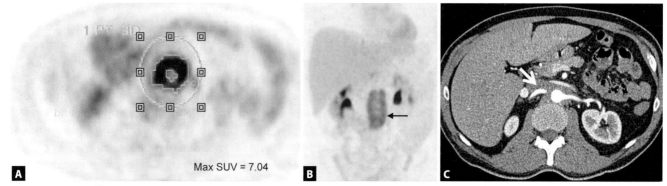

Figs 13.4A to C [18]FDG-PET-CT scanning in chronic periaortitis. (A) Intense FDG uptake is seen affecting the aortic wall and periadventitial tissue with a maximum SUV = 7.04; (B) The abnormal uptake is seen to be confined to the abdominal aorta (arrow); (C) The CT image reveals the inflammatory mass surrounding the aorta and extending along the proximal renal arteries (white arrow)

plasma cells and on occasion eosinophils. Both arteritis and periarteritis are a relatively frequent finding. FGD-PET/CT has a very high sensitivity for detection of active and untreated IgG4-RD. Recent data suggest that FDG-PET/CT may have various roles in the management of IgG4-RD.[69,70] First, it has a higher sensitivity for active organ involvement than conventional imaging methods, especially as far as arterial and periarterial involvement is concerned. This allows a more precise evaluation of disease extent and can help to guide diagnostic biopsies. Secondly, the pattern of FDG uptake is sometimes reasonably specific for IgG4-RD and it has been proposed as an additional diagnostic criteria. Lastly, FDG-PET uptake appears to rapidly abate after therapy, with the possible exception of monotherapy with rituximab. Thus, FDG-PET is a promising technique for assessment of many aspects of IgG4-RD.[69,70]

Assessment of Disease Activity and Response to Therapy

Giant cell arteritis: Since approximatively 50% of GCA patients experience a relapse during steroid tapering, PET has been investigated as a means for establishing disease activity. However, its role is still to be determined. In contrast to the changes seen with MR, the FDG-PET findings rapidly improve after therapy initiation.[14-16] However, FDG-PET has proven moderately insensitive for identifying smoldering, inflammation, and subsequent disease relapse.[17] Moreover, some arterial uptake may persist during clinical and serological remission, and it is unknown whether this represents persistent low-grade vascular inflammation or processes of tissue repair and remodeling. FDG-PET scans during clinical relapses reveal similar arterial involvement to that seen during quiescent disease.[17] Moreover, aortic uptake

while on treatment fails to predict late enlargement of the thoracic aorta.[18]

Takayasu arteritis: The vast majority of patients with TA have a chronic or relapsing course, and approximately 50% of subjects are refractory to first-line therapy with steroids and immunosuppressive agents. Thus, activity assessment is pivotal for the management of TA. Unfortunately, we still lack validated activity indices, as biomarkers have been found to be unreliable in up to 50% of cases.[31,32] Similarly, active inflammation in histology specimens and new vessel involvement in sequential angiographic studies were present in 44% patients and 61% of patients were thought to have inactive disease.[31] Different processes may underlie arterial progression, including inflammation, wall edema, arterial remodeling, and fibrotic scar formation. FDG-PET/CT can detect overt vascular inflammation, but its capability for identifying smoldering inflammation, or arterial remodeling is still unknown.

The inaccuracy in the reference methods used for activity assessment in most studies precludes drawing a precise picture of the performance of FDG-PET/CT in evaluating the status of disease activity in TA. Moreover, there is heterogeneity between studies in terms of assessment of arterial uptake, definition of positive uptake, percentage of patients undergoing immunological therapies, and results obtained. Individual studies and a meta-analysis report a sensitivity of ~70% and a specificity of ~75%, using the reference of NIH activity criteria.[37,38,40,41,71-74] However, another study did not confirm these results, failing to evidence an association between FDG-PET findings and other activity indices.[75] Thus, the role of FDG-PET/CT in the assessment of TA activity is still to be defined. Similarly, the presence of associations between PET results and inflammatory markers has not been fully ascertained. The effect of concurrent therapies on FDG-PET accuracy is still debated, although a recent study reported similar performances of PET independently from treatment status.[74] Despite these equivocal results from cross-sectional analysis of TA activity with FDG-PET/CT, repeated scans may be useful to monitor disease activity and response to treatment within the same patient.[36,38-40,72] Along with the expense of these scans, repeated radiation exposure in young patients is however of significant concern.

^{18}F-FDG/CT PET in Medium-Vessel Vasculitides

Kawasaki Disease

The experience of FDG-PET scanning for Kawasaki disease is mainly limited to assessment of myocardial viability.[76] Myocardial perfusion and coronary flow reserve have been evaluated by PET with other radiotracers.[77,78] An isolated case report shows that FDG-PET/CT can be of help in the assessment of aortic and coronary artery inflammation.[79]

Polyarteritis Nodosa

There are only isolated small reports suggesting that FDG-PET can identify patchy vascular inflammation in active polyarteritis nodosa.[80,81] The potential utility of FDG-PET in these patients is still to be assessed.

^{18}F-FDG/CT PET in Small-Vessel Vasculitides

Spatial resolution of current PET scanners prevents identification of the small inflammatory foci that are typical of small-vessel vasculitides. However, some ANCA-associated vasculitides, especially granulomatosis with polyangiitis (GPA), may have discrete granulomatous lesions or vasculitic inflammatory involvement sufficient to be identified with FDG-PET.

Granulomatosis with Polyangiitis

Only several case reports and two small case series have assessed the possible role of FDG-PET/CT in GPA. With a high sensitivity for detecting active untreated GPA, FDG-PET can help in cases where the diagnosis is unclear, guide the biopsy, and assess disease extent.[82,83] In particular, FDG-PET/CT may have a higher sensitivity than nonenhanced CT for detection of upper respiratory tract involvement.[82] FDG-PET/CT can accurately identify involvement of lung, heart, and lymphnodes, but not of skin, joint, eye, or peripheral nerves.[83] FDG-PET sensitivity for detecting kidney involvement is hampered by renal excretion of the radionucleotide.[82,83] Although PET can identify disease involvement at multiple sites, it seems not to increase detection over standard assessment methods and does not influence therapeutic decisions.[83] It has been reported that FDG activity decreases sharply after effective treatment and increases during flare involving sites easily evaluated by FDG-PET/CT, suggesting a possible role in assessing disease activity.[82-84]

Microscopic Polyangiitis and Eosinophilic GPA

Published experience of FDG-PET/CT in microscopic polyangiitis or eosinophilic GPA comes from a case series of six patients.[83] The frequent absence of ample inflammatory foci in these diseases results in low sensitivity of FDG-PET/CT for identifying active disease. However, FDG-PET/CT might be useful for individual difficult cases.

Thromboangiitis Obliterans

A single case series of 10 patients observed arterial uptake in only one subject at diagnosis and in another during follow-up, concluding that FDG-PET/CT is not a useful tool for diagnosis and activity assessment of thromboangiitis obliterans.[85]

FUTURE PROMISING TECHNICAL IMPROVEMENTS

Novel Radiotracers

Novel radiotracers other than FDG can target inflammation and may be promising for diagnosis or activity assessment of vasculitides. Among them, the only radiotracer that has been studied in vasculitides is ^{11}C-PK11195. PK11195 is a ligand of the translocator protein (also known as peripheral benzodiazepine receptor), a protein expressed on activated cells of the mononuclear phagocyte lineage. In one proof of concept study, PK11195-PET/CT identified vascular inflammation in 7/7 patients with active GCA or TA and in none of eight controls with inactive inflammatory diseases, including three patients with inactive TA.[86] In another report, PK11195-PET/CT showed uptake in the temporal arteries of a GCA patient.[87] In the rapidly evolving field of novel radiotracers targeting inflammation, these promising results deserve further confirmation in larger studies. It is worth noting that ^{11}C-labeled compounds require an onsite cyclotron facility, thus limiting their clinical applicability until ^{18}F-labeled radiotracers are available.

Combined PET-MR

Hybrid PET/MR systems are entering clinical use. Hybrid PET/MR scanners have had to overcome considerable technical problems due to interactions that potentially reduces the quality of both images. In the vasculitis field, advantages of integrated PET/MR over PET/CT are: (i) Magnetic resonance can provide anatomical information with much higher soft-tissue contrast and without the radiation dose from CT. (ii) Magnetic resonance can provide functional information, including perfusion, diffusion, and spectroscopy in addition to PET. However, it is worth noting that PET has a much higher sensitivity for functional analyses.[88] (iii) Sparing of radiation exposure associated with the CT scan, which may enable repeated examinations in young patients, for example with TA. At the time of submission, only a single case report describes a PET/MR scan in a patient with vasculitis.[89] The role, advantages, and indications of PET/MR for patients with vasculitides are still to be investigated.

KEY POINTS

- PET can provide sensitive functional information about specific biological processes.
- FDG targets active glucose metabolism. Inflamed tissues as well as many neoplasms and sites of infection are FDG-avid.
- PET/CT coregistration is a major technical advance and allows more precise localization of radiotracer uptake.
- FDG-PET/CT is a sensitive method for the diagnosis of patients with GCA prior to therapy initiation. FDG-PET/CT demonstrates the presence and extent of large-artery involvement in GCA, and may provide prognostic information about the risk of future aortic aneurysms.
- Initiation of therapy lowers the diagnostic accuracy of FDG-PET/CT scans.
- FDG-PET/CT is useful for the diagnosis of patients with TA, although it may be less sensitive than in patients with GCA.
- FDG-PET/CT may uncover mimics of the LVVs, including isolated PMR, some malignancies and periarterial fibrotic diseases. Active atherosclerosis is also FDG-avid.
- FDG-PET/CT may detect vascular as well as extravascular inflammation in conditions with multisystemic involvement.

- During follow-up after therapy initiation, FDG-PET/CT may be useful for evaluating disease activity, although accuracy is lower than in the diagnostic setting.
- Data from PET/CT in small-vessel vasculitides are limited and its use should be restricted to specific questions on an individual basis.
- Costs of FDG-PET scans and radiation exposure remain open issues.
- This is a rapidly evolving field: further improvements in the PET scanners and use of novel ligands might substantially change the role of PET in the vasculitis field.

ACKNOWLEDGMENTS

The authors acknowledge Drs Maria Picchio, Federico Fallanca, Elena Incerti, and Luigi Gianolli (San Raffaele Scientific Institute, Milan, Italy) for the PET scan images in Figure 13.2, and funding from EULAR (ET) and the Imperial College NIHR, Biomedical Resource Centre (JCM).

REFERENCES

1. Kapoor V, McCook BM, Torok FS. An introduction to PET-CT imaging. Radiographics. 2004;24:523-43.
2. Basu S, Kwee TC, Surti S, et al. Fundamentals of PET and PET/CT imaging. Ann N Y Acad Sci. 2011;1228:1-18.
3. Adams MC, Turkington TG, Wilson JM, et al. A systematic review of the factors affecting accuracy of SUV measurements. AJR Am J Roentgenol. 2010;195:310-20.
4. Boellaard R, O'Doherty MJ, Weber WA, et al. FDG PET and PET/CT: EANM procedure guidelines for tumour PET imaging: version 1.0. Eur J Nucl Med Mol Imaging. 2010;37:181-200.
5. Delbeke D, Coleman RE, Guiberteau MJ, et al. Procedure guideline for tumor imaging with 18F-FDG PET/CT 1.0. J Nucl Med. 2006;47:885-95.
6. Guttikonda R, Herts BR, Dong F, et al. Estimated radiation exposure and cancer risk from CT and PET/CT scans in patients with lymphoma. Eur J Radiol. 2014;83:1011-5.
7. Ball EL, Walsh SR, Tang TY, et al. Role of ultrasonography in the diagnosis of temporal arteritis. Br J Surg. 2010;97:1765-71.
8. Muratore F, Boiardi L, Restuccia G, et al. Comparison between colour duplex sonography findings and different histological patterns of temporal artery. Rheumatology (Oxford). 2013;52:2268-74.
9. Bley TA, Uhl M, Carew J, et al. Diagnostic value of high-resolution MR imaging in giant cell arteritis. AJNR Am J Neuroradiol. 2007;28:1722-7.
10. Fuchs M, Briel M, Daikeler T, et al. The impact of 18F-FDG PET on the management of patients with suspected large vessel vasculitis. Eur J Nucl Med Mol Imaging. 2012;39:344-53.

11. Lehmann P, Buchtala S, Achajew N, et al. 18F-FDG PET as a diagnostic procedure in large vessel vasculitis-a controlled, blinded re-examination of routine PET scans. Clin Rheumatol. 2011;30:37-42.

12. Besson FL, Parienti JJ, Bienvenu B, et al. Diagnostic performance of (1)(8)F-fluorodeoxyglucose positron emission tomography in giant cell arteritis: a systematic review and meta-analysis. Eur J Nucl Med Mol Imaging. 2011;38:1764-72.

13. Prieto-Gonzalez S, Depetris M, Garcia-Martinez A, et al. Positron emission tomography assessment of large vessel inflammation in patients with newly diagnosed, biopsy-proven giant cell arteritis: a prospective, case-control study. Ann Rheum Dis. 2014;73:1388-92.

14. Both M, Ahmadi-Simab K, Reuter M, et al. MRI and FDG-PET in the assessment of inflammatory aortic arch syndrome in complicated courses of giant cell arteritis. Ann Rheum Dis. 2008;67:1030-3.

15. Scheel AK, Meller J, Vosshenrich R, et al. Diagnosis and follow up of aortitis in the elderly. Ann Rheum Dis. 2004;63:1507-10.

16. Meller J, Strutz F, Siefker U, et al. Early diagnosis and follow-up of aortitis with [(18)F]FDG PET and MRI. Eur J Nucl Med Mol Imaging. 2003;30:730-6.

17. Blockmans D, de Ceuninck L, Vanderschueren S, et al. Repetitive 18F-fluorodeoxyglucose positron emission tomography in giant cell arteritis: a prospective study of 35 patients. Arthritis Rheum. 2006;55:131-7.

18. Blockmans D, Coudyzer W, Vanderschueren S, et al. Relationship between fluorodeoxyglucose uptake in the large vessels and late aortic diameter in giant cell arteritis. Rheumatology (Oxford). 2008;47:1179-84.

19. Dunphy MP, Freiman A, Larson SM, et al. Association of vascular 18F-FDG uptake with vascular calcification. J Nucl Med. 2005;46:1278-84.

20. Bural GG, Torigian DA, Basu S, et al. Atherosclerotic inflammatory activity in the aorta and its correlation with aging and gender as assessed by 18F-FDG-PET. Hell J Nucl Med. 2013;16:164-8.

21. Lee A, Luk A, Phillips KR, et al. Giant cell aortitis: a difficult diagnosis assessing risk for the development of aneurysms and dissections. Cardiovasc Pathol. 2011;20:247-53.

22. Burke AP, Tavora F, Narula N, et al. Aortitis and ascending aortic aneurysm: description of 52 cases and proposal of a histologic classification. Hum Pathol. 2008;39:514-26.

23. Wang H, Smith RN, Spooner AE, et al. Giant cell aortitis of the ascending aorta without signs or symptoms of systemic vasculitis is associated with elevated risk of distal aortic events. Arthritis Rheum. 2012;64:317-9.

24. Schmidt WA, Seifert A, Gromnica-Ihle E, et al. Ultrasound of proximal upper extremity arteries to increase the diagnostic yield in large-vessel giant cell arteritis. Rheumatology (Oxford). 2008;47:96-101.

25. Diamantopoulos AP, Haugeberg G, Hetland H, et al. Diagnostic value of color Doppler ultrasonography of temporal arteries and large vessels in giant cell arteritis: a consecutive case series. Arthritis Care Res (Hoboken). 2014;66:113-9.

26. Brack A, Martinez-Taboada V, Stanson A, et al. Disease pattern in cranial and large-vessel giant cell arteritis. Arthritis Rheum. 1999;42:311-7.

27. Hautzel H, Sander O, Heinzel A, et al. Assessment of large-vessel involvement in giant cell arteritis with 18F-FDG PET: introducing an ROC-analysis-based cutoff ratio. J Nucl Med. 2008;49:1107-13.

28. Besson FL, de Boysson H, Parienti JJ, et al. Towards an optimal semiquantitative approach in giant cell arteritis: an (18)F-FDG PET/CT case-control study. Eur J Nucl Med Mol Imaging. 2014;41:155-66.

29. Martinez-Rodriguez I, del Castillo-Matos R, Quirce R, et al. Comparison of early (60 min) and delayed (180 min) acquisition of 18F-FDG PET/CT in large vessel vasculitis. Rev Esp Med Nucl Imagen Mol. 2013;32:222-6.

30. Papathanasiou ND, Du Y, Menezes LJ, et al. 18F-Fludeoxyglucose PET/CT in the evaluation of large-vessel vasculitis: diagnostic performance and correlation with clinical and laboratory parameters. Br J Radiol. 2012;85:e188-94.

31. Kerr GS, Hallahan CW, Giordano J, et al. Takayasu arteritis. Ann Intern Med. 1994;120:919-29.

32. Maksimowicz-McKinnon K, Clark TM, Hoffman GS. Limitations of therapy and a guarded prognosis in an American cohort of Takayasu arteritis patients. Arthritis Rheum. 2007;56:1000-9.

33. Nazareth R, Mason JC. Takayasu arteritis: severe consequences of delayed diagnosis. QJM. 2011;104:797-800.

34. Mason JC. Takayasu arteritis—advances in diagnosis and management. Nat Rev Rheumatol. 2010;6:406-15.

35. Meller J, Grabbe E, Becker W, et al. Value of F-18 FDG hybrid camera PET and MRI in early takayasu aortitis. Eur Radiol. 2003;13:400-5.

36. Andrews J, Al-Nahhas A, Pennell DJ, et al. Non-invasive imaging in the diagnosis and management of Takayasu's arteritis. Ann Rheum Dis. 2004;63:995-1000.

37. Karapolat I, Kalfa M, Keser G, et al. Comparison of F18-FDG PET/CT findings with current clinical disease status in patients with Takayasu's arteritis. Clin Exp Rheumatol. 2013;31:S15-21.

38. Santhosh S, Mittal BR, Gayana S, et al. F-18 FDG PET/CT in the evaluation of Takayasu arteritis: an experience from the tropics. J Nucl Cardiol. 2014.

39. Bertagna F, Bosio G, Caobelli F, et al. Role of 18F-fluorodeoxyglucose positron emission tomography/computed tomography for therapy evaluation of patients with large-vessel vasculitis. Jpn J Radiol. 2010;28:199-204.

40. Kobayashi Y, Ishii K, Oda K, et al. Aortic wall inflammation due to Takayasu arteritis imaged with 18F-FDG PET coregistered with enhanced CT. J Nucl Med. 2005;46:917-22.

41. Webb M, Chambers A, A AL-N, et al. The role of 18F-FDG PET in characterising disease activity in Takayasu arteritis. Eur J Nucl Med Mol Imaging. 2004;31:627-34.

42. McAdam LP, O'Hanlan MA, Bluestone R, et al. Relapsing polychondritis: prospective study of 23 patients and a review of the literature. Medicine (Baltimore). 1976;55:193-215.

43. Damiani JM, Levine HL. Relapsing polychondritis—report of ten cases. Laryngoscope. 1979;89:929-46.

44. De Geeter F. Nuclear imaging in relapsing polychondritis. J Clin Rheumatol. 2013;19:55-6.

45. Wang J, Li S, Zeng Y, et al. 18F-FDG PET/CT is a valuable tool for relapsing polychondritis diagnose and therapeutic response monitoring. Ann Nucl Med. 2014;28:276-84.

46. Yamashita H, Takahashi H, Kubota K, et al. Utility of fluorodeoxyglucose positron emission tomography/computed tomography for early diagnosis and evaluation of disease activity of relapsing polychondritis: a case series and literature review. Rheumatology (Oxford). 2014.

47. Saadoun D, Wechsler B, Desseaux K, et al. Mortality in Behçet's disease. Arthritis Rheum. 2010;62:2806-12.

48. Cho SB, Yun M, Lee JH, et al. Detection of cardiovascular system involvement in Behçet's disease using fluorodeoxyglucose positron emission tomography. Semin Arthritis Rheum. 2011;40:461-6.

49. Trad S, Bensimhon L, El Hajjam M, et al. 18F-fluoro-deoxyglucose positron emission tomography scanning is a useful tool for therapy evaluation of arterial aneurysm in Behçet's disease. Joint Bone Spine. 2013;80:420-3.

50. Loh H, Yung G, Bui C, et al. Pulmonary artery aneurysm with false-positive FDG PET in a patient with Behçet disease. Clin Nucl Med. 2010;35:286-8.

51. Gluth MB, Baratz KH, Matteson EL, et al. Cogan syndrome: a retrospective review of 60 patients throughout a half century. Mayo Clin Proc. 2006;81:483-8.

52. Balink H, Bruyn GA. The role of PET/CT in Cogan's syndrome. Clin Rheumatol. 2007;26:2177-9.

53. Tsuno H, Takahashi Y, Yoshida Y, et al. Successful early treatment in a case of Cogan's syndrome. Nihon Rinsho Meneki Gakkai Kaishi. 2012;35:92-6.

54. Orsal E, Ugur M, Seven B, et al. The Importance of FDG-PET/CT in Cogan's Syndrome. Mol Imaging Radionucl Ther. 2014;23:74-5.

55. Blockmans D, De Ceuninck L, Vanderschueren S, et al. Repetitive 18-fluorodeoxyglucose positron emission tomography in isolated polymyalgia rheumatica: a prospective study in 35 patients. Rheumatology (Oxford). 2007;46:672-7.

56. Yamashita H, Kubota K, Takahashi Y, et al. Whole-body fluorodeoxyglucose positron emission tomography/computed tomography in patients with active polymyalgia rheumatica: evidence for distinctive bursitis and large-vessel vasculitis. Mod Rheumatol. 2012;22:705-11.

57. Camellino D, Cimmino MA. Imaging of polymyalgia rheumatica: indications on its pathogenesis, diagnosis and prognosis. Rheumatology (Oxford). 2012;51:77-86.

58. Cantini F, Niccoli L, Storri L, et al. Are polymyalgia rheumatica and giant cell arteritis the same disease? Semin Arthritis Rheum. 2004;33:294-301.

59. Katabathina VS, Restrepo CS. Infectious and noninfectious aortitis: cross-sectional imaging findings. Semin Ultrasound CT MR. 2012;33:207-21.

60. Balink H, Spoorenberg A, Houtman PM, et al. Early recognition of aortitis of the aorta ascendens with (1)(8)F-FDG PET/CT: syphilitic? Clin Rheumatol. 2013;32:705-9.

61. Vaglio A, Salvarani C, Buzio C. Retroperitoneal fibrosis. Lancet. 2006;367:241-51.

62. Moroni G, Castellani M, Balzani A, et al. The value of (18)F-FDG PET/CT in the assessment of active idiopathic retroperitoneal fibrosis. Eur J Nucl Med Mol Imaging. 2012;39:1635-42.

63. Salvarani C, Pipitone N, Versari A, et al. Positron emission tomography (PET): evaluation of chronic periaortitis. Arthritis Rheum. 2005;53:298-303.

64. Vaglio A, Greco P, Versari A, et al. Post-treatment residual tissue in idiopathic retroperitoneal fibrosis: active residual disease or silent "scar"? A study using 18F-fluorodeoxyglucose positron emission tomography. Clin Exp Rheumatol. 2005;23:231-4.

65. Nakajo M, Jinnouchi S, Tanabe H, et al. 18F-fluorodeoxyglucose positron emission tomography features of idiopathic retroperitoneal fibrosis. J Comput Assist Tomogr. 2007;31:539-43.

66. Bertagna F, Treglia G, Leccisotti L, et al. [(1)(8)F]FDG-PET/CT in patients affected by retroperitoneal fibrosis: a bicentric experience. Jpn J Radiol. 2012;30:415-21.

67. Guignard R, Simukoniene M, Garibotto V, et al. 18F-FDG PET/CT and contrast-enhanced CT in a one-stop diagnostic procedure: a better strategy for management of patients suffering from retroperitoneal fibrosis? Clin Nucl Med. 2012;37:453-9.

68. Piccoli GB, Consiglio V, Arena V, et al. Positron emission tomography as a tool for the 'tailored' management of retroperitoneal fibrosis: a nephro-urological experience. Nephrol Dial Transplant. 2010;25:2603-10.

69. Ebbo M, Grados A, Guedj E, et al. Usefulness of 2-[18F]-fluoro-2-deoxy-D-glucose-positron emission tomography/computed tomography for staging and evaluation of treatment response in IgG4-related disease: a retrospective multicenter study. Arthritis Care Res (Hoboken). 2014;66:86-96.

70. Zhang J, Chen H, Ma Y, et al. Characterizing IgG4-related disease with F-FDG PET/CT: a prospective cohort study. Eur J Nucl Med Mol Imaging. 2014.

71. Lee SG, Ryu JS, Kim HO, et al. Evaluation of disease activity using F-18 FDG PET-CT in patients with Takayasu arteritis. Clin Nucl Med. 2009;34:749-52.

72. Lee KH, Cho A, Choi YJ, et al. The role of (18)F-fluorodeoxyglucose positron emission tomography in the assessment of disease activity in patients with takayasu arteritis. Arthritis Rheum. 2012;64:866-75.

73. Cheng Y, Lv N, Wang Z, et al. 18-FDG-PET in assessing disease activity in Takayasu arteritis: a meta-analysis. Clin Exp Rheumatol. 2013;31:S22-7.

74. Tezuka D, Haraguchi G, Ishihara T, et al. Role of FDG PET-CT in Takayasu arteritis: sensitive detection of recurrences. JACC Cardiovasc Imaging. 2012;5:422-9.

75. Arnaud L, Haroche J, Malek Z, et al. Is (18)F-fluorodeoxyglucose positron emission tomography scanning a reliable way to assess disease activity in Takayasu arteritis? Arthritis Rheum. 2009;60:1193-200.

76. Hwang B, Liu RS, Chu LS, et al. Positron emission tomography for the assessment of myocardial viability in Kawasaki disease using different therapies. Nucl Med Commun. 2000;21:631-6.

77. Muzik O, Paridon SM, Singh TP, et al. Quantification of myocardial blood flow and flow reserve in children with a history of Kawasaki disease and normal coronary arteries using positron emission tomography. J Am Coll Cardiol. 1996;28:757-62.

78. Hauser M, Bengel F, Kuehn A, et al. Myocardial blood flow and coronary flow reserve in children with "normal" epicardial coronary arteries after the onset of Kawasaki disease assessed by positron emission tomography. Pediatr Cardiol. 2004;25:108-12.

79. Suda K, Tahara N, Kudo Y, et al. Persistent coronary arterial inflammation in a patient long after the onset of Kawasaki disease. Int J Cardiol. 2012;154:193-4.

80. Bleeker-Rovers CP, Bredie SJ, van der Meer JW, et al. F-18-fluorodeoxyglucose positron emission tomography in diagnosis and follow-up of patients with different types of vasculitis. Neth J Med. 2003;61:323-9.

81. Bleeker-Rovers CP, Bredie SJ, van der Meer JW, et al. Fluorine 18 fluorodeoxyglucose positron emission tomography in the diagnosis and follow-up of three patients with vasculitis. Am J Med. 2004;116:50-3.

82. Ito K, Minamimoto R, Yamashita H, et al. Evaluation of Wegener's granulomatosis using 18F-fluorodeoxyglucose positron emission tomography/computed tomography. Ann Nucl Med. 2013;27:209-16.

83. Soussan M, Abisror N, Abad S, et al. FDG-PET/CT in patients with ANCA-associated vasculitis: case-series and literature review. Autoimmun Rev. 2014;13:125-31.

84. Umemoto A, Ikeuchi H, Hiromura K, et al. Hydronephrosis caused by a relapse of granulomatosis with polyangiitis (Wegener's). Mod Rheumatol. 2012;22:616-20.

85. Hackl G, Milosavljevic R, Belaj K, et al. The value of FDG-PET in the diagnosis of thromboangiitis obliterans-a case series. Clin Rheumatol. 2014.

86. Pugliese F, Gaemperli O, Kinderlerer AR, et al. Imaging of vascular inflammation with [11C]-PK11195 and positron emission tomography/computed tomography angiography. J Am Coll Cardiol. 2010;56:653-61.

87. Gaemperli O, Boyle JJ, Rimoldi OE, et al. Molecular imaging of vascular inflammation. Eur J Nucl Med Mol Imaging. 2010;37:1236.

88. Disselhorst JA, Bezrukov I, Kolb A, et al. Principles of PET/MR Imaging. J Nucl Med. 2014;55:2S-10S.

89. Einspieler I, Thurmel K, Eiber M, et al. First experience of imaging large vessel vasculitis with fully integrated positron emission tomography/MRI. Circ Cardiovasc Imaging. 2013;6:1117-9.

CHAPTER 14

Cutaneous Vasculitis

Sunil Dogra, Vinay Keshavamurthy

INTRODUCTION

Cutaneous vasculitis (CV) is a heterogeneous group of disorders occurring either in isolation or as a part of systemic vasculitis. It can be broadly classified into primary CV, where there is no definitive trigger, and secondary CV, where the causative factors are known (autoimmune diseases, infections, and drugs). Skin is also a common organ involved in systemic vasculitides with a spectrum of lesions, the most common being palpable purpura. Skin is often the first or the predominant organ to be involved because of its abundant vascular supply in the dermis and subcutaneous tissue, hydrostatic pressure within these vascular beds, and proximity to environmental influences. Knowledge of cutaneous manifestations would alert the physician for prompt evaluation and diagnosis.

EPIDEMIOLOGY

The incidence of different vasculitis has shown variations because of nonuniformity in the classification and nomenclature used. Differences in incidence and prevalence may also reflect a different ethnic background, differences in trigger factors, different demography and different environmental factors.

A prevalence study from a multiethnic urban area reported that the prevalence of primary systemic vasculitis was twice as high in individuals of European descent as those of non-European.[1] The prevalence of granulomatosis with polyangiitis (GPA) is more than microscopic polyangiitis (MPA) in northern Europe and the United Kingdom. On the other hand, MPA is common than GPA in southern Europe.[2] Studies from Japan and the United Kingdom also found that GPA was common in the United Kingdom and MPA was common in Japan.[3] These differences were due to the

difference in the genetic makeup of the population, HLA B27 being more common in northern Europe predisposed to formation of proteinase (PR3)-antineutrophil cytoplasmic antibody (ANCA).[4] Certain vasculitides are common in children and in early adulthood. Immunoglobulin A (IgA) vasculitis, Kawasaki's disease, and Takayasu arteritis occur commonly in younger age group, whereas giant cell arteritis and ANCA-associated vasculitis (AAV) are common in the elderly. Other environmental factors such as latitude of residence and sun exposure may also influence the occurrence of different AAV.

In a 15-year prospective study by Watts et al,[5] the incidence of primary systemic vasculitis in a well-defined population in Norfolk between 1989 and 2003 was 19.6/million, GPA 10.2/million, MPA 5.8/million, and eosinophilic granulomatosis with polyangiitis (EGPA) 4.2/million. Cutaneous vasculitis as an idiopathic process limited to the skin was seen in 32–37% of adult patients and as a manifestation of a primary systemic vasculitis in 12–22% of patients.[6] In patients with secondary systemic vasculitis, the most common underlying causes were infections, drugs, and connective tissue diseases. Infections were a commoner cause in south-east Asia and Australia whereas connective tissue diseases were more common in Europe.[7]

CLASSIFICATION AND NOMENCLATURE OF VASCULITIS

Classification of vasculitis is required to group the diseases into homogeneous groups for uniformity in research. However, the classification of vasculitis is challenging and there is a lack of consensus among dermatologists, rheumatologists, and pathologists on a uniform classification system. This is due to multiple factors, including paucity of knowledge regarding etiologies, overlapping clinical features, and few "pathognomonic" or specific signs or symptoms of individual vasculitic disorders.[8]

Zeek in 1952 was the first to propose a classification for vasculitis.[9] Five distinct vasculitides—hypersensitivity angiitis, granulomatous allergic angiitis, rheumatic arteritis, periarteritis nodosa, and temporal arteritis—were described. On the foundation of Zeek's classification many classifications evolved based on etiology, pathogenesis, size of the vessel affected, type of inflammation, organ distribution, clinical manifestations, genetic predispositions, and distinctive demographic characteristics. One of the widely accepted classification systems was that established by the American College of Rheumatology (ACR) in 1990.[10] However, the ACR classification system had many limitations with a lot of overlap between various groups. Further, important disease groups like MPA were not included. With better understanding of the pathophysiology of various vasculitides and availability of accurate serological and imaging techniques, there is a need to update the classification and diagnostic criteria.

Because of the controversies surrounding the classification system, a nomenclature system was introduced. These were a set of definitions that define individual vasculitic group, but are often mistaken for classification or diagnostic criteria. There are currently no diagnostic criteria for the primary systemic vasculitides and physicians must rely on experience and disease definitions. The most commonly used and widely accepted nomenclature system is the Chapel Hill Consensus Conference Nomenclature 2012 (CHCC).[11] Cutaneous vasculitis is broadly divided into infective vasculitis, caused by direct vessel wall invasion by pathogens and noninfectious vasculitis. Noninfectious vasculitis is further classified depending on the size of the predominant vessels involved into large-vessel vasculitis, medium-vessel vasculitis (MVV), and small-vessel vasculitis (SVV). They are subclassified based on etiology (lupus vasculitis, hepatitis B- and C-associated vasculitis), pathogenesis (ANCA-associated versus immune complex SVV), pathology (MPA versus GPA), demographics (Takayasu arteritis versus giant cell arteritis), and clinical manifestations. In the CHCC 2012 nomenclature system, eponyms have been replaced with suitable noneponymous terminology. The recent nomenclature system is adopted in this chapter (Table 14.1).

PATHOGENESIS

The detailed consideration of the pathogenesis of systemic vasculitis is beyond the scope of this chapter. Depending on the disease pathogenesis, CHCC 2012 divides SVV into ANCA-associated SVV and immune complex-associated SVV. We limit our discussion to pathogenesis of these subgroups and single-organ vasculitis of the skin.

Table 14.1 Chapel Hill Consensus Conference 2012 nomenclature of vasculitides

- **Large-vessel vasculitis**
  Takayasu arteritis
  Giant cell arteritis
- **Medium-vessel vasculitis**
  Polyarteritis nodosa
  Kawasaki disease
- **Small-vessel vasculitis**
  – *Antineutrophil cytoplasmic antibody-associated vasculitis*
    Microscopic polyangiitis
    Granulomatosis with polyangiitis
    Eosinophilic granulomatosis with polyangiitis
  – *Immune complex SVV*
    Antiglomerular basement membrane disease
    Cryoglobulinemic vasculitis
    IgA vasculitis
    Hypocomplementemic urticarial vasculitis
- **Variable-vessel vasculitis**
  Behçet's disease
  Cogan's syndrome
- **Single-organ vasculitis**
  Cutaneous leukocytoclastic angiitis
  Cutaneous arteritis
  Primary central nervous system vasculitis
  Isolated aortitis
  Others
- **Vasculitis associated with systemic disease**
  Lupus vasculitis
  Rheumatoid vasculitis
  Sarcoid vasculitis
  Others
- **Vasculitis associated with probable etiology**
  Hepatitis C virus-associated cryoglobulinemic vasculitis
  Hepatitis B virus-associated vasculitis
  Syphilis-associated aortitis
  Drug-associated immune complex vasculitis
  Drug-associated ANCA-associated vasculitis
  Cancer-associated vasculitis
  Others

Pathogenesis of Pauci Immune SVV

Role of B-Cells and ANCA in Vasculitis

Antineutrophil cytoplasmic antibodies were first described by Davies in 1982 in a patient with systemic vasculitis and glomerulonephritis and was later recognized as a serological marker of GPA.[12] Two major types of ANCAs are identified:

1. PR3-ANCA also known as cytoplasmic ANCA
2. Myeloperoxidase (MPO) ANCA also known as perinuclear ANCA (P-ANCA).

PR3 and MPO are not the only autoantigens recognized by ANCAs. Antineutrophil cytoplasmic antibodies specific for other antigens like elastase, catalase, α-enolase, lactotransferrin, bactericidal permeability-increasing protein, and lysosomal associated membrane protein 2 also occur.[13]

Antineutrophil cytoplasmic antibodies are strongly associated with AAV. Conventional enzyme-linked immunosorbent assay (ELISA) using pathogenic linear epitopes shows a strong correlation between titers of P-ANCA and disease activity.[14] Factors that induce the development of pathogenic ANCA by B cells are varied and include genetic and environmental factors. Infections, drugs, and defective immune regulation can produce pathogenic ANCAs. Nasal colonization of *Staphylococcus aureus* is strongly associated with the development of GPA.[15] Molecular mimicry best explains the role of microorganisms, with the development of antibodies against shared complementary proteins that cross reacts with ANCA.[13] The other main environmental triggers are drugs, mainly propylthiouracil, levamisole, minocycline, and hydralazine. Drug-induced AAV frequently have ANCA against PR3, elastase and may also have anti-histone and anti-ds-DNA antibodies.[16] The mechanism of drug-induced AAV is speculative. Hydralazine being a non-nucleoside DNA methylation inhibitor inhibits reverse epigenetic silencing of PR3 and MPO, which could result in increased expression of both autoantigens.[16] No clear mechanisms are known for AAV caused due to propylthiouracil and levamisole, but reactive oxygen species formation has been proposed.[16]

In patients with AAV, there is activation of cytokine-primed neutrophils following which they express ANCA antigens PR3 and MPO on their cell surface. These antigens then interact with circulating ANCA IgG and generate a respiratory burst with production of toxic oxygen radicals, release destructive enzymes and extrude neutrophil extracellular traps.[17] Neutrophil extracellular traps comprising extracellular fibrillary material containing chromatin and granule proteins extruded by activated neutrophils are said to play an important role in the pathogenesis.[18] Histopathological findings in early stages of AAV show extensive neutrophilic infiltration that rapidly progresses to leukocytoclasia and fibrinoid necrosis.[13] These activated neutrophils cause endothelial injury and activate alternative complement pathway that further propagate the disease process by recruiting more neutrophils. Disruption of endothelium allows plasma to spill into vascular and perivascular tissue where activation of the coagulation cascade produces the fibrin strands of fibroid necrosis. Characteristically, immunohistochemistry reveals paucity, if not complete absence of immune complex. These features suggest cellular inflammation as the major pathogenic mechanism.

Role of Regulatory Cells

Dysfunction of T and B regulatory (reg) cells is implicated in the pathogenesis of AAV. Normally T reg cells negatively control the production of pathogenic ANCA by B cells. In patients with active disease, there is a decrease in the FOXP3 positive T reg cells, which normalizes during remission.[19] B cells that have high expression of CD5 and produce IL-10 also have regulatory capabilities. Patients with active AAV have a reduced percentage of circulating CD5$^+$ B cells, whereas most patients in remission have a normal percentage.[20]

Role of Eosinophils

Eosinophils are a part of inflammatory infiltrate in necrotizing small and MVV. Tissue and circulating eosinophilia are characteristic of EGPA and play a role in its pathogenesis. The eosinophil cause tissue damage through direct cytotoxic effects, or indirectly as a result of recruitment and activation of other inflammatory cells.[21] Eosinophilic cationic protein (ECP), CCL 11, CCL 26, and IL-25 secreted by eosinophils are associated with disease activity in EGPA.[21] These cytokines upregulate the Th2 immune response and ECP, TGF-β, and IL-1β are also profibrogenic.[22]

Eosinophilia is also a feature of other vasculitis including GPA and Kawasaki's disease. However, prominent tissue eosinophilia strongly suggests drug-induced vasculitis and helps to differentiate from other SVV.

Pathogenesis of Immune Complex Vasculitis

Immune complex vasculitis are characterized by the deposition of antigen-antibody complex in the vessel wall with subsequent activation of the complement system.[23] An additional pathomechanism is that of direct endothelial cell damage by antiendothelial cell antibodies. The triggers for immune complex are varied, including infections, vaccination, drugs, and tumor antigens. The prototype of immune complex vasculitis is serum sickness. Other disorders with immune complex deposition include IgA vasculitis, hepatitis B and C virus-induced vasculitis, urticarial vasculitis, and cryoglobulinemic vasculitis.

The circulating immune complexes mediating vasculitis interact with the complement system to generate C3a and C5a anaphylatoxins. They subsequently stimulate the production of chemotactic factors and release vasoactive amines and proinflammatory cytokines.[24] Endothelial cell retraction and detachment occur due to altered membrane integrity induced by vasoactive amines and probably by the membrane attack complex of complement.[24] The activated complement system and various other inflammatory cytokines (IL-1, TNFα, and INFγ) secreted cause chemotaxis of neutrophils. These neutrophils in an attempt to engulf the immune complex secrete lysosomal enzymes, ultimately causing inflammation and necrosis of the vessel wall.

APPROACH TO A PATIENT WITH VASCULITIS (FLOW CHART 14.1)

Clinical Presentation

Any suspected patient of CV should have a detailed history with review of systemic symptoms, complete clinical examination, and relevant investigation. Note should also be made of any precipitating factors such as recent infections, drug intake, or any preexisting medical condition. Extracutaneous manifestation of vasculitis such as asthma, allergic rhinitis, and nasal polyps (EGPA); sinusitis, otitis media, epistaxis, stuffiness of nose, and hemoptysis (GPA); hematuria (MPA, GPA, and EGPA); recurrent pain abdomen and previous episodes of bowel infarctions PAN; mononeuritis multiplex (PAN and MPA) should be asked for. Examination of a skin lesion should focus on the type of primary lesion, its

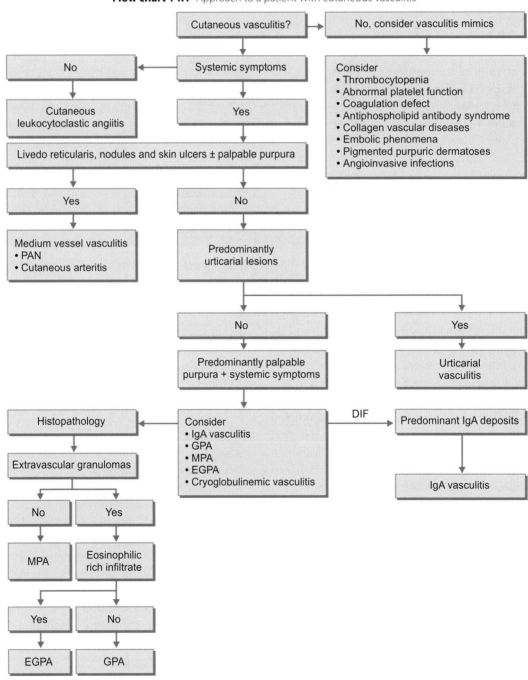

Flow chart 14.1 Approach to a patient with cutaneous vasculitis

distribution, and changes in the surrounding skin. Cutaneous vasculitis has varied presentation in the skin, depending on the type of blood vessel involved. Patients with MVV (PAN and cutaneous arteritis) show livedo reticularis, net-like cyanotic discoloration of skin with pale central areas; bilateral but asymmetrically distributed cutaneous nodules, usually along the blood vessels and punched-out tender skin ulcers. Vasculitis involving the small vessels (AAV and immune complex vasculitis) usually presents with crops of symmetrical palpable purpura over lower limbs and dependent parts of the body. These lesions are usually asymptomatic, but can be associated with itching, burning, and aching pain. Diascopy of purpuric lesions demonstrate partial blanching; the blanchable component indicates underlying inflammation, whereas the nonblanchable component represents hemorrhage (purpura).[25] Other cutaneous manifestations of SVV include vesicles, pustules, skin ulcers, urticarial, erythema multiforme like targetoid lesions and infarction.[26] The specific cutaneous manifestations of different vasculitides are described later in the chapter.

Histopathology

All clinical suspects of CV should have a skin biopsy from a fresh lesion (3–12 hours old) for histopathology and direct immunofluorescence (DIF). A punch skin biopsy will usually suffice when SVV is suspected. Histopathology of SVV classically reveals a polymorphonuclear infiltrate, primarily affecting postcapillary venules, with fibrinoid deposits in and around the vessel wall, endothelial swelling, and extravasation of red blood cells.[27] On the basis of the distribution of vascular inflammation and the presence or absence of granulomatosis and asthma, systemic AAV is categorized as MPA if there is vasculitis without any evidence of granulomatosis or asthma, GPA if there is granulomatosis but no asthma, EGPA if there is granulomatosis, asthma, and blood eosinophilia.[11] An incisional biopsy is required when MVV is suspected since medium-size vessels lie deep in the subcutis that is generally not sampled by punch biopsy. When skin nodules are present they should be preferably sampled. Lesions of PAN show features of leukocytoclastic vasculitis affecting the walls of medium-sized arteries and arterioles of septa in the upper portions of the subcutaneous fat. The involved vessels typically demonstrate a target-like appearance resulting from an eosinophilic ring of fibrinoid necrosis.[28]

Direct immunofluorescence testing in leukocytoclastic vasculitis shows deposits of IgG and/or C3 in vessel walls. Granular IgA deposits in the vessels are indicative of IgA vasculitis. Direct immunofluorescence can be negative in AAV (pauci immune type). Positive rates of DIF vary depending on the type of lesion sampled. The yield is highest when fresh lesions are biopsied.

Lab Evaluation

An isolated incident of CV without systemic symptoms usually follows a benign course and clinical observation without extensive diagnostic workup is a reasonable approach (Table 14.2). An extensive evaluation is warranted when systemic vasculitis is thought of. Serological testing for ANCA is necessary because of its diagnostic and prognostic implication. The international guidelines for ANCA testing recommend screening for ANCA by an indirect fluorescence test and positive test to be confirmed by the ELISA test as an obligatory minimum requirement.[29] In North America and Europe, patients with GPA more often have PR3-ANCA than MPO-ANCA; patients with MPA have similar frequency of MPO-ANCA, and PR3-ANCA, and EGPA; and renal-limited vasculitis patients have predominantly MPO ANCA.[4] In Asia, MPO-ANCA is more frequent than PR3-ANCA in patients with GPA as well as MPA.[30] Double positivity for MPO-ANCA and PR3-ANCA is seen in association with drug-induced vasculitis.[31] Other serological investigations like anti-nuclear antibody, ds-DNA, rheumatoid factor, and cryoglobulins are done when clinically indicated. All patients with suspected systemic vasculitis should have a baseline evaluation of renal parameters. Evaluation for other organ involvement should be guided by clinical suspicion.

Table 14.2 Investigations in cutaneous vasculitis
Initial laboratory screening
• Complete blood count, differential count, and peripheral smear
• Erythrocyte sedimentation rate
• Renal function test
• Liver function tests
• Urinalysis
• Chest radiography
• Stool for occult blood
• Skin biopsy
• Direct immunofluorescence
Targeted investigations
• Antineutrophil cytoplasmic antibodies
• Antinuclear antibody
• Hepatitis B and C serology
• Streptococcal antibodies
• Rheumatoid factor
• Complement levels (C3, C4, total)
• Cryoglobulins
• Serum monoclonal protein study
• Renal biopsy
• Nerve conduction studies
• CT/MR angiogram

Differential Diagnosis

Cutaneous vasculitis should be differentiated from nonpalpable purpura and petechiae associated with thrombocytopenia, abnormal platelet function, coagulation defects, antiphospholipid antibody syndrome, collagen vascular diseases, embolic phenomena, pigmented purpuric dermatoses, and angio invasive infections. Palpable purpura can also occur in conditions that are not vasculitis. This mimicry is apparent in antiphospholipid syndrome and disseminated intravascular coagulopathy presenting with palpable purpura.[32,33] However, skin biopsy of these entities will not show evidence of leukocytoclastic vasculitis.

CUTANEOUS LEUKOCYTOCLASTIC ANGIITIS (CLA, TABLE 14.3)

It is the most common type of CV commonly affecting the postcapillary venules. It is classified as single-organ vasculitis by CHCC 2014.[11] It is commonly caused due to drugs, infection, and connective tissue diseases, but is idiopathic in 50% of cases.[8] Like other SVV, the most common presentation of CLA is crops of symmetrically distributed palpable purpura over lower limb (Fig. 14.1). Cutaneous leukocytoclastic angiitis can preferentially affect the areas of pressure or friction, such as waistbands, belts, shoulder straps, or sock collars. Other cutaneous lesions include urticarial lesions, ulcers, pustules, and vesicobullous lesions (Fig. 14.2). Systemic manifestations like fever, malaise, and joint pain may be complained of, but

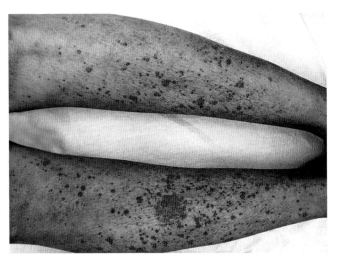

Fig. 14.1 Crops of symmetrically distributed palpable purpura over the lower limb in a case of CLA

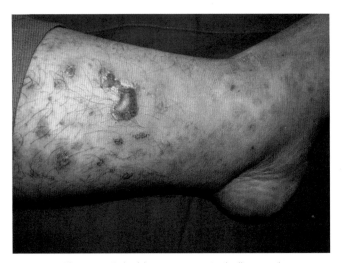

Fig. 14.2 Palpable purpura, vesicobullous and urticarial lesions in a case of CLA

Table 14.3 Etiology of cutaneous leukocytoclastic angiitis*

Drugs (10–15%)
- Antibiotics-β lactams, sulfonamides, and penicillins
- Diuretics
- Nonsteroidal anti-inflammatory drugs
- Anticonvulsants
- Antipsychotics
- TNF-α inhibitors
- Rituximab
- IFN β

Infections (15–20%)
- Viral (HBV, HCV, and HIV)
- Bacterial—staphylococci and streptococci
- Fungal—candida
- Protozoan

Connective tissue disease (15–20%)

Malignancy

Inflammatory bowel disease

Chronic active hepatitis

Idiopathic (50%)

*Source: Marzano AV, Vezzoli P, Berti E. Skin involvement in cutaneous and systemic vasculitis. Autoimmun Rev. 2013;12:467-76.

internal organ involvement is by definition uncommon and should prompt a search for other pathology. The key factor in evaluating CLA is to exclude systemic involvement and identify and remove the offending agent. The natural course is usually self-limiting and most lesions remit once the inciting factor is withdrawn. However, 10% of patients suffer from chronic relapsing and remitting course.[34]

IgA VASCULITIS

IgA vasculitis (IgAV) is an immune complex-type of SVV with predominant deposition of IgA1 in the vessel wall. Previously known as Henoch-Schonlein purpura, this eponym has been replaced by IgA vasculitis by CHCC 2012.[11] Consensus Conference Nomenclature 2012 describes IgAV as "often involving skin and gastrointestinal tract, and frequently causes

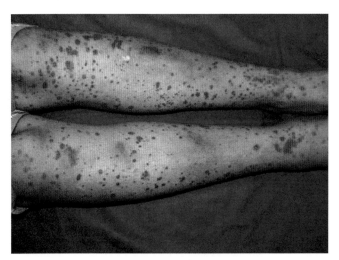

Fig. 14.3 A case of IgA nephropathy for 4 years developed crops of symmetrically distributed palpable purpura over the lower limb with arthritis. DIF showed deposits of IgA in the vessel wall, a feature of IgA vasculitis

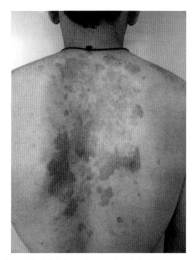

Fig. 14.4 Case of NUV showing urticarial plaques over the back subsiding with postinflammatory hyperpigmentation

arthritis. Glomerulonephritis indistinguishable from IgA nephropathy may occur."[11] In patients with IgAV, IgA1 in serum and in tissue deposits has reduced terminal glycosylation in the hinge region.[35] Also these patients have circulating abnormally glycosylated IgA. Glycan-specific IgG antibodies form IgA1–IgG anti-IgA1 immune complexes.[36] IgG antibodies directed against the abnormal glycosylation putatively bind to IgA1 molecules and localize in vessel walls, causing inflammation.

IgAV is usually a disease of children; most patients range in age from 4 to 7 years. It has a slight male predominance of 1.5:1. A seasonal variation with a peak incidence in spring has been noted. An upper respiratory tract infection can precede the development of IgAV. Though IgAV is characteristically described by the tetrad of palpable purpura, arthritis, bowel angina, and glomerulonephritis, most patients frequently exhibit only a subset of symptoms. Cutaneous involvement is virtually seen in all patients. Palpable purpura, symmetrically distributed, in a retiform pattern, involving the lower limbs and buttocks, is the usual cutaneous manifestation (Fig. 14.3). Lesions distributed above the waist and increasing age are risk factors for renal involvement.[37] Rarely IgAV can be confined to the skin and kidneys, without features of other organ involvement. The latter form is known as IgA nephropathy and should be considered as expressing limited form of the disease. Such patients can progress at any time to develop the full range of IgAV.

URTICARIAL VASCULITIS

It is a chronic remitting and relapsing disorder with predominant skin lesions being urticarial plaques. It

clinically presents with urticated plaques predominantly over proximal extremities frequently with associated angioedema. Of patients with chronic urticaria, approximately 5–10% have UV.[38] Distinguishing features of UV include the symptoms, duration, and resolution of the lesions. Unlike chronic spontaneous urticaria, these lesions last more than 24 hours, have burning/aching pain, show purpuric spots on blanching, and subside with postinflammatory hyperpigmentation (Fig. 14.4). Systemic features like fever, joint pain, and hematuria are common in UV. Urticarial vasculitis is strongly associated with some connective tissue diseases, having a prevalence of 32% in patients with Sjögren's syndrome and 20% in patients with SLE.[38] Two types of UV are described.[39]

1. Hypocomplementemic urticarial vasculitis (HUV)
2. Normocomplementemic urticarial vasculitis (NUV).

Urticarial vasculitis is an immune complex vasculitis. Hypocomplementemic urticarial vasculitis is caused due to anti-C1q antibodies directed against the collagen-like region of C1q.[40] The antigen-antibody complex thus formed gets deposited in the vessel wall, activate complement leading to CV. Glomerulonephritis (20–30%), arthritis, obstructive pulmonary disease (20%), and ocular inflammation (10%) are common features of HUV.[11,32] Normocomplementemic urticarial vasculitis is a self-limited process restricted to cutaneous tissues and carries a favorable prognosis.

CRYOGLOBULINEMIC VASCULITIS

Cryoglobulins are immunoglobulins that reversibly precipitate or gel in the cold. Brouet et al.[41] proposed the now standard classification of cryoglobulins into types I, II, and III. Type I cryoglobulins are monoclonal antibodies of IgG, IgM, and rarely IgA class. They are single proteins and do not form immune complexes. Type I cryoglobulins cause cryogelling and present with acral cyanosis, Raynaud's phenomena, occlusion, infarction, and gangrene. Unlike type I cryoglobulinemia, types II and III (known as mixed cryoglobulins) are multiple molecule proteins that bind to an antigen in the blood (commonly the Fc portion of IgG/IgM, rheumatoid factor) to form immune complex. Cryoglobulinemic vasculitis is caused by deposition of these immune complexes in the vessels. There is a strong association between HCV infection and presence of mixed cryoglobulins. Other infections like Lyme disease, subacute bacterial endocarditis, hepatitis A and B, human T-cell leukemia virus I and HIV, chronic inflammatory disease such as liver cirrhosis, and connective tissue disease are also associated with mixed cryoglobulins.[42,43]

The common cutaneous finding in cryoglobulinemic vasculitis is palpable purpura over the lower limbs, often extending till the buttocks. One-third of the patient may notice cold exacerbation of the lesions. Cutaneous nodules like those in PAN are seen in 20% of cases. Other internal manifestations include glomerulonephritis, arthritis, alveolitis, lung fibrosis, and peripheral neuropathy. A low complement C4 level is found in 90% and rheumatoid factor is positive in 70%.

ANCA-ASSOCIATED VASCULITIS

Antineutrophil cytoplasmic antibody-associated vasculitis (AAV) commonly affects the small vessels presenting as palpable purpura, pustules, vesicles, necrosis, and ulceration. Medium vessels can also be involved and presentation with livedo reticularis and skin nodules are not uncommon. The discussion of the protean manifestation of AAV is beyond the scope of this chapter. Thus, we limit the discussion to cutaneous manifestation of AAV.

Microscopic Polyangiitis

Microscopic polyangiitis commonly presents with palpable purpura over the dependent parts. Petechiae, purpuric macules, urticarial lesions, pustules, and vesicobullous lesions can be seen (Fig. 14.5). Constitutive symptoms like myalgia, arthralgia, fever, and weight loss are usually present. The characteristic systemic complications include necrotizing glomerulonephritis and lung involvement.

Granulomatosis with Polyangiitis

Previously known as Wegener's granulomatosis, this eponym has been replaced by GPA by CHCC 2012.[11] The

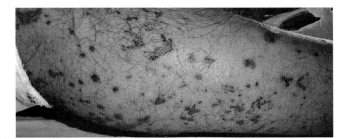

Fig. 14.5 Crops of purpuric macules with angulated margins over the lower limb in a case of MPA

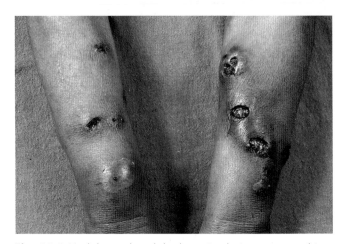

Fig. 14.6 Nodular and noduloulcerative lesions arranged in a linear fashion (along the vessels) in a case of granulomatosis with polyangiitis

CHCC defines GPA as a triad of necrotizing granulomatous inflammation of upper and lower respiratory tract, necrotizing vasculitis affecting small to medium vessels and necrotizing glomerulonephritis.[11] The initial manifestation usually affects respiratory tract with sinusitis, otitis media, epistaxis, hoarseness of voice, and stridor. Granulomatosis with polyangiitis can present with a locally aggressive midline destructive granuloma. Oral involvement manifests as nonspecific erosive/ulcerative lesions or rarely present with strawberry gingivitis, which is a hyperplastic granular gingivitis nearly pathognomonic of GPA.[44] Involvement of lower respiratory tract can present with chronic cough, hemoptysis, and cavitation mimicking tuberculosis. Cutaneous features are seen in 40% of patients and are the presenting feature in 13%.[45] Cutaneous manifestations include lower limb predominant palpable purpura, vesicles, petechiae, and large painful skin ulcer with violaceus, undermined margins, mimicking pyoderma gangrenosum.[46] Rarely, papulonecrotic and nodular and noduloulcerative lesions over extremities can be the presenting feature (Fig. 14.6).

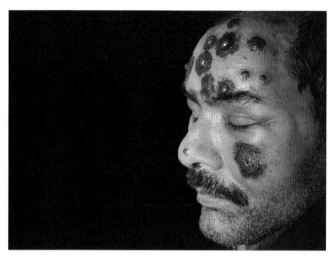

Fig. 14.7 Vesiculobullous, purpuric lesions with surrounding erythema over the head and neck area in a case of eosinophilic granulomatosis with polyangiitis

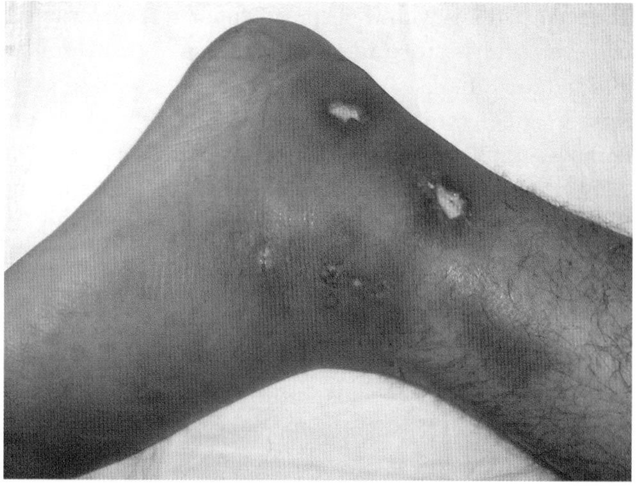

Fig. 14.8 Multiple inflammatory nodules arranged in a group over the ankle with few lesions showing ulceration in a case of PAN

Eosinophilic Granulomatosis with Polyangiitis

Eosinophilic granulomatosis with polyangiitis characteristically progress through three clinical stages.[47] The first phase is characterized by nasal polyps, allergic rhinitis, sinusitis, and asthma and can last up to 30 years. The second stage consists of peripheral blood and tissue eosinophilia leading to pneumonia and gastroenteritis. With an average of 3 years after the onset of asthmatic symptoms, the third phase ensues with systemic vasculitis and granulomatous inflammation. The initial manifestations are nonspecific myalgia, arthralgia, asthenia, and other constitutive symptoms. Palpable purpura distributed over lower limbs and scalp is the most common presentation, but vesicle, bullae, pustules, ulceration, and skin nodules can also be seen (Fig. 14.7).[47,48]

POLYARTERITIS NODOSA AND CUTANEOUS ARTERITIS

Polyarteritis nodosa and its skin limited form cutaneous arteritis predominantly affect the medium vessels, with variable involvement of small vessels. Involvement of internal organ system can present with isolated hypertension, ischemic nephropathy, bowel angina and infarction, testicular pain, myocardial infarction, myocardial infarction, peripheral neuropathy, and ruptured aneurysms. Constitutional symptoms like fever, myalgia, arthralgia, and weight loss are quite common. Cutaneous manifestations are present in nearly 50% of the patients.[32] Characteristic presentations include livedo reticularis and tender inflammatory nodules involving the extremities (Fig. 14.8). These nodules are usually multiple, asymmetrical, and in proximity to a medium-sized vessel. Typical sites involved are the shin, knee, and ankle. Nodules can ulcerate to form punched-out ulcers. Palpable purpura is the most common cutaneous manifestation. Gangrene, infarction, pustules, vesicle, and bullae can also be present. Cutaneous arteritis, previously known as cutaneous PAN, shares similar cutaneous features of PAN, but extra cutaneous involvement is limited to adjacent muscles, nerves, and joints.[49]

TREATMENT

Treatment of various systemic vasculitis is discussed in relevant chapters. We limit our discussion to treatment of single-organ vasculitis of the skin.

In patients of CLA, the primary aim is identification and removal of any precipitating factor. Efforts to minimize stasis, such as use of compression hosiery and elevation of dependent areas, should be encouraged. Nonsteroidal anti-inflammatory drugs and antihistamines can be used to alleviate symptoms associated with cutaneous lesions and arthralgias, but they have little impact on the course of the disease.[23,50]

Treatments depend on the severity and extend of the disease. Since most patients have self-limiting disease, conservative treatment is favored.[26] Patients with extensive cutaneous involvement, severe symptomatic, ulcerative, and necrotic disease and those with chronic disease warrant systemic treatment.[26] A short course of systemic steroids (0.5–1 mg/kg/day) in tapering doses over 2–4 weeks can be given for patients with widespread cutaneous involvement or severe constitutive features. Patients with ulcerative and necrotic disease, chronic disease, who require long-term treatment and those who recur after short course of corticosteroids are treated with steroid-sparing adjuvants. The commonly used steroid-sparing adjuvants include dapsone (2–3 mg/kg/day) and colchicine (0.5 mg twice daily).[33,51] However, the only randomized controlled study to date for colchicine use in vasculitis did not demonstrate efficacy.[52] In patients with disease refractory to these agents, cytotoxic and immunomodulatory drugs like azathioprine, methotrexate, cyclophosphamide, cyclosporine, and mycophenolate mofetil are used.[8,50] Patients with persistent ulceration may benefit from treatment with intravenous immunoglobulin.[53] Rituximab, an anti-CD 20 monoclonal antibody, is tried in recalcitrant cases.[54] Anakinra, IL-1 receptor antagonist, and canakinumab, a long-acting fully humanized monoclonal anti-IL-1β antibody, are reported to be effective in treating UV.[55,56] The evidence for the use of these newer treatment modalities is limited and warrants further evaluation.

KEY POINTS

- Cutaneous vasculitides can occur either in isolation or as a part of systemic vasculitis.
- A spectrum of lesions can occur with palpable purpura being the most common.
- Knowledge of cutaneous manifestations is necessary for early diagnosis and treatment of various vasculitides.

REFERENCES

1. Mahr A, Guillevin L, Poissonnet M, et al. Prevalences of polyarteritis nodosa, microscopic polyangiitis, Wegener's granulomatosis, and Churg–Strauss syndrome in a French urban multiethnic population in 2000: a capture-recapture estimate. Arthritis Rheum. 2004;51:92-9.
2. Watts RA, Gonzalez-Gay MA, Lane SE, et al. Geoepidemiology of systemic vasculitis: comparison of the incidence in two regions of Europe. Ann Rheum Dis. 2001;60:170-2.
3. Fujimoto S, Watts RA, Kobayashi S, et al. Comparison of the epidemiology of anti-neutrophil cytoplasmic antibody-associated vasculitis between Japan and the U.K. Rheumatology (Oxford). 2011;50:1916-20.
4. Scott DG, Watts RA. Epidemiology and clinical features of systemic vasculitis. Clin Exp Nephrol. 2013;17:607-10.
5. Watts RA, Mooney J, Lane SE, et al. The incidence of primary systemic vasculitis—unchanged over 15 years. Arthritis Rheum. 2004;50:S270.
6. Garcia-Porrua C, Gonzalez-Gay MA. Comparative clinical and epidemiological study of hypersensitivity vasculitis versus Henoch–Schonlein purpura in adults. Semin Arthritis Rheum. 1999;28:404-12.
7. Pina T, Blanco R, Gonzalez-Gay MA. Cutaneous vasculitis: a rheumatologist perspective. Curr Allergy Asthma Rep. 2013;13:545-54.
8. Fiorentino DF. Cutaneous vasculitis. J Am Acad Dermatol. 2003;48:311-40.
9. Zeek PM. Periarteritis nodosa; a critical review. Am J Clin Pathol. 1952;22:777-90.
10. Bloch DA, Michel BA, Hunder GG, et al. The American College of Rheumatology 1990 criteria for the classification of vasculitis. Patients and methods. Arthritis Rheum. 1990;33:1068-73.
11. Jennette JC, Falk RJ, Bacon PA, et al. 2012 revised International Chapel Hill Consensus Conference Nomenclature of Vasculitides. Arthritis Rheum. 2013;65:1-11.
12. Davies DJ, Moran JE, Niall JF, et al. Segmental necrotising glomerulonephritis with antineutrophil antibody: possible arbovirus aetiology? Br Med J (Clin Res Ed). 1982;285:606.
13. Jennette JC, Falk RJ. Pathogenesis of antineutrophil cytoplasmic autoantibody-mediated disease. Nat Rev Rheumatol. 2014;10:463-73.
14. Roth AJ, Ooi JD, Hess JJ, et al. Epitope specificity determines pathogenicity and detectability in ANCA-associated vasculitis. J Clin Invest. 2013;123:1773-83.
15. Laudien M, Gadola SD, Podschun R, et al. Nasal carriage of *Staphylococcus aureus* and endonasal activity in Wegener's granulomatosis as compared to rheumatoid arthritis and chronic Rhinosinusitis with nasal polyps. Clin Exp Rheumatol. 2010;28:51-5.
16. Pendergraft WF 3rd, Niles JL. Trojan horses: drug culprits associated with antineutrophil cytoplasmic autoantibody (ANCA) vasculitis. Curr Opin Rheumatol. 2014;26:42-9.
17. Falk RJ, Terrell RS, Charles LA, et al. Antineutrophil cytoplasmic autoantibodies induce neutrophils to degranulate and produce oxygen radicals in vitro. Proc Natl Acad Sci USA. 1990;87:4115-9.
18. Abreu-Velez AM, Smith JG Jr, Howard MS. Presence of neutrophil extracellular traps and antineutrophil cytoplasmic antibodies associated with vasculitides. N Am J Med Sci. 2009;1:309-13.
19. Rimbert M, Hamidou M, Braudeau C, et al. Decreased numbers of blood dendritic cells and defective function of regulatory T cells in antineutrophil cytoplasmic antibody-associated vasculitis. PLoS One. 2011;6:e18734.
20. Morgan MD, Day CJ, Piper KP, et al. Patients with Wegener's granulomatosis demonstrate a relative deficiency and functional impairment of T-regulatory cells. Immunology. 2010;130:64-73.
21. Khoury P, Grayson PC, Klion AD. Eosinophils in vasculitis: characteristics and roles in pathogenesis. Nat Rev Rheumatol. 2014;10:474-83.
22. Zagai U, Dadfar E, Lundahl J, et al. Eosinophil cationic protein stimulates TGF-beta1 release by human lung fibroblasts in vitro. Inflammation. 2007;30:153-60.
23. Lotti T, Ghersetich I, Comacchi C, et al. Cutaneous small-vessel vasculitis. J Am Acad Dermatol. 1998;39:667-87; quiz 88-90.

24. Claudy A. Pathogenesis of leukocytoclastic vasculitis. Eur J Dermatol. 1998;8:75-9.

25. Piette WW. The differential diagnosis of purpura from a morphologic perspective. Adv Dermatol. 1994;9:3-23; discussion 4.

26. Goeser MR, Laniosz V, Wetter DA. A practical approach to the diagnosis, evaluation, and management of cutaneous small-vessel vasculitis. Am J Clin Dermatol. 2014;15:299-306.

27. Russell JP, Gibson LE. Primary cutaneous small-vessel vasculitis: approach to diagnosis and treatment. Int J Dermatol. 2006;45:3-13.

28. Elder DE, Elenitsas R, Johnson BL, et al. Lever's Histopathology of the Skin, 10th edition. Philadelphia: Lippincott; 2008. pp. 185-206.

29. Savige J, Gillis D, Benson E, et al. International consensus statement on testing and reporting of antineutrophil cytoplasmic antibodies (ANCA). Am J Clin Pathol. 1999;111:507-13.

30. Xu PC, Chen M, Zhao MH. Antineutrophil cytoplasmic autoantibody-associated vasculitis in Chinese patients. Clin Exp Nephrol. 2013;17:705-7.

31. McGrath MM, Isakova T, Rennke HG, et al. Contaminated cocaine and antineutrophil cytoplasmic antibody-associated disease. Clin J Am Soc Nephrol. 2011;6:2799-805.

32. Marzano AV, Vezzoli P, Berti E. Skin involvement in cutaneous and systemic vasculitis. Autoimmun Rev. 2013;12:467-76.

33. Callen JP. A clinical approach to the vasculitis patient in the dermatologic office. Clin Dermatol. 1999;17:549-53.

34. Crowson AN, Mihm MC Jr, Magro CM. Cutaneous vasculitis: a review. J Cutan Pathol. 2003;30:161-73.

35. Suzuki H, Kiryluk K, Novak J, et al. The pathophysiology of IgA nephropathy. J Am Soc Nephrol. 2011;22:1795-803.

36. Suzuki H, Fan R, Zhang Z, et al. Aberrantly glycosylated IgA1 in IgA nephropathy patients is recognized by IgG antibodies with restricted heterogeneity. J Clin Invest. 2009;119:1668-77.

37. Tancrede-Bohin E, Ochonisky S, Vignon-Pennamen MD, et al. Schonlein–Henoch purpura in adult patients. Predictive factors for IgA glomerulonephritis in a retrospective study of 57 cases. Arch Dermatol. 1997;133:438-42.

38. Black AK. Urticarial vasculitis. Clin Dermatol. 1999;17:565-9.

39. Wisnieski JJ. Urticarial vasculitis. Curr Opin Rheumatol. 2000;12:24-31.

40. Wisnieski JJ, Jones SM. IgG autoantibody to the collagen-like region of Clq in hypocomplementemic urticarial vasculitis syndrome, systemic lupus erythematosus, and 6 other musculoskeletal or rheumatic diseases. J Rheumatol. 1992;19:884-8.

41. Brouet JC, Clauvel JP, Danon F, et al. Biologic and clinical significance of cryoglobulins. A report of 86 cases. Am J Med. 1974;57:775-88.

42. Trejo O, Ramos-Casals M, Garcia-Carrasco M, et al. Cryoglobulinemia: study of etiologic factors and clinical and immunologic features in 443 patients from a single center. Medicine (Baltimore). 2001;80:252-62.

43. Bonnet F, Pineau JJ, Taupin JL, et al. Prevalence of cryoglobulinemia and serological markers of autoimmunity in human immunodeficiency virus infected individuals: a cross-sectional study of 97 patients. J Rheumatol. 2003;30:2005-10.

44. Stewart C, Cohen D, Bhattacharyya I, et al. Oral manifestations of Wegener's granulomatosis: a report of three cases and a literature review. J Am Dent Assoc. 2007;138:338-48; quiz 96, 98.

45. Hoffman GS, Kerr GS, Leavitt RY, et al. Wegener granulomatosis: an analysis of 158 patients. Ann Intern Med. 1992;116:488-98.

46. Patten SF, Tomecki KJ. Wegener's granulomatosis: cutaneous and oral mucosal disease. J Am Acad Dermatol. 1993;28:710-8.

47. Noth I, Strek ME, Leff AR. Churg–Strauss syndrome. Lancet. 2003;361:587-94.

48. Guillevin L, Cohen P, Gayraud M, et al. Churg–Strauss syndrome. Clinical study and long-term follow-up of 96 patients. Medicine (Baltimore). 1999;78:26-37.

49. Morgan AJ, Schwartz RA. Cutaneous polyarteritis nodosa: a comprehensive review. Int J Dermatol. 2010;49:750-6.

50. Boehm I, Bauer R. Low-dose methotrexate controls a severe form of polyarteritis nodosa. Arch Dermatol. 2000;136:167-9.

51. Callen JP. Colchicine is effective in controlling chronic cutaneous leukocytoclastic vasculitis. J Am Acad Dermatol. 1985;13:193-200.

52. Sais G, Vidaller A, Jucgla A, et al. Colchicine in the treatment of cutaneous leukocytoclastic vasculitis. Results of a prospective, randomized controlled trial. Arch Dermatol. 1995;131:1399-402.

53. Ong CS, Benson EM. Successful treatment of chronic leucocytoclastic vasculitis and persistent ulceration with intravenous immunoglobulin. Br J Dermatol. 2000;143:447-9.

54. Chung L, Funke AA, Chakravarty EF, et al. Successful use of rituximab for cutaneous vasculitis. Arch Dermatol. 2006;142:1407-10.

55. Botsios C, Sfriso P, Punzi L, et al. Non-complementaemic urticarial vasculitis: successful treatment with the IL-1 receptor antagonist, anakinra. Scand J Rheumatol. 2007;36:236-7.

56. Krause K, Mahamed A, Weller K, et al. Efficacy and safety of canakinumab in urticarial vasculitis: an open-label study. J Allergy Clin Immunol. 2013;132:751-4.e5.

CHAPTER **15**

Retinal Vasculitis

Reema Bansal, Mohit Dogra, Amod Gupta

INTRODUCTION

Retinal vasculitis, an inflammatory disease of the vessel walls primarily of the retinal veins, is a sight-threatening condition that, on fundus fluorescein angiography, in the initial stages is characterized, by staining of the vessel walls and nonperfusion of the retina in more severe cases. The clinical appearance of retinal vasculitis is highly variable and may involve focal, segmental, or diffuse perivascular infiltrates with evidence of inflammatory cells in the vitreous body or the aqueous humor.[1] These patients of retinal (peri) vasculitis need to be differentiated from ocular involvement in true systemic vasculitic diseases such as systemic lupus erythematosus (SLE), polyarteritis nodosa (PAN), or temporal arteritis that do not show perivascular infiltrates but may cause occlusion of retinal arterioles or posterior ciliary arteries. They do not show signs of intraocular inflammation.

Retinal vasculitis may be due to primary ocular inflammations or secondarily due to systemic inflammatory or infectious diseases and can be classified as follows.

Primary Retinal Vasculitis

Herein, the primary target of inflammation is the retinal vessels and can be further categorized as follows:
- Localized to the eye
  – Idiopathic
  – Intermediate uveitis of the pars planitis type
  – Frosted branch angiitis
  – Idiopathic retinal vasculitis, aneurysms, and neuroretinitis
- Involving the eye and other organs (primary systemic associations)

- Giant cell arteritis
- Takayasu arteritis
- PAN
- Granulomatosis with polyangiitis (Wegener's granulomatosis)

Eosinophilic granulomatosis with polyangiitis (Churg-Strauss syndrome), essential cryoglobulinemic vasculitis, and cutaneous leukocytoclastic angiitis are rare systemic associations.

Secondary Retinal Vasculitis

Herein, the retinal vasculitis is a prominent feature but is secondary to an inflammatory process not primarily directed against the retinal vessels.
- Localized to the eye
  – Ocular sarcoidosis
  – Birdshot chorioretinopathy
  – Necrotic herpetic retinopathies (*Herpes simplex* virus, and *varicella zoster* virus)
  – Toxoplasmic retinochoroiditis
  – Tuberculosis (TB)
  – Diffuse unilateral subacute neuroretinitis (DUSN)
  – Primary vitreoretinal lymphoma
- Involving the eye and systemic inflammatory disease/others
  – Sarcoidosis
  – Behçet's disease
  – Multiple sclerosis
  – SLE
  – Spondyloarthritis with HLA-B27-associated uveitis
  – Inflammatory bowel diseases
  – Relapsing polychondritis
  – TB

– Syphilis
– Lyme disease
– Viral (Cytomegalovirus[CMV], HIV, and West Nile)
– *Toxocara canis*
– Intravenous immunoglobulins
– Inhalation of methamphetamine
– Cancer associated retinopathy
– Oculocerebral lymphoma

Susac's syndrome, Sjögren's syndrome, rheumatoid arthritis, juvenile idiopathic arthritis, Whipple' disease, and rickettsial diseases are some of the rare systemic associations.

CLINICAL FEATURES

Patients with retinal vasculitis may present with a painless decrease in vision, floaters, metamorphopsia (change in shape of an object) in case of macular involvement, or altered color perception. However, the patients may be asymptomatic if the retinal vasculitis is localized to the retinal periphery.

Fundus examination typically reveals sheathing (whitish–yellow cuffing of blood vessels) of the affected retinal vessels. Retinal hemorrhages are usually present around the areas of involvement (Fig. 15.1). Vitreous inflammation may be present in varying degrees. Vasculitis may be focal when it involves noncontiguous portions of the vessel, or may be diffuse in case of widespread involvement. Systemic inflammatory diseases such as SLE may present as cotton-wool spots due to occlusion of retinal arterioles. Additional evidence of ocular inflammation such as cells in the aqueous humor may accompany retinal vasculitis. Cystoid macular edema (CME) may commonly complicate inflammation in

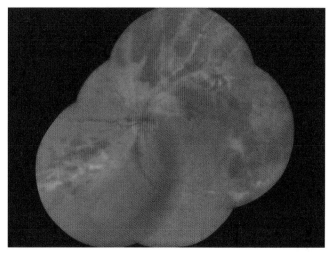

Fig. 15.1 Left eye fundus showing sheathing of retinal vessels with perivascular cuffing and extensive retinal hemorrhages suggestive of active retinal vasculitis

such eyes and lead to reduced vision. Inflammation may involve retinal arteries, veins or capillaries, but peripheral venous involvement is commonly recognized in the fundus.[2] Neovascularization in the retina commonly occurs consequent to significant retinal capillary nonperfusion. Vitreous hemorrhage and tractional retinal detachment are responsible for severe visual loss.

Fluorescein angiography plays a significant role in confirming the diagnosis. Active vasculitis is seen as leakage of fluorescein dye due to breakdown of blood–retinal barrier, and vessel wall staining. More widespread retinal vasculitis is revealed on fluorescein angiography (FA) than clinical examination (Figs 15.2A and B). Areas of capillary nonperfusion are detected on FA that need laser photocoagulation to prevent subsequent retinal neovascularization (Figs 15.3A to C). Optical coherence tomography (OCT) aids in quantitative monitoring of CME during treatment (Figs 15.4A to C).

DIAGNOSTIC WORK-UP

The laboratory evaluation should include a tailored approach, directed by a careful history and physical examination. A relevant systemic evaluation is needed to rule out systemic associations, if any. Random screening with full battery of tests is rarely productive and can be misleading.

Besides subjecting every patient of retinal vasculitis to fundus photography and FA, we perform the following ancillary tests as and when indicated:
• OCT
• Ultrasonography
• Indocyanine green angiography
• Ultrasound biomicroscopy

Laboratory studies that should be done in all patients with isolated retinal vasculitis include:
• Full blood counts
• Erythrocyte sedimentation rate
• Mantoux test
• Chest X-ray to rule out sarcoidosis or TB (Computed tomography if required)
• Syphilis serology (*Treponema pallidum* hemagglutination test)

When strongly suspecting a specific etiology, the following tests are ordered in relevance to the particular disorder:
• Toxoplasma serology
• HIV
• Lyme disease serology
• X-ray of the sacroiliac joints
• C-reactive protein
• Serum angiotensin-converting-enzyme

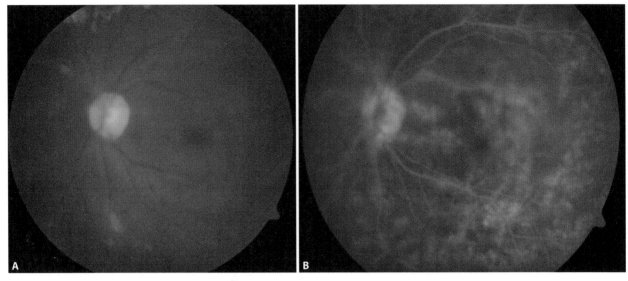

Figs 15.2A and B Fundus photograph showing retinal vasculitis (A) and fluorescein angiogram (FA) showing more widespread retinal vasculitis on FA as seen by vascular leakage (B)

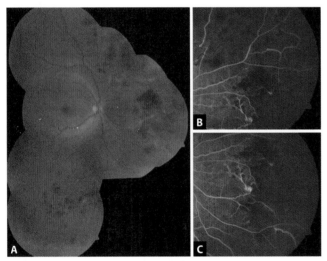

Figs 15.3A to C Right eye retinal vasculitis (A) with areas of capillary nonperfusion as seen on fluorescein angiogram (B and C)

- Human leukocyte antigen typing
  B51 for Behçet's disease, DR3 for SLE, and A29 for Birdshot chorioretinopathy; although Behçet's disease is associated with the HLA-B51 locus, not all patients have this genotype:[3]
- Rheumatoid factor
- Antinuclear antibody for juvenile idiopathic arthritis
- Antineutrophil cytoplasmic antibody
- Polymerase chain reaction (PCR) of intraocular fluids (suspected tubercular or viral etiology)
- Vitreous biopsy (suspected vitreoretinal lymphoma)
- Magnetic resonance imaging
- Cerebrospinal fluid analysis—cytology and cell count

A repeat evaluation and follow-up may be required in cases where laboratory test results do not yield any

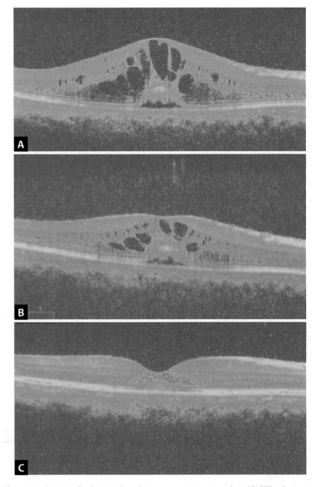

Figs 15.4A to C Optical coherence tomography (OCT) showing cystoid macular edema due to retinal vasculitis at baseline (A). Following initiation of therapy, the OCT showed resolution of edema at 2 days (B), and at 3 months (C)

positive information. A large majority of cases still remain undiagnosed by the routinely available laboratory tests and continue to be labeled as idiopathic.[2]

Certain tests such as liver function and renal function tests are ordered before initiating antimicrobial drugs or during the course of treatment before considering immunosuppressive therapy or while evaluating the adverse effects of some of the treating agents.

Although no signs are pathognomonic of a particular etiology, we discuss some of the common causes of retinal vasculitis, their manifestations, and management.

TUBERCULOSIS

Mycobacterium tuberculosis is considered a common cause of retinal vasculitis in an endemic setting. Presence of a perivascular choroiditis/scar is highly predictive of tubercular etiology (Fig. 15.5).[3] Typically, vasculitis is occlusive that is seen on FA as areas of capillary nonperfusion with or without neovascularization in the fundus (Figs 15.6A and B).

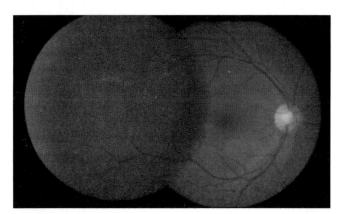

Fig. 15.5 Fundus photograph showing a perivascular choroiditis scar that is highly predictive of tubercular etiology of retinal vasculitis

Consequently, if left untreated, these eyes develop vitreous hemorrhage or tractional retinal detachment (Fig. 15.7).

Diagnosis is made in the presence of typical clinical signs and an evidence of TB infection. Molecular diagnostic techniques like PCR from the vitreous, or less commonly from the aqueous, have been in use since long to confirm the diagnosis.[4] Tuberculin skin test (TST), interferon gamma release assays, chest X-rays and high-resolution CT scans of the chest are done to look for systemic evidence of TB. However, most often, tubercular retinal vasculitis occurs without any concurrent systemic TB. Treatment comprises of oral steroids (1 mg/kg/day) and antitubercular therapy (ATT). Four-drug ATT that includes isoniazid, rifampicin, ethambutol, and pyrazinamide is given for 2 months. Isoniazid and rifampicin are continued thereafter for another 10 months. Liver functions should be routinely monitored. Scatter laser photocoagulation of the ischemic retina should be done to prevent development of new vessels. Vitreous surgery may be required for sight threatening complications such as vitreous hemorrhage or tractional retinal detachment (Figs 15.7 and 15.8). Prognosis is good, and recurrence of inflammation is prevented by the administration of ATT.[5]

HERPES VIRUSES

Herpes simplex virus and *Varicella zoster* virus may be associated with retinal vasculitis, typically with acute retinal necrosis. Necrotizing retinitis and occlusive vasculitis of the arterioles are common clinical presentations in viral retinal vasculitis (Figs 15.9A and B).[6] A significant inflammatory reaction is seen in the vitreous and anterior chamber. The PCR for viruses from ocular fluids helps to confirm the diagnosis. Treatment includes intravenous acyclovir (20–30 mg/kg)

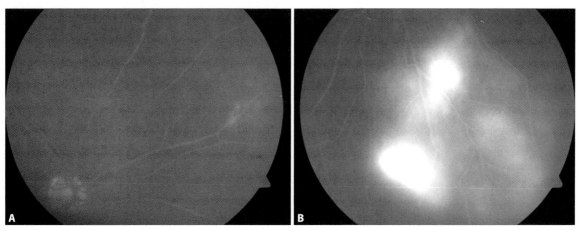

Figs 15.6A and B Fluorescein angiogram showing leakage of fluorescein dye in active retinal vasculitis (A), with neovascularization in peripheral retina (B)

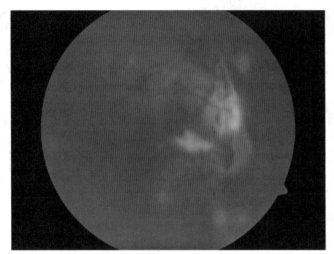

Fig. 15.7 Fundus photograph showing vitreous hemorrhage and tractional retinal detachment following retinal vasculitis

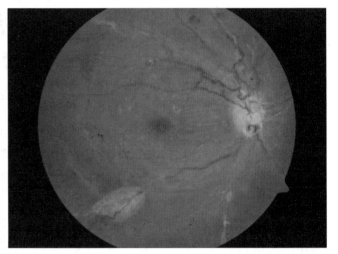

Fig. 15.8 Fundus photograph of the same eye as in Figure 15.7 after pars plana vitreous surgery

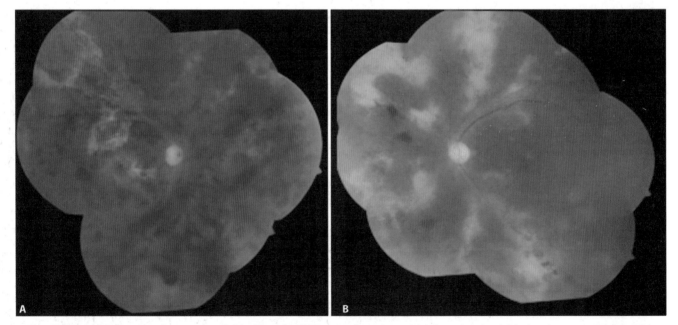

Figs 15.9A and B Fundus photographs of right (A), and left (B), eyes of a patient with bilateral viral retinitis showing extensive vasculitis

three times a day for 14 days, followed by oral antivirals, along with oral corticosteroids. Prognosis is generally poor, as retinal detachment and optic atrophy occur despite treatment. Retinal detachment requires vitreous surgery with silicone oil tamponade.

CYTOMEGALOVIRUS

Cytomegalovirus virus usually causes ocular infection in patients of AIDS or other immunocompromised states. Retinal periphlebitis with retinal necrosis and retinal hemorrhages are the main presenting signs (Fig. 15.10).[7,8] This appearance is also known as the "pizza–pie" appearance. Extensive vasculitis causing a frosted branch angiitis may also be seen.

Prognosis is guarded. HAART along with intravenous ganciclovir and biweekly injections of intravitreal ganciclovir are given, with clinical monitoring of ocular lesions and systemic monitoring of CD4 counts. Maintenance therapy includes oral valganciclovir for 3 months. Retinal detachment may occur, requiring vitreous surgery.

TOXOPLASMOSIS

This parasitic infection is caused by *Toxoplasma gondii*, an obligate intracellular parasite. It occurs due to contamination of food with cat feces. While the cat is a definitive host, humans act as incidental hosts. Retina is commonly involved as a patch of necrotizing retinitis or retinochoroiditis, usually adjacent to a scar of congenital toxoplasmosis.[9] Dense vitritis overlying the lesion is seen. Retinal periphlebitis is seen either surrounding the lesion or in the midperiphery

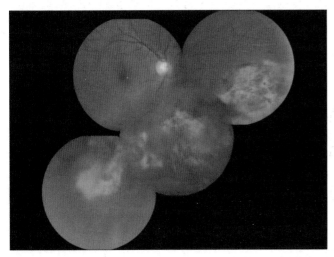

Fig. 15.10 Fundus photograph showing retinal vasculitis in a case of cytomegalovirus retinitis

(Figs 15.11A and B). Focal perivascular exudates simulating arterial emboli (Kyrieleis' arteriolitis) may be seen around or distant to the area of retinitis. Serum IgG and IgM levels of antitoxoplasma antibodies help to corroborate the diagnosis. Vitreous fluid PCR for toxoplasma confirms the diagnosis.

The most commonly used treatment combinations are clindamycin and corticosteroids; or pyrimethamine, sulfadiazine, and corticosteroids. Oral corticosteroids are used to limit the damaging effects of inflammation. Recommended regimen includes tablet clindamycin 300 mg four times daily (3–4 weeks) along with tablet septran-DS 960 mg daily (960 mg sulfamethoxazole and 160 mg trimethoprim) for 3–4 weeks. In recent years, intravitreal clindamycin 1 mg/0.1 mL given twice a week have been found to be highly effective in resolving the toxoplasmic retinitis lesions. Oral corticosteroids (1–1.5 mg/kg/day) are started 48 hours after starting antitoxoplasma therapy, and tapered according to the clinical response. Other drugs that have been used in ocular toxoplasmosis are atovaquone and spiramycin.

SYPHILIS

Syphilis is a sexually transmitted disease caused by a spirochete *Treponema pallidum*. Though ocular involvement is rare, it can mimic any other uveitic entity due to its protean manifestations, thus giving it the name of "great masquerader." Chorioretinitis, macular edema, intermediate uveitis, vitritis, and optic neuritis may occur.[10] Syphilitic retinal vasculitis involves the arterioles mainly, but may involve veins as well.

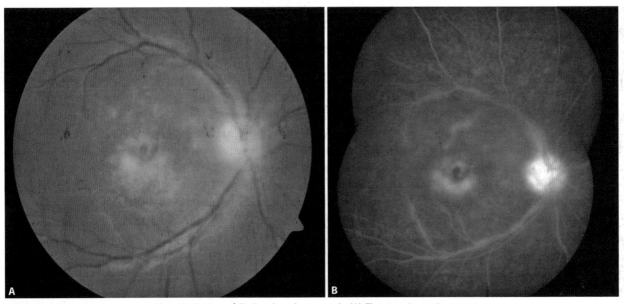

Figs 15.11A and B Fundus photograph: (A) Fluorescein angiogram; (B) Retinal vasculitis in case of toxoplasmic retinochoroiditis

Inflammatory venous or arterial occlusions may occur and leads to neovascularization of the disc and retina. In all cases of retinal vasculitis, syphilis needs to be ruled out to avoid misdiagnosis and timely appropriate therapy.

If ocular syphilis is suspected, CSF tap for VDRL must be done to look for neurosyphilis. HIV status should be checked. Penicillin remains the standard treatment for ocular syphilis.[11] The recommended regimen for treatment of ocular syphilis is the same as that for neurosyphilis, i.e. intravenous crystal penicillin G 12–18 million units/day for 10–14 days, followed by supplementary intramuscular penicillin G 2.4 million units weekly for 3–4 weeks. If the patient is allergic to penicillin, then oral tetracycline 500 mg four times a day for 4–6 weeks is a good alternative.

BEHÇET'S DISEASE

It is a multisystem vasculitis, which affects the skin, eyes, and genitalia. Ocular involvement may be seen as anterior uveitis, with or without hypopyon, vitritis, non-necrotizing retinitis, occlusive retinal vasculitis, or optic disc vasculitis. The criteria laid down by the International Study Group for Behçet's Disease (1990) are used for diagnosis.[12] Retinal vasculitis affects the veins and causes large areas of avascular retina that may cause neovascularization and its sequelae. The FA shows diffuse vasculitis of small capillaries with a "fern like pattern" (Figs 15.12A to F). Optic atrophy may occur due to optic disc vasculitis (Fig. 15.13). Severe sheathing of the vessels may occur and can present as a frosted branch angiitis. HLA-B51 is strongly associated with this disorder.

Although the vasculitis associated with Behçet's disease responds well to systemic corticosteroids, it presents with multiple relapses of inflammation. The long-term consequences of corticosteroids are unacceptable and they are not always suitable as a monotherapy for maintaining remission of vasculitis due to adverse side effects. Often it becomes necessary to add immunosuppressive drug as a steroid-sparing agent.

Cyclosporine A (3–5 mg/kg/day) and azathioprine (2.5 mg/kg/day) are known to effectively control intraocular inflammation, to maintain visual acuity, and to prevent onset or progression of eye disease in ocular Behçet's disease.[13] Recently, novel biologic drugs, including interferon alpha and tumor necrosis factor-alpha antagonists, have been introduced in the treatment of ocular Behçet's disease with very promising results and seem for the first time to improve the prognosis of the disease. Unfortunately, these new drugs are very expensive and therefore they may be not universally available in countries with a low economic status.

SARCOIDOSIS

It is a multisystem granulomatous disease, which affects the lymph nodes, lungs, skin, and eyes. Ocular involvement may be seen as acute or chronic anterior uveitis, intermediate uveitis, multifocal choroiditis, optic disc granuloma, or retinal vasculitis.[14-16] Vasculitis appears as sheathing of vessels and profuse perivascular leakage of fluid and hard exudates, resembling the "melted wax of a candle." Vasculitis is segmental, usually nonocclusive, and involves larger retinal veins than in Behçet's disease (Fig. 15.14). Occlusive vasculitis is less common, unlike tubercular vasculitis. Optic nerve head involvement is more commonly associated with sarcoidosis than in TB. Choroiditis, if present, tends to be more multifocal and peripheral, as opposed to tubercular vasculitis. Diagnosis is by clinical features, a negative TST, chest X-ray, or CT chest suggestive of involvement of mediastinal lymph nodes and lung parenchyma. A transbronchial biopsy or needle aspiration is done to confirm the diagnosis by demonstrating noncaseating granulomas. Serum ACE levels and lysozyme levels may be raised in some cases.

Oral steroids are the mainstay of treatment and are administered in consultation with the pulmonologist. Immunosuppressant therapy is rarely needed. Prognosis for visual recovery is good.

SYSTEMIC VASCULITIS GRANULOMATOSIS WITH POLYANGIITIS (WEGENER'S GRANULOMATOSIS), POLYARTERITIS NODOSA, AND TAKAYASU'S ARTERITIS

These are life-threatening systemic necrotizing vasculitic entities with multisystem involvement. Wegener's granulomatosis affects the upper and lower respiratory tract, eyes and kidneys. Ocular involvement is severe and includes necrotizing scleritis, corneal involvement as peripheral ulcerative keratitis (PUK), or retinal artery or vein occlusion, or optic nerve vasculitis.[17]

Ocular involvement in PAN may involve inflammation of orbital vessels, scleritis, PUK, papillitis, or ischemic optic neuropathy.[18] Retinal vasculitis mainly affects the arteries, and may cause central retinal artery occlusion. Choroidal vessels may also be affected.

Prognosis is guarded and warrants high dose pulse steroids with intravenous cyclophosphamide in consultation with the rheumatologist.

Typically a chronic granulomatous necrotizing vasculitis mainly affecting the large- and medium-sized arteries, Takayasu's arteritis is due to inflammation around the vasa

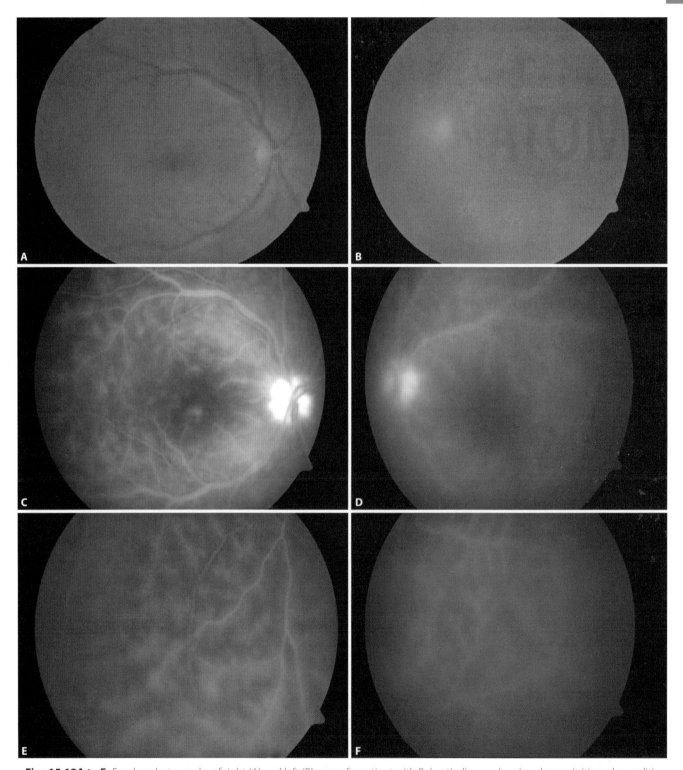

Figs 15.12A to F Fundus photographs of right (A) and left (B) eyes of a patient with Behçet's disease showing dense vitritis and vasculitis. Fluorescein angiography shows vascular leakage in posterior pole (C and D) and peripheral retina (E and F)

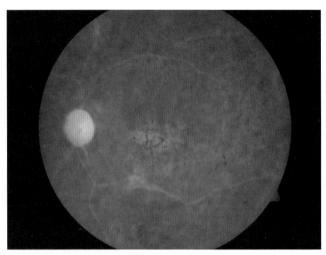

Fig. 15.13 Fundus photograph showing optic atrophy following optic disc vasculitis in a case of Behçet's disease

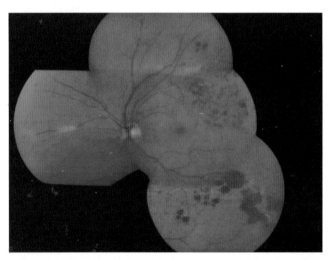

Fig. 15.14 Fundus photograph showing segmental perivascular cuffing with active retinal vasculitis in a case of sarcoidosis

vasorum. Ophthalmic manifestations, though rare, are caused by ocular hypotension secondary to carotid artery involvement, or ocular hypertension secondary to renal artery involvement.[19] Visual morbidity results from ischemic retinopathy and branch retinal artery occlusions.

FROSTED BRANCH ANGIITIS

This is a morphological description of extensive perivascular sheathing of vessels, giving the appearance of frosted branches of a tree. It may be seen in CMV retinitis, sarcoidosis, toxoplasmosis, leukemia, or Behçet's disease. Treatment is that of the underlying cause.

Idiopathic Retinal Vasculitis, Aneurysms and Neuroretinitis

It is a rare syndrome, which affects young females more commonly than males, without any systemic association. It is characterized by bilateral retinal vasculitis, multiple aneurysmal dilatations of the retinal arterioles, and neuroretinitis. Extensive peripheral retinal vascular occlusion is seen. Massive exudative response and neovascular sequelae of retinal ischemia produce visual loss. The characteristic "light bulb" appearance of the arteriolar aneurysms is diagnostic on FA. Scatter laser of peripheral nonperfusion areas with immunosuppressive therapy is indicated.

Complications of Retinal Vasculitis

- *Macular edema:* It is the most common cause of vision loss in retinal vasculitis. Oral corticosteroids, or more recently, sustained release intravitreal dexamethasone implants (Ozurdex) are effective in treating macular edema.
- *Vitreous hemorrhage and/or tractional retinal detachment:* These are the neovascular sequelae of retinal ischemia seen in many forms of occlusive retinal vasculitis. They cause severe vision loss. Intravitreal injections of antivascular growth factor are effective in some patients of vitreous hemorrhage. Others require vitreous surgery for nonresolving vitreous hemorrhage or retinal detachment (tractional or combined). Despite anatomic success, the functional outcome in these eyes with retinal detachment is generally poor.
- *Epiretinal membrane:* Surgical intervention is needed for these membranes causing macular edema and visual loss.
- *Neovascular glaucoma:* End stage of all untreated occlusive retinal vasculitis is neovascular glaucoma with anterior segment neovascularization. These eyes have poor vision and high intraocular pressures. Prognosis for vision is extremely poor.

KEY POINTS

- The treatment of retinal vasculitis has two main goals:
  - To prevent vision-threatening complications
  - When feasible, to treat the underlying disease.
- Identification of infectious or noninfectious systemic associations warrants initiation of specific therapy, besides conventional corticosteroids.
- The prognosis for patients with retinal vasculitis is variable, reflecting the heterogeneous nature of this group of disorders.

REFERENCES

1. Graham E, Spalton DJ, Sanders MD. Immunological investigations in retinal vasculitis. Trans Ophthalmol Soc U K. 1981;101:12-6.
2. Sanders MD. Duke-elder lecture. Retinal arteritis, retinal vasculitis and autoimmune retinal vasculitis. Eye. (Lond) 1987;1:441-65.
3. Gupta A, Bansal R, Gupta V, et al. Ocular signs predictive of tubercular uveitis. Am J Ophthalmol. 2010;149:562-70.
4. Gupta A, Gupta V, Arora S, et al. PCR-positive tubercular retinal vasculitis: clinical characteristics and management. Retina. 2001;21:435-44.
5. Bansal R, Gupta A, Gupta V, et al. Role of anti-tubercular therapy in uveitis with latent/manifest tuberculosis. Am J Ophthalmol. 2008;146:772-9.
6. Tran TH, Stanescu D, Caspers-Velu L, et al. Clinical characteristics of acute hsv-2 retinal necrosis. Am J Ophthalmol. 2004;137:872-9.
7. Culbertson WW. Infections of the retina in aids. Int Ophthalmol Clin. 1989;29:108-18.
8. Spaide RF, Vitale AT, Toth IR, et al. Frosted branch angiitis associated with cytomegalovirus retinitis. Am J Ophthalmol. 1992;113:522-8.
9. Theodossiadis P, Kokolakis S, Ladas I, et al. Retinal vascular involvement in acute toxoplasmic retinochoroiditis. Int Ophthalmol. 1995;19:19-24.
10. Tamesis RR, Foster CS. Ocular syphilis. Ophthalmology. 1990;97:1281-7.
11. Browning DJ. Posterior segment manifestations of active ocular syphilis, their response to a neurosyphilis regimen of penicillin therapy, and the influence of human immunodeficiency virus status on response. Ophthalmology. 2000;107:2015-23.
12. ISGBD. Criteria for diagnosis of Behçet's disease. Lancet. 1990;335:1078-80.
13. Okada AA. Drug therapy in Behçet's disease. Ocul Immunol Inflamm. 2000;8:85-91.
14. Jabs DA, Johns CJ. Ocular involvement in chronic sarcoidosis. Am J Ophthalmol. 1986;102:297-301.
15. Obenauf CD, Shaw HE, Sydnor CF, et al. Sarcoidosis and its ophthalmic manifestations. Am J Ophthalmol. 1978;86:648-55.
16. Rothova A. Ocular involvement in sarcoidosis. Br J Ophthalmol. 2000;84:110-6.
17. Bullen CL, Liesegang TJ, McDonald TJ, et al. Ocular complications of Wegener's granulomatosis. Ophthalmology. 1983;90:279-90.
18. Morgan CM, Foster CS, D'Amico DJ, et al. Retinal vasculitis in polyarteritis nodosa. Retina. 1986;6:205-9.
19. Chun YS, Park SJ, Park IK, et al. The clinical and ocular manifestations of Takayasu arteritis. Retina. 2001;21:132-40.

CHAPTER 16

Cardiac Manifestations

Rajesh Vijayvergiya, Saujatya Chakraborty

INTRODUCTION

Systemic vasculitis is basically an inflammatory disease of arteries involving various organ system. Cardiac involvement is not a predominant presentation in most of the cases. Prevalence of primary cardiac involvement varies depending upon type of vasculitis. It is rare in giant cell arteritis (GCA) and microscopic polyangiitis while frequently seen in Churg-Strauss syndrome, Kawasaki's, and Takayasu's disease. Cardiac manifestations can be secondary to drugs, such as glucocorticoids and disease modifying agents, or as a consequence to other diseases, such as hypertension, diabetes mellitus, renal failure, and obesity, which is frequently observed with progression and chronicity of systemic vasculitis. All cardiac components such as pericardium, myocardium, cardiac valves, endocardium, and coronary arteries can be involved. As cardiac manifestation is subtle, a high clinical suspicion is required for early diagnosis and management.

PATHOGENESIS

Cardiac involvement is explained by multiple inter-related pathogenetic pathways. Each pathway is described in the following paragraphs.

Autoimmune Pathway

Antineutrophil cytoplasmic antibodies (ANCA) are directed against antigens present in neutrophil granules. Neutrophils which are primed with cytokines and tumor necrosis factor-α (TNFα) expresses proteinase 3 antigens on their surface. These antigen expressed neutrophils are then targeted by ANCA. Activated neutrophils then become adherent to endothelial surface and lyse it with nitric oxide, reactive oxygen species, and lytic molecules such as elastase.[1] Neutrophil apoptosis is also dysregulated in ANCA-associated vasculitis, resulting in their accumulation at damaged endothelial surface.[2] Neutrophil bound myeloperoxidase and proteinase help in endothelial adherence and apoptosis.[3] An increased number of circulating necrotic endothelial cells are found in active ANCA-positive vasculitis, compared to patients in relapse or ANCA-negative vasculitis.[4] Progression of vascular injury is also mediated by T-cell-mediated pathways, which is activated by neutrophilic myeloperoxidase and protease.[3]

Cytokines also play an important role in activating endothelial cells to express adhesion molecules which then attract neutrophils. This aspect is well studied in pathogenesis of GCA.[5] Two important cytokine clusters interleukin-6–interleukin-17 axis and the interleukin-12–interferon-γ axis have been identified, which activate various inflammatory cell types like T_H1, T_H17, NK cells, macrophages, and dendritic cells. These activated cells travel via the vasa vasorum to the adventitial-medial interface and initiate cellular damage.[5] Cytokines also act as chemoattractants for neutrophils and stimulate fibrosis via transforming growth factor β.

Deposition of circulating immune complexes in the vessel wall and microvasculature is another mechanism, which is prominently seen in cryoglobulinemic and immunoglobulin A associated vasculitis.[6] It leads to chemotaxis of neutrophils and complement activation.

Accelerated Atherosclerosis

Chronic inflammation plays an important role in pathogenesis of atherosclerosis. Atherosclerosis is initiated by endothelial injury and expression of various adhesion molecules, similar to an observation in systemic vasculitis. Endothelial dysfunction is seen in both the diseases. This leads to plaque formation and progression in vasculitic lesions.[7] Following initial process of endothelial injury and recruitment of inflammatory cells, a proinflammatory prothrombotic milieu in intima-media section of the vessel wall is prominent in atherosclerosis. Autoantibodies such as antiendothelial cell antibodies (ANCA), and antiphospholipid antibodies are known to cause endothelial injury in the systemic vasculitis. Subsequent chemotaxis is mediated by chemokines, which are elevated in vasculitis. Important chemokines, such as CCL-2/MCP-1 and CCL5 which are implicated in atherosclerosis, are also elevated in the systemic vasculitis.[8] The next important step in atherosclerosis is conversion of monocytes to macrophages and foam cells. Toll-like receptors on macrophages which increases in infection-related vasculitis, helps in uptake of oxidized low-density lipoprotein.[9] Another important inflammatory cells found in both the processes are T-lymphocytes. Activation of proinflammatory T-cells such as CD4+, CD28 - T-cells and diminished number of regulatory T-cells is seen in both types of lesions.[10] Increased intimal medial thickness and elevated inflammatory serum markers have been found in Wegener's granulomatosis.[11] Aortic calcification is frequently observed in Takayasu's aortoarteritis.[12] Atherosclerotic lesions are more common in Takayasu's aortoarteritis than controls.[13] Endothelial dysfunction as assessed by brachial artery reactivity and pulse wave velocity has been demonstrated in Kawasaki's disease,[14,15] though other studies do not support it.[15] These findings are suggestive of a common and overlapped mechanism for both vasculitis and atherosclerosis.

Iatrogenic Causes

Prolonged glucocorticoid therapy is known to accelerate coronary artery disease. It causes dyslipidemia, impaired glucose tolerance, and hypertension.[16] Anthracycline analogs are known to cause acute myocarditis and cardiomyopathy.[17] However, both therapies also control the cardiovascular manifestation in active state. Steroids are known to improve endothelial dysfunction in vasculitic states.[18,19] Multiple cardiovascular risk factors, such as diabetes mellitus, hypertension, renal dysfunction, decreased physical activity, and weight gain, which develop during the course of disease also affect the cardiovascular system.[20]

SPECIFIC VASCULITIS

Giant Cell Arteritis

Giant cell arteritis is a granulomatous affection of the aorta and its major branches, with a predilection for the carotid arteries and their branches. It is a well-known entity in northern Europe but has been occasionally reported in India.[21] Limited case reports are available regarding cardiac involvement in GCA. There are few published reports of pericarditis and pericardial effusion in GCA.[22] Pericardial disease can be due to vasculitic process, but the relative rarity of this manifestation necessitates evaluation for more common causes such as infection or drugs.[22] Coronary arteritis manifesting as myocardial infarction and sudden cardiac death is also reported. A recent cohort study found incidence rate of myocardial infarction, cerebrovascular accident, and peripheral arterial disease as 10.0, 8.0, and 4.2 per 1000 patient-years, respectively.[23] Older patients with GCA may have concomitant risk factors contributing to obstructive, atherosclerotic coronary artery disease. It is important to differentiate atherosclerosis from active vasculitis, as treatment strategy is different in both. Myocarditis in GCA is extremely rare and limited to case reports.[24] Increased levels of immunosuppression are usually effective as treatment.

POLYARTERITIS NODOSA

Cardiac involvement is not frequent in polyarteritis nodosa (PAN). The clinical presentation is secondary to coronary arteritis, cardiomyopathy, and pericarditis. Coronary arteritis can present with myocardial infarction and sudden cardiac death.[25] There can be stenosis or aneurysm formation following arteritis.[26] Cardiomyopathy is frequently seen, specifically in those with hepatitis B-associated PAN.[27]

GRANULOMATOSIS WITH POLYANGIITIS (WEGENER'S)

All cardiac structures and conduction tissue can be involved in Wegener's granulomatosis. Though clinically silent, pathological involvement is more common and found in about one-third of patients.[28] Coronary arteries and pericardium are predominantly involved.[29] Coronary arteritis leads to ischemia and systolic dysfunction, which responds well to immunosuppression.[30-32] Pericardial involvement usually presents with acute pericarditis and effusion.[33] Fibrinous constrictive pericarditis is occasionally reported.[34,35] Inflammatory valvulitis can lead to mitral and aortic regurgitation.[36] Atrial tachycardia and atrioventricular conduction block can be there with associated myocarditis.[29,37,38]

EOSINOPHILIC GRANULOMATOSIS WITH POLYANGIITIS (CHURG-STRAUSS SYNDROME)

Cardiac involvement is frequently seen in Churg-Strauss syndrome. Six out of ten autopsy cases showed cardiac involvement in initial description of syndrome.[39] Recent imaging studies have also shown frequent cardiac involvement in it.[40] In one of the study, while clinical symptoms were present in 25% of patients, echocardiography and MRI revealed cardiac involvement in 50% and 62% patients, respectively. Forty percent of asymptomatic patients were found to have cardiac involvement.[40] Both gadolinium-enhanced cardiac MRI and positron emission tomography may reflect cardiac fibrosis and inflammation during disease course.[41,42] Clinically, cardiac involvement is seen in 16%–47% of cases.[37,43] Cardiomyopathy is a common clinical presentation. Symptoms of dyspnea because of cardiomyopathy should be differentiated from disease process of lung or naso-oropharyngeal region. Cardiomyopathy is usually associated with ANCA negativity and higher eosinophil counts.[44] Eosinophilic infiltration leads to myocardial cell loss and fibrosis.[45] Cardiomyopathy is a common cause of mortality and its onset leads to poor prognosis.[37,46,47] A pericardial involvement can present with pericardial effusion and acute or chronic pericarditis.[40,48] Valvular involvement is in form of mitral or aortic regurgitation, which may not be clinically apparent.[40] Cardiac masses have been reported due to granulomatous inflammation or thrombus formation.[49] Conduction blocks and ventricular arrhythmias are also reported.[50] Coronary arteritis is rarely seen, presented with stenosis or aneurysm formation.[51,52]

MICROSCOPIC POLYANGIITIS

Cardiac involvement is not thoroughly assessed in this relatively newer entity. In the French Vasculitis study, about 18% and 10% of patients developed heart failure and pericarditis, respectively. According to the data from same group, 2.4% of patients had coronary ischemia and myocardial infarction in microscopic polyangiitis.[53] Unusual presentations include acute heart failure,[54] aortic valve insufficiency,[55] and giant coronary artery aneurysm.[56]

CRYOGLOBULINEMIC VASCULITIS

Symptomatic cardiac involvement is rare in this infrequently diagnosed disease. In one of the study, 7 out of 165 patients developed cardiac manifestations.[57] Cardiac manifestations are in form of the right or the left heart failure, pericardial effusion, and hypertrophic cardiomyopathy. Patients with cardiac involvement had more skin and gastrointestinal involvement with greater risk of developing B-cell non-Hodgkin's lymphoma.[57] In an another study, 4 out of 49 patients had myocardial infarction.[58] Other manifestations can be pericarditis and mitral regurgitation.[58] Coronary

vasculitis has also been found reported in postmortem studies.[59]

KAWASAKI'S DISEASE

Kawasaki's disease is inflammatory vasculitis of medium- and small-sized arteries with special predilection to coronary arteries. Its etiopathogenesis is not very clear. Though, disease occurs during childhood, its undiagnosed coronary sequelae usually present in adulthood as acute coronary event. In acute stage, Kawasaki's disease can involve all the three layers of heart along with coronary arteries. About 50% of patients have myocardial involvement in acute phase.[60] Many a times, it resolves without any sequelae.[61] Pericarditis usually resolved without a long-term sequelae.[62] Mitral or aortic regurgitation can also be noticed in acute phase.[63] Coronary arteries are involved in about 20% of all cases. Coronary arteritis can be demonstrated by increased echogenicity of proximal segment of coronary arteries during acute phase of the disease.[64] Coronary artery dilatation, ectasia, or aneurysm can be demonstrated during initial 3–4 weeks of illness. Echocardiographic evaluation of proximal coronary segments, mid-distal right coronary artery, and posterior descending artery are of use to demonstrate coronary aneurysm during acute phase of illness.[65] Untreated patients during acute phase are more likely to develop coronary aneurysm. Early institution of intravenous immunoglobulin therapy has a salutary effect on retarding the progress of such lesions.[63] In the later phase, coronary aneurysm can further progress, developed stenosis or occlusion, and even can totally regress. Kato H ST, et al. had shown that 55% coronary aneurysms regresses over 10–21 years follow-up, while ischemic heart disease and myocardial infarction develops in 4.7% and 1.9%, respectively.[66] Computed tomography or conventional coronary angiography is needed for exact extent of coronary disease and in the presence of certain lesions such as stenosis, thrombosis, occlusion, or medium- to large-sized aneurysms. Cardiac MRI is a promising method of surveillance in patients with permanent sequelae, especially when it can be combined with functional assessment.[67]

TAKAYASU ARTERITIS

Cardiac involvement is common in Takayasu's arteritis. Obstructive coronary artery disease, aortic regurgitation, and left ventricular systolic dysfunction are few of the common manifestations. In one of the study of 225 patients of Takayasu's arteritis, 12% had coronary involvement.[68] Coronary ostia along with ascending aorta are typically involved, though diffuse proximal disease of both the right and the left coronary artery is also reported (Fig. 16.1).[68,69] Along with arteritis, accelerated atherosclerosis also contribute in lesion progression in coronary arteries.[13] Calcification is frequently noticed in these lesions.[12] Spontaneous coronary dissections can also be seen (Fig. 16.2). The clinical presentation can be stable angina, myocardial infarction, and even sudden cardiac death. Aortic regurgitation is found up to one-third of patients.[70] Aortic regurgitation is either because of annulus dilatation secondary to hypertension, aortoannulus ectasia, aneurysm formation or following valvulitis

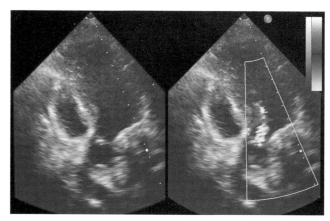

Fig. 16.3 Two-dimensional echo in a case of Takayasu's arteritis showing thickened aortic valve with mild aortic regurgitation

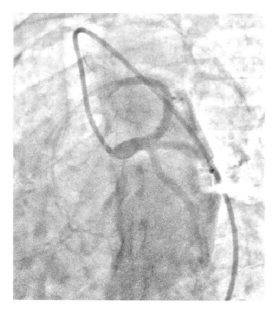

Fig. 16.1 The left main coronary artery osteal stenosis in a 29-year-old girl with Takayasu's arteritis

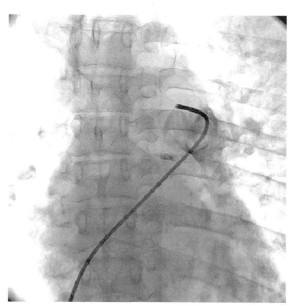

Fig. 16.4 The right pulmonary artery origin block in a 32-year-old girl having pulmonary artery systolic pressure of 62 mm Hg

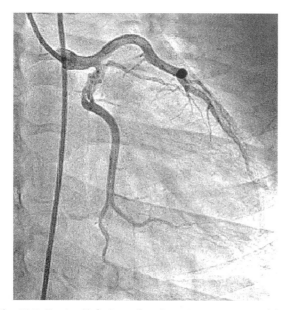

Fig. 16.2 Proximal left circumflex dissection in a 15-year-old girl with Takayasu's arteritis

and fibrous retraction of aortic leaflets (Fig. 16.3).[71] Left ventricular systolic dysfunction is common and is secondary to prolonged hypertension, ischemic heart disease, or following myocarditis. Inflammation of the myocardium with lymphocyte/mononuclear cell infiltration and nonspecific changes of dilated cardiomyopathy have been reported.[72,73] Pulmonary artery hypertension secondary to raised left heart filling pressure or pulmonary artery occlusion is frequently reported (Fig. 16.4).[74,75]

BEHÇET'S DISEASE

Behçet's disease is inflammatory perivasculitis of both arteries and veins. Cardiac involvement is present in less than 10% of cases.[76] Most of the cases have pericarditis, though myocarditis, valvular insufficiency, coronary arteritis, intracardiac thrombus, and endomyocardial fibrosis is also being reported.[77] A venous involvement can lead to deep vein thrombosis and pulmonary thromboembolism.[78]

KEY POINTS

- Cardiac involvement is common in systemic vasculitides.
- Most of the cases have subtle presentation or over-lapped by clinical presentation of other affected systems. Pericarditis, coronary arteritis, and ventricular systolic dysfunction are few of the common presentation.
- Accelerated atherosclerosis played an important role, in addition to inflammatory vasculitis in pathogenesis of disease process.
- Immunosuppression is the mainstay of the treatment. Percutaneous or surgical intervention is required in selected cases.

REFERENCES

1. Kallenberg CG, Heeringa P, Stegeman CA. Mechanisms of disease: pathogenesis and treatment of ANCA-associated vasculitides. Nat Clin Pract Rheumatol. 2006;2:661-70.
2. Abdgawad M, Pettersson A, Gunnarsson L, et al. Decreased neutrophil apoptosis in quiescent ANCA-associated systemic vasculitis. PLoS One. 2012;7:e32439.
3. Kamesh L, Harper L, Savage CO. ANCA-positive vasculitis. J Am Soc Nephrol. 2002;13:1953-60.
4. Woywodt A, Streiber F, de Groot K, et al. Circulating endothelial cells as markers for ANCA-associated small-vessel vasculitis. Lancet. 2003;361:206-10.
5. Weyand CM, Goronzy JJ. Immune mechanisms in medium and large-vessel vasculitis. Nat Rev Rheumatol. 2013;9:731-40.
6. Ferri C, Giuggioli D, Cazzato M, et al. HCV-related cryoglobulinemic vasculitis: an update on its etiopathogenesis and therapeutic strategies. Clin Exp Rheumatol. 2003;21:S78-84.
7. Shoenfeld Y, Gerli R, Doria A, et al. Accelerated atherosclerosis in autoimmune rheumatic diseases. Circulation. 2005;112:3337-47.
8. Dhawan V, Mahajan N, Jain S. Role of C-C chemokines in Takayasu's arteritis disease. Int J Cardiol. 2006;112:105-11.
9. Ward JR, Wilson HL, Francis SE, et al. Translational mini-review series on immunology of vascular disease: inflammation, infections and toll-like receptors in cardiovascular disease. Clin Exp Immunol. 2009;156:386-94.
10. Tervaert JW. Translational mini-review series on immunology of vascular disease: accelerated atherosclerosis in vasculitis. Clin Exp Immunol. 2009;156:377-85.
11. de Leeuw K, Sanders JS, Stegeman C, et al. Accelerated atherosclerosis in patients with Wegener's granulomatosis. Ann Rheum Dis. 2005;64:753-9.
12. Seyahi E, Ucgul A, Cebi Olgun D, et al. Aortic and coronary calcifications in Takayasu arteritis. Semin Arthritis Rheum. 2013;43:96-104.
13. Seyahi E, Ugurlu S, Cumali R, et al. Atherosclerosis in Takayasu arteritis. Ann Rheum Dis. 2006;65:1202-7.
14. Lee SJ, Ahn HM, You JH, et al. Carotid intima-media thickness and pulse wave velocity after recovery from Kawasaki disease. Korean Circ J. 2009;39:264-9.
15. McCrindle BW, McIntyre S, Kim C, et al. Are patients after Kawasaki disease at increased risk for accelerated atherosclerosis? J Pediatr. 2007;151:244-8.
16. Ericson-Neilsen W, Kaye AD. Steroids: pharmacology, complications, and practice delivery issues. Ochsner J. 2014;14:203-7.
17. Lange RA HL. Toxins and the heart. In: Bonow RO MD, Zipes DP, Libby P (Eds). Braunwald's Heart Disease, 9th edition. Philadelphia: Elsevier Sanders; 2012. pp. 1628-37.
18. Gonzalez-Juanatey C, Llorca J, Garcia-Porrua C, et al. Steroid therapy improves endothelial function in patients with biopsy-proven giant cell arteritis. J Rheumatol. 2006;33:74-8.
19. Raza K, Thambyrajah J, Townend JN, Exley AR, Hortas C, Filer A, et al. Suppression of inflammation in primary systemic vasculitis restores vascular endothelial function: lessons for atherosclerotic disease? Circulation. 2000;102:1470-2.
20. Johannsson G, Ragnarsson O. Cardiovascular and metabolic impact of glucocorticoid replacement therapy. Front Horm Res. 2014;43:33-44.
21. Laldinpuii J, Sanchetee P, Borah AL, et al. Giant cell arteritis (temporal arteritis): a report of four cases from north east India. Ann Indian Acad Neurol. 2008;11:185-9.
22. Bablekos GD, Michaelides SA, Karachalios GN, et al. Pericardial involvement as an atypical manifestation of giant cell arteritis: report of a clinical case and literature review. Am J Med Sci. 2006;332:198-204.
23. Tomasson G, Peloquin C, Mohammad A, et al. Risk for cardiovascular disease early and late after a diagnosis of giant-cell arteritis: a cohort study. Ann Intern Med. 2014;160:73-80.
24. Pugnet G, Pathak A, Dumonteil N, et al. Giant cell arteritis as a cause of acute myocarditis in the elderly. J Rheumatol. 2011;38:2497.
25. McWilliams ET, Khonizy W, Jameel A. Polyarteritis nodosa presenting as acute myocardial infarction in a young man: Importance of invasive angiography. Heart. 2013;99:1219.
26. Chung DC, Choi JE, Song YK, et al. Polyarteritis nodosa complicated by chronic total occlusion accompanying aneurysms on all coronary arteries. Korean Circ J. 2012;42:568-70.
27. Pagnoux C, Seror R, Henegar C, et al. Clinical features and outcomes in 348 patients with polyarteritis nodosa: a systematic retrospective study of patients diagnosed between 1963 and 2005 and entered into the french vasculitis study group database. Arthritis Rheum. 2010;62:616-26.
28. Fauci AS, Wolff SM. Wegener's granulomatosis: studies in eighteen patients and a review of the literature. 1973. Medicine. 1994;73:315-24.

29. Goodfield NE, Bhandari S, Plant WD, et al. Cardiac involvement in Wegener's granulomatosis. Br Heart J. 1995;73:110.

30. Sarlon G, Durant C, Grandgeorge Y, et al. [Cardiac involvement in Wegener's granulomatosis: report of four cases and review of the literature]. Rev Med Interne. 2010;31:135-9.

31. Davenport A, Goodfellow J, Goel S, et al. Aortic valve disease in patients with Wegener's granulomatosis. Am J Kidney Dis. 1994;24:205-8.

32. Morelli S, Gurgo Di Castelmenardo AM, Conti F, et al. Cardiac involvement in patients with Wegener's granulomatosis. Rheumatol Int. 2000;19:209-12.

33. Florian A, Slavich M, Blockmans D, et al. Cardiac involvement in granulomatosis with polyangiitis (Wegener granulomatosis). Circulation. 2011;124:e342-4.

34. Schiavone WA, Ahmad M, Ockner SA. Unusual cardiac complications of Wegener's granulomatosis. Chest. 1985;88:745-8.

35. Robinson VM, Joshi NV, Japp AG, et al. A case of constrictive pericarditis in a patient with granulomatosis and polyangiitis (Wegener's granulomatosis). J Am Coll Cardiol. 2014;63(12_S).

36. Lacoste C, Mansencal N, Ben m'rad M, et al. Valvular involvement in ANCA-associated systemic vasculitis: a case report and literature review. BMC Musculoskele Disord. 2011. pp.12-50.

37. Comarmond C, Pagnoux C, Khellaf M, et al. Eosinophilic granulomatosis with polyangiitis (Churg–Strauss): clinical characteristics and long-term follow-up of the 383 patients enrolled in the French Vasculitis Study Group cohort. Arthritis Rheum. 2013;65:270-81.

38. Allen DC, Doherty CC, O'Reilly DP. Pathology of the heart and the cardiac conduction system in Wegener's granulomatosis. Br Heart J. 1984;52:674-8.

39. Churg J, Strauss, L. Allergic granulomatosis, allergic angiitis, and periarteritis nodosa. Am J Pathol. 1951;27:277.

40. Dennert RM, van Paassen P, Schalla S, et al. Cardiac involvement in Churg–Strauss syndrome. Arthritis Rheum. 2010;62:627-34.

41. Marmursztejn J, Guillevin L, Trebossen R, et al. Churg–Strauss syndrome cardiac involvement evaluated by cardiac magnetic resonance imaging and positron-emission tomography: a prospective study on 20 patients. Rheumatology. 2013;52:642-50.

42. Marmursztejn J, Cohen P, Duboc D, et al. Cardiac magnetic resonance imaging in Churg–Strauss-syndrome. Impact of immunosuppressants on outcome assessed in a prospective study on 8 patients. Clin Exp Rheumatol. 2010;28:8-13.

43. Lanham JG, Cooke S, Davies J, et al. Endomyocardial complications of the Churg–Strauss syndrome. Postgrad Med J. 1985;61:341.

44. Neumann T, Manger B, Schmid M, et al. Cardiac involvement in Churg–Strauss syndrome: impact of endomyocarditis. Medicine. 2009;88:236-43.

45. Moosig F, Richardt G, Gross WL. A fatal attraction: eosinophils and the heart. Rheumatology. 2013;52:587-9.

46. Neumann T, Manger B, Schmid M, et al. Cardiac involvement in Churg–Strauss syndrome: impact of endomyocarditis. Medicine. 2009;88:236-43.

47. Moosig F, Bremer JP, Hellmich B, et al. A vasculitis centre based management strategy leads to improved outcome in eosinophilic granulomatosis and polyangiitis (Churg–Strauss, EGPA): monocentric experiences in 150 patients. Ann Rheum Dis. 2013;72:1011-7.

48. Azzopardi C, Montefort S, Mallia C. Cardiac involvement and left ventricular failure in a patient with the Churg-Strauss syndrome. Adv Exp Med Biol. 1999;455:547-9.

49. Leon-Ruiz L, Jimenez-Alonso J, Hidalgo-Tenorio C, et al. Churg-Strauss syndrome complicated by endomyocardial fibrosis and intraventricular thrombus. Importance of the echocardiography for the diagnosis of asymptomatic phases of potentially severe cardiac complications. Lupus. 2002;11:765-7.

50. Fong C, Schmidt G, Cain N, et al. Churg–Strauss syndrome, cardiac involvement and life threatening ventricular arrhythmias. Aust N Z J Med. 1992;22:167-8.

51. Hellemans S, Dens J, Knockaert D. Coronary involvement in the Churg–Strauss syndrome. Heart. 1997;77:576-8.

52. Riksen NP, Gehlmann H, Brouwer AE, et al. Complete remission of coronary vasculitis in Churg–Strauss syndrome by prednisone and cyclophosphamide. Clin Rheumatol. 2013;32(Suppl 1):S41-2.

53. Guillevin L, Durand-Gasselin B, Cevallos R, et al. Microscopic polyangiitis: clinical and laboratory findings in eighty-five patients. Arthritis Rheum. 1999;42:421-30.

54. Sendoh W, Higami K, Harigai M, et al. A case of microscopic polyangiitis with severe cardiac and respiratory muscle involvement. Ryumachi. 1999;39:757-62.

55. Kim BK, Park SY, Choi CB, et al. A case of microscopic polyangiitis associated with aortic valve insufficiency. Rheumatol Int. 2013;33:1055-8.

56. Kobayashi H, Yokoe I, Murata S, et al. A case of microscopic polyangiitis with giant coronary aneurysm. J Rheumatol. 2011;38:583-4.

57. Terrier B, Karras A, Cluzel P, et al. Presentation and prognosis of cardiac involvement in hepatitis C virus-related vasculitis. Am J Cardiol. 2013;111:265-72.

58. Rieu V, Cohen P, Andre MH, et al. Characteristics and outcome of 49 patients with symptomatic cryoglobulinaemia. Rheumatology. 2002;41:290-300.

59. Maestroni A, Caviglia AG, Colzani M, et al. Heart involvement in essential mixed cryoglobulinemia. Ric Clin Lab. 1986;16:381-3.

60. Rowley AH, Shulman ST. Kawasaki syndrome. Clin Microbiol Rev. 1998;11:405-14.

61. Yoshikawa H, Nomura Y, Masuda K, et al. Four cases of Kawasaki syndrome complicated with myocarditis. Circ J. 2006;70:202-5.

62. Soncagi A, Devrim I, Karagoz T, et al. Septated pericarditis associated with Kawasaki disease: a brief case report. Turk J Pediatr. 2007;49:312-4.

63. Singh S, Kansra S. Kawasaki disease. Natl Med J India. 2005;18:20-4.

64. Harada K, Kato H, et al. Guidelines for diagnosis and management of cardiovascular sequelae in Kawasaki disease. Pediatr Int. 2005;47:711-32.

65. Newburger JW, Takahashi M, Gerber MA, et al. Diagnosis, treatment, and long-term management of Kawasaki disease: a statement for health professionals from the committee on rheumatic fever, endocarditis and Kawasaki disease, council on cardiovascular disease in the young, American Heart Association. Circulation. 2004;110:2747-71.

66. Kato H, Sugimura T, Akagi T, et al. Long-term consequences of Kawasaki disease. A 10- to 21-year follow-up study of 594 patients. Circulation. 1996;94:1379-85.

67. Tacke CE, Kuipers IM, Groenink M, et al. Cardiac magnetic resonance imaging for noninvasive assessment of cardiovascular disease during the follow-up of patients with Kawasaki disease. Circ Cardiovasc Imaging. 2011;4:712-20.

68. Panja M, Sarkar C, Kar AK, et al. Coronary artery lesions in Takayasu's arteritis—clinical and angiographic study. J Assoc Physicians India. 1998;46:678-81.

69. Sun T, Zhang H, Ma W, et al. Coronary artery involvement in Takayasu arteritis in 45 chinese patients. J Rheumatol. 2013;40:493-7.

70. Bicakcigil M, Aksu K, Kamali S, et al. Takayasu's arteritis in Turkey—clinical and angiographic features of 248 patients. Clin Exp Rheumatol. 2009;27:S59-64.

71. Acar J, Leurent B, Slama M, et al. Aortic insufficiency and Takayasu disease. Ann Med Interne. 1983;134:606-13.

72. Talwar KK, Kumar K, Chopra P, et al. Cardiac involvement in nonspecific aortoarteritis (Takayasu's arteritis). Am Heart J. 1991;122:1666-70.

73. Ghosh S, Sinha DP, Ghosh S, et al. Dilated cardiomyopathy in non-specific aortoarteritis. Indian Heart J. 1999;51:527-31.

74. Panja M, Kar AK, Dutta AL, et al. Cardiac involvement in non-specific aorto-arteritis. Int J Cardiol. 1992;34:289-95.

75. Sharma S, Kamalakar T, Rajani M, et al. The incidence and patterns of pulmonary artery involvement in Takayasu's arteritis. Clin Radiol. 1990;42:177-81.

76. Cocco G, Jerie P. Cardiac pathology and modern therapeutic approach in Behçet disease. Cardiol J. 2014;21:105-14.

77. Geri G, Wechsler B, Thi Huong du L, et al. Spectrum of cardiac lesions in Behçet disease: a series of 52 patients and review of the literature. Medicine. 2012;91:25-34.

78. Seyahi E, Yurdakul S. Behçet's syndrome and thrombosis. Mediterr J Hematol Infect Dis. 2011;3:e2011026.

CHAPTER 17

Pulmonary Manifestations

SK Jindal

INTRODUCTION

The respiratory system, particularly the lungs, possesses a large vascular bed. There is an extensive anastomotic network due to the existence of dual blood supply by the systemic and pulmonary circulations. It is therefore, not surprising to find the pulmonary involvement in a large number of systemic vasculitides. Lungs are also directly exposed to the environment through the airways, which makes them vulnerable to a large number of direct inhalational insults to the pulmonary epithelial as well as the endothelial surfaces. Some such insults may manifest purely with pulmonary manifestations while others may involve other parts of body as well.

Lungs are frequently involved in systemic vasculitides, also because of the presence of a favorable milieu for inflammatory and immunological types of injuries.[1] Almost any systemic vasculitis can involve the respiratory system. The site, extent, and type of pulmonary involvement may vary depending upon the type of systemic vasculitis (Table 17.1). Most commonly, the lungs are involved in small-vessel antineutrophil cytoplasmic antibody (ANCA)-associated vasculitides that include granulomatosis with polyangiitis (GPA), eosinophilic granulomatosis with polyangiitis (EGPA, previously Churg–Strauss syndrome), microscopic polyangiitis (MPA), and idiopathic pauci-immune pulmonary capillaritis.[2] Diffuse alveolar hemorrhage (DAH) is the most important clinical presentation of several different vasculitides.

CLINICAL MANIFESTATIONS

Diffuse Alveolar Hemorrhage

Diffuse alveolar hemorrhage, characterized by intra-alveolar bleeding due to pulmonary capillary destruction, is a

Table 17.1 Pulmonary involvement depending upon the site in different systemic vasculitides

Site of involvement	Type of vasculitis
Tracheobronchial tree	• Granulomatosis with polyangiitis (Wegener's)–GPA • Infections––tuberculosis, fungal, or bacterial
Large pulmonary arteries	• Behçet's disease • Takayasu's arteritis
Lung parenchyma - small vessels	• Infections (Bacterial, TB, fungal) • GPA (Wegener's) • Systemic lupus erythematosus (SLE) • Allergic granulomatous polyangiitis or Churg–Strauss syndrome • Microscopic polyangiitis (MPA)

life-threatening condition.[3,4] A review of 9 studies undertaken between 1985 and 2012 on 207 total patients reported the mean age at presentation as 57 years with a similar distribution amongst male and female patients.[5] Hemoptysis, which is often massive, is the most common symptom. It results in a rapid fall of hemoglobin, may also progress to hypoxemic respiratory failure due to alveolar filling and low hemoglobin. Hemoptysis can be scanty or absent in up to one-third of cases who may manifest with only pallor, breathlessness, and radiological infiltrates.

Alveolar bleeding can also occur in the absence of capillaritis (i.e. bland hemorrhage), for example, due to a coagulation disorder, mitral stenosis, Goodpasture's syndrome, or idiopathic pulmonary hemosiderosis (Table 17.2). Characteristically, however, DAH results from capillaritis due to ANCA-associated disorders (Table 17.3) that pose difficulties of diagnosis and management.

Table 17.2 Causes of bland alveolar hemorrhage (without capillaritis)

- Mitral stenosis
- Coagulopathy
- Pulmonary venous hypertension
- Cytotoxic drugs
- Sepsis
- Radiation
- Bone marrow transplantation
- Lung transplantation
- Antiphospholipid antibody syndrome
- Idiopathic pulmonary hemosiderosis

Table 17.3 Causes of diffuse alveolar hemorrhage due to capillaritis

- Granulomatosis with polyangiitis (Wegener's)
- Churg–Strauss syndrome
- Microscopic polyangiitis
- Isolated pauci-immune pulmonary capillaritis
- Primary immune complex-mediated vasculitis
  - Goodpasture's syndrome
  - Henoch–Schönlein purpura
- Connective tissue diseases
  - Systemic lupus erythematosus
  - Rheumatoid arthritis
  - Antiphospholipid antibody syndrome
  - Polymyositis/dermatomyositis
- Behçet's disease
- Lung infections—bacterial, viral, or tubercular
- Drug induced capillaritis
- *Miscellaneous causes:* Inhalational toxins, cryoglobulinemia, autologous bone marrow transplantation, and acute lung transplantation rejection

Diagnosis

The cardinal symptoms of DAH include the history of hemoptysis, and rapidly developing pallor due to a fall in hematocrit. Diffuse alveolar hemorrhage may present with acute or subacute form of variable severity. Sometimes, it is repetitive for a few days or weeks. The diagnosis is corroborated by the presence of alveolar infiltrates seen on a chest skiagram and/or a computed tomography (CT) scan. The radiological pattern is generally diffuse but may be patchy, and sometimes unilateral. Occasionally, the alveolar bleeding is chronic that keeps on happening over months or years. This type of chronic DAH can present as pulmonary fibrosis.

Bronchoscopy with bronchoalveolar lavage (BAL) is required for diagnosis of alveolar infiltrates in the absence of hemoptysis. Bronchoalveolar lavage in such a case may show progressive hemorrhagic fluid. Presence of >5% hemosiderin-laden macrophages in the BAL fluid may point to the occurrence of an insidious onset or recurrent hemorrhage. These can be demonstrated by Perls' Prussian blue staining of the centrifuge from the BAL fluid.

After establishing the presence of DAH, it is important to look for its underlying etiology.[6,7] A variety of investigations are required for this purpose.

History and Clinical Features

A number of causes of DAH with and without capillaritis have been listed earlier (Tables 17.2 and 17.3). Most causes of bland hemorrhage (Table 17.2) are easily recognizable. A careful history and a good physical examination are helpful to make the diagnosis. However, a battery of tests may be needed for the differential diagnosis of DAH with capillaritis.

Laboratory Investigations

Presence of an infection and/or sepsis needs exclusion with hematological (total and differential counts and blood film) and microbiological (sputum examination and blood cultures) investigations. Assessment of coagulation parameters is required for diagnosis of a suspected coagulopathy. Electrocardiography and echocardiography are done whenever a cardiac problem is the likely cause of hemorrhage. Radiology is essential for diagnosis of DAH as well as to look for a cardiac abnormality.

Chest X-ray and CT findings are generally nonspecific to suggest the etiology of DAH. Chest X-ray, however, is a sensitive investigation that shows rapidly changing opacities with a perihilar distribution. Presence of diffuse ground-glass opacities or extensive consolidation with air bronchograms may be seen on high-resolution CT scans even in the presence of a normal chest roentgenogram.[8] Presences of nodular opacities that sometimes show cavitation suggests the diagnosis of underlying vasculitis. Lymph node enlargement may point to the diagnosis of an infection or malignancy.[9,10] Other investigations that suggest the possibility of alveolar blood include the increased diffusion capacity to carbon monoxide on lung function tests and delayed clearance of the radioisotope C^{150} from the lung fields.[11]

Routine biochemical assessment for liver and renal functions is required in all cases. Urine examination is particularly helpful in suspected cases of pulmonary–renal syndromes such as Goodpasture's syndrome, GPA, and MPA. Microscopic hematuria and proteinuria are commonly seen in most of these patients.

Immunological Investigations

Serological testing is required for the underlying vasculitic disorder responsible for DAH. Antineutrophil cytoplasmic antibodies are present in most cases of GPA (Wegener's). Presence of antiglomerular basement membrane (GBM) antibodies points to Goodpasture's syndrome while antinuclear antibodies, anti-dsDNA antibodies, and antiphospholipid antibodies are detected in patients with systemic lupus erythematosus (SLE). Some connective tissue disorders (CTDs) are associated with specific laboratory abnormalities such as anti-Jo1 and U1 RNP positivity. Elevated total IgE and low complement (C_3 and C_4) levels help to establish the diagnosis of EGPA and SLE, respectively.

Histological Examination

Lung biopsy is important for the demonstrating presence of occult blood and to document small-vessel vasculitis. While filling of alveoli with red blood cells is seen in an acute DAH, chronic DAH is diagnosed by the presence of hemosiderin-laden interstitial alveolar macrophages, which may also be seen in the BAL fluid.[5,12]

GRANULOMATOSIS WITH POLYANGIITIS (WEGENER'S)

Granulomatosis with polyangiitis was earlier known by the eponym Wegener's granulomatosis, which was later abandoned after the Nazi association of Friedrich Wegener came to be known.[13,14] Granulomatosis with polyangiitis along with MPA and allergic GPA are together listed as ANCA-associated small-vessel vasculitis. As per the original Chapel Hill Consensus Nomenclature that is widely followed, GPA was defined as the granulomatosis involving the respiratory tract and necrotizing vasculitis affecting small-to-medium-sized vessels (i.e. capillaries, venules, arterioles, and arteries).[15]

Clinical Features

Characteristically, GPA involves the upper respiratory tract, the lungs, the eyes, sometimes the kidneys, and other organs. Nose is most commonly affected in the upper respiratory tract with manifestations of serosanguinous secretions or nasal bleeding. Sinonasal involvement is also a common cause of nasal crusting and blockade.[16] Destruction of nasal septum may result in saddle nose deformity. Pan sinusitis, stomatitis, gingivitis, otitis media, and mastoiditis may also occur. There is frequent super infection with staphylococci that is sometimes considered as the cause of disease relapses.[17]

Pulmonary Involvement

Clinical symptoms of GPA commonly include fever, cough, hemoptysis, nasal blockade, and/or discharge. Lung involvement is most commonly seen in the form of single or multiple pulmonary nodules or masses that may frequently cavitate (Figs 17.1A and B) and mimic a lung abscess or even lung cancer. Less commonly, the disease may present with reticular or reticulonodular opacities, atelectasis, and consolidation. Lymph node enlargement and pleural

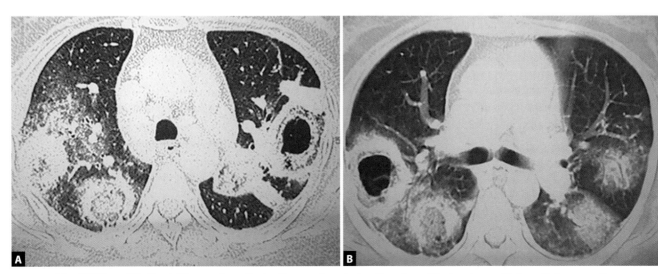

Figs 17.1A and B Chest CT scan of a patient with granulomatosis with polyangiitis showing multiple cavitating opacities

effusion are very rare. A review of a cohort of 131 completely resected, histologically unexplained pulmonary necrotizing granulomas between 1994 and 2004 revealed GPA as a cause of 15 of 79 cases in whom a cause could be determined; 64 of 79 had one or the other infection as the underlying cause.[18] Airway involvement may result in subglottic stenosis following mucosal inflammation and ulceration.[19,20] Symptoms of hoarseness, cough, breathlessness, and wheezing are quite distressing in such cases. Occasionally, the patient may present with severe and progressive respiratory distress.[3,20,21]

Eye and Ear Involvement

Granulomatosis with polyangiitis commonly involves the eyes in the form of scleritis, episcleritis, and conjunctivitis presenting with red eyes. Keratitis and uveitis can cause blurred vision and visual impairment. Optic perineuritis and hypertrophic pachymeningitis responsible for loss of vision have been described.[22] Occasionally, exophthalmos results due to retro-orbital granulomatous inflammation. Both middle and inner ear involvement may occur producing earache, tinnitus, and ear discharge. Hearing loss and deafness may occur in late stages.

Other Organ Involvement

Renal involvement is demonstrable in up to 80% of patients at one or the other point during the course of GPA. Glomerulonephritis, unless treated in the early stages may soon progress to renal failure before the symptoms develop. Presence of hematuria and erythrocyte casts that are often microscopic points to the underlying glomerulonephritis.

Granulomatosis with polyangiitis may also involve other organs in different patients. Skin involvement is seen in the form of leukocytoclastic vasculitis, purpura, or ulcers in about one-third of patients. Arthritis of small, medium, or large joints may manifest with arthralgias, myalgia, and painful movements. Cardiac conduction abnormalities, mononeuritis multiplex, polyneuropathy, and gastrointestinal bleeding are occasionally seen.

Diagnosis

The diagnosis of GPA as of other forms of vasculitides requires a multipronged approach. No single test is pathognomonic.[23,24] While clinical features and radiology are of great help in suspecting the diagnosis, it is essentially established on the antibody presence and histopathological demonstration of

characteristic features. Antineutrophil cytoplasmic antibody positivity is seen in >80% of patients. Of the three different patterns of ANCA on indirect immunofluorescent staining (i.e. cytoplasmic, perinuclear, and atypical), the C-ANCA is considered as more specific. The PR3-ANCA (i.e. antibodies reacting with proteinase 3) with C-ANCA combination and the MPO-ANCA (myeloperoxidase ANCA) with P-ANCA (perinuclear ANCA) combination show good sensitivity and specificity for ANCA-associated vasculitides.[25] In ANCA-negative patients, a single algorithm based on an evaluation of autoantibodies and 18-F-FDG-PET-CT scanning has been suggested.[24] Although FDG-PET/CT accurately identifies the localization of lesions, it has no additional benefit to the usual organ screening in vasculitides other than GPA.[26]

False positive C-ANCA/PR3 has been reported in conditions such as infective endocarditis.[27] It is positive in over half of the patients of MPA and EGPA in whom it is p-ANCA/anti-MPO positive.[28] There is some association between ANCA titers and disease activity but the use of serial measurements for follow-up assessments and disease-relapse is not clearly established.[29] A comprehensive assessment of clinical, radiological, and laboratory parameters is important for prediction of relapses and retreatment.

Histopathological demonstration of features of necrotizing vasculitis with granuloma formation is necessary for differential diagnosis, since, a large number of clinical conditions can present not only with similar clinical and radiological features, but also with a false positive or negative ANCA results. Histopathological specimens such as lung biopsy can be obtained with bronchoscopy, thoracoscopy, and sometimes with open thoracic surgery. Kidney biopsy may be needed whenever there is suspicion of MPA.

BEHÇET'S DISEASE

Like GPA, Behçet's disease involves multiple organs primarily with pulmonary manifestations. Unlike GPA, it is characterized by large-vessel vasculitis involving medium-sized or large-sized arteries. It is commonly described from the Far East and Middle East countries along the ancient Silk route. It mostly involves young adults with no particular gender preference.

Behçet's disease is diagnosed on the basis of criteria proposed by the International Study Group for Behçet's disease.[30] Recurrent oral ulcers are essential with at least two or more features that comprise of skin lesions, eye lesions, recurrent genital ulcers, and a positive pathergy test demonstrated by the formation of a papule or a pustule following skin prick by needle.

Pathologically, the disease is characterized by multiple arterial aneurysms, vascular thrombosis, pulmonary infarcts, and hemorrhages. Recurrent pulmonary infections, organizing bronchiolitis, and pleurisy may also occur.[31] Hemoptysis in Behçet's is not uncommon, occasionally, it may present with DAH and massive bleeding.[32,33] Bleeding generally occurs from erosion or bronchial walls, bronchial wall–arterial fistulae, or rupture of arterial aneurysms. Fever, anemia, raised ESR, and pulmonary infiltrates are other clinical features that are sometimes seen. The disease in ethnic groups with higher prevalence is reported to follow a more severe course.[33]

Diagnosis of Behçet's disease requires the clinical criteria and radiological assessment with the help of chest X-rays, CT, and MRI angiography. Round or lobular opacities seen on chest X-ray represent aneurysms that can be confirmed on helical CT scanning with contrast. Biopsy is occasionally required. Major histocompatibility complex antigen HLA-B5 is present in a large number of patients.

EOSINOPHILIC GRANULOMATOSIS WITH POLYANGIITIS (CHURG–STRAUSS SYNDROME)

Eosinophilic granulomatosis with polyangiitis also known as Churg-Strauss syndrome, is an ANCA-associated vasculitis with p-ANCA-MRO positivity in most cases. Asthma is the most important feature of respiratory tract involvement while pulmonary infiltrates and pleural effusion can rarely occur.[34] Peripheral blood eosinophilia and necrotizing vasculitis involving small- and medium-sized vessels are other important manifestations. Systemic features may include those related to peripheral nerves (mononeuritis or polyneuritis multiplex), skin, heart, gastrointestinal, and central nervous system. Eosinophilic granulomatosis with polyangiitis resembles a nonallergic eosinophilic asthma phenotype, and is sometimes difficult to distinguish from other hypereosinophilic syndromes.[35] Diffuse alveolar hemorrhage does not usually occur in EGPA. Diagnosis is confirmed on histological examination of biopsies from lungs, peripheral nerves, or skin.

CONNECTIVE TISSUE DISORDERS

Of various connective tissue disorders, SLE is more commonly associated with vasculitis and rarely with life-threatening DAH. Pulmonary capillaritis can also occur with other CTDs such as polymyositis, rheumatoid arthritis, and mixed connective tissue disease. Pulmonary involvement in polyarteritis nodosa (PAN) is very rare. It has been occasionally described in anecdotal reports. Diffuse alveolar hemorrhage in SLE occurs due to immune complex deposition and carries a high mortality rate.[36] General constitutional symptoms, cough, breathlessness, and hemoptysis are important symptoms in patients with pulmonary vasculitis. Pulmonary infiltrates, consolidation, or diffuse alveolar filling may be seen on chest X-ray and/or CT scans. Bronchoscopic lavage is required for diagnosis of alveolar infiltrates in doubtful cases. Presence of siderophages in BAL fluid will strongly support the diagnosis of alveolar bleeding and pulmonary capillaritis in GPA (Wegener's).

MISCELLANEOUS VASCULITIDES WITH PULMONARY MANIFESTATIONS

Large- and medium-vessel vasculitides such as giant cell arteritis (GCA) and Takayasu's arteritis do not commonly involve the lungs. Chronic obstructive pulmonary disease and other comorbidities such as hypertension, diabetes, and coronary heart disease were seen to be associated with a higher risk of GCA in a large nationwide cohort reported from Sweden.[37] Pulmonary complications in GCA include the interstitial or nodular pulmonary infiltrates and occasionally, pleural effusions. Pulmonary vessels are involved in over half the patients of Takayasu's arteritis though clinically significant disease is much less common, i.e. <5% of patients. Clinical symptoms include the presence of cough, dyspnea, chest pain, and hemoptysis; while angiographic findings include pulmonary artery narrowing and pulmonary hypertension.

A wide spectrum of pulmonary involvement including large- and small-vasculitis with thrombosis and/or DAH has also been described in patients with antiphospholipid syndrome.[38] An early diagnosis is important for timely intervention. Vessel wall necrotizing inflammation can occur in an infective lesion in the lungs, for example, a necrotizing pneumonia, septic infarct, or lung abscess. Occasionally, it may result in aneurysmal dilatation and/or rupture of the vessel within a cavity (Figs 17.2A and B). Drugs, inhalational toxins, and immunological insults in patients with organ transplantation are sometimes responsible for secondary vasculitis. Anecdotal reports are also available on rare pulmonary manifestations such as phenytoin-induced allergic reaction and clinical pulmonary disease, pulmonary silicosis-induced ANCA positivity, and asthma with increased arterial inflammation.[39-41] Such reports only emphasize the wide and yet poorly understood spectrum of pulmonary vasculitides.

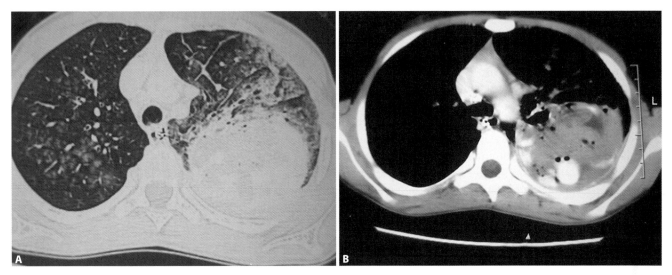

Figs 17.2A and B Chest CT scan of a patient with necrotizing pneumonic consolidation with an intracavitary aneurysm showing contrast enhancement

PULMONARY RENAL SYNDROME

Occurrence of both renal and respiratory failures due to autoimmune-mediated glomerulonephritis and alveolar bleeding together constitute the pulmonary renal syndrome.[42] Goodpasture's syndrome that consists of rapidly progressive glomerulonephritis (RPGN) and DAH is the most important cause of pulmonary renal syndrome. Rapidly progressive glomerulonephritis occurs due to deposition of GBM antibodies. The clinical features consist of hematuria that may be detected on microscopic examination and hemoptysis, which may sometimes be massive and fatal. While DAH and RPGN with anti-GBM antibodies occur together in 60–80% of cases, the disease is limited to the lungs in about 10% of patients.[43] The diagnosis rests on the demonstration of anti-GBM antibodies along with RPGN and alveolitis. There is a strong genetic association with HLA-DRBI 1501 and DRBI 1502.[44]

Other causes of pulmonary renal syndrome include the presence of anti-GBM disease with other ANCA-associated vasculitis, i.e. the GPA and the MPA that preferentially involve the lungs and the kidneys, respectively. Microscopic polyangiitis is a necrotizing vasculitis with few or no immune deposits in which necrotizing GN is very common.[45] Pulmonary capillaritis and DAH can sometimes occur in MPA as well.[46]

MANAGEMENT OF PULMONARY VASCULITIS

The general approach to management of pulmonary vasculitis is similar to the management of systemic vasculitis, primarily directed to control inflammation with effective immunosuppressive therapy. Supportive therapy is required to maintain oxygenation in the presence of respiratory failure. Maintenance of blood pressure and blood replacement are needed in cases of DAH, wherever there is a massive alveolar hemorrhage.

Besides systemic corticosteroids, a host of immunosuppressant and cytotoxic drugs are available for use in these patients. (The drugs have been discussed in details in separate chapters). The initial treatment for induction of remission is aggressive depending upon the grade of disease severity. Maintenance treatment to maintain a remission is required to be continued for a longer period, but not as intense as the initial therapy.

The primary regimen for induction consists of combined therapy with intravenous administration of cyclophosphamide and methylprednisolone. Induction treatment is continued for 3–6 months or longer depending upon the initial disease activity and response to the therapy. Cyclophosphamide given as a pulse therapy is associated with lesser side effects and greater efficacy.[47] Methotrexate is considered as an alternative to cyclophosphamide in the presence of limited disease. Rituximab-based regimens are shown to be more effective than the cyclophosphamide-based regimen for relapsing disease.[48] Mycophenolate mofetil is another relatively safer alternative to cyclophosphamide.

Maintenance treatment is required for 18 months to 2 years. Azathioprine, methotrexate, and mycophenolate along with oral corticosteroids are some of the recommended drugs used to maintain remission.[49]

In summary, the lungs are involved in several different vasculitic disorders either as the primary site or as one of the several systemic manifestations. Diffuse alveolar hemorrhage is the most severe manifestation that can prove to be life-threatening. Granulomatosis with polyangiitis and EGPA represent the most common vasculitides that present with lung manifestations. A battery of investigations including the demonstration of autoantibodies helps to establish the diagnosis. Treatment of pulmonary manifestations follows the general principles of management of vasculitides discussed elsewhere in this book.

KEY POINTS

- The respiratory system is an important site of involvement in several vasculitic disorders such as granulomatosis with polyangiitis (Wegener's) and eosinophilic granulomatosis with polyangiitis.
- Diffuse pulmonary hemorrhage is the most dreaded manifestation presenting with massive hemoptysis and a rapid fall in hemoglobin.
- Several connective tissue diseases that can manifest with pulmonary findings of vasculitic involvement include SLE and PAN.
- Most of these forms of disorders are classified as ANCA-associated vasculitides.
- Pulmonary renal syndromes that include Goodpasture's syndrome and other ANCA-associated vasculitis present with both alveolar bleeding and autoimmune mediated glomerulonephritis.
- Diagnosis of pulmonary vasculitides is made on the basis of clincoradiological features, demonstration of antibodies and histopathological findings.
- The immunosuppressive treatment is the primary mode of management.

REFERENCES

1. Shukla A. Lung in systemic vasculitis. Pulmonary and critical care medicine: pulmonary manifestations of the systemic diseases. 2014;2:293.
2. Frankel SK, Schwarz MI. The pulmonary vasculitides. Am J Respir Crit Care Med. 2012;186:216-24.
3. Collard HR, Schwarz MI. Diffuse alveolar hemorrhage. Clin Chest Med. 2004;25:583-92, vii.
4. Siogoki E, Polychronopoulos V. Diffuse alveolar hemorrhage syndromes, Wegener's granulomatosis. Textbook Pulm Crit Care Med. 2011.pp.1523-34.
5. West S, Arulkumaran N, Ind PW, et al. Diffuse alveolar haemorrhage in ANCA-associated vasculitis. Intern Med. 2013;52:5-13.
6. Ioachimescu OC, Stoller JK. Diffuse alveolar hemorrhage: diagnosing it and finding the cause. Cleve Clin J Med. 2008;75:258, 260, 264-255 passim.
7. Park MS. Diffuse alveolar hemorrhage. Tuberc Respir Dis (Seoul). 2013;74:151-62.
8. Cortese G, Nicali R, Placido R, et al. Radiological aspects of diffuse alveolar haemorrhage. Radiol Med. 2008;113:16-28.
9. Brown KK. Pulmonary vasculitis. Proc Am Thorac Soc. 2006;3:48-57.
10. Specks U. Diffuse alveolar hemorrhage syndromes. Curr Opin Rheumatol. 2001;13:12-7.
11. Ewan PW, Jones HA, Rhodes CG, et al. Detection of intrapulmonary hemorrhage with carbon monoxide uptake. Application in goodpasture's syndrome. N Engl J Med. 1976;295:1391-6.
12. Gaudin PB, Askin FB, Falk RJ, et al. The pathologic spectrum of pulmonary lesions in patients with anti-neutrophil cytoplasmic autoantibodies specific for anti-proteinase 3 and anti-myeloperoxidase. Am J Clin Pathol. 1995;104:7-16.
13. Falk RJ, Gross WL, Guillevin L, et al. Granulomatosis with polyangiitis (Wegener's): an alternative name for Wegener's granulomatosis. Arthritis Rheum. 2011;63:863-4.
14. Jindal SK. Nazi eponyms in medicine (ed). J Postgrad Ed Res. 2012;46:v-vi.
15. Jennette JC, Falk RJ, Andrassy K, et al. Nomenclature of systemic vasculitides. Proposal of an international consensus conference. Arthritis Rheum. 1994;37:187-92.
16. Kohanski MA, Reh DD. Chapter 11: granulomatous diseases and chronic sinusitis. Am J Rhinol Allergy. 2013;27:S39-41.
17. Stegeman CA, Tervaert JW, Sluiter WJ, et al. Association of chronic nasal carriage of *Staphylococcus aureus* and higher relapse rates in Wegener granulomatosis. Ann Intern Med. 1994;120:12-7.
18. Mukhopadhyay S, Wilcox BE, Myers JL, et al. Pulmonary necrotizing granulomas of unknown cause: clinical and pathologic analysis of 131 patients with completely resected nodules. Chest. 2013;144:813-24.
19. Gomez-Gomez A, Martinez-Martinez MU, Cuevas-Orta E, et al. Pulmonary manifestations of granulomatosis with polyangiitis. Reumatol Clin. 2014:Doi:S1699-1258X(1614)00008-00004 [pii].
20. Polychronopoulos VS, Prakash UB, Golbin JM, et al. Airway involvement in Wegener's granulomatosis. Rheum Dis Clin North Am. 2007;33:755-75, vi.
21. Toma C, Belaconi I, Dumitrache-Rujinski S, et al. Rapidly progressive pattern of granulomatosis with polyangiitis (Wegener's)-clinical case. Chest. 2014;145:223A.
22. Takazawa T, Ikeda K, Nagaoka T, et al. Wegener granulomatosis-associated optic perineuritis. Orbit. 2014;33:13-6.
23. Casian A, Jayne D. Current modalities in the diagnosis of pulmonary vasculitis. Expert Opin Med Diagn. 2012;6:499-516.
24. Cohen Tervaert JW. What to do when you suspect your patient suffers from pulmonary vasculitis? Expert Opin Med Diagn. 2013;7:1-4.

25. Russell KA, Wiegert E, Schroeder DR, et al. Detection of anti-neutrophil cytoplasmic antibodies under actual clinical testing conditions. Clin Immunol. 2002;103:196-203.

26. Soussan M, Abisror N, Abad S, et al. Fdg-pet/ct in patients with anca-associated vasculitis: case-series and literature review. Autoimmun Rev. 2014;13:125-31.

27. Choi HK, Lamprecht P, Niles JL, et al. Subacute bacterial endocarditis with positive cytoplasmic antineutrophil cytoplasmic antibodies and anti-proteinase 3 antibodies. Arthritis Rheum. 2000;43:226-31.

28. Frankel SK, Cosgrove GP, Fischer A, et al. Update in the diagnosis and management of pulmonary vasculitis. Chest. 2006;129:452-65.

29. Finkielman JD, Merkel PA, Schroeder D, et al. Antiproteinase 3 antineutrophil cytoplasmic antibodies and disease activity in Wegener granulomatosis. Ann Intern Med. 2007;147:611-9.

30. International study group for Behçet's disease. Criteria for diagnosis of Behçet's disease. Lancet. 1990;335:1078-80.

31. Erkan F, Gul A, Tasali E. Pulmonary manifestations of Behçet's disease. Thorax. 2001;56:572-8.

32. Grosso V, Boveri E, Bogliolo L, et al. Diffuse alveolar hemorrhage as a manifestation of Behçet disease. Reumatismo. 2013;65:138-41.

33. Hatemi G, Yazici Y, Yazici H. Behçet's syndrome. Rheum Dis Clin North Am. 2013;39:245-61.

34. Keogh KA, Specks U. Churg–Strauss syndrome: clinical presentation, antineutrophil cytoplasmic antibodies, and leukotriene receptor antagonists. Am J Med. 2003;115:284-90.

35. Mahr A, Moosig F, Neumann T, et al. Eosinophilic granulomatosis with polyangiitis (Churg–Strauss): evolutions in classification, etiopathogenesis, assessment and management. Curr Opin Rheumatol. 2014;26:16-23.

36. Santos-Ocampo AS, Mandell BF, Fessler BJ. Alveolar hemorrhage in systemic lupus erythematosus: presentation and management. Chest. 2000;118:1083-90.

37. Zoller B, Li X, Sundquist J, et al. Occupational and socio-economic risk factors for giant cell arteritis: a nationwide study based on hospitalizations in Sweden. Scand J Rheumatol. 2013;42:487-97.

38. Kanakis MA, Kapsimali V, Vaiopoulos AG, et al. The lung in the spectrum of antiphospholipid syndrome. Clin Exp Rheumatol. 2013;31:452-7.

39. Fukuhara A, Tanino Y, Sato S, et al. Systemic vasculitis associated with anti-neutrophil cytoplasmic antibodies against bactericidal/permeability increasing protein. Intern Med. 2013;52:1095-9.

40. Kheir F, Daroca P, Lasky J. Phenytoin-associated granulomatous pulmonary vasculitis. Am J Ther. 2013.

41. Vijayakumar J, Subramanian S, Singh P, et al. Arterial inflammation in bronchial asthma. J Nucl Cardiol. 2013;20:385-95.

42. West SC, Arulkumaran N, Ind PW, et al. Pulmonary-renal syndrome: a life threatening but treatable condition. Postgrad Med J. 2013;89:274-83.

43. Salama AD, Levy JB, Lightstone L, et al. Goodpasture's disease. Lancet. 2001;358:917-20.

44. Hellmark T, Segelmark M. Diagnosis and classification of Goodpasture's disease (anti-gbm). J Autoimmun. 2014;48-49:108-12.

45. Jennette JC, Falk RJ, Bacon PA, et al. 2012 Revised International Chapel Hill Consensus Conference Nomenclature of vasculitides. Arthritis Rheum. 2013;65:1-11.

46. Kallenberg CG. The diagnosis and classification of microscopic polyangiitis. J Autoimmun. 2014;48-49:90-3.

47. de Groot K, Harper L, Jayne DR, et al. Pulse versus daily oral cyclophosphamide for induction of remission in antineutrophil cytoplasmic antibody-associated vasculitis: a randomized trial. Ann Intern Med. 2009;150:670-80.

48. Jones RB, Tervaert JW, Hauser T, et al. Rituximab versus cyclophosphamide in ANCA-associated renal vasculitis. N Engl J Med. 2010;363:211-20.

49. Pagnoux C, Mahr A, Hamidou MA, et al. Azathioprine or methotrexate maintenance for ANCA-associated vasculitis. N Engl J Med. 2008;359:2790-803.

CHAPTER 18

Renal Manifestations

Manish Rathi, Aman Sharma, Ritambhra Nada

INTRODUCTION

The systemic vasculitides (SV) are important group of rheumatological disorders that commonly affect kidneys. The renal manifestations may vary from asymptomatic urinary abnormalities to severe life-threatening rapidly progressive renal failure. The renal involvement can develop either in an established case or can be the presenting manifestations of the SV.[1] In some cases, the manifestations of vasculitis can remain confined to the kidneys for many years and this entity is thus appropriately known as renal-limited vasculitis. However, in most cases, occurrence of renal involvement denotes the severity of disease and warrants urgent immunosuppressive treatment. Although all forms of vasculitides have the potential to involve kidneys, it happens in variety of ways. The large- and medium-vessel vasculitis involves the larger renal vessels leading to hypertension, renal artery stenosis, and ischemic nephropathy. On the other hand, the small-vessel vasculitis commonly involves the glomerular capillaries leading to proliferative glomerulonephritis.[2] The common forms of renal involvement in various SV are summarized in Table 18.1. Below we will discuss some of the important causes and forms of renal involvement in SV.

LARGE-VESSEL VASCULITIS

Takayasu Arteritis

Takayasu arteritis: It is the prototypic large-vessel vasculitis that causes granulomatous inflammation of the aorta and its major branches. It usually involves patients <40 years age, and predominantly females. The involvement of the aorta around the area of renal ostia or the proximal one third of the renal arteries can lead to renal artery stenosis (RAS). This involvement of the renal arteries is often

Table 18.1 Renal involvement in different types of vasculitis

Type of vasculitis	Incidence	Common renal manifestation
Large-vessel vasculitis		
Takayasu arteritis	20–90%	Renal artery stenosis
Giant cell arteritis	Rare	Asymptomatic urinary abnormalities
Medium-vessel vasculitis		
Polyarteritis nodosa	50–75%	Renal artery microaneurysms, renal infarcts, renal parenchymal bleed, and hypertension
Small-vessel vasculitis		
Antineutrophil antibody-associated vasculitis	50–90%	Pauci-immune proliferative glomerulonephritis
Henoch-Schönlein purpura	33–66%	Proliferative IgA dominant glomerulonephritis
Cryoglobulinemic vasculitis	30–50%	Mesangioproliferative glomerulonephritis
Systemic lupus erythematosus	0.5–24%	Uncomplicated immune deposits, noninflammatory necrotising vasculopathy, thrombotic microangiopathy, true vasculitis

bilateral and results in renovascular hypertension.[3] In many countries, TA is the most common cause of renovascular hypertension, though in the western world, it is superseded by atherosclerosis.[4] Glomerular diseases, such as mesangial proliferative glomerulonephritis, membranoproliferative GN (MPGN), minimal change disease, immunoglobulin A (IgA) nephropathy (IgAN), fibrillary GN, crescentic GN, and amyloidosis have been described rarely. In addition, ischemic nephropathy resulting from RAS can also be seen. The disease process occurs in two stages: an acute inflammatory stage and a chronic fibrotic stage. Patients in acute stage can have constitutional symptoms such as fever and carotid artery tenderness (carotidynia), while there may not be any symptoms other than hypertension in the chronic stage.[5] The hypertension due to RAS may be difficult to control, can have associated recurrent flash pulmonary edema, or can develop worsening of renal dysfunction with the use of either angiotensin-converting enzyme inhibitors (ACEI) or angiotensinogen receptor blockers (ARB). The later condition develops in bilateral RAS or RAS occurring in solitary functioning kidney. Long standing uncontrolled hypertension results in ischemic nephropathy manifested by development of renal dysfunction. The treatment of disease in acute stage is with a course of oral steroids (1 mg/kg/day tapered to 5 mg/day over 3 months). Second line agents include methotrexate, cyclophosphamide (CYC), and azathioprine. The chronic fibrotic stage usually does not require any immunosuppressive treatment. The hypertension can be treated with the usual antihypertensive medications with the precaution to avoid ACEI or ARBs in cases of bilateral RAS or RAS in solitary functioning kidney. Balloon angioplasty of renal arteries with or without stenting, surgical bypass, and renal autotransplantation has been successfully used at the later stage of fibro-occlusive disease, though the effect of these procedures in comparison to medical therapy alone over the long-term is inconclusive.[6]

Giant Cell Arteritis

Giant cell arteritis: It is another granulomatous large-vessel vasculitis involving aorta and its major branches with a predilection to involve extracranial branches of the carotid and vertebral arteries.[2] In contrast to TA, it occurs more commonly in elderly population and is frequently associated with polymyalgia rheumatic. The renal involvement is rare and may happen in form of asymptomatic urinary abnormalities. The renal dysfunction due to acute or rapidly progressive renal failure has been described occasionally.[7] Rarely, a combination of GCA with crescentic glomerulonephritis due to antineutrophilic cytoplasmic antibodies (ANCAs)-associated vasculitis has been described in literature.[8]

MEDIUM-VESSEL VASCULITIS

Polyarteritis Nodosa

The classical medium-vessel vasculitis involving kidneys is polyarteritis nodosa (PAN). This is a necrotising vasculitis associated with aneurysmal nodules along the walls of medium-sized muscular arteries and is the condition classically described by Kussmaul and Maier in 1866.[9] The incidence is around 2.0–9.0 per million with predominance in adults and males. The renal involvement has been reported in up to two-thirds of cases.[10] In these cases, PAN causes segmental involvement of medium-sized vessels leading to skip lesions with eccentric inflammation of the vessel wall.[11] These areas of necrosis of the vessel wall results in the aneurysm formation, which can rupture causing parenchymal or perirenal hematomas, presenting as gross hematuria and flank pain. Rarely, patients may present with spontaneous perirenal hematomas as the presenting manifestation.[12] In addition, there may be thrombotic occlusion of the vessels that can lead to renal infarcts. Hypertension is common finding in patients with PAN and can occur at any time during the illness.[10] The perirenal hematoma and renal infarcts can be diagnosed by ultrasonography and computed tomography, but angiography (either conventional or digital subtraction angiography) is the modality of choice.[11] Other nonspecific investigations include elevated inflammatory markers such as erythrocyte sedimentation rate and C-reactive protein. An association with hepatitis B infection has been described in up to half of the cases,[10] while associated hepatitis C is rare. The renal histology shows ischemic changes in glomeruli and rarely proliferative GN. Therapy of PAN has not been described well. In severe cases, like those with associated renal involvement, a course of high-dose corticosteroids given orally or as pulses with or without CYC has been used with variable success.

SMALL-VESSEL VASCULITIS

The most common group of vasculitides associated with renal involvement are the small-vessel vasculitis, particularly, the ANCA-associated vasculitis (AAV).[1]

ANCA-Associated Vasculitis

The AAV includes granulomatosis with polyangiitis (GPA, previously Wegener's granulomatosis), microscopic polyangiitis (MPA), and eosinophilic granulomatosis with polyangiitis (EGPA or Churg-Strauss syndrome).[2] These disorders are characterized by inflammation and destruction of the small arteries, arterioles, capillaries, venules, and veins. As the name suggests, these diseases are commonly associated with the positivity of ANCA, although the type and positivity rates vary according to the disease. While the GPA is usually associated with cytoplasmic (c-) ANCA, the MPA is associated with perinuclear (p-) ANCA. The c-ANCA is also synonymous with Proteinase-3 ANCA, while the p-ANCA is synonymous with myeloperoxidase (MPO) ANCA.

The negativity of ANCA in these cases is <5–10%; however, significant ANCA negativity has been reported in patients with renal-limited vasculitis or in studies where only biopsy proven pauci-immune glomerulonephritis patients are included. The EGPA is associated with MPO-ANCA in 55–60% cases and PR3-ANCA in about 10% cases.[13]

The renal disease has been reported to be more frequent in MPA; however, recurrences are more in GPA. In studies from the National Institutes of Health, the renal involvement occurs in about 18% of patients at presentation,[14] while it subsequently develops in up to 77–85% cases, and it usually happens within the first 2 years of disease onset.[14,15] The renal involvement in different types of AAV manifests in a similar fashion and includes microscopic hematuria, subnephrotic proteinuria, and rapidly progressive renal failure. ANCA-associated vasculitis is the most common cause of rapidly progressive glomerulonephritis in Western countries, while in developing countries it is superseded by postinfectious GN (PIGN).[16] At least 50% of patients with ANCA-associated glomerulonephritis have pulmonary disease. Massive pulmonary hemorrhage affects about 10% of patients with ANCA glomerulonephritis, and is associated with an elevated risk of death.[17] Constitutional signs and symptoms, such as fever, myalgias, arthralgias, and malaise, often accompany small-vessel vasculitis. Vessels in the skin, respiratory tract, kidneys, gut, peripheral nerves, and skeletal muscle are often involved, but the frequencies vary among different phenotypes of small blood vessel vasculitis.[18,19] The renal biopsy is essential in majority of cases as sometimes there may not be clinic-pathological correlation. One can see severe histological involvement in cases of asymptomatic urinary abnormalities. The renal histology also helps in determining the appropriate treatment and prognostication of the patients. Histologically, these diseases are characterized by focal segmental necrotizing glomerulonephritis and crescents. In addition, interstitial granulomas may be found in GPA, while eosinophilic interstitial infiltrate can be found in EGPA. The identification of actual vasculitis in the kidney biopsy is rare. The immunofluorescence typically shows <2+ staining for immunoglobulin or complement deposits, thus giving the term "pauci-immune GN." Though the histological findings are largely similar in different types of AAV, the extra-renal manifestations and serological findings are different and help in classifying them. Recently, a histological classification has been proposed for these diseases, where the pauci-immune GN is divided into four classes, namely focal, crescentic, mixed, and sclerotic.[20] This classification depends on the predominance (i.e. >50% of the glomeruli in the biopsy) of either focal involvement, crescent involvement, or sclerotic involvement in the kidney biopsy. If none of

these three lesions predominate, then the biopsy is labeled as mixed class (Figs 18.1A to D). Subsequently, many studies around the world, including the one done at our center have validated this classification.[20,21] These studies have shown that this classification has an influence on the renal as well as patient outcome of these subjects. The focal class has the best prognosis and treatment outcomes, followed by crescentic and mixed class, while the sclerotic class is the worst.[20-22] Rarely, the kidney biopsy may show isolated interstitial inflammation or vasculitis in absence of pauci-immune glomerulonephritis. Some patients have combination of AAV and antiglomerular basement membrane (GBM) disease, in which case, the biopsy will show linear deposition of immunoglobulin along the GBM. These patients are older, have more severe renal disease and are more likely to have pulmonary involvement than just ANCA-associated renal vasculitis.[16] An association between AAV and systemic lupus erythematosus (SLE) has also been described, where one can observe immune complex deposition along with features of both lupus nephritis and necrotizing glomerulonephritis in the biopsy. Other reported associations include MGN, IgAN, and PIGN.[16]

Sometimes, the vasculitic process remains limited to the kidneys and is known as renal-limited vasculitis. This entity has similar clinical and histological manifestations of the kidneys and is usually associated with MPO-ANCA.[16] Their patients have symptoms related to renal involvement only; however, there may also be presence of constitutional symptoms in addition. These patients are treated in similar manner as to AAV. The relapses are known to occur and the disease may evolve into SV usually MPA, even after many years.[23,24]

In majority of these cases, renal involvement depicts the severity of illness and warrants immediate immunosuppressive therapy. The therapy is determined by the severity of renal failure and the associated extra-renal symptoms. The therapy is usually divided into an initial aggressive induction therapy to induce remission, followed by less aggressive maintenance therapy to prevent relapses.[25] Based on the evidence, the current standard of treatment includes pulse steroids and CYC or rituximab as induction therapy followed by azathioprine for maintenance treatment.[26-28] Cyclophosphamide is administered at 15 mg/kg or 750 mg/m^2 intravenous pulse (dose modified for age and renal function) every 2 weeks for three doses followed by three CYC pulse every 3 weeks. Oral CYC, which was being used previously, has now been substituted by this intravenous regimen in majority of centers.[28-30] In addition, most patients are also subjected to 3–5 intravenous methylprednisolone pulses. Addition of plasmapheresis is required if the serum

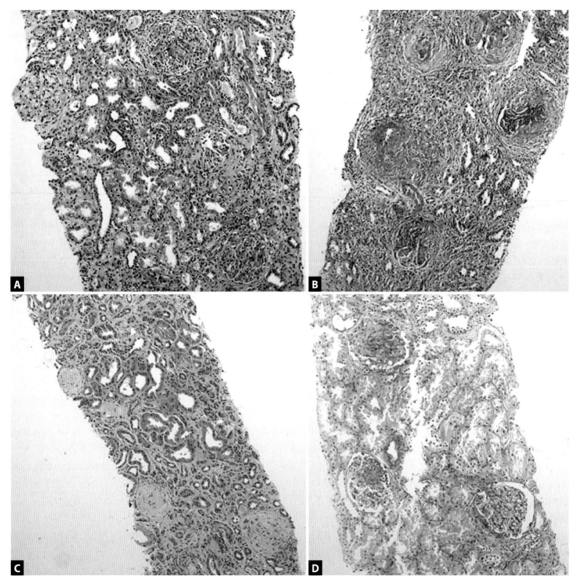

Figs 18.1A to D Representative photomicrographs of the four histopathological classes in ANCA-associated vasculitis. (A) Focal; (B) Crescentic; (C) Sclerotic; and (D) Mixed

creatinine is >5.5 mg/dL or if there is associated pulmonary hemorrhage.[31-34] Rituximab has been compared with intravenous CYC in the recent randomized controlled trials (RITUXIVAS and RAVE trial) as an induction therapy with comparable efficacy and no difference in adverse events.[35,36] The duration of induction therapy is usually 3–6 months and is followed by the maintenance therapy with oral azathioprine (1.5–2 mg/kg/day) along with low-dose steroids.[37] The period of the maintenance therapy is debatable but most centers treat them for at least 2 years after achieving remission.[25] With this regimen, one can expect a remission rate between 80–100% and a mortality rate of <10%.[38,39] Other therapies, such as mycophenolate mofetil (MMF), leflunomide, methotrexate,

anti-CD52 therapy alemtuzumab, antitumor necrosis factor therapies such as infliximab and etanercept, antithymocyte globulin, and intravenous immunoglobulin have also been used but are not established in cases with significant renal failure.[16] In fact, use of methotrexate is contraindicated in patients with serum creatinine of 1.5–2.0 mg/dL. A recent study in China compared MMF and CYC as induction therapy in 35 patients, with serum creatinine >5.5 mg/dL. The study revealed higher rates of remission and maintenance of normal renal function in the MMF group (44%) compared with the CYC group (15%) at 6 months.[40] The EUVAS MYCYC trial is comparing MMF and CYP for induction of remission but has yet to report the findings. Although there are no clinical trials about the efficacy of calcineurin inhibitors in AAV, we have recently reported a successful outcome in a case of GPA with renal involvement with the use of tacrolimus.[41]

Relapses are known to occur, especially with GPA. The relapse can be identified by reappearance of active sediments in urine, development or worsening of renal dysfunction, symptoms of vasculitis in other organ system such as the lung, increase in inflammatory markers such as erythrocyte sedimentation rate and increase in ANCA titers.[16] A repeat renal biopsy is indicated only even the renal relapse is in doubt. The relapses are treated in similar manner as to the new disease with either CYC or rituximab. If the patient has received CYC in past, then rituximab is a good alternative. Refractory disease leading to end-stage renal disease has been reported in 10–26% cases, depending on the length of follow-up and the initial severity of renal failure.[38,39] The survival of these patients either on dialysis or transplant is comparable to those with any other cause.[42,43] The renal transplant is usually performed if the disease is quiescent for at least 6 months with stable or declining ANCA titers. The immunosuppressive regimen is similar and the recurrence after transplant occurs in <10% cases.[44]

OTHER VASCULITIS

Henoch-Schönlein Purpura

Henoch-Schönlein purpura is a small-vessel vasculitis, which is characterized by predominant deposition of IgA along with complements in the involved vessels. Due to this characteristic feature of predominant deposition of IgA, HSP has been renamed as IgA vasculitis (IgAV) in the most recent classification of vasculitis.[2] The disease usually affects skin and gut, while involvement of kidneys occurs in about 20–100% of cases.[45] Symptoms include constitutional symptoms, arthritis, palpable skin purpura over extensor aspects of the limbs, and bloody diarrhea. The renal manifestations include recurrent episodes of microscopic hematuria, variable degree of proteinuria, and renal insufficiency.[45,46] The renal involvement occurs in about one-third of children and two-thirds of adult patients,[47] and usually manifests days to weeks after onset of systemic symptoms. The patient can also have single-organ vasculitis limited to either skin or kidneys. Histologically, the pattern of renal injury is indistinguishable from IgAN, characterized by mesangial and endocapillary proliferation on light microscopy, and dominance or co-dominance of IgA on immunofluroscence.[48] The disease is usually self-limiting and the treatment is mainly supportive. However, the development of rapidly progressive renal failure, older age, and other severe systemic manifestations warrants treatment with steroids or other immunosuppressant drugs such as CYC. The renal prognosis of HSP is usually favorable, except in adults, where about 10–15% cases develop decreased glomerular filtration rate over long-term.[49]

Cryoglobulinemic Vasculitis

The CV is a small-vessel vasculitis characterized by deposition of cryoglobulins along the arterioles, venules, and capillaries along with presence of cryoglobulins and decreased complement levels C3 and C4 in the circulation.[2] There are various causes of cryoglobulinemia including malignancies and associated hepatitis C virus (HCV) infection. However, the vast majority is idiopathic or essential cryoglobulinemia. The CV can involve the kidneys in about one third of cases.[1] These symptoms include microscopic or gross hematuria, variable degree of proteinuria, and renal insufficiency. The most common renal histology is MPGN, while the specific features include presence of hyaline thrombi and organized tubular deposits.[1] Immunofluorescence will reveal presence of immunoglobulin M, G, C1q, and C3. In addition, vasculitis of small- and medium-sized arteries may also be seen.[50] The therapy includes antiviral therapy in cases of HCV-associated CV[51] or immunosuppressant such as steroids, CYC, rituximab, and plasma exchange in other cases.[52]

Lupus-associated Vasculitis

Lupus nephritis is the most common cause of renal involvement in patients with SLE.[1] Although vascular lesions are less common cause of renal involvement, these are often an ignored component of renal involvement in kidneys.[53] Even the most recent classification of lupus nephritis does not pay much importance to these lesions in the kidney biopsy of patients with SLE.[54] There may be a variety of vascular lesions in SLE and includes uncomplicated immune deposits, noninflammatory necrotizing vasculopathy, thrombotic microangiopathy, arteriosclerosis, and true vasculitis (Fig. 18.2). Isolated true vasculitis is extremely rare and often occurs in combination with other vascular lesions or lupus nephritis. The renal manifestations are similar to that of severe class IV lupus nephritis with microscopic hematuria, subnephrotic proteinuria, hypertension, and renal dysfunction. Associated thrombotic microangiopathy may manifest with microangiopathic hemolytic anemia and thrombocytopenia. The treatment is similar to that of class IV lupus nephritis. Addition of plasmapheresis to the treatment has been shown to improve the outcome. Although MMF

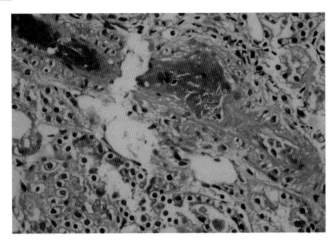

Fig. 18.2 Thrombotic microangiopathy in a case of systemic lupus erythematosus

has been used successfully in lupus-associated vasculitis (LV),[55] there are reports of development of LV while patient is receiving MMF.[56]

KEY POINTS

- Kidneys are one of the most important organs to be involved in SVs.
- Although AAV is the most common form of vasculitis involving kidneys and rapidly progressive renal failure is the most common presentation, attention should also be paid to other forms of renal presentation, and the fact that kidneys may also be affected in other forms of vasculitis.
- Development of renal involvement is associated with significant morbidity and mortality, and thus this should be identified early and treated aggressively.

REFERENCES

1. Mittal T, Rathi M. Rheumatological disease and kidneys: a nephrologist's perspective. Int J Rheum Dis. 2014 Jun 21. doi: 10.1111/1756-185X.12424.
2. Jennette JC, Falk RJ, Bacon PA, et al. 2012 revised International Chapel Hill Consensus Conference Nomenclature of Vasculitides. Arthritis Rheum. 2013;65:1-11.
3. Chaudhry MA, Latif F. Takayasu's arteritis and its role in causing renal artery stenosis. Am J Med Sci. 2013;346:314-8.
4. Jain S, Kumari S, Ganguly NK, et al. Current status of Takayasu arteritis in India. Int J Cardiol. 1996;54:S111-6.
5. Mwipatayi BP, Jeffery PC, Beningfield SJ, et al. Takayasu arteritis: clinical features and management: report of 272 cases. ANZ J Surg. 2005;75:110-7.
6. Perera AH, Youngstein T, Gibbs RG, et al. Optimizing the outcome of vascular intervention for Takayasu arteritis. Br J Surg. 2014;101:43-50.
7. Klien RG, Hunder GG, Stanson AW, et al. Large artery involvement in giant cell (temporal) arteritis. Ann Intern Med. 1975;83:806.
8. Logar D, Rozman B, Vizjak A, et al. Arteritis of both internal carotid arteries in a patient with focal crescentic glomerulonephritis and antineutrophilic cytoplasmic antibodies (c-ANCA). Br J Rheumatol. 1994;33:167-9.
9. Kussmaul A, Maier R. Über eine bisher nicht beschriebene eigenthümliche Arterienerkrankung (Periarteriitis nodosa), die mit Morbus Brightii und rapid fortschreitender allgemeiner Muskellähmung einhergeht. Dtsch Arch Klin Med. 1866;1:484-518.
10. Pagnoux C, Seror R, Henegar C, et al. French Vasculitis Study Group. Clinical features and outcomes in 348 patients with polyarteritis nodosa: a systematic retrospective study of patients diagnosed between 1963 and 2005 and entered into the French Vasculitis Study Group Database. Arthritis Rheum. 2010;62:616-26.
11. Ozaki K, Miyayama S, Ushiogi Y, et al. Renal involvement of polyarteritis nodosa: CT and MR findings. Abdom Imaging. 2009;34:265-70.
12. Mukhopadhyay P, Rathi M, Kohli HS, et al. Polyarteritis nodosa presenting with spontaneous perirenal hematoma. Indian J Nephrol. 2012;22:295-7.
13. Nachman PH, Jennette JC, Falk RJ. Vasculitic diseases of the Kidney. In: Shrier WR, Gottoschalk WC (Eds). Diseases of the Kidney & Urinary tract. 8. 2. Philadelphia: Lippincott Williams & Wilkins; 2007. pp. 1748-75.
14. Hoffman GS, Kerr GS, Leavitt RY, et al. Wegener granulomatosis: an analysis of 158 patients. Ann Intern Med. 1992;116:488.
15. Fauci AS, Haynes BF, Katz P, et al. Wegener's granulomatosis: prospective clinical and therapeutic experience with 85 patients for 21 years. Ann Intern Med. 1983;98:76.
16. Galesic K, Ljubanovic D, Horvatic I. Treatment of renal manifestations of ANCA associated Vasculitis. J Nephropathol. 2013;2:6-19.
17. Sugimoto T, Deji N, Kume S, et al. Pulmonary-renal syndrome, diffuse pulmonary hemorrhage and glomerulonephritis, associated with Wegener's granulomatosis effectively treated with early plasma exchange therapy. Intern Med. 2007;46:49-53.
18. Samarkos M, Loizou S, Vaiopoulos G, et al. The Clinical Spectrum of Primary Vasculitis. Semin Arthritis Rheum. 2005;35:95-111.
19. Ozaki S. ANCA-associated vasculitis: diagnostic and therapeutic strategy. Allergol Int. 2007;56:87-96.
20. Berden AE, Ferrario F, Hagen EC, et al. Histopathologic classification of ANCA-associated glomerulonephritis. J Am Soc Nephrol. 2010;21:1628-36.
21. Naidu GS, Sharma A, Nada R, et al. Histopathological classification of pauci-immune glomerulonephritis and its impact on outcome. Rheumatol Int. 2014 May 18. [Epub ahead of print].
22. Chang DY, Wu LH, Liu G, et al. Re-evaluation of the histopathologic classification of ANCA-associated glomerulonephritis: a study of 121 patients in a single center. Nephrol Dial Transplant. 2012;27:2343-9.

23. Seo P, Stone JH. The antineutrophil cytoplasmic antibody-associated vasculitides. Am J Med. 2004;117:39.

24. Woodworth TG, Abuelo JG, Austin HA 3rd, et al. Severe glomerulonephritis with late emergence of classic Wegener's granulomatosis. Report of 4 cases and review of the literature. Medicine (Baltimore). 1987;66:181.

25. Mukhtyar C, Guillevin L, Cid MC, et al. EULAR recommendations for the management of primary small- and medium-vessel vasculitis. Ann Rheum Dis. 2009;68:310-7.

26. Specks U, Merkel PA, Seo P, et al. Efficacy of remission-induction regimens for ANCA-associated vasculitis. N Engl J Med. 2013;369:417-27.

27. Walters GD, Willis NS, Craig JC. Interventions for renal vasculitis in adults. A systematic review. BMC Nephrol. 2010;24:11-12.

28. Guillevin L, Cordier JF, Lhote F, et al. A prospective, multicenter, randomized trial comparing steroids and pulse cyclophosphamide versus steroids and oral cyclophosphamide in the treatment of generalized Wegener's granulomatosis. Arthritis Rheum. 1997;40:2187-98.

29. Haubitz M, Schellong S, Göbel U, et al. Intravenous pulse administration of cyclophosphamide versus daily oral treatment in patients with antineutrophil cytoplasmic antibody-associated vasculitis and renal involvement: a prospective, randomized study. Arthritis Rheum. 1998;41:1835-44.

30. de Groot K, Harper L, Jayne DR, et al. Pulse versus daily oral cyclophosphamide for induction of remission in antineutrophil cytoplasmic antibody-associated vasculitis: a randomized trial. Ann Intern Med. 2009;150:670-80.

31. Jayne DR, Gaskin G, Rasmussen N, et al. Randomized trial of plasma exchange or high-dosage methylprednisolone as adjunctive therapy for severe renal vasculitis. J Am Soc Nephrol. 2007;18:2180-8.

32. Klemmer PJ, Chalermskulrat W, Reif MS, et al. Plasmapheresis therapy for diffuse alveolar hemorrhage in patients with small-vessel vasculitis. Am J Kidney Dis. 2003;42:1149-53.

33. Walsh M, Catapano F, Szpirt W, et al. Plasma exchange for renal vasculitis and idiopathic rapidly progressive glomerulonephritis: a meta-analysis. Am J Kidney Dis. 2011;57:566-74.

34. Walsh M, Casian A, Flossmann O, et al. Long-term follow-up of patients with severe ANCA-associated vasculitis comparing plasma exchange to intravenous methylprednisolone treatment is unclear. Kidney Int. 2013;84:397-402.

35. Jones RB, Tervaert JW, Hauser T, et al. Rituximab versus cyclophosphamide in ANCA-associated renal vasculitis. N Engl J Med. 2010;363:211-20.

36. Stone JH, Merkel PA, Spiera R, et al. Rituximab versus cyclophosphamide for ANCA-associated vasculitis. N Engl J Med. 2010;363:221-32.

37. Hiemstra TF, Walsh M, Mahr A, et al. Mycophenolate mofetil vs azathioprine for remission maintenance in antineutrophil cytoplasmic antibody-associated vasculitis: a randomized controlled trial. J Am Med Assoc. 2010;304: 2381-8.

38. Slot MC, Tervaert JW, Franssen CF, et al. Renal survival and prognostic factors in patients with PR3-ANCA associated vasculitis with renal involvement. Kidney Int. 2003;63:670.

39. Booth AD, Almond MK, Burns A, et al. Outcome of ANCA-associated renal vasculitis: a 5-year retrospective study. Am J Kidney Dis. 2003;41:776.

40. Hu W, Liu C, Xie H, et al. Mycophenolate mofetil versus cyclophosphamide for inducing remission of ANCA vasculitis with moderate renal involvement. Nephrol Dial Transplant. 2008;23:1307-12.

41. Ramachandran R, Tiwana S, Prabhakar D, et al. Successful induction of granulomatosis with polyangiitis with tacrolimus. Indian J Nephrol. In Press.

42. Lionaki S, Hogan SL, Jennette CE, et al. The clinical course of ANCA small-vessel vasculitis on chronic dialysis. Kidney Int 2009;76:644.

43. Moroni G, Torri A, Gallelli B, et al. The long-term prognosis of renal transplant in patients with systemic vasculitis. Am J Transplant. 2007;7:2133.

44. Gera M, Griffin MD, Specks U, et al. Recurrence of ANCA-associated vasculitis following renal transplantation in the modern era of immunosuppression. Kidney Int. 2007;71:1296.

45. Chang WL, Yang YH, Wang LC, et al. Renal manifestations in Henoch–Schönlein purpura: a 10-year clinical study. Pediatr Nephrol. 2005;20:1269-72.

46. Mir S, Yavascan O, Mutlubas F, et al. Clinical outcome in children with Henoch–Schönlein nephritis. Pediatr Nephrol. 2007;2:64-70.

47. Pillebout E, Thervet E, Hill G, et al. Henoch–Schönlein purpura in adults: outcome and prognostic factors. J Am Soc Nephrol. 2002;13:1271-8.

48. Poterucha TJ, Wetter DA, Gibson LE, et al. Histopathology and correlates of systemic disease in adult Henoch–Schönlein purpura: a retrospective study of microscopic and clinical findings in 68 patients at Mayo Clinic. J Am Acad Dermatol. 2013;68:420-4.

49. Dudley J, Smith G, Llewelyn-Edwards A, et al. Randomised, double-blind, placebo-controlled trial to determine whether steroids reduce the incidence and severity of nephropathy in Henoch–Schönlein purpura (HSP). Arch Dis Child. 2013;98:756-63.

50. D'Amico G, Colasanti G, Ferrario F, et al. Renal involvement in essential mixed cryoglobulinemia. Kidney Int. 1989;35:1004.

51. Cacoub P, Terrier B, Saadoun D. Hepatitis C virus-induced vasculitis: therapeutic options. Ann Rheum Dis. 2014;73:24-30.

52. Terrier B, Krastinova E, Marie I, et al. Management of noninfectious mixed cryoglobulinemia vasculitis: data from 242 cases included in the CryoVas survey. Blood. 2012;119:5996-6004.

53. Radic M, Martinovic Kaliterna D, Radic J. Vascular manifestations of systemic lupus erythematosis. Neth J Med. 2013;71:10-16.

54. Weening JJ, D'Agati VD, Schwartz MM, et al. The classification of glomerulonephritis in systemic lupus erythematosus revisited. Kidney Int. 2004;65:521-30.

55. Rathi M, Nada R. Mycophenolate mofetil in the treatment of lupus vasculopathy. Lupus. 2014;Jun 4. pii: 0961203314539027

56. Gonzalez-Suarez ML, Waheed AA, Andrews DM, et al. Lupus vasculopathy: Diagnostic, pathogenetic and therapeutic considerations. Lupus. 2014;23:421-7.

CHAPTER 19

Neurological Manifestations

Manish Modi, Manoj Goyal

INTRODUCTION

The neurological manifestions in vasculitic disorders can be due to direct consequences of the vasculitis or secondary to other organ involvement or to the therapy. Many factors like hypertension, uremia, other metabolic derangements, drug toxicity, and opportunistic infections contribute to neurological disorders seen in vasculitis. Any part of the nervous system (central or peripheral) may be involved in vasculitis[1] either simultaneously or individually in diverse ways (Table 19.1). Although the neurological complications of vasculitis are sporadic manifestations of these uncommon illnesses, these inflammatory diseases are often treatable and merit consideration in the differential diagnosis of many neurological presentations. Often a thorough medical history, general physical examination, and basic laboratory work provides the first clue that a patient with a neurological presentation actually has a systemic illness.

Table 19.1 Neurological manifestations of vasculitis

Central nervous system disorders:
- Headache
- Meningitis
- Cerebrovascular disease
- Movement disorders
- Seizures
- Acute confusional state
- Cognitive dysfunction
- Affective or psychotic disorders
- Myelopathy

Peripheral nervous system syndromes:
- Cranial neuropathy
- Myopathies
- Peripheral neuropathies

CENTRAL NERVOUS SYSTEM SYNDROMES

Headache

Vasculitis may cause headache by varied mechanisms ranging from benign disorders like migraine to more serious causes like meningitis, arteritis, intracranial hemorrhage or venous sinus thrombosis (discussed later on in this chapter). Nearly, one-third of the patients of systemic sclerosis have been reported to have migraine. When patients have chronic recurrent headache consistent with migraine or tension headache, treatment is often symptomatic and no specific evaluation or anti-inflammatory treatment may be needed. These benign headaches need to be differentiated from more serious conditions.

Headache is characteristic of temporal arteritis (TA) and is the presenting symptom in one-third of the patients.[2] Temporal arteritis is part of the differential diagnosis of new headache patterns in those older than 50 years. Characteristically patients of TA have associated jaw claudication and one-half of these patients have associated polymyalgia rheumatica (PMR). Patients of TA have scalp pain ranging from non-localized tenderness to enlarged, nodular, painful scalp arteries, particularly the temporal artery. The diagnosis of TA can be proven by temporal artery biopsy, which may reveal granulomatous arterial inflammation with giant cells located between intima and media.

Patients with systemic inflammatory disease and headache also need assessment for acute causes like stroke or meningitis. There are reported associations of intracranial hypertension and Behçet's syndrome, systemic lupus erythematosus (SLE), or Sjögren's syndrome; in these patients, cerebral sinus thrombosis must be excluded, especially in those with Behçet's syndrome.[3,4]

Meningitis

Acute episodes of aseptic meningitis classically present with fever, headache and neck stiffness and are difficult to differentiate from other common causes of acute meningitis. Cerebrospinal fluid (CSF) studies are needed to exclude an infectious cause, especially in immunosuppressed patients who are at risk of opportunistic infections. Cerebrospinal fluid analysis in aseptic meningitis classically shows mononuclear pleocytosis with raised proteins and normal sugars and no evidence of infection by culture, PCR or serology. Acute, recurrent, or chronic aseptic meningitis is an infrequent complication of SLE, Sjögren's syndrome, Behçet's syndrome, primary angiitis of central nervous system (CNS), and systemic necrotizing vasculitis. Patients with Behçet's or Sjögren's syndrome occasionally have more neutrophils in the CSF. In all patients with inflammatory diseases and meningitis, a high priority is excluding infectious causes, especially in patients vulnerable to opportunistic infections. Drug-induced meningitis is another important diagnostic consideration.[5]

Pachymeningitis (inflammation of duramater) is visible on MRI as thickened, gadolinium-enhancing dura.[6] Patients may be asymptomatic or have headache, cranial neuropathies, focal brain dysfunction, or seizures. Pachymeningitis is a rare late complication of rheumatoid arthritis[7] and has also been reported in patients with granulomatosis with polyangiitis (GPA), Behçet's syndrome, Sjögren's syndrome, MCTD, and TA.[6,8] Some cases of pachymeningitis are idiopathic, but infections and neoplasia must be excluded.[8]

Cerebrovascular Disease

Patients with vasculitis are at increased risk of both ischemic and hemorrhagic strokes. Ischemic strokes may be caused by accelerated atherosclerosis, cardiogenic emboli, arteriolar disease, prothrombotic state with antiphospholipid antibodies or *per se* by vasculitis.

Cardiac causes of ischemic stroke in patients with vasculitis range from nonbacterial endocarditis, myocardial infarction, valvular disease, or atrial fibrillation. Patients with SLE or with primary antiphospholipid antibody syndrome are prone to nonbacterial endocarditis. Patients with vasculitis can develop myocardial infarction leading to secondary mural thrombosis or arrhythmia.

Intracranial arteriolar disease can arise from secondary hypertension, cerebral vasculopathy (e.g., in lupus), or cerebral vasculitis (e.g., in PACNS). Polyarteritis nodosa (PAN) affects arterioles and small arteries in meninges and brain parenchyma and is responsible for stroke in approximately

11% of cases suffering from PAN.[9] Stroke or TIA can affect almost 5% of patients suffering from temporal arteritis (TA) and can even be a presenting manifestation of TA. In patients presenting with a first stroke, the cause is unlikely to be due to vasculitis. Among 891 first ischemic strokes recorded in a registry, four patients had PACNS, three patients had lupus, one had systemic necrotizing vasculitis, and one had TA.[10]

In a study of 234 patients with SLE, 5.6% had stroke or TIA's.[11] More than half of the events occurred within 5 years of diagnosis of SLE. Patients with SLE are at increased risk of atherosclerotic disease of the carotid and other major arteries. Patients of SLE may also have antiphospholipid antibodies (Lupus anticoagulant or anticardiolipin antibodies) that predispose to endovascular thrombosis and cerebral infarction.[12] Approximately 30% of patients with SLE with these antibodies have thrombotic events. These antibodies reportedly inhibit protein C activity and prostacyclin and antithrombin III activity and may affect platelet membranes. Stroke may also be related to cryoglobulinemia seen in SLE, Sjögren's syndrome, rheumatoid arthritis. Stroke may result when blood vessels in the nervous system are injured by mixed cryoglobulin deposition that may cause an immune-complex-mediated vasculitis. Stroke may also be related to hyper viscosity, cold agglutination of erythrocytes, defective clotting and platelet function.[13] *Takayasu's arteritis* can lead to vertebral or carotid artery stroke. A very unusual cause of vertebral artery stroke is arterial distortion due to cervical ligamentous laxity in a patient with long-standing rheumatoid arthritis.[14]

Intracranial hemorrhage and sub-arachnoid hemorrhage, with varied underlying mechanisms like hypertension, coagulopathy, use of anticoagulants, can be seen as an unusual complication of SLE, Behçet's syndrome, primary angiitis of CNS, systemic necrotizing vasculitis, Sjögren's syndrome, or large-vessel vasculitis.[15]

Cerebral venous thrombosis (CVT) is one of its major neurological manifestations of Behçet's disease (BD), a chronic inflammatory multisystem disorder that can involve the central nervous system (CNS). The incidence of CVT in BD per 1,000 person-years is approximately 3 (95% CI: 1–8), being higher among patients with neurologic involvement (15.1/1,000 person-years). Intracranial hypertension syndrome is a frequent presentation of CVT in BD. The most frequent sites of occlusion are the superior sagittal and the transverse sinus.[16] When treated, BD associated CVT bears a good prognosis. In a series of 48 patients with cerebral venous thrombosis (CVT), five had BD, two had SLE, and one had GPA.[17,18]

The SLE, primary antiphospholipid antibody syndrome, and Sjögren's syndrome can cause relapsing-remitting multifocal CNS syndromes that might be confused with MS. Neuro-Behçet's syndrome can also have episodic recurrences. Rarely, primary angiitis of the CNS can also follow a relapsing-remitting pattern.[19] However, evidence of systemic disease, associated peripheral neuropathy, a spinal MRI showing lesions that span more than two spinal segments, or a brain MRI that is atypical for MS with gray matter lesions or sparing of the corpus callosum gives a clue to the diagnosis of a systemic vasculitis. In Behçet's syndrome, the MRI often shows large confluent lesions involving the brainstem or basal ganglia.[20]

Movement Disorders

Many movement disorders like chorea, athetosis, dystonia, Parkinsonism can be a presenting manifestation of vasculitis or can occur any time during the course of the disease. Three possible mechanisms are postulated for movement disorders in vasculitis. An antibody generated cerebral vasculitis may cause ischemic injury to the basal ganglia. Secondly antibodies may stimulate or inhibit basal ganglia epitopes directly, resulting in dysfunction of neuronal circuitry. Finally, non-immune systemic metabolic disturbances in vasculitic disorders may also play a role. The best-known association between movement disorders and systemic inflammatory disease is chorea that can occur in SLE or primary antiphospholipid antibody syndrome. In SLE choreo-athetosis is seen in 1–2% of patients and may be a presenting feature.[21] In most cases, chorea occurs before the age of 30 years and tends to manifest during lupus flare.[12] Chorea is also a rare occurrence in Sjögren's syndrome, PAN, Behçet's syndrome, or Primary CNS vasculitis.[22-25] Parkinsonism is not a common manifestation due to vasculitis and is usually seen in patients with subcortical white matter disease.[26-28] Some cases are responsive to dopaminergic therapy, yet reversible with anti-inflammatory treatment.[29]

Seizures

Patients with systemic inflammatory disease or vasculitis are at increased risk of seizures, ranging from single episodes, often attributable to secondary metabolic derangements or infection, to recurrent focal or generalized seizures, especially in patients who have had strokes or other focal brain lesions. Seizures have been reported in 4–5% of patients suffering from PAN, GPA, SLE and other vasculitis. When seizures occur in this setting, management requires characterizing the seizure type and investigating metabolic and structural causes. Detailed work-up includes metabolic profile, imaging (including MRI), CSF analysis and EEG. At times, 2 or more etiological factors may be responsible for seizures in a patient of vasculitis.

A number of anticonvulsants, including phenytoin, carbamazepine, valproic acid, and lamotrigine, can cause drug-induced lupus;[30] however, drug-induced lupus rarely causes CNS disease. The use of these drugs is probably not contraindicated in patients with SLE.[31]

Acute Confusional State

Delirium and other manifestations of encephalopathy can complicate a number of diseases. Sometimes the pathogenesis is directly related to the inflammatory disease through stroke or focal brain lesions. However, a number of other mechanisms, such as electrolyte disturbance, hepatic or renal failure, hypertensive encephalopathy, seizures, hypoxia, opportunistic infections, or drug toxicity, must be considered, as each requires specific treatment.

Some unusual causes of encephalopathy in vasculitic disorders also merit consideration as they require specific management. *Reversible posterior leukoencephalopathy*, which can cause headache, delirium, seizures, visual or motor deficits, and characteristic white matter changes on brain CT or MRI, can be precipitated by severe hypertension, renal failure, or medications such as cyclosporine, cyclophosphamide, and corticosteroids and has affected patients with SLE, systemic sclerosis, and GPA.[32,33] Treatment includes blood pressure control and discontinuing offending drugs.

Systemic lupus erythematosus (SLE) can be complicated by TTP (*Thrombotic thrombocytopenic purpura*), which is characterized by encephalopathy, fever, renal failure, microangiopathic hemolytic anemia, and thrombocytopenia.[34] TTP can also present in patients with systemic necrotizing vasculitis, systemic sclerosis, rheumatoid arthritis, or Sjögren's syndrome. Primary treatment of TTP is plasmapheresis and high-dose pulse corticosteroids.[35]

Progressive multifocal leukoencephalopathy (PMLE) usually causes insidious rather than acute changes in mental status. In addition, patients often have visual, motor, sensory, or speech deficits. A number of cases have been reported in patients treated with corticosteroids or other immunosuppressants for treatment of vasculitis.[36-38]

Cognitive Dysfunction

Waxing and waning subtle cognitive dysfunction is frequent in patients with SLE or Sjögren's syndrome. More severe dementia can occur in these illnesses, Behçet's syndrome, or vasculitis, particularly in primary angiitis of CNS. Dementia is one of the protean presentations of TA and can improve with corticosteroid therapy.[39]

Affective or Psychotic Disorders

Systemic lupus erythematosus (SLE) is the prototype of a systemic inflammatory disease that can cause depression, anxiety, or psychosis. One fifth of patients will experience a major depression during their lives and many more will have difficulty with mood and anxiety. Depression is also common in patients with rheumatoid arthritis, systemic sclerosis, or Sjögren's syndrome.[40-44] Depression can be a prominent aspect of polymyalgia rheumatica. There is ongoing debate on the relative roles of organic brain disease and of reaction to serious illness as the cause of affective disorders in many of these patients.[40] These disorders are usually treated with routine psychiatric drugs like selective serotonin reuptake inhibitors (SSRIs) and benzodiazepines rather than immunosuppressive therapy.

Patients of lupus are also at increased risk of psychosis, which may be due to CNS inflammation or secondary to uremia, hypertension, drugs, etc. In psychotic patients on steroids, differentiating lupus psychosis from steroid psychosis is a key to planning treatment.

Myelopathy

Lesions localized to spinal cord are one of the common presenting manifestations of systemic vasculitis. The myelopathy can evolve slowly or acutely; can be generalized or localized; can be complete or incomplete transverse myelopathy (like partial Brown-Sequard syndrome). Some patients of vasculitis have a history of optic neuritis and are classified as having Devic's syndrome. Acute or subacute myelopathy is a rare occurrence in SLE, antiphospholipid antibody syndrome, Sjögren's syndrome, Behçet's syndrome, and vasculitis. In a study of patients presenting with acute myelitis, 6% were associated with SLE, 1% with antiphospholipid antibody syndrome and 9% with Sjögren's syndrome, compared to 43% caused by MS.[41] Transverse myelitis is seen in 1–2% of patients with SLE; 20 of 29 usually these patients have thoracic cord involvement with paraparesis, thoracic sensory level and sphincter disturbance. Patients with systemic inflammatory disease usually have a CSF pleocytosis and mild protein elevation; one-sixth may have CSF oligoclonal bands. The spinal MRI is often helpful in distinguishing the myelitis of systemic inflammatory disease from the myelitis of MS, because in the former, intramedullary lesions causing T2 bright signal on MRI often span two of more spinal segments. Sometimes the cord is swollen and some lesions may enhance on contrast administration. In patients with large-vessel vasculitis, anterior spinal artery infarction is sometimes responsible for acute transverse myelopathy.[42,43]

Patients with rheumatoid arthritis and atlantoaxial joint dislocation are especially vulnerable to compression of the high cervical spinal cord. Cervical myelopathy caused by atlanto axial subluxation/dislocation and by a soft tissue pannus is a feared late complication of rheumatoid arthritis. Subluxation, caused by laxity of inflamed ligament, is usually anterior but can occur in any direction. It is rare in the first year of rheumatoid arthritis, but develops in more than one fourth of patients with disease duration of ≥ 15 years.[44] Patients of high cervical instability are at particular risk of spinal cord injury during intubation and anesthesia. Every patient with myelopathy needs spinal imaging to exclude cord compression.

PERIPHERAL NERVOUS SYSTEM SYNDROMES

Cranial Neuropathy

Optic neuritis can occur in patients with SLE, antiphospholipid antibody syndrome, Behçet's syndrome, Sjögren's syndrome, systemic sclerosis, and systemic necrotizing vasculitis, but the association is uncommon. About 1% of patients with SLE or Behçet's syndrome develop optic neuritis. Conversely, of 457 patients in the optic neuritis treatment trial, only two had a connective tissue disease.[45] Clinically, the visual findings do not distinguish systemic inflammatory cases from idiopathic or demyelinating optic neuritis. MRI shows enlargement and enhancement of segments of the optic nerve in some cases, but this finding can also be seen in idiopathic optic neuritis.[46] In some patients, vision improves after treatment with cyclophosphamide.[47]

Patients with vasculitis, particularly those with TA, risk sudden visual loss from acute ischemic optic neuropathy (AION). The usual mechanism is occlusion of posterior ciliary artery causing acute anterior ischemic optic neuropathy. Mono-ocular blindness may be sudden or occur over few days. Patients with sudden vision loss must be treated urgently as the contralateral eye may be affected within days.[2] Cases of AION have also been reported in association with rheumatoid arthritis or antiphospholipid antibody syndrome. Patients with Wegener's granulomatosis can also develop optic neuropathy from granuloma compressing the nerve or within the nerve.[48,49]

Ophthalmoparesis, characterized by diplopia and ptosis is rare in patients with systemic inflammatory diseases. The etiology may vary from brainstem affliction in SLE or Behçet's disease to cranial nerve III, IV, or VI palsy due to SLE, Behçet's syndrome, Sjögren's syndrome, GPA and other vasculitides. Orbital inflammation and orbital pseudotumor can cause diplopia due to mechanical reasons in GPA. Rarely Brown's syndrome, i.e., superior oblique tendinitis can cause diplopia in Rheumatoid arthritis, Sjögren's syndrome, SLE. A careful neuro-ophthalmological and imaging examination is needed to identify the localization and cause.

Trigeminal neuropathy, characterized by impaired sensation usually in the maxillary or mandibular divisions without involving the motor functions, can evolve acutely or sub acutely in vasculitis. Trigeminal sensory neuropathy, unilateral or bilateral, is particularly associated with Sjögren's syndrome, systemic sclerosis, and MCTD. Most cases of trigeminal neuropathy are not attributable to systemic inflammatory disease.[50,51] However, in patients with painless, purely sensory neuropathy of the lower face, connective tissue disease deserves more consideration.[52]

Ischemic cranial mononeuropathies, especially of the facial nerve, are unusual complications of SLE or vasculitis. The annual incidence of Bell's palsy is far higher than the prevalence of SLE, and cranial neuropathies occur in < 1% of lupus patients. Most patients with isolated cranial mononeuropathies do not need extensive evaluation for vasculitis or connective tissue disease, unless there are other clues to suggest systemic illness.

Single or multiple cranial neuropathies are frequent in patients with GPA where local granulomatous disease of the ear, sinuses or orbit can lead to focal nerve inflammation or compression of optic, ocular motor nerves, Vth, VIIth and VIIIth nerves.[53-55] Multiple cranial nerve involvement was observed in 15 out of 114 cases of PAN in one series.[23]

Vertical atlanto-axial subluxation in patients of long standing rheumatoid arthritis can lead to brainstem and lower cranial nerve involvement causing bulbar palsy, trigeminal sensory loss, ophthalmoparesis, nystagmus, etc.[44,56]

Myopathies

A large number of diseases like SLE, systemic sclerosis, Sjögren's syndrome, MCTD, rheumatoid arthritis may be associated with inflammatory myopathies. The inflammatory myopathies are dermatomyositis (DM), polymyositis (PM), and inclusion-body myositis (IBM).[57] Both DM and PM cause subacute, predominantly immunopathogenesis, and relation to other connective tissue diseases.

Dermatomyositis (DM)

It can affect either children or adults. It is usually accompanied by characteristic skin changes: heliotrope upper eyelid discoloration with swelling and an erythematous rash on the face, neck, anterior chest, back and shoulders, and extensor surfaces of extremity joints. On the fingers, a papular, reddish purple keratotic rash can involve the knuckles but spare the phalanges (Gottron's papules). Fingernails may show dilated capillaries under the bases and distorted cuticles. In DM inflammatory changes concentrate around blood vessels and in the perifasicular connective tissue. Perifasicular atrophy of myocytes is characteristic. The inflammatory cells are predominantly CD4+. The DM affects about one-eighth of patients with systemic sclerosis and probably occurs in more than one-half of patients with MCTD.[58]

Polymyositis (PM)

It rarely occurs before the age of 18 years. Weakness develops insidiously and is not associated with rash. The PM occurs in 5–8% of patients with SLE and has a lower prevalence in patients with rheumatoid arthritis or Sjögren's syndrome. Serum creatine kinase (CK) is elevated up to 50 times normal. Electromyography (EMG) shows brief, low-amplitude, easily recruited motor unit potentials, often accompanied by fibrillation potentials or positive-sharp waves. Antisynthetase autoantibodies are present in up to one-fourth of patients with DM or PM; anti-Jo 1 is the most common of these. Muscle biopsy sample shows inflammatory infiltrates, predominantly CD8+ lymphocytes, invading muscle fibers. However, muscle biopsy samples of some patients with myositis and MCTD have a combination of perivascular CD4+ cells and endomysial CD8+ cells.[59]

Myositis

It is not the only form of muscle dysfunction seen in those with inflammatory diseases. Patients with advanced rheumatoid arthritis often have diffuse weakness. The EMG and serum CK are normal. Muscle biopsy shows type II atrophy, the same pattern that can be seen with disuse. Similarly, patients with Sjögren's syndrome may have mild weakness with normal serum CK levels. Severe hypokalemia due to distal renal tubular acidosis is a rare cause of weakness in patients with Sjögren's syndrome.[60] Most patients with systemic sclerosis have some proximal weakness. These patients have normal or slightly elevated serum CK, sometimes mildly decreased duration or increased polyphasia of motor unit potentials by EMG, and nonspecific changes, such as type II atrophy, on muscle biopsy specimen.[61-63]

Drug toxicity is another cause of muscle disease in patients being treated for connective tissue diseases. Corticosteroid myopathy is a common cause of proximal weakness, especially in patients on high doses or chronic therapy.[64,65]

Treatment with cyclosporine or chloroquine may rarely cause myalgias and weakness.[66] Penicillamine can cause myositis.[67]

Myasthenia Gravis

Patients with myasthenia gravis have an increased incidence of other autoimmune diseases. The prevalence of rheumatoid arthritis in patients with myasthenia gravis may be 2 or 4%.[68-70] The prevalence of SLE is also increased in patients with myasthenia.[71] Case reports link SLE and Lambert–Eaton syndrome.[68] Myasthenia can be a toxic effect of penicillamine or chloroquine.[71,72]

Peripheral Neuropathy

A large number of primary and secondary vasculitic disorders affect the peripheral nerves at the level of radicles, plexus, individual nerves, or diffusely in the form of symmetrical peripheral neuropathy. These disorders are discussed in greater detail in chapter on vasculitic neuropathies. Broadly, the peripheral nervous system can be affected in following ways:

Acute and Chronic Inflammatory Demyelinating Polyradiculoneuropathy

Patients with SLE or rheumatoid arthritis and other connective tissue disorders have an increased incidence of Guillain–Barré syndrome. An association is plausible because of the tendency of autoimmune diseases to overlap.[73-75] Antiphospholipid antibodies can appear transiently in patients with Guillain-Barré syndrome and are not by themselves diagnostic of antiphospholipid antibody syndrome. An alternative but uncommon explanation for acute ascending paralysis in patients with lupus or vasculitis is fulminant vasculitic neuropathy. Chronic inflammatory demyelinating polyneuropathy is also linked to systemic inflammatory diseases in case reports.[76,77]

Autonomic Neuropathy

Autonomic neuropathy is characterized by orthostatic hypotension, impotence, impaired sweating, constipation or diarrhea and abnormal cardiac reflexes. It may or may not be associated with sensory neuropathy or neuronopathy and may complicate a number of connective tissue diseases, including rheumatoid arthritis, SLE, Sjögren's syndrome, and systemic sclerosis.[78] In these illnesses autonomic deficits are more likely to be found on physiological testing than to be symptomatic. In an occasional patient of Sjögren's syndrome, more severe autonomic dysfunction is the predominant neurological problem.[79]

Mononeuropathy and Mononeuritis Multiplex

Carpal tunnel syndrome is the most common neurological manifestation of rheumatoid arthritis and is seen in almost one-half of the patients.[80] Ulnar nerve compression in the ulnar groove, peroneal and posterior nerve compression by Baker's cyst in the popliteal region, tarsal tunnel syndrome and digital neuropathies may affect patients with rheumatoid arthritis.[81]

Vasculitis is a common cause of mononeuritis multiplex. About one-fourth of patients with mononeuropathy multiplex have nonsystemic vasculitis neuropathy and another one-fourth have some form of systemic necrotizing vasculitis.[82] Diabetic amyotrophy, diabetic radiculopathy, and other manifestations of multifocal asymmetric diabetic neuropathy are often associated with vasculitis in the affected nerves, a pattern that is unusual in diabetics whose neuropathy is limited to the more common distal symmetric pattern.[83] Mononeuritis multiplex is unusual in patients with SLE or Sjögren's syndrome.

Polyneuropathy

Distal symmetric axonal polyneuropathy can accompany many of the vasculitic disorders like SLE or Sjögren's syndrome and rheumatoid arthritis. Vasculitic neuropathy in NSVN or systemic necrotizing vasculitis sometimes causes a distal relatively symmetric clinical pattern. Neuropathy occurs much less frequently in patients with systemic sclerosis, Behçet's syndrome, or TA. Some of the drugs used in treatment of inflammatory diseases, including gold, chloroquine, colchicine, and penicillamine, can cause neuropathy. In patients with multifocal CNS disease, concomitant peripheral neuropathy does not rule out MS but can alert the clinician to check carefully for SLE, Sjögren's syndrome, and vasculitis.

Distal sensory or sensori-motor neuropathy is the most common peripheral neuropathy in patients with Sjögren's syndrome and is seen in up to one-fifth of patients. It usually presents as asymmetric dysfunction of small and large sensory fibers. There is impaired touch, pain, temperature and joint position senses. There may be depressed reflexes, pseudoathetosis and sensory ataxia on examination in advanced disease. Pathologically sural nerve biopsy shows axonal loss in large and small fibers and only few cases show evidence of vasculitis and lymphocytic infiltration. Dorsal root ganglia may show neuronal destruction and lymphocytic infiltration.

Treatment

There is a paucity of class I data on treatment of the neurological manifestations of vasculitis. The rarity and diversity of these syndromes makes it difficult to design prospective, randomized, controlled treatment trials. Therefore, the more extensive experience in treating systemic vasculitis is often extrapolated to treating neurological disease. Glucocorticoids and cyclophosphamide are the therapeutic mainstays. Other immunosuppressants such as azathioprine, methotrexate, or cyclosporine are used at times. Newer approaches to immunomodulation, like rituximab, infliximab, etanercept are sometimes tried. The choice of therapy depends more on the severity of the neurological complication than on underlying systemic diagnosis. Thus, mononeuritis multiplex, myelitis, symptomatic focal brain lesions, or optic neuritis often warrant aggressive immunosuppression, while mild peripheral neuropathy, recurrent headache, or subtle cognitive problems might be treated symptomatically. Syndromes such as myasthenia gravis and Guillain-Barré syndrome, in which antibodies play a direct pathogenic role, often respond to plasmapheresis or IVIg.

KEY POINTS

- Any part of the central or peripheral nervous system can be involved in systemic vasculitis. The suspicion is strong when both central and peripheral nervous system are involved simultaneously in a patient.
- Suspicion of vasculitis is strong when multiple organ systems are involved in addition to neurological disorder.
- Although the neurological complications of vasculitis are sporadic manifestations of these uncommon illnesses, these inflammatory diseases are often treatable and merit consideration in the differential diagnosis of many neurological presentations.
- Diagnosis has to be established quickly in certain diseases like mononeuritis multiplex, as the delay may lead to catastrophic consequences and early aggressive treatment can be gratifying.
- Although no class I evidence exists for use of newer agents these drugs may have promising future in better management of neurological disorders in vasculitis.

REFERENCES

1. Jennekens FG, Kater L. The central nervous system in systemic lupus erythematosus. Part 1. Clinical syndromes: A literature investigation. Rheumatology (Oxford). 2002;41:605-18.
2. Younge BR, Cook BE, Jr, Bartley GB, et al. Initiation of glucocorticoid therapy: Before or after temporal artery biopsy? Mayo Clin Proc. 2004;79:483-91.
3. Sbeiti S, Kayed DM, Majuri H. Pseudotumour cerebri presentation of systemic lupus erythematosus: More than an association. Rheumatology (Oxford). 2003;42:808-10.
4. Stanescu D, Bodaghi B, Huong DL, et al. Pseudotumor cerebri associated with sjögren's syndrome. Graefes Arch Clin Exp Ophthalmol. 2003;241:339-42.
5. Moris G, Garcia-Monco JC. The challenge of drug-induced aseptic meningitis. Arch Intern Med. 1999;159:1185-94.
6. Kupersmith MJ, Martin V, Heller G, et al. Idiopathic hypertrophic pachymeningitis. Neurology. 2004;62:686-94.
7. Cellerini M, Gabbrielli S, Maddali BS, et al. MRI of cerebral rheumatoid pachymeningitis: report of two cases with follow-up. Neuroradiology. 2001;43:147-50.
8. Fujimoto M, Kira J, Murai H, et al. Hypertrophic cranial pachymeningitis associated with mixed connective tissue disease; a comparison with idiopathic and infectious pachymeningitis. Intern Med. 1993;32:510-12.
9. Malamud N, Foster DB. Periarteritis nodosa: A clinico-pathologic report, with special reference to the central nervous system. Archives of Neurology and Psychiatry. 1942;47:828-38.
10. Bogousslavsky J, Van MG, Regli F. The Lausanne stroke registry: Analysis of 1,000 consecutive patients with first stroke. Stroke. 1988;19:1083-92.
11. Kitagawa Y, Gotoh F, Koto A, et al. Stroke in systemic lupus erythematosus. Stroke. 1990;21:1533-9.
12. Cervera R, Asherson RA, Font J, et al. Chorea in the antiphospholipid syndrome. Clinical, radiologic, and immunologic characteristics of 50 patients from our clinics and the recent literature. Medicine (Baltimore). 1997;76:203-12.
13. Abramsky O, Slavin S. Neurologic manifestations in patients with mixed cryoglobulinemia. Neurology. 1974;24:245-9.
14. Snelling JP, Pickard J, Wood SK, et al. Reversible cortical blindness as a complication of rheumatoid arthritis of the cervical spine. Br J Rheumatol. 1990;29:228-30.
15. Futrell N, Millikan C. Frequency, etiology, and prevention of stroke in patients with systemic lupus erythematosus. Stroke. 1989;20:583-91.
16. Aguiar de Sousa D, Mestre T, Ferro JM. Cerebral venous thrombosis in Behçet's disease: A systematic review. J Neurol. 2011;258:719-27.
17. Bousser MG, Chiras J, Bories J, et al. Cerebral venous thrombosis: a review of 38 cases. Stroke. 1985;16:199-213.
18. Enevoldson TP, Russell RW. Cerebral venous thrombosis: New causes for an old syndrome? Q J Med. 1990;77:1255-75.
19. Ropper AH, Ayata C, Adelman L. Vasculitis of the spinal cord. Arch Neurol. 2003;60:1791-4.
20. Tali ET, Atilla S, Keskin T, et al. MRI in Neuro-Behçet's disease. Neuroradiology. 1997;39:2-6.
21. Edwards MJ, Dale RC, Church AJ, et al. A dystonic syndrome associated with anti-basal ganglia antibodies. J Neurol Neurosurg Psychiatry. 2004;75:914-6.

22. Delalande S, de Seze J, Fauchais AL, et al. Neurologic manifestations in primary sjogren syndrome: A study of 82 patients. Medicine (Baltimore). 2004;83:280-91.

23. Ford RG, Siekert RG. Central nervous system manifestations of periarteritis nodosa. Neurology. 1965;15:114-22.

24. Kuriwaka R, Kunishige M, Nakahira H, et al. Neuro-Behçet's disease with chorea after remission of intestinal Behçet's disease. Clin Rheumatol. 2004;23:364-7.

25. Sigal LH. The neurologic presentation of vasculitic and rheumatologic syndromes. A review. Medicine (Baltimore). 1987;66:157-80.

26. Budzilovich GN, Feigin I, Siegel H. Granulomatous angiitis of the nervous system. Arch Pathol. 1963;76:250-6.

27. Mayo J, Arias M, Leno C, et al. Vascular parkinsonism and periarteritis nodosa. Neurology. 1986;36:874-5.

28. Nishimura H, Tachibana H, Makiura N, et al. Corticosteroid-responsive parkinsonism associated with primary Sjögren's syndrome. Clin Neurol Neurosurg. 1994;96:327-31.

29. Lee PH, Joo US, Bang OY, et al. Basal ganglia hyperperfusion in a patient with systemic lupus erythematosus-related parkinsonism. Neurology. 2004;63:395-6.

30. Sarzi-Puttini P, Panni B, Cazzola M, et al. Lamotrigine-induced lupus. Lupus. 2000;9:555-7.

31. Futrell N, Schultz LR, Millikan C. Central nervous system disease in patients with systemic lupus erythematosus. Neurology. 1992;42:1649-57.

32. Min L, Zwerling J, Ocava LC, et al. Reversible posterior leukoencephalopathy in connective tissue diseases. Semin Arthritis Rheum. 2006;35:388-95.

33. Shin KC, Choi HJ, Bae YD, et al. Reversible posterior leukoencephalopathy syndrome in systemic lupus erythematosus with thrombocytopenia treated with cyclosporine. J Clin Rheumatol. 2005;11:164-6.

34. Aleem A, Al-Sugair S. Thrombotic thrombocytopenic purpura associated with systemic lupus erythematosus. Acta Haematol. 2006;115:68-73.

35. Allford SL, Hunt BJ, Rose P, et al. Guidelines on the diagnosis and management of the thrombotic microangiopathic haemolytic anaemias. Br J Haematol. 2003;120:556-73.

36. Ahmed F, Aziz T, Kaufman LD. Progressive multifocal leukoencephalopathy in a patient with systemic lupus erythematosus. J Rheumatol. 1999;26:1609-12.

37. Case records of the Massachusetts Feneral Hospital. Weekly clinicopathological exercises. Case 20-1995. A 66-year-old man with a history of rheumatoid arthritis treated with adrenocorticosteroids, with the development of aphasia and right-sided weakness. N Engl J Med. 1995;332:1773-80.

38. Warnatz K, Peter HH, Schumacher M, et al. Infectious CNS disease as a differential diagnosis in systemic rheumatic diseases: Three case reports and a review of the literature. Ann Rheum Dis. 2003;62:50-7.

39. Caselli RJ. Giant cell (temporal) arteritis: A treatable cause of multi-infarct dementia. Neurology. 1990;40:753-5.

40. Malinow KL, Molina R, Gordon B, et al. Neuropsychiatric dysfunction in primary Sjögren's syndrome. Ann Intern Med. 1985;103:344-50.

41. de Seze J, Stojkovic T, Breteau G, et al. Acute myelopathies: Clinical, laboratory and outcome profiles in 79 cases. Brain. 2001;124:1509-21.

42. Gibb WR, Urry PA, Lees AJ. Giant cell arteritis with spinal cord infarction and basilar artery thrombosis. J Neurol Neurosurg Psychiatry.1985;48:945-8.

43. Nair KR, Bhaskaran R, Retnakumari S, et al. Ischemic myelopathy in Takayasu's disease. J Assoc Physicians India. 1985;33:735-6.

44. Naranjo A, Carmona L, Gavrila D, et al. Prevalence and associated factors of anterior atlantoaxial luxation in a nation-wide sample of rheumatoid arthritis patients. Clin Exp Rheumatol. 2004;22:427-32.

45. Beck RW, Cleary PA, Anderson MM, Jr., et al. A randomized, controlled trial of corticosteroids in the treatment of acute optic neuritis. The optic neuritis study group. N Engl J Med. 1992;326:581-8.

46. Sklar EM, Schatz NJ, Glaser JS, et al. Mr of vasculitis-induced optic neuropathy. AJNR Am J Neuroradiol. 1996;17:121-8.

47. Rosenbaum JT, Simpson J, Neuwelt CM. Successful treatment of optic neuropathy in association with systemic lupus erythematosus using intravenous cyclophosphamide. Br J Ophthalmol. 1997;81:130-2.

48. Bullen CL, Liesegang TJ, McDonald TJ, et al. Ocular complications of Wegener's granulomatosis. Ophthalmology. 1983;90:279-90.

49. Drachmann DA. Neurological complications of Wegener's granulomatosis. Arch Neurol. 1963;8:45-55.

50. Blau JN, Harris M, Kennett S. Trigeminal sensory neuropathy. N Engl J Med. 1969;281:873-6.

51. Spillane JD, Wells CE. Isolated trigeminal neuropathy. A report of 16 cases. Brain. 1959;82:391-416.

52. Lecky BR, Hughes RA, Murray NM. Trigeminal sensory neuropathy. A study of 22 cases. Brain (Pt 6). 1987;110:1463-85.

53. Anderson JM, Jamieson DG, Jefferson JM. Non-healing granuloma and the nervous system. Q J Med. 1975;44:309-23.

54. Fauci AS, Haynes BF, Katz P. Wegener's granulomatosis: Prospective clinical and therapeutic experience with 85 patients for 21 years. Ann Intern Med. 1983;98:76-85.

55. Nishino H, Rubino FA, DeRemee RA, et al. Neurological involvement in Wegener's granulomatosis: an analysis of 324 consecutive patients at the mayo clinic. Ann Neurol. 1993; 33:4-9.

56. Clark CR, Goetz DD, Menezes AH. Arthrodesis of the cervical spine in rheumatoid arthritis. J Bone Joint Surg Am. 1989;71:381-92.

57. Dalakas MC, Hohlfeld R. Polymyositis and dermatomyositis. Lancet. 2003;362:971-82.

58. Hall S, Hanrahan P. Muscle involvement in mixed connective tissue disease. Rheum Dis Clin North Am. 2005;31:509-517, vii.

59. Vianna MA, Borges CT, Borba EF, et al. Myositis in mixed connective tissue disease: A unique syndrome characterized by immunohistopathologic elements of both polymyositis and dermatomyositis. Arq Neuropsiquiatr. 2004;62:923-34.

60. Christensen KS. Hypokalemic paralysis in Sjögren's syndrome secondary to renal tubular acidosis. Scand J Rheumatol. 1985;14:58-60.

61. Clements PJ, Furst DE, Campion DS, et al. Muscle disease in progressive systemic sclerosis: Diagnostic and therapeutic considerations. Arthritis Rheum. 1978;21:62-71.

62. Hausmanowa-Petrusewicz I, Jablonska S, Blaszczyk M, et al. Electromyographic findings in various forms of progressive systemic sclerosis. Arthritis Rheum. 1982;25:61-65.

63. Ringel RA, Brick JE, Brick JF, et al. Muscle involvement in the scleroderma syndromes. Arch Intern Med. 1990;150:2550-2.

64. Askari A, Vignos PJ Jr, Moskowitz RW. Steroid myopathy in connective tissue disease. Am J Med. 1976;61:485-92.

65. Khaleeli AA, Edwards RH, Gohil K, et al. Corticosteroid myopathy: A clinical and pathological study. Clin Endocrinol (Oxford). 1983;18:155-66.

66. Noppen M, Velkeniers B, Dierckx R, et al. Cyclosporine and myopathy. Ann Intern Med. 1987;107:945-6.

67. Doyle DR, McCurley TL, Sergent JS. Fatal polymyositis in d-penicillamine-treated rheumatoid arthritis. Ann Intern Med. 1983;98:327-30.

68. Deodhar A, Norden J, So Y, et al. The association of systemic lupus erythematosus and lambert-eaton myasthenic syndrome. J Rheumatol. 1996;23:1292-4.

69. Oosterhuis HJ, de Haas WH. Rheumatic diseases in patients with myasthenia gravis. An epidemiological and clinical investigation. Acta Neurol Scand. 1968;44:219-27.

70. Thorlacius S, Aarli JA, Riise T, et al. Associated disorders in myasthenia gravis: Autoimmune diseases and their relation to thymectomy. Acta Neurol Scand. 1989;80:290-5.

71. Kuncl RW, Pestronk A, Drachman DB, et al. The pathophysiology of penicillamine-induced myasthenia gravis. Ann Neurol. 1986;20:740-4.

72. Robberecht W, Bednarik J, Bourgeois P, et al. Myasthenic syndrome caused by direct effect of chloroquine on neuromuscular junction. Arch Neurol. 1989;46:464-8.

73. Leneman F. The Guillain-Barre syndrome. Definition, etiology, and review of 1,100 cases. Arch Intern Med. 1966;118:139-44.

74. Laidlaw DA, Smith PE, Hudgson P. Orbital pseudotumour secondary to giant cell arteritis: An unreported condition. BMJ. 1990;300:784.

75. Mochizuki H, Kamakura K, Masaki T, et al. Motor dominant neuropathy in Sjögren's syndrome: Report of two cases. Intern Med. 2002;41:142-6.

76. Barnes D, Hammans SR, Legg NJ. Chronic relapsing inflammatory polyneuropathy complicating sicca syndrome. J Neurol Neurosurg Psychiatry. 1988;51:159-60.

77. Rechthand E, Cornblath DR, Stern BJ, et al. Chronic demyelinating polyneuropathy in systemic lupus erythematosus. Neurology. 1984;34:1375-7.

78. Louthrenoo W, Ruttanaumpawan P, Aramrattana A, et al. Cardiovascular autonomic nervous system dysfunction in patients with rheumatoid arthritis and systemic lupus erythematosus. QJM. 1999;92:97-102.

79. Mori K, Iijima M, Koike H, et al. The wide spectrum of clinical manifestations in Sjögren's syndrome-associated neuropathy. Brain. 2005;128:2518-34.

80. Fleming A, Dodman S, Crown JM, et al. Extra-articular features in early rheumatoid disease. Br Med J. 1976;1:1241-3.

81. Gray RG, Gottlieb NL. Hand flexor tenosynovitis in rheumatoid arthritis. Prevalence, distribution, and associated rheumatic features. Arthritis Rheum. 1977;20:1003-8.

82. Collins MP, Periquet MI. Nonsystemic vasculitic neuropathy. Curr Opin Neurol. 2004;17:587-98.

83. Said G, Lacroix C, Lozeron P, et al. Inflammatory vasculopathy in multifocal diabetic neuropathy. Brain. 2003;126:376-85.

CHAPTER 20

Vasculitic Neuropathy

Manoj Goyal, Manish Modi

INTRODUCTION

Vasculitides are a group of disorders that are clinically, pathologically, and etiologically diverse, with the presence of inflammation in the blood vessels resulting in vessel wall injury being the common link. Accordingly, most of the vasculitides affect multiple organs either simultaneously or sequentially.[1] However, in some patients, vasculitis may be restricted to a single organ, tissue, or body region, including peripheral nervous system.[2] Clinical manifestations of vasculitis are protean depending upon the location and size of affected vessels, degree of inflammation, and associated comorbid conditions such as diabetes, etc. Vasculitic neuropathy (VN) results from affection of vasa nervosum or epineurial capillary blood vessels by the inflammatory process resulting in decreased blood supply, necrosis of blood vessels, and ischemic injury to the nerves. Vasculitic neuropathies are aggressive and result in significant morbidity, but they typically improve following treatment. Thus, the importance of early diagnosis of vasculitic neuropathies cannot be overemphasized. In some cases, diagnosis is straightforward, e.g. a patient present with mononeuritis multiplex in context of multiorgan involvement. However, at other times, it may be difficult more so when clinical picture is more of a generalized symmetric neuropathy. Thus, it is imperative that clinicians should develop a rational approach to a patient with peripheral neuropathy, keeping in mind the possibility of underlying vasculitis.[3]

CLASSIFICATION

Last two decades have seen increase in complexity of classification of vasculitic neuropathies in part because of better understanding of vasculitis and in part because of addition of other disorders. There are several ways to classify the vasculitic neuropathies. These can be classified in terms of clinical characteristics (organ involvement, disease association), histopathological features (size of involved vessels), and underlying mechanisms. Most widely accepted classification schemes for vasculitic neuropathies include 2012 Chapel Hill Consensus Conference (CHCC 2012) classification, peripheral nerve society task force classification, and classification based on the size of the involved vessels.[4]

The first classification of vasculitic neuropathies came from American College of Rheumatology (ACR) in 1990, which published classification criteria for diagnosis of primary systemic vasculitis. A major limitation of these criteria was that these did not distinguish vasculitis from nonvasculitic conditions, though these were useful for classifying already diagnosed patients of primary systemic vasculitic neuropathies. Later, CHCC proposed nomenclature of vasculitis based on size and histopathology of involved vessels. Large vessels were primarily targeted by giant cell arteritis (GCA) and Takayasu arteritis; small-to-medium-sized arteries were primarily targeted by polyarteritis nodosa (PAN) and Kawasaki disease while vasculitides such as granulomatosis with polyangiitis (previously Wegener's), eosinophilic granulomatosis with polyangiitis (previously Churg Strauss syndrome), microscopic polyangiitis (MPA), Henoch-Schönlein purpura (HSP), cryoglobulinemia, and cutaneous angiocytoclastic angiitis affect the microvasculature.[5]

These classification/nomenclature systems had some inherent problems. These often yield incoherent results when applied to same cohort of patients. Both these systems are not useful for classifying de novo patients, and both these do not use antineutrophilic cytoplasmic antibodies (ANCAs) for classification. Cytoplasmic ANCAs (cANCAs) directed against proteinase 3 and perinuclear ANCAs (pANCAs) directed against myeloperoxidase are specific for primary systemic vasculitides affecting small- and medium-sized vessels. In addition, there is some evidence to suggest that ANCAs play a direct role in pathogenesis of small-vessel vasculitis and their presence is an independent predictor of higher chance of relapse. Thus, efforts were made ongoing to incorporate ANCAs' status into new classification schemes.[5]

Chapel Hill Consensus Conference classification scheme (2012) gave better understanding of vasculitic neuropathies. In this classification, vasculitic neuropathies were categorized using knowledge of etiology, pathogenesis, pathology, demographics, and clinical markers.[6] The main change that has occurred in CHCC 2012 compared to 1994 version is subcategorization of small-vessel vasculitides based on the presence of immunoglobulin deposition in the vessel wall. The group without immunoglobulin deposition is ANCA-associated vasculitis (AAV), which includes MPA, WG (renamed as granulomatosis with angiitis) and CSS (renamed as eosinophilic granulomatosis with polyangiitis [EGPA]). Small-vessel vasculitis associated with deposition of immune complexes includes cryoglobulinemic vasculitis.

Vasculitic neuropathies are classified into three main groups by a peripheral nerve society task force: (a) primary systemic vasculitis, (b) secondary systemic vasculitis, and (c) nonsystemic vasculitic neuropathies. While in primary systemic vasculitis, there is an absence of an obvious cause that can account for vasculitis, secondary systemic vasculitis includes vasculitis that results from immune-mediated damage, triggered by infections or drugs or malignancy or is associated with predisposing autoimmune conditions such as connective tissue disorders. The term nonsystemic VN (NSVN) implies localized vasculitis restricted to peripheral nervous system.[7] In this classification, diabetic lumbosacral and cervical radiculoplexus neuropathy has been categorized as nonsystemic or localized vasculitis, and nondiabetic radiculoplexus neuropathy has been categorized under NSVN.

Another simpler method of classification of neuropathies is based on the size of involved blood vessels—namely nerve large arteriole vasculitis and nerve microvasculitis.[4] While nerve large arteriole vasculitis (rheumatoid vasculitis, PAN, WG, CSS) primarily affects epineurial and perineurial vessels, 75–400 μm in diameter, nerve microvasculitis (classic NSVN, Sjögren's syndrome, neuropathy associated with sicca syndrome, some virus-associated vasculitic neuropathies) primarily affects smallest arterioles (<40 μm), endometrial microvessels (capillaries), and venules. The systemic vasculitides affecting large nerve arteriole can be subclassified into small-vessel predominant vasculitic neuropathies (CSS), medium-vessel predominant vasculitic

Table 20.1 Classification of vasculitic neuropathies

- **Primary systemic vasculitides**
  - Predominant small-vessel involvement
    - Microscopic polyangiitis (ANCA related)
    - EGPA (eosinophilic granulomatosis with polyangiitis) (ANCA related)
    - GPA (granulomatosis with polyangiitis) (ANCA related)
    - HCV-related essential mixed cryoglobulinemia
    - Henoch-Schönlein purpura (IgA vasculitis)
  - Predominant medium-vessel involvement
    - Polyarteritis nodosa
  - Predominant large-vessel involvement
    - Giant cell arteritis
- **Secondary systemic vasculitides**
  - Connective tissue disease: rheumatoid arthritis, systemic lupus erythematosus, Sjögren syndrome, systemic sclerosis, dermatomyositis, and mixed connective tissue disease
  - Sarcoidosis
  - Behçet syndrome
  - Infections (hepatitis B virus, hepatitis C virus, *cytomegalovirus*, leprosy, lyme disease, etc.)
  - Drugs
  - Malignancy
  - Inflammatory bowel disease
- **Nonsystemic/localized vasculitis**
  - Nonsystemic vasculitic neuropathy
    - Nondiabetic radiculoplexus neuropathy
    - Wartenberg migrant sensory neuritis
  - Diabetic lumbosacral and cervical radiculoplexus neuropathy

Source: Collins et al. (2010).

neuropathies (PAN), and large-vessel predominant vasculitic neuropathies (GCA). It is important to note that even medium- and large-vessel vasculitides can affect large nerve arterioles that are actually categorized as small vessels as per vasculitic nomenclature. Secondary causes of systemic vasculitides include connective tissue disorders, drugs, and malignancies. In general, nerve large arteriole vasculitis is associated with more aggressive course and severe systemic manifestations than nerve microvasculitis and needs to be treated more aggressively.[4]

The classification of vasculitic neuropathies is summarized in Table 20.1.

EPIDEMIOLOGY

The annual incidence of systemic vasculitides is estimated to be about 14/1 lakh adults.[8] The most common systemic vasculitides are GCA and predominant cutaneous vasculitis followed by rheumatoid, GPA, and MPA. Approximately 60–70% of systemic vasculitides affect peripheral nervous system, and 30% of elderly people with a progressive, disabling, and painful neuropathy have VN.[9] Most commonly encountered vasculitic neuropathies include NSVN (26%),

MPA/PAN (25%), rheumatoid vasculitis (12%), and EGPA (10%). Though VN is not a predictor of death or relapse in primary small-vessel or medium-vessel vasculitis, it does affect quality of life significantly.[10] Women are more affected than men (60 versus 40%), and mean age at time of diagnosis is about 60 years.

PATHOGENESIS AND PATHOLOGY

There is ample evidence to suggest that vasculitic neuropathies are immune-mediated diseases, resulting in endothelial dysfunction and vessel wall damage. At the site of inflammation, activated endothelial cells and leukocytes release chemokines and cytokines which result in recruitment, adhesion, and extravasation of circulating leukocytes. During normal life, a critically balanced interaction between proinflammatory and anti-inflammatory factors controls invading pathogens and their harmful effects, promotes vascular repair, and ascertains that inflammatory process is transient.[11] An uncontrolled cascade of events, whereby leukocytes are recruited and activated disproportionately, adhere to the endothelial cell surface followed by complement activation, endothelial cell apoptosis, and further extravasation of leucocytes, results in severe inflammation and vasculitis. The disruption of normal endothelial cell-leukocyte homeostasis is influenced by both pathogen-specific factors as well as host-specific and genetic factors.

Immune pathways that have been implicated in pathogenesis include (a) antigen-induced formation of immune complexes and their deposition in vessel wall; (b) antigen personation by endothelial cells; (c) pathogen-induced alteration of antigenic expression on endothelial cells; (d) autoantibodies such as ANCA, antiendothelial cell, or anti-HSP60 antibodies; (e) cell-mediated immune responses through CD4+ and CD8+-activated T cells, CD 68+ macrophages and neutrophils that release matrix metalloproteinases and other proteolytic enzymes, induce complement activation, and induce endothelial cell apoptosis.[12-14] Studies on nerve pathology support a main role for cellular immune response in pathogeneses of VN, as suggested by predominance of activated CD8+ and CD4+ T cells and macrophages in epineurial vascular infiltrates while there is paucity of B cells, natural killer cells, and polymorphonuclear cells. In addition, antigen-presenting cells (macrophages, neutrophils, Schwann cells) show increased expression of MHC class I and class II molecules that present antigens to CD8+ cytotoxic and CD4+ helper T cells. Immunological studies also reveal a wide range of inflammatory mediators expressed by endothelial cells or inflammatory cells, which include chemokines and cytokines (TNFα, IL1, IL2, IL6, nuclear factor kappa B), cellular adhesion molecules, ligands and receptors (ICAM-1, ICAM-2, VCAM-1, selectins, β2-integrins), oxidative and hypoxic stress-induced proteins, metalloproteinases, perforins, and Fas receptors, suggestive of cytotoxic T cell-inducible apoptosis.[9] Commensurate with these changes, there is an upregulation of immune genes related T cell and macrophage activation as well as for all the inflammatory mediators, as discussed in previous paragraph.[9]

Humoral mechanisms may also be operative in pathogenesis of VN as suggested by deposition of immunoglobulins and complement in wall of epineurial blood vessels. Also, there is marked upregulation of immunoglobulin genes in vasculitic neuropathies. Thus, humoral immune response might constitute another mechanism of vascular damage in vasculitic neuropathies.[5]

Peripheral nerves are supplied by a rich anastomotic network of two integrated blood systems. This rich blood supply coupled with the fact that peripheral nerves are resistant to effects of ischemia makes peripheral nerves resistant to chronic ischemic damage. Only when there is extensive involvement of vasa nervosum, damage occurs in the peripheral nerves and usually regions of poorest blood supply are affected, i.e. central regions of large fascicles in watershed zones of proximal and middle portions of extremity nerves.[15-18]

Nerve biopsy in vasculitic neuropathies usually reveals evidence of axonal degeneration, which tends to be centrofascicular in proximal nerve, but tends to be multifocal in distal nerves due to intermingling of descending fibers. There is evidence of loss of myelinated nerve fibers, Wallerian degeneration, and regenerating axonal clusters on nerve biopsy. While systemic vasculitis predominantly affects vessel 50–300 μm in diameter, NSVN typically affects vessels less than 100 μm in diameter, though not exclusively. In one study, Morozumi et al.[19] analyzed nerve pathology in eight cases of MVA-associated systemic VN. They found diffuse involvement of epineurium throughout the nerve along with severe involvement of nutrient arteries. There was marked loss of myelinated fibers in middle segments of the nerves that correspond to distal arm and thigh. Axonal degeneration was prominent in distal parts of nerves, whereas proximal segments revealed myelin wrinkling and mild demyelination/remyelination. They concluded that systemic vasculitis affects peripheral nerves diffusely but causes maximal damage in proximal and middle portion of extremity nerves corresponding to border zones of perfusion.

CLINICAL FEATURES

The clinical presentation of VN varies as per the site and severity of blood vessel involvement.[5] Though neuropathy may be heralding feature in up to 25% of patients with PAN or AAV, usually signs and symptoms that predominate in both primary and secondary SVN are related to renal, gastrointestinal, or other organ systems. Even in NSVC, which by definition is restricted to PNS, fatigue, weight loss, and myalgias occur in up to 30% and fever in up to 10% of patients.[7] As a rule, SVN tends to be more severe and aggressive as compared to NSVN. The type of presentation varies. While most of the patients have a subacute onset ranging from weeks to months, a few may prevent fulminantly, while a few run a chronic indolent progression over years. The median delay in diagnosis ranges from 2–8 months from onset of symptoms. Most patients experience acute attacks, while approximately 33% run a chronic slowly progressive course.[5,7,20-26] Most patients present with both motor as well sensory deficits, but approximately 15% of patients present with sensory deficits predominantly, secondary to cutaneous nerve involvement.[5] The sensory disturbance usually involve all modalities. Less common presentations include sensory ataxic neuropathy, small fiber neuropathy, and radiculoplexus neuropathy. Pure motor or autonomic presentations are exceptional, but do occur. Cranial nerves are involved in approximately 10% of patients. Most of the vasculitic neuropathies (up to 80%) are painful.[7]

The most characteristic phenotype is that of multiple mononeuropathy (45%), characterized by involvement (sequential or simultaneous) of multiple individual nerves, followed by asymmetric polyneuropathy (35%) and distal symmetric polyneuropathy (20%). However, symmetric phenotype is rare, and most of these patients will show evidence of minor asymmetry if examined carefully.[7] A chronic, slowly progressive, distal symmetric presentation over years is unlikely to result from VN. Vasculitis tends to affect some nerves more than other depending upon the amount of collateral blood supply. Common peroneal nerve and distal peroneal part of sciatic nerve as well as ulnar nerve are prone to be affected by vasculitic process.[5] These are followed by tibial, sural, median, and radial nerves in that order. The cranial nerves are most commonly affected in GPA or EGPA. Most commonly affected cranial nerves include second, third, fifth, sixth, and seventh cranial nerves.[9]

Diagnosis of probable VN should be considered in the presence of following features: acute or subacute onset and a progressive or intermittently progressive course, sensory or sensorimotor involvement, asymmetrical or multifocal pattern with distal involvement, predominant affection of lower limbs and pain. The clinical diagnosis is much more likely in the presence of sign and symptoms of multiorgan involvement. However, in the presence of appropriate clinical features, diagnosis of NSVN should always be considered, and appropriate investigations should be carried out including nerve muscle biopsy.[7]

TYPES OF VASCULITIC NEUROPATHIES

Primary Medium- and Small-vessel Systemic Vasculitides

The illnesses under this category are potentially life-threatening diseases that tend to affect peripheral nerves along with other organs. Their annual incidence ranges from 10 to 20/million.[27-29] These include PAN, MPA, EGPA, GPA, IgA vasculitis, antiglomerular basement membrane disease, and hypocomplementemic urticarial vasculitis.[6] The AAVs (GPA, MPA and EGPA) have a predilection for small vessels and potential to cause rapidly progressive glomerulonephritis and pulmonary capillaritis.[5]

Polyarteritis Nodosa

Polyarteritis nodosa is a systemic vasculitis which has a predilection for small- and medium-sized arteries. Traditionally, it was considered as the most common form of small- and medium-vessel vasculitis and is the commonest cause of VN. It is characterized pathologically by focal, segmental, necrotizing vasculitis of small- and medium-sized vessels and clinically by renal arteritis (renal infarcts, hypertension) and presence of visceral microaneurysms on angiography. Granulomas and eosinophilic infiltrates are seen occasionally. Hepatitis B surface antigen may be positive in PAN (20–30%) as can be HCV (5–10%). After CHCC 2012 criteria that included demonstration of microvessel involvement on pathological examination as the exclusion criteria, MPA has become more prevalent. It is also excluded by presence of pulmonary vasculitis, glomerulonephritis, cryoglobulins, or ANCAs.[7,30] Polyarteritis nodosa typically affects people between 40 and 70 years of age with subacute (weeks to months) onset of constitutional symptoms. Fever and weight loss occurs in 60–70% of patients with evidence of disease process in peripheral nervous system, joints (50%), skin (55–60%), kidneys (40–50%), muscles, GI tract (30%), heart (10–15%), and testis (2–29%). Neuropathies occur in 60–70% of patients and are the presenting feature in 30% of cases. These typically occur in the form of mononeuritis multiplex affecting limb nerves. Cranial nerve involvement is seen in <5% of cases. Commonest cause of death is mesenteric vascultis.[30-34]

Laboratory abnormalities commonly described in PAN include elevated erythrocyte sedimentation rate (ESR) (85%), leukocytosis (70%), anemia (60%), and thrombocytosis (60%). Antinuclear antibodies (ANAs) (15%), rheumatoid factor (RF) (30%), and decreased complement levels (25%) are observed occasionally. Approximately 66% of patients show evidence of microaneurysms in renal, hepatic, and mesenteric arteries on visceral angiography, while nonspecific occlusive changes are seen in 98%.[35]

Microscopic Polyangiitis

Microscopic polyangiitis, primarily affecting arterioles, capillaries, and venules, with an annual incidence of 3–10 per million in Europe. Mean age at time of diagnosis ranges from 60–71 years. The clinical course of MPA is similar to PAN except for presence of rapidly progressive glomerulonephritis (80%), lung involvement (35–50%) (alveolar hemorrhage in 20%), and MPO-pANCAs (50–70%) as well as PR3-cANCAs (20–30%) and absence of hepatitis B surface antigen and visceral microaneurysms. Other common clinical features include skin involvement (30–60%), (palpable purpura), joint involvement (40–50%), ENT (20–30%), cardiac involvement (10–20%), and abdominal pain. Erythrocyte sedimentation rate is elevated in more than 90% of patients and ANAs are positive in about 20–30% of patients. Rheumatoid factor is positive in 20–30% of patients. Complement levels are usually normal. The commonest causes of death in MPA include renal failure, alveolar hemorrhage, or infection. Peripheral neuropathy occurs in up to 45% of patients with MPA. The most common form of PNS involvement is mononeuritis multiplex and it can be presenting feature in up to 10–15% of cases. Sural nerve biopsies show evidence of necrotizing vasculitis in up to 80% of cases.[4,5,7,9,36-40]

Eosinophilic Granulomatosis with Polyangiitis (Churg-Strauss Syndrome)

It is yet another pauci-immune ANCA-associated syndrome that occurs in about 30–40% of cases (usually MPO-ANCAs). The mean age at diagnosis ranges from 48 to 52 years, and it is the least common among AAVs with annual incidence of 1–3 per million. The clinical diagnostic criteria for EGPA include presence of asthma, eosinophilia of >1500/mm^3, and evidence of vasculitis affecting two or more extra pulmonary sites.[41] The salient histopathological alteration in EGPA includes eosinophilic tissue infiltration, extravascular granulomas, and vasculitis. The classification criteria agreed by ACR require presence of four out of the following: asthma, blood eosinophilia of >10%, fleeting pulmonary infiltrates, mononeuropathy or polyneuropathy, paranasal sinus abnormality, and extravascular eosinophilic infiltration on biopsy specimens.[4] The clinical course of EGPA is characterized by three phases. In the first phase, patient usually develops atopic features such as asthma or allergic rhinosinusitis. During the next phase, there is peripheral blood eosinophilia with eosinophilic tissue infiltration, and the third phase is characterized by systemic vasculitis, typically 5–10 years after the onset of asthma. The clinical features that distinguish EGPA from PAN include asthma (100%), pulmonary infiltrates (50–75%), allergic rhinosinusitis (60–80%), glomerulonephritis (15–30%), and congestive cardiac failure (30–50%). Other clinical manifestations include cutaneous involvement in 50–70%, GI tract involvement in 35–50%, and joint involvement in 30–50%. In contrast to MPA, renal failure is rare in EGPA. Most common cause of death in EGPA is heart failure that accounts for up to 50% of deaths. Peripheral neuropathy occurs in majority of patients and can be a presenting manifestation in 20–65% of cases. [42-47]

The characteristic laboratory abnormalities include peripheral blood eosinophilia in all, elevated ESR in 85%, elevated IgE levels in 75%, positive ANCA in 30–40%, ANA in 10%, and RF in 40–50%. There is no association with HBV or HCV. Nerve biopsies reveal evidence of necrotizing vasculitis in 30%, eosinophilic infiltrates in 35%, and granulomas in 10%.[48,49]

Granulomatosis with Polyangiitis (Wegener Granulomatosis)

The third pauci-immune AAV is GPA characterized by granulomatous inflammation, necrosis and vasculitis affecting small- and medium-sized arteries and veins primarily affecting lungs and kidneys. Mean age at diagnosis ranges from 50–68 years, with annual incidence of 2–11 per million. It usually starts as localized involvement, often of respiratory tract, resulting in chronic sinusitis with blood-stained or purulent nasal discharge, nasal ulceration or perforation, otitis with conductive hearing loss, and nasal deformities. In the next phase, generalized vasculitis occurs affecting upper respiratory tract (90–95%), lungs (65–85%), glomeruli (60–70%), eyes (50–60%), skin (25–50%), joints (50–60%), heart (5–10%), and GI tract (5–10%). Neuropathy develops in 20–40% of patients and can be a presenting feature in 25%. The neuropathy occurs more commonly in men, elderly, and in patients who have renal involvement, severe disease, and high titers of ANCA. Among AAVs, WG is the one that is associated most commonly with cranial neuropathy (15%). Usual causes of death include involvement of lung or kidneys.[50-54]

The common laboratories abnormalities include positive ANCA in 80–90% (PR3 in 70–80% and MPO in 10–15%), elevated ESR in 85%, anemia in 75%, thrombocytosis in 55%, and leukocytosis in 25%. Rheumatoid factor is positive in 50–60% and ANA in 25%. Diagnostic yield depends on the site, with method of biopsy with open lung biopsies giving confirmatory diagnosis in 90% of cases.[55,56]

Predominant Large-vessel Primary Systemic Vasculitides

Giant Cell Arteritis

This granulomatous vasculitis, that has predilection for branches of aortic arch and extracranial carotid arteries, is the most common primary vasculitis (17–19/1 lakh adults over 50 years) in the west, affecting primary adults (women > men) aged above 50 years with a peak in eighth decade.[57] The most common clinical features include headache, weight loss, fever, and polymyalgia rheumatica (50%). Vestibular dysfunction (90%), hearing loss (60%), and visual loss due to anterior ischemic optic neuropathy (15–20%) are other common symptoms. Neuropathy in form of focal or multifocal neuropathy occurs in 6% of cases affecting predominantly distal median nerve, C5/6 roots, or upper brachial plexus.[58-61] Though self-limited, relapses are common in GCA, and median duration of treatment is 2 years.

Most common laboratory abnormalities include high ESR and CRP as well as IL-6. Anemia occurs in 55% of cases, and leukocytosis is seen in 25% of patients. Temporal artery ultrasonography reveals the characteristic halo sign (dark, hypoechoic, circumferential thickening around the lumen suggestive of edema), and superficial temporal artery biopsy reveals characteristic granulomatous inflammation.[5,62,63]

Secondary Systemic Vasculitides Associated with Neuropathy

Rheumatoid vasculitis: It affects small-to-medium-sized vessels occurring as a late manifestation of severe seropositive rheumatoid arthritis (RA). It is important to remember that all neuropathies in RA are not vasculitic and in fact the commonest cause of neuropathies in RA is entrapment neuropathies and neuropathies related to drug treatment. However, some of the neuropathies associated with RA are truly vasculitic. When RA progresses to rheumatoid vasculitis, any of systemic accompaniments of vasculitis may accompany. PNS is involved in 40–50% of cases. On an average, vasculitic neuropathies occur in 10% of cases of RA.[4,5,7]

Sjögren's syndrome: This is an autoimmune disease with predilection for involvement of exocrine glands (salivary and lacrimal), resulting in dry eyes and dry mouth. The diagnosis of this syndrome is based on characteristic lymphocytic infiltrates on minor salivary gland biopsy, positive ANAs (especially anti-SSA or SSB), and ophthalmological signs of keratoconjunctivitis sicca. Incidence of PNS involvement in Sjögren's syndrome ranges from 2 to 4%, with trigeminal neuropathy, distal sensorimotor neuropathy, small or large fiber neuropathy, or autonomic neuropathy being the most common manifestations. Multiple mononeuropathy as part of VN accounts for only 15% of Sjögren's-related neuropathies. Nerve biopsies reveal epineurial vascular inflammation with necrotizing vasculitis occasionally, but these patients do not develop other features of systemic vasculitis. [64-66]

Hepatitis C-related cryoglobulinemic neuropathy: The cryoglobulins are proteins that precipitate at cold temperatures (4°C). These can be monoclonal or polyclonal. Types II and III are considered mixed, as they contain a combination of polyclonal immunoglobulins. When these immunoglobulins are not associated with any other underlying disorder, these are called essential mixed cryoglobulinemia (EMC), which is associated with HCV in 80–90% of cases. Essential mixed cryoglobulinemia is also associated with systemic vasculitic disorder. On the contrary, HCV itself is associated with EMC in only 50% of cases, and only 15% develop symptomatic EMC. The clinical features include cutaneous symptoms (95%) such as purpura, leg ulcers, arthritis (70–90%), glomerulonephritis (30%), Raynaud phenomenon (25–30%), GI tract involvement with abdominal pain (10–20%), and sicca complex (30%). Peripheral neuropathy that occurs in 65% of patients can present either as distal symmetrical or asymmetrical polyneuropathy or as multiple mononeuropathy. Laboratory investigations reveal high ESR (70%), positive RF (70–90%), low complement (70–90%), positive ANA (55%), and anemia (70%). Occasionally (5%), patients have positive hepatitis B surface antigen.[67-70] Recently, series of HCV-positive, cryoglobulin-negative peripheral neuropathy patients have been reported. The pattern is of small fiber neuropathy, and nerve biopsies reveal epineurial vasculitic in both cryoglobulin-positive and negative patients.[71,72] HCV is also associated with a PAN like illness with VN in about 19% of cases, which is much more severe than EMC.[68]

HIV-related vasculitic neuropathy: A rare entity occurring in <1% of HIV patients usually once CD4 cell counts are in range of 200–500/μL. It results from immune complex deposition rather than as a direct result of HIV infection. In addition, HIV infection can cause neuropathies in several other ways such as drugs, CMV related when CD4 cell count falls to < 50/µL, hepatitis B-associated PAN and MPA etc.[73-75]

Paraneoplastic vasculitic neuropathies: Though rare, these can present as painful sensorimotor neuropathy or as multiple mononeuropathy. These usually occur in association with lymphoma, small cell lung cancer. Most of these patients have vasculitis restricted to peripheral nervous system, including muscle and nerve. Serums anti-Hu (ANNA-2) antibodies have been described in association with paraneoplastic vasculitic neuropathies.[76-78]

Vasculitic neuropathies associated with infections other than HCV: Almost any infection can induce vasculitis by acting as antigenic stimulus, thereby inducing the formation of immune complexes. Other mechanisms through which infections can produce vasculitis include direct invasion of vessel wall (CMC, varicella zoster virus), release of toxins, and induction of immune responses against vascular autoantigens via molecular mimicry. Among the bacterial infections, only Lyme disease has strong association with VN, while among the viruses, HBV, HCV, HIV, and parvovirus B19 have strongest association. The most well-characterized infectious vasculitis among all these is HBV-related PAN, which occurs in about 1–5% of chronic HBV patients, occurring secondary to immune complex deposition. The clinical features, though similar to idiopathic PAN, differ in lower incidence of cutaneous manifestations and higher incidence of neuropathy (85%), hypertension, orchitis, and abdominal pain in HBV-related PAN. Vasculitis usually occurs in early stages of HBV infection and follows a self-limited course. Relapses are uncommon.[70,78-82]

Single-organ Vasculitides

Nonsystemic Vasculitic Neuropathy

Nonsystemic vasculitic neuropathy is the commonest cause of VN. The clinical presentation of NSVN is similar to that of SVN in terms of age of presentation (mean 60 years) and female preponderance. However, in contrast to SVN, NSVN is restricted to nerve and muscle, NSVN progress slowly with less frequent attacks, is not fatal, and is associated with constitutional symptoms (weight loss in 30% and fever in 10–15%) of much lesser severity. The clinical picture in classic NSVN is that of a slowly progressive, asymmetrical, or multifocal neuropathy, with superimposed acute attacks. Clinically, approximately 45% patients have multiple mononeuropathy, 30% have asymmetrical polyneuropathy, and 25% have distal symmetrical polyneuropathy. Usually, neuropathy is sensorimotor, but up to 15% have pure sensory

neuropathy. Pain is a frequent symptom, occurring in up to 95% of patients. Most patients remain ambulant and independent in activities of daily living, but approximately 60% complain of chronic pain.[4,5,20,83,84]

The diagnosis of NSVN usually depends on evidence of definite or probable vasculitis on nerve biopsy without any clinical evidence of systemic involvement. The peripheral nerve society guideline group has released diagnostic criteria for NSVN.[7] Patients are required to have pathologically definite or clinically probable VN and are then evaluated for clinical/laboratory evidence of systemic vasculitis that should be absent. Other features that exclude the diagnosis for NSVN include involvement of organs other than PNS; presence of visceral aneurysms, ANCAs, cryoglobulins; ESR ≥100 mm first hour; pathological evidence of vasculitis in non-neuromuscular tissues, underlying infection, presence of medical condition or drug intake that predisposes to vasculitis. Constitutional symptoms, diabetes mellitus, and muscle vasculitis are compatible with diagnosis of NSVN.

Approximately 10% of patients of NSVN change into SVN, and this fact led some researchers to hypothesize NSVN as a part of continuum of SVN (MPA and PAN). Although there are points in favor and against both the hypotheses, it is difficult to conclude at this point, if these represent two ends of spectrum of a common disease or are different diseases.

NSVN Variants

These include diabetic lumbosacral radiculoplexus neuropathy (DLRPN), nondiabetic LRPN, diabetic cervical radiculoplexus neuropathy (DCRPN), and painless diabetic motor neuropathy. Diabetic lumbosacral radiculoplexus neuropathy occurs in approximately 1% of patients with NIDDM. Though classically monophasic, it often results in profound disability. Typically middle-aged individuals are affected more often, and usually DLRPN occurs in individuals with good glycemic control and no other complications of diabetes. Most patients also complain of loss of weight. The illness usually starts with severe pain in the hip/thigh followed several days to weeks later by weakness. The pain can be sharp, lancinating, deep aching, burning, or consistent with allodynia. The onset is often so acute that patients remember the exact day of onset. At the beginning, usually proximal weakness is more than distal, but weakness often spreads to affect more than one segments of lower limb, often affecting the entire lower limb. Pain and weakness typically begin unilaterally, but spread to contralateral side in 80–90%. In one prospective study, nearly all patients needed support for ambulation, and 50% became wheelchair bound.[85] Approximately 50% develop new autonomic dysfunction (orthostatic hypotension, sexual dysfunction, and change in bladder or bowel habits). The clinical deficits affect multiple thigh and leg muscles conforming to distribution of lumbosacral plexus and as paraspinal muscles show evidence of denervation, the condition is actually a radiculoplexus neuropathy (involvement of roots, plexus, and nerves). Symptoms typically progress over weeks to months and then may slowly improve over 1–2 years, but relapses occur in about 10–15%. Most of the patients are left with residual deficits, with foot drop being the commonest sequalae. These patients may also have evidence of thoracic or abdominal radiculopathy, upper limb mononeuropathy (33%), and cervical radiculoplexus neuropathy (10%).[85,86]

The underlying pathology of DLRPN is microvasculitis resulting in peripheral nerve ischemia. In one series, all nerve biopsies showed evidence of inflammation, and 50% of biopsies were consistent with diagnosis of microvasculitis.[86]

Recently, an upper limb variant of diabetic radiculoplexus neuropathy termed DCRPN has been described.[87] The clinical picture is similar to DLPRN, with mean age being 60 years. Weight loss is common. Pain is the commonest symptom, which disappears as soon as weakness appears, so that at time of evaluation, weakness predominates. The clinical picture is more acute than DLRPN, with peak deficits usually reached within a week in > 50% of cases. The upper, middle, and lower plexus are affected almost equally with entire plexus involved in 30% (DD—brachial neuritis in which involvement of upper plexus predominates). More than 50% of patients have involvement of at least one additional body segment (contralateral cervical, thoracic, lumbosacral), suggesting that pathology in these condition is widespread. Nerve biopsies reveal evidence of inflammation and ischemic injury similar to DLRPN. Based on these facts, it is reasonable to conclude that DLRPN, DCRPN, and diabetic thoracic radiculoplexus neuropathy are regional manifestations of a more widespread and multifocal syndrome of diabetic radiculoplexus neuropathy resulting from microvasculitis, which can affect upper limbs, lower limbs, and trunk in variable proportions. Lumbosacral radiculoplexus neuropathy is a similar syndrome to DLRPN that occurs in the absence of diabetes.

Occasionally, DLRPN can be painless (painless diabetic motor neuropathy). This complication also occurs in patients with good glycemic control and without other complications related to diabetes. Usually, the duration of diabetes is 5–6 years, and most patients complain of weight loss. In contrast to DLRPN, deficits are more severe and 50% of patients are wheelchair bound at presentation. Also, distal muscles were affected more severely compared to proximal nature of weakness in DLRPN. 66% have bilateral deficits at presentation and >90% develop bilateral disease over course of time. Almost all patients have sensory symptoms and approximately 40% complain of autonomic dysfunction. CSF protein is elevated in most. On biopsy, there is evidence of ischemic injury and microvasculitis in contrast to CIDP, where onion bulbs and demyelination are more common. Also, a number of these patients improve subsequently, suggesting a monophasic course. Thus, this syndrome has been separated from CIDP and put in subcategory of DLRPN.[88]

Another variant of NSVN is Wartenberg migrant sensory neuritis, which is defined by episodic, migratory attacks of pure sensory symptoms in distribution of individual cutaneous nerves. It begins with transient pain and tingling which is followed by sensory loss that persists. Usually, limbs nerves are involved, but truncal and trigeminal nerves may also get involved in 30% of cases. The clinical course is benign but may extend for years.[5]

DIAGNOSIS

The first and most important step for reaching at diagnosis of VN is prompt clinical suspicion. Vasculitis should not be considered only in differential diagnosis of acute or subacute multifocal neuropathies, but also in differentials of "slowly progressive sensorimotor or sensory polyneuropathies", especially if painful, distal predominant, and asymmetric.[5]

Laboratory Testing

Laboratory tests in suspected VN include complete blood count, metabolic panel, urine examination, ESR, CRP, ANA, ANCA, RF, angiotensin-converting enzyme levels, serum protein electrophoresis, glucose tolerance test, glycosylated hemoglobin (HbA_{1C}), cryoglobulins, complement, hepatitis B surface antigen (HbsAg), hepatitis C antibodies, HIV, chest radiographs.[7] Depending upon the clinical scenario, computed tomography of chest and abdomen, and testing for CMV, VZV, Lyme disease, and porphyria can be performed. Though ESR is mildly elevated in NSVN also, an elevation of >100 mm is considered as diagnostic of SVN. Antineutrophilic cytoplasmic antibodies, by definition, rule out diagnosis of NSVN. CSF examination is not very helpful, as moderate protein elevation occurs in both SVN and NSVN as well in several other disorders including multifocal acquired demyelinating sensory motor neuropathy. However, it may in ruling out other causes of mononeuritis multiplex such as neurolymphomatosis and may help in ruling out other associated conditions such as arachnoiditis. Lumbar puncture should be carried out in patients with clinical features suggestive of root involvement, in patients with electrophysiological evidence of demyelination, or when meningeal pathology is being suspected.[5,7]

Electrodiagnostic Studies

Electromyography (EMG) and nerve conduction studies (NCSs) help to identify (a) if the neuropathy is focal, multifocal, or diffuse? (b) is the neuropathy length dependent or not? (c) if the neuropathy is dominantly sensory or sensorimotor or motor? (d) if the neuropathy is characterized by dominant large or small fiber involvement or both? (e) if the neuropathy is dominantly axonal or demyelinating or both? Both these tests also help in selecting the nerve for biopsy.[89,90]

The usual findings on NCSs in vasculitic neuropathies include decreased amplitudes of sensory nerve action potentials (SNAPs) and compound muscle action potentials with normal or mildly reduced conduction velocities, consistent with axonal degeneration. Electromyography shows an active denervation in 70% of cases, decreased recruitment and evidence of large polyphasic motor unit potentials consistent with chronic reinnervation. Findings of axonal loss in asymmetric distribution are consistent with diagnosis of VN. On the contrary, symmetric length-dependent findings reduce the likelihood of VN. Conduction block occurs in approximately 15% of cases and reflects nerve infarction. However, if conduction studies are repeated after 2 weeks, these conduction blocks give way to axonal degeneration and do not persist, unlike CIDP. Significantly reduced conduction velocities or persistent conduction blocks should raise doubts about alternate diagnoses such as multifocal acquired demyelinating motor and sensory neuropathy.[24,91,92]

Nerve Biopsy

As vasculitic neuropathies often require strong immunosuppression, it is mandatory that their diagnosis is confirmed by nerve biopsy. One possible exemption to this rule is when a patient with known systemic vasculitic develops a peripheral neuropathy that is consistent with VN. On the contrary, it is not always required to perform nerve biopsy in all patients with idiopathic axonal neuropathy. This is especially true if illness has been progressing very slowly over decades, as likelihood of a nerve biopsy to yield a positive result in unexplained distal, symmetric, polyneuropathy is only 4%.[90,93] This low diagnostic yield should be compared with risks of nerve biopsy such as permanent sensory loss, pain, delayed wound healing or nonhealing, and wound infection. Likelihood of identifying vasculitis is increased in the presence of asymmetric/multifocal pattern, acute or subacute course, elevated ESR or CRP, positive ANCAS, elevated β_2-microglobulin, and elevated VEGF.[93-97]

Commonly biopsied nerves include superficial peroneal that has advantage of peroneus brevis muscle biopsy through same incision, sural nerve, dorsal cutaneous branch of ulnar nerve, and superficial radial nerve. However, the selection of the nerve should be guided by electrophysiological studies.[22] If required, sural nerve biopsy may be combined with muscle biopsy from quadriceps or gastrocnemius or even tibialis anterior muscle, depending upon the clinical examination and electrophysiological studies. Concomitant muscle biopsy increases the diagnostic yield by 15%.[5,98] However, this may not be true for proximal muscle biopsy such as quadriceps, as suggested by one study.[24] On the contrary, biopsy of distal limb muscles such as gastrocnemius, peroneus brevis increases diagnostic yield of definite vasculitis in 25% of patients with NSVN from 20% with nerve biopsy alone.[5]

Pathological diagnosis of VN: The peripheral nerve society guidelines on NSVN provide diagnostic criteria for definite and probable VN.[10.] These results are summarized in Table 20.2. The overall sensitivity for finding of definite vasculitis in sural nerve biopsy alone is 50–55%, whereas that for combined superficial peroneal nerve/peroneus brevis muscle or for combined sural nerve/distal leg muscles is 60%. The yield is more in SVN as compared to NSVN.[5]

DIFFERENTIAL DIAGNOSIS

Differential diagnosis of vasculitic neuropathies is broad and is tabulated in Table 20.3. As is evident from the table, the differential diagnosis is broad and for the same reason, most of the patients with suspected VN undergo nerve muscle biopsy as well as other investigations (discussed under previous sections) to confirm the diagnosis.

MANAGEMENT

The first step in management of vasculitic neuropathies, as is true for most of other diseases of medicines, is to identify the precipitating cause and if possible, elimination of the same. However, in most of the cases, triggering agent cannot be identified and management is restricted to use of nonspecific immunomodulation.

Aim of treatment: It should be clearly defined from the beginning and discussed with the patient and caregivers. It should be kept in mind that most of times, vasculitis results in axonal degeneration and recovery of sensorimotor function,

Table 20.2 Criteria for diagnosis of vasculitic neuropathies[10]

Pathologically definite vasculitic neuropathy requires both intramural inflammation and vessel wall damage as given:

Active lesion

Nerve biopsy should show collection of inflammatory cells in vessel wall and one or more signs of acute vascular damage which are:

- Fibrinoid necrosis
- Loss/disruption of endothelium
- Fragmentation of internal elastic lamina
- Loss/fragmentation of smooth muscle cells in media (can be highlighted with antismooth muscle actin staining)
- Acute thrombosis
- Vascular/perivascular hemorrhage or
- Leukocytoclasia

Chronic lesion with signs of healing/repair

Nerve biopsy should show collection of mononuclear inflammatory cells in vessel wall and one or more signs of chronic vascular damage with repair which are:

- Intimal hyperplasia
- Fibrosis of media
- Adventitial/periadventitial fibrosis
- Chronic thrombosis with recanalization

Note: There should be no evidence of any other primary disease process that could be confused with vasculitic neuropathy such as lymphoma, lymphomatoid granulomatosis, or amyloidosis.

Pathologically probable vasculitic neuropathy can be diagnosed by following criteria:

- Nonsatisfaction of criteria for pathologically definite vasculitic neuropathy
- Predominant axonal changes
- Perivascular inflammation accompanied by signs of active or chronic vascular damage; perivascular or vascular inflammation and at least one additional class II or III pathological predictor of definite vasculitic neuropathy:
  - Vascular deposition of complement, IgM, or fibrinogen by direct immunofluorescence
  - Hemosiderin deposits
  - Asymmetric nerve fiber loss or degeneration
  - Prominent active axonal degeneration
  - Myofiber necrosis, regeneration or infarcts in peroneus brevis muscle biopsy (not explained by underlying myopathy)

Note: Additional alterations used by some authorities as supportive of vasculitis but lacking in evidence include (a) neovascularization (class II and III evidence suggests that this findings is not suggestive of vasculitis), (b) endoneurial purpura (one class III positive and one class II negative study), (c) focal perineurial inflammation, degeneration, and thickening (class IV evidence), (d) injury neuroma and microfasciculation (class IV evidence), (e) swollen axons filled with organelles (nonconvincing negative class II study), and other experimental changes of acute ischemia such as attenuated axons, flattened myelin profiles, tubular profiles, and axonal cytolysis.

even after successful treatment may not be complete. Thus, the short-term goal of treatment is to stabilize the deficits and prevent further worsening. In this regard, it is important to look for clinical and biochemical markers of disease activity and avoid overtreating the patient. The long-term aim is to achieve improvement in neurological status and proper rehabilitation, while recognizing the fact that recovery may not be complete. Management of vasculitic neuropathies is summarized in Table 20.4.

Management of Infectious Vasculitides

In chronic viral infections, removal of antigenic stimulus is of utmost importance, more so as immunosuppression may worsen underlying infection.[70] For example, corticosteroids worsen the HBV-related liver disease, and thus cornerstone of therapy in HBV-PAN is antiviral agents. In a protocol designed by French group, patients with HBV-PAN were treated with antiviral agents, plasma exchange to remove circulating immune complexes, and a 2-week course of steroids. This protocol induced complete remission in 80–90% with a seroconversion rate of 50% for hepatitis B e antigen.[70,99]

In HCV-related mixed cryoglobulinemia, interferon alpha and ribavirin have been used with success, but rituximab (monoclonal antibody against CD20 that selectively depletes B cells) may be more effective in severe cryoglobulinemic neuropathies. Thus, while antiviral therapy alone is used for mild cryoglobulinemic neuropathies, rituximab combined with antiviral therapy is the treatment of choice for severe neuropathies.[10,100,101] In CMV-related vasculitis, treatment is based on antiviral agents (ganciclovir, valganciclovir, foscarnet, or cidofovir). For non-CMV VN in HIV patients, treatment is similar to

Table 20.3 Differential diagnosis of vasculitic neuropathies[5,10]

Asymmetric or multifocal neuropathy:

- Ischemic neuropathies: (a) peripheral nerve vasculitis, (b) livedoid vasculopathy, (c) sickle cell anemia, (d) cholesterol emboli, (e) atrial myxoma, (f) thrombophilic states
- Inflammatory/immune-mediated neuropathies: (a) sarcoidosis, (b) multifocal acquired demyelinating sensory motor neuropathy (MADSAM), (c) multifocal motor neuropathy, (d) multifocal variants of Guillain-Barré syndrome, (e) neuralgic amyotrophy, (f) neuropathy with eosinophilic disorders (occasionally associated with vasculitic neuropathy), (g) neuropathy with gastrointestinal disorders (inflammatory bowel disease) (occasionally associated with vasculitis), (h) chronic graft versus host disease, (i) sensory perineuritis (occasionally associated with vasculitis)
- Infectious/ toxic neuropathies (occasionally associated with vasculitis): (a) leprosy, (b) Lyme disease, (c) viruses (HCV, HBV, HIV, HTLV-1, VZV,CMV, EBV, parvovirus 19, West Nile virus), (d) other (infective endocarditis, leptospirosis, tuberculosis, sporotrichosis, meningococcus, group A beta hemolytic *Streptococcus*, *Mycoplasma*, *Salmonella*, *Pseudomonas*, trichinosis, ascariasis, scrub typhus, relapsing fever)
- Drug related (occasionally associated with vasculitis): (a) montelukast and other leukotriene receptor antagonists, (b) interferon alpha, (c) tumor necrotic factor alpha inhibitors (infliximab, adalimumab, etanercept), (d) antibiotics (penicillin, minocycline, sulfonamides, cycline), (e) leflunomide, (f) drugs of abuse (amphetamines, cocaine, heroin), (g) others (cromolyn, cimetidine, thiouracil, allopurinol, amantadine, naproxen, piroxicam, valacyclovir, mesalazine, rituximab, masitinib, gasoline sniffing)
- Genetic neuropathies: (a) hereditary neuropathy with liability to pressure palsies, (b) hereditary neuralgic amyotrophy, (c) Charcot-Marie-Tooth neuropathy, (d) porphyria, (e) familial amyloid polyneuropathy, (f) Tangier disease, (g) Krabbe disease, (h) mitochondrial disorders
- Neuropathies related to neoplastic disease: (a) direct infiltration of nerves by tumor, (b) paraneoplastic (vasculitic and nonvasculitic), (c) multifocal peripheral nerve tumors with external/internal compression, (d) neurofibromatosis 2, (e) lymphomatoid granulomatosis (routinely associated with vasculitis), (f) intravascular large B cell lymphoma, (g) neoplastic meningitis, (h) primary AL amyloidosis
- Mechanical neuropathies: (a) multiple peripheral nerve injuries or burns, (b) multiple entrapment neuropathies, (c) Wartenberg migrant sensory neuritis.
- Intraneural hemorrhage: (a) idiopathic thrombocytopenic purpura, (b) acute leukemia, (c) hemophilia
- Degenerative: motor neuron disease with sensory involvement

Rapidly progressive symmetric, sensorimotor or sensory neuropathy:

(1) Vasculitis, (2) axonal variant of Guillain-Barré syndrome, (3) critical illness neuropathy, (4) acute alcohol-nutritional deficiency neuropathy, (5) other causes of nutritional deficiency (beriberi, hyperemesis gravidarum, repeated vomiting after gastric resection surgery), (6) toxins/drugs, (7) acute painful diabetic neuropathy, (8) high-grade neoplastic infiltrative neuropathies

HBV-PAN with antiviral agents and plasma exchanges and steroids.[102,103]

Management of Noninfectious Vasculitides

Management of Primary Small-vessel or Medium-vessel Vasculitides

This group includes PAN, MPA, EGPA, and GPA. The standard immunosuppressive regimen consists of corticosteroids combined with another immunosuppressive agent.

For fear of serious side effects (bladder cancer, lymphoma) associated with use of cyclophosphamide, though it is a cheap and highly effective, its use is avoided in patients with mild disease. For patients with localized or mild generalized disease without any organ-threatening manifestations, high-dose corticosteroids are used with methotrexate (MTX) 15–25 mg per week while recognizing the fact that relapse rates are higher when MTX is used for induction instead of cyclophosphamide.[104-106] Prednisone is started at 1 mg/kg per day for 1 month and then tapered to 10 mg per day after 6 months and then stopped or continued at

5–7.5 mg daily depending upon the clinical condition. There is clear cut evidence that low-dose steroid reduce relapse rate if continued.[107] Methotrexate is stopped after 18–24 months. In the presence of moderate-to-severe generalized disease, steroids are given with cyclophosphamide (2 mg/kg per day or 0.6–0.7 g/m^2 every 2-3 weeks). Cyclophosphamide is given for 3–6 months, by that time the disease usually remits, and is replaced by either azathioprine (1.5–2 mg/kg per day) or MTX 20–25 mg per week. Maintenance therapy is continued for at least 18–24 months. In elderly patients and those with renal disease, lower doses of cyclophosphamide are used. In patients with severe renal disease or alveolar hemorrhage, plasma exchange is used with corticosteroids and cyclophosphamide.[108]

Recently, two RCTs have shown that rituximab/steroids are not inferior to cyclophosphamide/steroids for inducing remission and may be even better in prevention of relapses. Thus, rituximab is currently the drug of choice for inducing remission, but there are safety concerns as rate of infections is high with this regimen (22–42%).[109,110] In our institute, cyclophosphamide is used as initial choice, failing which rituximab is used.

Table 20.4 Management of vasculitic neuropathies

Primary small-vessel or medium-vessel vasculitides (PAN, MPA, EGPA and GPA):

1. Localized or mild generalized disease (no organ-threatening manifestations)	High-dose corticosteroids (1 mg/kg day for 1 month and then tapered to 10 mg per day after 6 months and then stopped or continued at 5–7.5 mg daily depending upon the clinical condition) + Methotrexate (MTX) 15–25 mg per week, stopped after 18–24 months
2. Moderate-to-severe generalized disease	Steroids + Cyclophosphamide (2 mg/kg per day or 0.6–0.7 g/m² every 2–3 weeks for 3–6 months) followed by either azathioprine (1.5–2 mg/kg per day) or MTX 20–25 mg per week for at least 18–24 months

SVN—same as for primary small-vessel or medium-vessel vasculitides:

• NSVN

1. NSVN might decrease relapse further.	Prednisone(1 mg/kg per day tapered to 25 mg per day at 3 months, 15–30 mg per day at 4 months and 10 mg at 6 months. May be continued at 5–7.5 mg per day for 6–18 months)
2. Severe rapidly progressive NSVN or NSVN that progresses on steroid monotherapy	Prednisolone + Either cyclophosphamide (0.6 g/m² every 2 weeks for 3 doses, then 0.7 g/m² every 3 weeks for 3–6 doses for 3–6 months followed by MTX 20–25 mg per day or azathioprine 1–2 mg/kg per day for at least 18–24 months) or MTX (started at 15 mg per week and is titrated to 25 mg per week over 1–2 months) for at least 18–24 months or Azathioprine (1.5–2 mg/kg per day) for at least 18–24 months
• Refractory disease	If previously not received cyclophosphamide, start cyclophosphamide If received cyclophosphamide, consider IVIG pulses, rituximab, or plasma exchange

Management of SVN and NSVN

While there is no doubt that most of the patients with these disorders require treatment, one needs to address certain important issues related to treatment before actually starting treatment. These include whether the treatment should be started with corticosteroids alone or in combination with a cytotoxic agent? How long an induction treatment needs to be continued before replacing it with less toxic maintenance treatment? Which agents will be used for induction and maintenance? And finally, how long maintenance treatment will be administered?

For SVNs, treatment rules are generally the same as for primary small- and medium-vessel vasculitides. There is evidence to suggest that neuropathic manifestations improve hand in hand with other non-neurologic manifestations.[7]

As NSVN is milder as compared to SVN, less aggressive protocols may be used for management.[23,24,111] However, there is evidence to suggest that combination therapy is more effective than steroids alone in inducing sustained remission and improving disability.[20,21] As per Peripheral Nerve

Society Task Force recommendations[7], start treatment with prednisone 1 mg/kg per day tapered to 25 mg per day at 3 months, 15–30 mg per day at 4 months, and 10 mg at 6 months. Continuation of low-dose prednisolone 5–7.5 mg day for 6–18 months might decrease relapse further.[107] With severe rapidly progressive NSVN, pulse intravenous methylprednisolone is used. For rapidly progressive NSVN and for patients who progress on steroid monotherapy, combination therapy is used. The options available include MTX, azathioprine, and cyclophosphamide. Cyclophosphamide is preferred in severe cases and is usually given in pulses (0.6 g/m² every 2 weeks for three doses, then 0.7 g/m² every 3 weeks for 3–6 doses) to decrease cumulative dose. The dose is decreased in elderly and in patients with renal disease. Methotrexate is started at 15 mg per week and is titrated to 25 mg per week over 1–2 months. Azathioprine is used in doses of 1.5–2 mg/kg day. Once clinical remission (no worsening by any objective measure for 6 months and some improvement in at least one objective measure over 6 months) is achieved, patient can be started on maintenance doses of MTX (20–25 mg per week) or azathioprine (1–2 mg/kg per day).

Management of DLRPN and LRPN

Immunotherapy should be strongly considered for DLRPN and LRPN, if a patient presents early in the course of disease or is progressing. In one randomized controlled trial,[112] there was greater degree of symptom improvement with intravenous methylprednisolone compared to placebo. Neuropathy symptoms and change subscores were significantly better in methylprednisolone group. There are no controlled trials assessing effects of IVIG, but case series suggest that IVIG does improve pain and strength.[113] For LRPN, treatment recommendations are same as for NSVN. In one case series, five patients of DLRPN were treated with plasma exchange and all of them improved.[114]

Treatment of Resistant Disease

Treatment resistance is defined as unchanged or increased disease activity after 4–6 weeks of therapy with cyclophosphamide and corticosteroids or improved but persistent disease activity after 8 weeks of treatment. The Peripheral Nerve Society Guideline Group reviewed 16 studies (only one was class I). The class I study was double-blind RCT comparing IV immunoglobulin (2 g/kg over 5 days in divided doses) versus placebo in refractory MPA or GPA. The other studies were mostly class III investigating different agents. The group concluded from these studies that IVIG and rituximab were the safest; survival over 1–2 years was high with all drugs, but reduced with mycophenolate and alemtuzumab; complete remission rates were lowest with antithymocyte globulin and 15-deoxyspergualin; relapse rates were highest with mycophenolate, antithymocyte globulin, and alemtuzumab.

Thus, patients with refractory NSVN, not already treated with cyclophosphamide, should receive pulse IV or oral cyclophosphamide. In case there is no response, reconsider the diagnosis. If diagnosis s reconfirmed, IVIG and rituximab should be tried. In case of response, retreatment with these agents may be required to prevent relapse.[7]

Nonpharmacological Strategies

These include management of pain, rehabilitation, counseling, and education. Pain relief may require judicious use of tricyclic antidepressants, gabapentine, pregabalin, carbamazepine, tramadol, topical lidocaine, topical capsaicin, and even narcotics. Physical and occupation therapy should be initiated as soon as the pain subsides. It helps to maintain strength and range of movement, prevent contractures, limit osteoporosis, and disuse myopathy. Occupational

therapy helps to maximize functions and helps to maintain independence in activities of daily livings. Walking aids or wheelchair may be required for mobility. Counseling and psychological support form the essential part of treatment. Patients with VN are often depressed because of several reasons such as chronic pain, physical limitations, uncertain prognosis, and exposure to drugs such as corticosteroids.

Follow-up

One of the most difficult aspects in management of vasculitic neuropathies is absence of any easy way to monitor disease. Subjective responses of patient are important, but these cannot always be relied upon, especially in painful neuropathies, as relief of pain due to symptomatic treatment often improves the well-being of the patient. Thus, objective assessment is important. Some of the ways to assess the progression of disease include manual testing of power and sensory functions, amplitudes of SNAPs and CMPAs on NCSs, EMG findings, and use of disability scales. Re-emergence only of pain, in absence of other signs, is usually not taken as a criterion for need to intensify immunomodulation.[5]

Treatment of VN continues for at least 1 year, and during this period, clinician should assess the patient periodically once every 4–8 weeks and on an as and when required basis. A detailed neurological examination should be carried out at each visit to ensure that patient is not worsening and in case of any doubt, electrophysiological studies can be performed as well. New motor or sensory deficits appearing while patient is on treatment may necessitate change of drug or use of higher doses. Quite often, patients do not improve during the initial weeks or months of therapy and improve only later. During this period, temptation to increase immunosuppression should be resisted, and any increase should be made only if there is documented worsening or appearance of new deficits.[5]

CONCLUSION

Vasculitis affecting peripheral nerves is commonly seen in patients with primary systemic vasculitides, connective tissue disorders, viral infections, or malignancies. In about 30%, vasculitis is restricted to peripheral nervous system (NSVN). DLRPN, LRPN, DCRPN, and painless diabetic motor neuropathy are considered as spectrum of NSVNs. Although knowledge of pathogenesis and pathology of vasculitic neuropathies has reached an advanced stage, more need to be learnt especially with regards to radiculoplexus neuropathies. Also, the treatment protocols remain to be defined for most of vasculitic neuropathies and well-designed randomized controlled trials should be carried out to define these protocols in a more definitive manner.

KEY POINTS

- Vasculitic neuropathies are aggressive but treatable disorders, which result in considerable morbidity if not diagnosed and managed early.
- It is essential for a clinician to develop rational approach to peripheral neuropathy and consider possibility of underlying vasculitis in every patient who presents with peripheral neuropathy.

REFERENCES

1. Langford CA, Fauci AS. The vasculitic syndrome. In: Longo DL (Ed). Harrison's Principles of Internal Medicine, 18th edition. New York: McGraw-Hill; 2012.
2. Hernandez-Rodriguez J, Hoffman GS. Updating single organ vasculitis. Curr Opin Rheumatol. 2012;24:38-45.
3. Lacomis D, Zivkovic SA. Approach to vasculitic neuropathies. J Clin Neuromuscul Dis. 2007;9:265-76.
4. Gwathmey KG, Burns TD, Collins MP, et al. Vasculitic neuropathies. Lancet Neurol. 2014;13:67-82.
5. Collins MP, Arnold WD, Kissel JT. The neuropathies of vasculitis. Neurol Clin. 2013;31:557-95.
6. Jennette J, Falk R, Bacon P, et al. 2012 revised International Chapel Hill Consensus Conference nomenclature of vasculitides. Arthritis Rheum. 2013;65:1-11.
7. Collins MP, Dyck PJ, Gronseth GS, et al. Peripheral nerve society guideline of the classification, diagnosis, investigation, and immunosuppressive therapy of non-systemic vasculitic neuropathy: executive summary. J Peripher Nerv Syst. 2010;15:176-84.
8. Gonzalez-Gay MA, Gracia-Porrua C. Systemic vasculitic in adults in northwestern Spain, 1988–1997. Clinical and epidemiological aspects. Medicine. 1999;78:292-308.
9. Vrancken AFJE, Said G. Vasculitic neuropathy. Handbook Clin Neurol. 2013;115:463-63.
10. Collins MP. Vasculitic neuropathies: an update. Curr Opin Neurol. 2012;25:753-85.
11. Maugeri N, Rovere-Querini P, Baldini M, et al. Translational mini-review series on immunology of vascular disease: mechanisms of vascular inflammation and remodeling in systemic vasculitis. Clin Exp Immunol. 2009;156:395-404.
12. Alard JE, Dueymes M, Youinou P, et al. HSP60 and anti-HSP60 antibodies in vasculitis: they are two of a kind. Clin Rev Allergy Immunol. 2008;35:66-71.
13. Ball GV, Bridges SL Jr. Pathogenesis of vasculitis. In: GV Ball, SL Bridges (Eds). Vaculitis, 2nd edition, chapter 7. New York:Oxford University Press. pp. 67-68.
14. Szekanecz Z, Koch AE. Biology of endothelial cells. In: GV Ball, SL Bridges (Eds). Vaculitis, 2nd edition, chapter 4. New York: Oxford University Press. pp. 35-45.
15. Lundborg G. Structure and function of the intraneural microvessels as related to trauma, edema formation and nerve function. J Bone Joint Surg Am. 1975;57:938-48.
16. Kissel JT, Collins MP, Mendell JR. Vasculitic neuropathy. In: Mendell JR, Kissel JT, Comblath DR, (Eds). Diagnosis and management of peripheral nerve disorders. New York. Oxford University Press; 2001. pp. 202-32.
17. Low PA, Lagerlund TD, McManis PG. Nerve blood flow and oxygen delivery in normal, diabetic and ischemic neuropathy. Int Rev Neurobiol. 1989;31:355-438.
18. Nukada H, Dyck PJ. Microsphere embolization of nerve capillaries and fiber degeneration. Am J Pathol. 1984;115:275-87.
19. Morozumi S, Koike H, Tomita M, et al. Spatial distribution of nerve fiber pathology and Vasculitis in microscopic polyangiitis- associated neuropathy. J Neuropathol Exp Neurol. 2011;70:340-48.
20. Collins MP, Periquet MI, Mendell JR, et al. Nonsystemic vasculitic neuropathy: insights from a clinical cohort. Neurology. 2003;61:623-30.
21. Davies L, Spies JM, Pollard JD, et al. Vasculitis confined to peripheral nerves. Brain. 1996;119:1441-48.
22. Collins MP, Mendell JR, Periquet MI, et al. Superficial peroneal nerve/peroneus brevis muscle biopsy in vasculitic neuropathy. Neurology. 2000;55:636-43.
23. Sugiura M, Koike H, Lijima M, et al. Clinicopathological features of nonsystemic vasculitic neuropathy and microscopic polyangiitis associated neuropathy. J Neurol Sci. 2006;241:31-37.
24. Bennett DL, Groves M, Blake J, et al. The use of nerve and muscle biopsy in the diagnosis of vasculitis: a 5 year retrospective study. J Neurol Neurosurg Psychiatry. 2008;79:1376-81.
25. De Toni Franceschini L, Amadio S, Scarlato M, et al. A fatal case of Churg–Strauss syndrome presenting with acute polyneuropathy mimicking Guillain–Barre syndrome. Neurol Sci. 2011;32:937-40.
26. Cassereau J, Baguenier-Desormeaux C, Letournel F, et al. Necrotizing vasculitis revealed in a case of multiple mononeuropathy after a 14-year course of spontaneous remissions and relapses. Clin Neurol Neurosurg. 201;114:290-3.
27. Langford CA. Vsculitis. J Allergy Clin Immunol. 2010;125: S216-25.
28. Ntatsaki E, Watts RA, Scott DG. Epidemiology of ANCA-associated vasculitis. Rheum Dis Clin North Am. 2010;36:447-61.
29. Reinhold-Keller E, Herlyn K, Wagner-Bastmeyer R, et al. No difference in the incidence of vasculitides between north and south Germany: first results of Germany vasculitis register. Rheumatology. 2002;41:540-9.
30. Pagnoux C, Seror R, Henegar C, et al. Clinical features and outcomes in 348 patients with polyarteritis nodosa: a systemic retrospectives study of patients diagnosed between 1993 and 2005 and entered into French vasculitis study database. Arthritis Rheum. 2010;62:616-26.
31. Stone JH. Polyarteritis nodosa. JAMA. 2002;288:1632-9.
32. Lightfoot RW, Michel BA, Bloch DA, et al. The American College of Rheumatology 1990 criteria for classification of polyarteritis nodosa. Arthritis Rheum. 1990;33:1088-93.

33. Ball GV, Bridges SL. Polyarteritis nodosa. In: Koopman WJ, Moreland LW (Eds). Arthritis and Related Conditions, 15th edition. Philadelphia: Lippincott Williams & Wilkins; 2005.
34. Collins MP, Kissel JT. Neuropathies with systemic vasculitis. In: Dyck PJ, Thomas PK (Eds). Peripheral Neuropathy. Philadelphia: Elsevier Saunders; 2005. pp. 2335-404.
35. Stanson AW, Friese JL, Johnson CM, et al. Polyarteritis nodosa: spectrum of angiographic findings. Radiographics. 2001;21:151-9.
36. Serra A, Cameron JS, Turner DR, et al. Vasculitis affecting the kidney: presentation, histopathology and long term outcome. Q J Med. 1984;53:181-207.
37. Adu D, Howie AJ, Scott DG, et al. Polyarteritis and the kidney. Q J Med. 1987;62:221-37.
38. Cisternas M, Soto L, Jacobelli S, et al. Clinical features of Wegener's granulomatosis and microscopic polyangiitis in Chilean patients. Rev Med Chil. 2005;133:273-8.
39. Villiger PM, Guillevin L. Microscopic polyangiitis: clinical presentation. Autoimmun Rev. 2010;9:812-9.
40. Ahn JK, Hwang JW, Lee J, et al. Clinical features and outcomes of microscopic polyangiitis under a new consensus algorithm of ANCA-associated vasculitides in Korea. Rheumatol Int. 2012;32:2979-86.
41. Lanham JG, Elkon KB, Pusey CD, et al. Systemic vasculitis with asthma and eosinophilia: a clinical approach to the Churg-Strauss syndrome. Medicine. 1984;63:65-81.
42. Keogh KA, Specks U. Churg-Strauss syndrome: clinical presentation, anti-neutrophil cytoplasmic antibodies and leukotriene receptor antagonists. Am J Med. 2003;115:284-90.
43. Sinico RA, Di Toma L, Maggiore U, et al. Prevalence and clinical significance of antineutrophil cytoplasmic antibodies in Churg-Strauss syndrome. Arthritis Rheum. 2005;52:2926-35.
44. Baldini C, Della Rossa A, Grossi S, et al. Churg–Strauss syndrome: outcome and long term follow up of 38 patients from a single Italian center. Reumatismo. 2009;61:118-24.
45. Vinit J, Muller G, Bielefeld P, et al. Churg-Strauss syndrome: retrospective study in Burgundian population in France in past 10 years. Rheumatol Int. 2011;3:587-93.
46. Comarmond C, Pagnoux C, Khellaf M, et al. Eosinophilic granulomatosis with polyangiitis (Churg-Strauss syndrome): clinical characteristics and long term follow up of 383 patients enrolled in FVSG cohort. Arthritis Rheum. 2013;65:270-81.
47. Moosig F, Bremer JP, Hellmich B, et al. A vasculitis centre based management strategy leads to improved outcome in eosinophilic granulomatosis and polyangiitis (Churg-Strauss, EGPA): homocentric experience in 150 patients. Ann Rheum Dis. 2013;72:1011-7.
48. Oka N, Kawasaki T, Matsui M, et al. Two subtypes of Churg-Strauss syndrome with neuropathy: the role of eosinophils and ANCA. Mod Rheumatol. 2011;21:290-5.
49. Shimoi T, Shojima K, Murota A, et al. Clinical and pathologic features of Churg-Strauss syndrome among a Japanese population: a case series of 18 patients. Asian Pac J Allergy Immunol. 2012;30:61-70.
50. Hoffman GS, Kerr GS, Leavitt RY, et al. Wegener's granulomatosis: an analysis of 158 patients. Ann Intern Med. 1992;116:488-96.
51. Mahr AD. Epidemiological features of Wegener's granulomatosis and microscopic polyangiitis: two diseases or one 'one anti-neutrophil cytoplasmic antibody associated vascultis' entity? APMIS Suppl. 2009;127:41-47.
52. Mohammad AJ, Jacobsson LT, Westman KW, et al. Incidence and survival rates in Wegener's granulomatosis, microscopic polyangiitis, Churg-Strauss syndrome and polyarteritis nodosa. Rheumatology. 2009;48:1560-5.
53. Holle JU, Gross WL, Latza U, et al. Improve outcome in 445 patients with Wegener's granulomatosis in a German vasculitis center over four decades. Arthritis Rheum. 2011;63:257-66.
54. Nishino H, Rubino FA, DeRemee RA, et al. Neurological involvement in Wegener's granulomatosis: an analysis of 324 consecutive patients at the Mayo clinic. Ann Neurol. 1993;33:4-9.
55. Devaney KO, Travis WD, Hoffman G, et al. Interpretation of head and neck biopsies in Wegener's granulomatosis. A pathologic study of 126 biopsies in 70 patients. Am J Surg Pathol. 1990;14:555-64.
56. Travis WD, Hoffman GS, Leavitt RY, et al. Surgical pathology of lung in Wegener's granulomatosis. Review of 87 open lung biopsies from 67 patients. Am J Surg Pathol. 1991;15:315-33.
57. Gonzalez-Gay MA, Vazquez-Rodriguez TR, Lopez-Diaz MJ, et al. Epidemiology of giant cell arteritis and polymyalgia rheumatic. Arthritis Rheum. 2009;61:1454-61.
58. Caselli RJ, Hunder GG, Whisnant JP. Neurologic disease in biopsy proven giant (temporal) cell arteritis. Neurology. 1988;38:352-9.
59. Burton EA, Winer JB, Barber PC. Giant cell arteritis of cervical radicular vessels presenting with diaphragmatic weakness. J Neurol Neurosurg Psychiatry. 1999;67:223-6.
60. Nesher G. Neurologic manifestations of giant cell arteritis. Clin Exp Rheumatol. 200;18:S24-26.
61. Proven A, Gabriel SE, Orces C, et al. Glucocorticoid therapy in giant cell arteritis: duration and adverse outcomes. Arthritis Rheum. 2003;49:703-8.
62. Gonzalez-Gay MA, Lopez-Diaz MJ, Barros S, et al. Giant cell arteritis: laboratory tests at the time of diagnosis in a series of 240 patients. Medicine. 2005;84:277-90.
63. Weyand CM, Fulbright JW, Hunder GG, et al. Treatment of giant cell arteritis: interleukin-6 as a marker of disease activity. Arthritis Rheum. 2000;43:1041-8.
64. Rosenbaum R. Neuromuscular complications of connective tissue disease. Muscle Nerve. 2001;24:154-69.
65. Mori K, Lijima M, Koike H, et al. The wide spectrum of clinical manifestations in Sjögren's syndrome associated neuropathy. Brain. 2005;128:2518-34.
66. Grant IA, Hunder GG, Homburger HA, et al. Peripheral neuropathy associated with sicca complex. Neurology. 1997;48:855-62.
67. Ferri C. Mixed cryoglobulinemia. Orphanet J Rare Dis. 2008;3:25.
68. Saadoun D, Terrier B, Semoun O, et al. Hepatitis C virus associated polyarteritis nodosa. Arthritis Care Res. 2011;63:427-35.

69. Migliaresi S, Di Iorio G, Ammendola A, et al. Peripheral nervous system involvement in HCV-related mixed cryoglobulinemia. Reumatismo. 2001;53:26-32.

70. Pagnoux C, Cohen P, Guillevin L. Vasculitides secondary to infections. Clin Exp Rheumatol. 2006;24:S71-81.

71. Yoon M-S, Obermann M, Dockweiler C, et al. Sensory neuropathy in patients with cryoglobulin negative hepatitis C infection. J Neurol. 2011;258:80-88.

72. Nemni R, Sanvito L, Quattrini A, et al. Peripheral neuropathy in hepatitis C infection with or without cryoglobulinemia. J Neurol Neurosurg Psychiatry. 2003;74:1267-71.

73. Calabrese LH. Vasculitis and infection with human immunodeficiency virus. Rheum Dis Clin North Am. 1991;17:131-47.

74. Johnson RM, Barbarinin G, Barbaro G. Kawasaki like syndrome and other vasculitic syndromes in HIV-infected patients. AIDS. 2003;17:S77-82.

75. Roullet E, Assuerus V, Gozlan J, et al. Cytomegalovirus multifocal neuropathy in AIDS: analysis of 15 consecutive cases. Neurology. 1994;44:2174-82.

76. Rudnicki SA, Dalmau J. Paraneoplastic vasculitis of the peripheral nerves. Curr Opin Neurol. 2005;18:598-603.

77. Oh SJ. Paraneoplastic vasculitis of the peripheral nervous system. Neurol Clin. 1997;15:849-63.

78. Eggers C, Hagel C, Pfeiffer G. Anti-Hu associated paraneoplastic sensory neuropathy with peripheral nerve demyelination and microvasculitis. J Neurol Sci. 1998;155:178-81.

79. Lidar M, Lipschitz N, Langevitz P, et al. The infectious etiology of vasculitis. Autoimmunity. 2009;42:432-8.

80. Chretien F, Gray F. Lescs MC, et al. Acute varicella-zoster virus ventriculitis and meningo-myelo-radiculitis in acquired immunodeficiency syndrome. Acta Neuropathol. 1993;86:659-65.

81. Schafers M, Neukirchen S, Toyka KV, et al. Diagnostic value of sural nerve biopsy in patients with suspected Borrelia neuropathy. J Peripher Nerv Syst. 2008;13:81-91.

82. Lenglet T, Haroche J, Schnuriger A, et al. Mononeuropathy multiplex associated with acute parvovirus B19 infection: characteristics, treatment and outcome. J Neurol. 2011;258:1321-6.

83. Dyck PJ, Benstead TJ, Conn DL, et al. Nonsystemic vasculitic neuropathy. Brain. 1987;110:843-53.

84. Agadi JB, Raghav G, Mahadevan A, et al. Usefulness of superficial peroneal nerve/peroneus brevis muscle biopsy in the diagnosis of vasculitic neuropathy. J Clin Neurosci. 2012;19:1392-6.

85. Dyck PJB, Windebank AJ. Diabetic and nondiabetic lumbosacral radiculoplexus neuropathies: new insights into pathophysiology and treatment. Muscle Nerve. 2002;25:477-91.

86. Dyck PJB, Norell JE, Dyck PJ. Microvasculitis and ischemia in diabetic lumbosacral radiculoplexus neuropathy. Neurology. 1999;53:2113-21.

87. Katz JS, Saperstein DS, Wolfe G, et al. Cervicobrachial involvement in diabetic radiculoplexopathy. Muscle Nerve. 2001;24:794-98.

88. Garces Sanchez M, Laughlin RS, Dyck PJB, et al. Painless diabetic motor neuropathy: a variant of diabetic lumbosacral radiculoplexus neuropathy? Ann Neurol. 2011;69:1043-54.

89. Zivkovic SA, Ascherman D, Lacomis D. Vasculitic neuropathy-electrodiagnostic findings and association with malignancies. Acta Neurol Scand. 2007;115:432-6.

90. Claussen GC, Thomas TD, Goyne C, et al. Diagnostic value of nerve and muscle biopsy in suspected vasculitic cases. J Clin Neuromuscul Dis. 2000;1:117-23.

91. McCluskey L, Feinberg D, Cantor C, et al. "Pseudo-conduction blocks" in vasculitic neuropathy. Muscle Nerve. 1999;22:1361-6.

92. Jamieson PW, Giuliani MJ, Martinez AJ. Necrotizing angiopathy presenting with multifocal conduction blocks. Neurology. 1991;41:442-4.

93. Rappaport WD, Valente J, Hunter GC, et al. Clinical utilization and complications of sural nerve biopsy. Am J Surg. 1993;166:252-6.

94. Sakai K, Komai K, Yanase D, et al. Plasma VEGF as a marker for the diagnosis and treatment of vasculitic neuropathy. J Neurol Neurosurg Psychiatry. 2005;76:296.

95. Terrier B, Lacroix C, Guillevin L, et al. Diagnostic and prognostic relevance of neuromuscular biopsy in primary Sjögren's syndrome related neuropathy. Arthritis Rheum. 2007;57:1520-9.

96. Vrancken AF, Notermans NC, Jansen GH, et al. Progressive idiopathic axonal neuropathy—a comparative clinical and histopathological study with vasculitic neuropathy. J Neurol. 2004;251:269-78.

97. Chalk CH, Homburger HA, Dyck PJ. Anti-neutrophil cytoplasmic antibodies in vasculitic peripheral neuropathy. Neurology. 1993;43:1826-7.

98. Vrancken AF, Gathier CS, Cats EA, et al. The additional yield of combined nerve/muscle biopsy in vasculitic neuropathy. Eur J Neurol. 2011;18:49-58.

99. Guillevin L, Mahr A, Callard P, et al. Hepatitis B virus-associated polyarteritis nodosa: clinical characteristics, outcome and impact of treatment in 115 patients. Medicine. 2005;84:313-22.

100. De Vita S, Quartuccio L, Isola M, et al. A randomized controlled trial of rituximab for the treatment of severe cryoglobulinemic vasculitis. Arthritis Rheum. 2012;64:843-53.

101. Sneller MC, Hu Z, Langford CA. A randomized controlled trial of rituximab following failure of antiviral therapy for hepatitis C virus-associated cryoglobulinemic vasculitis. Arthritis Rheum. 2012;64:835-42.

102. Ahmed A. Antiviral treatment of cytomegalovirus infection. Infect Disord Drug Targets. 2011;11:475-503.

103. Patel N, Patel N, Khan T, et al. HIV infection and clinical spectrum of associated vasculitides. Curr Rheumatol Rep. 2011;13:506-12.

104. Lapraik C, Watts R, Bacon P, et al. BSR and BHPR guidelines for the management of adults with ANCA associated vasculitis. Rheumatology. 2007;46:1615-6.

105. Mukhtyar C, Guillevin L, Cid MC, et al. EULAR recommendations for the management of primary small and medium vessel vasculitis. Ann Rheum Dis. 2009;68:310-7.

106. Faurschou M, Westman K, Rasmussen N, et al. Brief report: long term outcome of randomized clinical trial comparing methotrexate to cyclophosphamide for remission induction in early systemic antineutrophil cytoplasmic antibody-associated vasculitis. Arthritis Rheum. 2012;64:3472-7.

107. Walsh M, Merkel PA, Mahr A, et al. Effects of duration of glucocorticoid therapy on relapse rate in antineutrophil cytoplasmic antibody-associated vasculitis: a meta-analysis. Arthritis Care Res. 2010;62:1166-73.

108. Walsh M, Catapano F, Szpirt, et al. Plasma exchange for renal vasculitis and idiopathic rapidly progressive glomerulonephritis: a meta-analysis. Am J Kidney Dis. 2011;57:566-74.

109. Jones RB. Tervaert JW, Hauser T, et al. Rituximab versus cyclophosphamide in ANCA associated renal vasculitis. N Engl J Med. 2010;363:211-20.

110. Stone JH, Merkel PA, Spiera R, et al. Rituximab versus cyclophosphamide for ANCA associated vasculitis. N Engl J Med. 2010;363:221-32.

111. Vital C, Vital A, Canron C, et al. Combined nerve and muscle biopsy in diagnosis of vasculitic neuropathy. A 16 year retrospective study or 202 cases. J Peripher Nerv Syst. 2006;11:20-29.

112. Dyck PJB, O'Brien P, Bosch P, et al. the multi-center double-blind controlled trial of IV methylprednisolone in diabetic lumbosacral radiculoplexus neuropathy. Neurology. 2006;66:A191.

113. Tamburin S, Zanette G. Intravenous immunoglobulin for the treatment of diabetic lumbosacral radiculoplexus neuropathy. Pain Med. 2009;10:1476-80.

114. Pascoe MK, Low PA, Windebank AJ, et al. Subacute diabetic proximal neuropathy. Mayo Clin Proc. 1997;72:1123-32.

CHAPTER 21

Gastrointestinal Manifestations

Saroj K Sinha, Raghavendra Prasada, Rakesh Kochhar

INTRODUCTION

Vasculitis refers to inflammation of the vessel walls, which may lead to alteration in blood supply to the dependent organ and its subsequent damage. It is categorized into large-, medium-, and small-vessel vasculitis.[1] Vasculitis involving gastrointestinal (GI) system may be systemic or localized. The spectrum of GI manifestations ranges from ulcer, submucosal edema, aneurysm formation, hemorrhages to paralytic ileus, mesenteric ischemia, bowel obstruction, and perforation.[2] Gastrointestinal vasculitis is seen mostly as a part of systemic inflammatory process. It is well recognized in patients with medium- and small-vessel vasculitis. Gastrointestinal complications generally indicate a severe disease and they adversely affect the prognosis[3] (Flow chart 21.1).

GASTROINTESTINAL TRACT INVOLVEMENT IN LARGE-VESSEL VASCULITIS

Takayasu Arteritis

In Takayasu arteritis (TA), there is granulomatous inflammation of aorta and its major branches, and the disease classically involves aortic arch and its branches, particularly the subclavian arteries. Abdominal aorta and its branches are frequently involved in Indian patients, occurring in 79% of patients, and it is a common cause of renovascular hypertension.[4] However, mesenteric involvement, per se, is rare.[5] There are occasional reports of inflammatory bowel disease and TA, though the association is not clear.[6,7] Ischemic bowel disease can occur due to involvement of origin of celiac axis, superior mesenteric artery, or inferior mesenteric artery. This can be treated by endovascular intervention like placement of metal stents to open the stenotic segment.

Giant Cell Arteritis

Giant cell (temporal) arteritis (GCA) is a form of granulomatous arteritis of the aorta and its major branches, with a predilection for the extracranial branches of the carotid artery.[1] The most common symptom is headache, while perhaps the most specific is jaw claudication. Gastrointestinal involvement is rare and there are isolated case reports of mesenteric ischemia and infarction.[8] Giant cell arteritis should be considered in the differential diagnosis in a setting of fever, GI symptoms, and raised ESR in those >50 years presenting with acute abdomen when no cause is apparent. Autopsy series show mesenteric involvement in approximately 20% cases. Liver function abnormalities, most commonly elevated alkaline phosphatase, are seen in one-third to one half of patients with GCA. Transaminases, ALT and AST can be mildly elevated in 10–40% of patients.[9] Symptomatic liver involvement is extremely rare.

GASTROINTESTINAL TRACT INVOLVEMENT IN MEDIUM-VESSEL VASCULITIS

Polyarteritis Nodosa (Table 21.1)

- Gastrointestinal involvement is common and occurs in about 50% of polyarteritis nodosa (PAN) patients.
- Patients of PAN with GI involvement have poorer prognosis.
- Acute abdomen is common among those patients of PAN who have GI involvement. However, the most common symptom remains pain abdomen which occurs in 60–97% cases.
- Gastrointestinal tract (GIT) involvement is more common with HBV-related PAN.

Flow chart 21.1 Approach to GI vasculitis

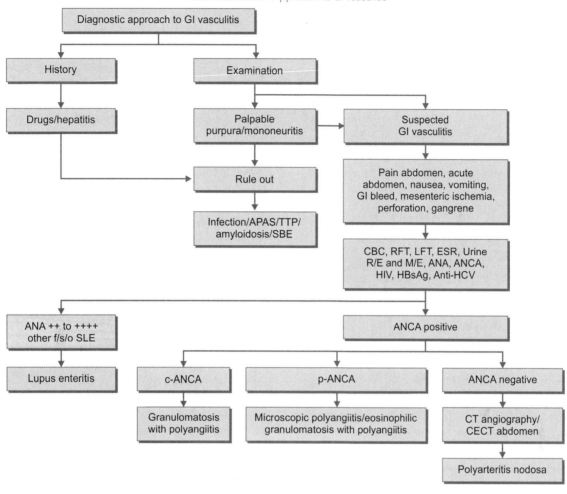

Table 21.1 Gastrointestinal tract manifestations of polyarteritis nodosa[16,27]

GI manifestations	Frequency
Abdominal pain	37/38 (97%)
Nausea/vomiting	12/38 (32%)
Diarrhea	6/38 (16%)
Hematochezia/melena	3–5
Hematemesis	3/38 (8%)
Esophageal ulceration	5/38 (13%)
Gastroduodenal ulceration	12/38 (32%)
Colorectal ulceration	2/38 (5%)
Surgical abdomen/peritonitis	14–32

- CT angiography is used as a primary modality to diagnose PAN and is helpful in more than two-thirds of cases. The classic finding is string of beads appearance, with aneurysm up to 1 cm in diameter.
- The five-factor score (FFS) of ≥1 indicates poor prognosis.
- Outcome of medical treatment with corticosteroids and immunosuppressive is good.

Polyarteritis nodosa is necrotizing focal segmental inflammation of medium-sized or small-sized arteries, with usually no involvement of arterioles, capillaries, or venules. It is not associated with antineutrophil cytoplasmic antibodies (ANCAs). As per the largest series of PAN patients, the most frequent manifestations are general symptoms which are seen in 93.1% of patients, followed by neurologic manifestations in 79%, skin involvement in 49.7%, abdominal pain in 35.6%, and hypertension in 34.8%.[10]

The symptoms due to GI involvement usually occur as a result of mesenteric ischemia. The transmural necrotizing inflammation of the medium-sized arteries results in fibrinoid necrosis of arterial wall and infiltration by polymorphonuclear leukocytes. Injury to the arterial wall results in weakening of wall, aneurysmal dilatation with potential to rupture, stenosis of vessels, and thrombosis resulting in ischemia of the organ. This can lead to ulcerations along the GIT, infarcts or gangrene, and ischemic atrophy.

Clinical presentation of PAN is extremely variable, and delay in diagnosis is common. Classification criteria of PAN have been discussed in Chapter on PAN. Gastrointestinal involvement occurs in 14–65% of patients with PAN and is a major cause of morbidity and mortality. Patients with severe GI involvement carry a poor prognosis.[11,12] Most patients with GIT involvement have systemic symptoms and other organ involvement also. When there is isolated involvement of GIT, the small intestine and the gall bladder are most frequently involved.[13,14] The most common symptom is abdominal pain, which occurs in 60–97% of patients, usually has features suggestive of abdominal angina and becomes worse after meals.[15,16] Other manifestations include nausea or vomiting, gastroduodenal ulcerations, surgical abdomen in the form of GI infarction, perforation or peritonitis, diarrhea, GI bleeding in the form of hematemesis, hematochezia, or melena.[16] Bowel ischemia may result in bowel gangrene and perforation peritonitis, requiring urgent surgical intervention. Acute abdomen is not uncommon in PAN. In fact, in a series of 54 patients, 24(44%) had GIT involvement.[12] Of these, 13 had acute surgical abdomen, either at presentation or on follow-up, and 11 had other GI symptoms. Of the 13 patients who developed acute abdomen but did not have bowel infarctions or perforations, acute cholecystitis and gallbladder infarction were the most common diagnoses (five cases). There were eight episodes of bowel infarction or perforation (four large bowel, four small bowel) and four aneurysmal ruptures (two involving hepatic arteries, one involving the splenic artery, and one involving the renal artery). Two patients suffered colonic perforations during colonoscopy. Risk of bowel perforation during colonoscopy is said to be higher in the setting of PAN, this is probably related to ischemic changes in bowel.

Liver involvement occurs in 16–56% of patients but patients may not have symptoms related to hepatic involvement.[17] Angiography reveals hepatic artery to be frequently involved, with microaneurysms and caliber changes in the form of corkscrew appearance. Hepatic arterial involvement may result in atrophy of a liver lobe, liver infarction, acute liver failure, nodular regenerative hyperplasia, or hemobilia. Rarely, biliary strictures, sclerosing cholangitis, and acalculous cholecystitis can also occur. Pancreatic involvement is also frequently seen on autopsy but clinically overt pancreatic symptoms are uncommon.

Polyarteritis nodosa is associated with HBV infection in about 7–35% cases.[10,18] But clinically overt PAN occurs in less than 1% of patients with HBV infection. HBV PAN is an early postinfectious disease with HBV infection occurring within 12 months preceding PAN. Hepatitis is silent in most cases with a mild transaminase level increase in 50% of patients.[19-22]

Gastrointestinal involvement is more common in HBV-related PAN patients than in non-HBV-related PAN patients. However, survival does not differ amongst these two groups.[15,23] Relapses are less common in HBV-related PAN than in those without HBV. When ischemia is limited to the mucosa or submucosa, it may lead to ulceration and bleeding, but when transmural ischemia occurs, there may be necrosis of the bowel wall leading to perforation and infarction, which is associated with a poor prognosis.[16,24]

Polyarteritis nodosa-like disease can rarely be seen with familial Mediterranean fever, leukemias, bronchogenic carcinoma, carcinoma stomach, carcinoma colon, inflammatory bowel disease, *Yersinia enterocolitis,* amebic colitis, and chronic parvovirus infection.

The five factor score (FFS) which includes (i) severe GI disease (GI bleeding, perforation, infarction, or pancreatitis); (ii) renal insufficiency (serum creatinine level >1.58 mg/dL); (iii) proteinuria >1 g/day; (iv) involvement of the central nervous system (CNS); and (v) cardiac involvement (infarction or heart failure), with one score for each.[23] A score of ≥1 is associated with poorer outcome.[16] Raised transaminases are observed in patients with PAN without much clinical significance though there may be a trend toward protective effect.[25] Polyarteritis nodosa can rarely manifest as acute pancreatitis.[26]

CT angiography is used as a primary modality to diagnose PAN and can be diagnostic in more than two-thirds of the patients.[12,16] Aneurysms ≤1 cm in diameter can be seen in renal, mesenteric, and hepatic vasculature. The classical finding of "string-of-beads" appearance, as well as areas of irregular stenosis and aneurysmal areas can be seen. Usually, upper GI tract biopsies are unyielding, whereas colonoscopic biopsy may demonstrate vasculitis in histological specimens.[16]

Histopathological demonstration of vascular inflammation in medium-sized or small-sized arteries is important in establishing the diagnosis of vasculitis and in excluding other disorders. In order to achieve the good diagnostic yield, biopsies need to be performed at symptomatic sites (e.g. muscle, sural nerve, skin, or testicle). In a large series of patients with PAN, combined muscle and nerve biopsies in symptomatic patients provided histological confirmation of vasculitis in 83% of cases. In case liver or kidney biopsy is planned, it is preferable to perform under USG guidance to reduce the risk of bleeding in these patients due to vascular changes.

Age >65 years, hypertension, and GI manifestations requiring surgery or at least consultation with a surgeon are independent predictors of death among patients with PAN, and patients with cutaneous manifestations or non-HBV-related PAN have a higher risk of relapse.[10]

Details of treatment of PAN are discussed in the other chapter of the book. Immunosuppression with corticosteroid, cyclophosphamide, or other immunosuppressive agents is the mainstay of therapy. HBV-related PAN is treated with short course (2–4 weeks) of steroid followed by rapid tapering. Steroids are used to contain the inflammatory process which causes the organ damage in PAN but long-term use of steroid may be associated with increased replication of HBV and associated risk of chronic liver disease. Rapid withdrawal of steroid may trigger e-antigen seroconversion. In severe cases, plasmapheresis has been tried with the aim of removal of immune complexes which have a role in the pathogenesis of PAN. Antiviral agents such as interferon alpha as well as oral agents like lamivudine have been used for the treatment of chronic HBV infection in the setting of PAN. HBeAg seroconversion occurs in almost two-thirds of the patients treated with interferon alpha or lamivudine, and HBsAg loss occurs in 30–50% cases, both figures are higher than other patients with chronic HBV infection. Published experience with other newer oral antivirals like tenofovir and entecavir is limited but they are likely to be efficacious. Contrary to idiopathic or primary PAN, relapses are rare in HBV-related PAN and never occur when viral replication has ceased and seroconversion has been achieved.[27]

Prognosis of untreated PAN is poor but with treatment, 5-year survival is 70–85%.[18] Poor prognostic factors include proteinuria, renal insufficiency, cardiomyopathy, severe GI manifestations, and CNS involvement. Gastrointestinal causes of death include GI bleeding, bowel gangrene, peritonitis, and acute pancreatitis. Details of the medical treatment are included in other chapters of the book.

Kawasaki's Disease

Kawasaki's disease (KD) is arteritis associated with the "mucocutaneous lymph node syndrome". It predominantly affects medium and small arteries. Development of coronary artery abnormalities is the hallmark of KD and accounts for most morbidity and mortality associated with the disease. Typically in KD, the diagnostic criteria include an illness unexplained by another disease, fever (at least 5 days), and four of the five following conditions: bilateral nonpurulent conjunctival injection, oral mucosal changes, peripheral extremity changes, truncal rash, and cervical lymphadenopathy (over 1.5 cm). Patients who fulfil the criteria for KD with a clinical feature that is not usually seen with KD constitute atypical KD. In a large cohort of KD patients, it was found that approximately 4.6% of them (10 out of 219) presented with an acute surgical abdomen.[28] The diagnosis included gallbladder hydrops with cholestasis in five,

paralytic ileus in three, and vasculitis leading to appendicitis in one, and to hemorrhagic duodenitis in one. Half of these patients with atypical presentation also had coronary artery involvement despite early intravenous immunoglobulin (IV Ig) therapy.

Treatment of choice is IV Ig and aspirin. In case of IV Ig resistance, a repeat IV Ig dose is given. If patients still do not respond, the options include methylprednisolone and infliximab.[29]

GASTROINTESTINAL TRACT INVOLVEMENT IN SMALL-VESSEL VASCULITIS

Granulomatosis with Polyangiitis (Wegener's)

Granulomatosis with polyangiitis (GPA) is characterized by granulomatous vasculitis of the upper and lower respiratory tracts, glomerulonephritis, and small-to-medium-vessel vasculitis. Gastrointestinal involvement is uncommon and usually detected in autopsy studies and resected surgical specimens. Different series quote GI involvement in 0–20% cases. The small bowel is the most common site of GI involvement. Gastrointestinal complications include esophageal ulceration, cholecystitis, gallbladder infarction, pancreatitis and pancreatic mass, bloody diarrhea, bowel infarction, small and large bowel perforation, spontaneous splenic hemorrhage, etc.[30] Clinical features include abdominal pain, being most common, diarrhea, nausea or vomiting, hematochezia or melena, and gastroduodenal ulcers.[16] Rarely, GPA may mimic inflammatory bowel disease. Untreated GPA has a 2-year mortality of around 80%. The survival has improved to 80% at 5 years after the introduction of cyclophosphamide and steroids. Details of medical treatment are included in the chapter on GPA.

Eosinophilic Granulomatosis with Polyangiitis (Churg-Strauss)

Churg–Strauss syndrome (CSS) is a form of granulomatous inflammation involving the respiratory tract and necrotizing vasculitis affecting small-to-medium-sized vessels and is associated with asthma and eosinophilia. Gastrointestinal manifestations are seen in one-third to 50% of patients.[15,31,32] Gastrointestinal involvement increases the risk of relapse in CSS.[33] Clinical presentations include abdominal pain in 22–97% of patients, diarrhea in 9–33%, hematochezia or melena in 6–18%, and a surgical abdomen in 9–34% patients.[16,31,34] Mechanisms of GI involvement include mesenteric vasculitis which is the most common, whereas obstructive symptoms or diarrhea due to bowel wall infiltration by eosinophils is rare. Unusual presentation can be in the form of odynophagia with esophageal involvement causing "congestive esophagitis" and esophageal thickening.[35] Intestinal involvement may be in the form of isolated or multiple ulcerations, both in small intestine and colon which may lead on to perforations more often in the former.[36] Most commonly, the ulcers are shallow with erythematous hallows. Other rare GI manifestations include hepatomegaly, ascites, Budd–Chiari syndrome, omental nodules, omental hematoma, etc. Angiography may reveal stenotic lesions in 33% and microaneurysms in 30% cases.[31] Vasculitis in tissue is usually diagnosed only in resected specimens and endoscopic biopsies are unyielding, as they require deeper submucosal sample.

Corticosteroids have greatly improved the prognosis of CSS with about 90% achieving remission. The results of a meta-analysis showed that cyclophosphamide in addition to corticosteroids improved outcome only for those patients who had FFS of two or greater in patients with microscopic polyangiitis (MPA), PAN, and CSS.[30] Myocardial involvement and severe GI disease secondary to mesenteric ischemia are significantly associated with a poor clinical outcome.

Microscopic Polyangiitis

Microscopic polyangiitis is necrotizing vasculitis predominantly affecting small vessels (i.e. capillaries, venules, or arterioles) with few or no immune deposits.[1] Pulmonary capillaritis and necrotizing glomerulonephritis are common. Men are affected slightly more often than women. Main clinical symptoms include renal manifestations that occur in 78%, weight loss in 72%, skin involvement in 62%, fever in 55%, mononeuritis multiplex in 57%, arthralgias in 50%, myalgias in 48%, hypertension in 34%, GI involvement in 30%, lung involvement in 24%, and cardiac failure in 17%.[37] The most commonly reported gastrointestinal symptom in MPA patients is abdominal pain, which can occur in 30–58% of patients, GI bleeding occurs in 29% of patients.[36] Other rare GI manifestations include bowel perforation, cholecystitis, and pancreatitis. The biochemical abnormality in liver functions can be seen in up to 11% cases.[37] Unlike PAN, findings in CT angiography in MPA are usually normal and do not reveal microaneurysms.[2]

IgA VASCULITIS (HENOCH-SCHÖNLEIN PURPURA)

- HSP typically affects young children 6 months to less than 20 years. About three-fourths of patients are less than 40 years of age.

- Gastrointestinal tract is most common organ system affected after skin. In the GIT, small bowel is most commonly affected.
- Pain abdomen is usually a prominent symptom, occurring in up to 98% of cases.
- Only small percentage of patients (<5%) develop bowel infarct, perforation, and irreducible intussusceptions. Surgical intervention may be required for these complications.
- The endoscopic lesions include mucosal erythema, petechiae, hemorrhagic erosions, and multiple ulcers. Second part of duodenum is the most commonly involved site of GIT.
- Adults more frequently have nephritis than children and have worse prognosis compared to children.
- The disease usually resolves spontaneously, particularly in children. However, steroids early in the course may alleviate pain abdomen early and reduce development of persistent renal dysfunction.

IgA vasculitis (IgAV) is characterized by IgA immune deposits, affecting small vessels (predominantly capillaries, venules, or arterioles). IgA vasculitis often involves the skin and GIT, joints, and kidneys.[1] Any part of the GI system can be affected, but small bowel involvement is the most common. Typically, it affects young children from 6 months to young adults of less than 20 years. Recent large series showed three fourths of the affected patients were younger than 20 and rest one-fourth were adults.[38]

As a first presentation, GI manifestations are seen in 14% patients, third most common organ system to be involved. Once the disease is established, GI system constitutes the second most common organ system involved next only to skin, being affected in 64–78% of cases.[38-40] In a series of 417 patients with HSP, at onset, the disease was characterized by the presence of skin lesions in 55.9%, GI involvement in 13.7%, joint symptoms in 9.1%, nephropathy in 24%, and fever in 6.2%.[38] However, during the clinical course, cutaneous lesions were observed in 100% of patients, joint manifestations (mainly arthralgia) occurred in 63.1% of patients, and GI involvement was present in 64.5% of patients. The main GI manifestations were a typical colicky abdominal pain (64.5%), nausea and vomiting (14.4%), melena and/or rectorrhagia (12.9%), and positive stool guaiac test (10.3%). Thus, among GI manifestations of HSP, the most common symptom is pain abdomen occurring in approximately 65–98% cases followed by nausea or vomiting (40%), GI bleeding (21%), and diarrhea (7%).[40] The abdominal pain is typically characterized as colicky and diffuse, the abdomen can be tender and quite distended. Pain is localized to epigastric area in 56%, right lower abdomen in 15%, periumbilical area in 11%, right upper abdomen in 6%, and uncommonly in left upper abdomen or diffusely in whole abdomen.[39] Less than 5% patients develop bowel infarct, perforation, or irreducible intussusception. Intussusceptions in two-thirds involve only the small bowel and half of the patients usually have a palpable mass. More than half of these intussusceptions are of the ileoileal type.[40] Adults have lesser frequency of abdominal pain, fever, and a higher frequency of arthritis, raised ESR, and nephritis compared with children, and hence more severe clinical syndrome in adults.[41] About 2–6% of patients with HSP may require surgical intervention for these complications.[42,43] Reasons for surgical intervention include bowel ischemia and infarction secondary to vasculitis, bowel perforation, irreducible intussusception, gastrointestinal bleeding, and acute appendicitis. Of these, intussusception is the most common cause of surgery, with an estimated incidence of 3.5%.[44] Bowel perforations in HSP typically result from vasculitis leading to ischemia and subsequent necrosis

of the bowel. In contrast, spontaneous bowel perforation that occurs mostly in the ileum is relatively rare, with an estimated incidence of 0.38%.[45] Although corticosteroids have been widely used in managing acute abdominal pain in children with HSP, systemic corticosteroid therapy may mask the signs of intra-abdominal surgical complications. Vasculitic involvement of the ileum or ascending colon may produce signs which mimic acute appendicitis and lead to unnecessary appendicectomy. Acute appendicitis including gangrenous appendicitis has been reported in patients with HSP (Table 21.2).[46]

The endoscopic lesions include mucosal erythema, petechiae, hemorrhagic erosions, multiple ulcers, nodular changes, and hematoma-like protrusions (Figs 21.1 to 21.4). The ulcers caused by HSP are usually small, irregular, superficial, and clean based. In the upper GI tract, the second portion of the duodenum is the most frequently involved area and it is usually most severely involved (52.9%). Other

Table 21.2 Clinical manifestations of HSP

Clinical and laboratory parameters	Frequency			
	Reference 38	Reference 51	Reference 52	Reference 53
No. of cases	417	122	102	87
Children	75.5%	68.8%	80.4%	74.7%
Adults	24.5%	31.2%	19.6%	25.3%
Cutaneous lesions	100%	100%	100%	100%
Palpable purpura	97.6%			
Others	20.6%			
Gastrointestinal involvement	64.5%	85.2%	59.8%	60%
Abdominal pain	64.5%			
Nausea and/or vomiting	14.4%			
Melena and/or rectorrhagia	12.9%			
Positive stool guaiac test	10.3%			
Joint involvement	63.1%	54%	67.6%	70%
Arthralgia	43.8%			
Arthritis	37.4%			
Nephropathy	41.2%	36.8%	59.8%	30%
Mild	34.1%	23.7%	55.9%	20.7%
Severe	7.1%	–	3.9%	9.2%
Renal insufficiency	4.8%	5.7%	2.9%	6.9%
Peripheral neuropathy	1.9%			
Laboratory findings				
Leukocytosis	36.7%	63.9%	19.6%	47.1%
Anemia	8.9%	–		2.3%
Increased ESR	80.1%	–		–
Increased IgA levels	31.7%	52.4%		30.2%
Positive rheumatoid factor	4.9%			
Positive antinuclear antibodies	14.2%			
Positive ANCAs	0%			
Cryoglobulins	20.4%			
Low C3 and/or C4	7.9%			

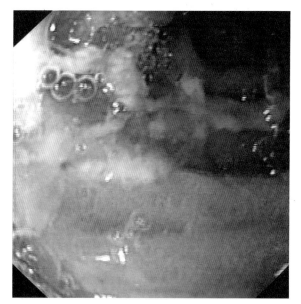

Fig. 21.1 Enteroscopy image showing jejunal ulcers with lots of exudates in a case of Henoch–Schönlein purpura

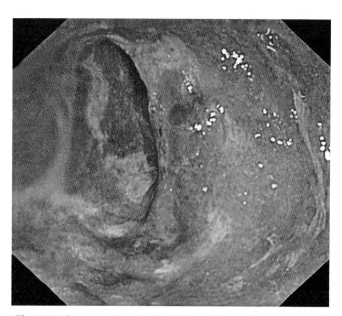

Fig. 21.2 Ileoscopy showing ileal ulcers with exudates in a case of small-vessel vasculitis of GIT

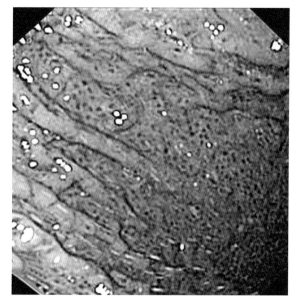

Fig. 21.3 Gastroscopy showing purpura like lesion in stomach in a case of Henoch–Schönlein purpura

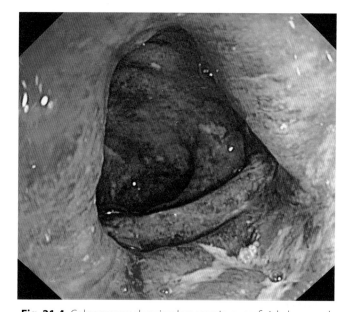

Fig. 21.4 Colonoscopy showing hyperemia, superficial ulcers, and exudates in colon in a case of small-vessel vasculitis of GIT

involved locations in upper GIT include duodenal bulb in 41.3%, gastric body in 25.4%, gastric antrum in 23.1%, gastric fundus in 3.8%, and esophagus in 3%.[39] In the lower GI tract, the rectum is frequently involved; however, the most severe lesions occur in the terminal ileum.[39] The most prominent endoscopic finding is severe hemorrhagic erosive duodenitis. It may be regarded as a typical but nonpathognomonic endoscopic finding of HSP. Rarely, severe GI complications such as bowel infarction, perforation, fistula, intussusception

(ileoileal), hemorrhagic ascites, pancreatitis, and portal vein thrombosis can occur.

Imaging modalities include ultrasound and CT scan. Ultrasound can detect bowel dilatation, mural wall thickening, ascitic fluid, and complications such as intussusception without any additional radiation exposure; it is the modality of choice in evaluating the bowel manifestations of HSP.[47] Findings from CT scan include bowel wall thickening with the target sign, engorgement of mesenteric vessels with comb sign, mesenteric edema and nonspecific lymphadenopathy.[48]

Leukocytoclastic vasculitis (LCV) is a characteristic feature of HSP. The frequency of LCV in biopsies correlates with the severity of duodenitis on endoscopy. The endoscopic finding, hematoma-like protrusion, seems to represent intramucosal hemorrhage due to vasculitis.[49] However, vasculitic changes may not be apparent on endoscopic or colonoscopic biopsies. In fact, in one series, all the endoscopic biopsies were reported as nonspecific inflammation.[39]

Overall prognosis of HSP is good in both children and adults; in one study, complete recovery occurred in 94% of children and 89% of adults.[41] Recovery typically occurs spontaneously in most of the children with only supportive care. In contrast, immunosuppressive therapy may be required in up to 63% of adult cases. A systematic review of 15 studies found that early intervention with steroids reduces symptomatic abdominal pain within the first 24 hours and reduces the odds of developing persistent renal disease.[50] Despite the good prognosis in majority of cases, patients with nephritis were associated with worse outcome than those without renal involvement. In a series of 417 patients of HSP, 35% patients received steroids, and cytotoxic drugs were given to 5% of patients, either as corticosteroid-sparing agents or as an additional therapy for patients with severe renal involvement.[38] Indications for use of steroid included persistent skin lesions or visceral involvement, including severe abdominal pain, GI bleeding, or nephropathy. The median duration of corticosteroid therapy was 1 month (range 0.5–4 months), and the median initial prednisone or equivalent dose was 30 mg/day. After a median follow-up of 12 months, complete recovery was observed in 83.2%. Persistent nephropathy (renal sequelae) was found in 7.7% patients.

VASCULITIS ASSOCIATED WITH SYSTEMIC DISEASE

Systemic Lupus Erythematosus

- Gastrointestinal symptoms occur in 50% of SLE patients, mostly secondary to adverse drug reaction or infections.
- Lupus mesenteric vasculitis (LMV) occurs in less than 10% SLE cases in Asia and even lesser in the West.
- Lupus mesenteric vasculitis is a common cause of acute abdominal pain in SLE.
- Leukopenia, hypoalbuminemia, and elevated serum amylase in the SLE vasculitis are associated with serious complications.
- Endoscopic biopsies are usually unyielding and are rarely helpful in diagnosing LMV.

- Barium enema may show "thumbprinting" suggestive of ischemic bowel, whereas the modality of choice is contrast-enhanced CT scan of abdomen which shows changes suggestive of mesenteric ischemia despite patent vessels (engorgement of mesenteric vessels, bowel wall thickening, layering of bowel wall, target sign, Coomb's sign, etc.).
- All lupus enteritis patients require corticosteroids and more than two-third patients require additional immunosuppression with cyclophosphamide.
- Remission can be obtained in up to 85% with medical treatment alone. Relapse of LMV occurs in about 25% of patients. Bowel wall thickness of more than 8 mm is a risk factor for relapse.

Gastrointestinal manifestations are common in SLE patients. Nausea and vomiting occur in approximately 50% of these patients. Most of the GI symptoms are related to adverse reactions to drugs and intercurrent infections. Symptoms directly attributable to the disease vary widely between 1–27%, oral lesions being the most common.[54] Though less common than lupus nephritis and often neglected, GI manifestations can be life threatening if not recognized promptly and treated with immunosuppressant. No specific antibody is associated with GI involvement.

Lupus Mesenteric Vasculitis

Vasculitis in SLE is not uncommon and the reported prevalence ranges between 11% and 36 %.[55] However, LMV also known as lupus enteritis is an uncommon but serious gastrointestinal complication in SLE patients. Its prevalence ranges from 0.2 to 9.7% in SLE patients and from 29 to 65% in patients presenting with acute abdominal pain.[56] The prevalence of intestinal vasculitis in SLE is 2.2–9.7% in Asia, whereas it is lesser in West.[57] SLE-related vasculitis commonly involves small vessels, and medium-sized vessels are involved only in small percentage of patients (86 and 14%, respectively) but involvement of medium-sized vessels may have more serious consequences like bowel ischemia and bowel gangrene.[58] The incidence of abdominal pain in SLE patients varies between 8 and 40% with a large series showing 22% incidence.[54,59] Lupus enteritis is a common cause of acute abdominal pain in SLE patients, its prevalence being 29–65%.[56,60] Other leading causes of pain abdomen among them include acute pancreatitis, pseudoobstruction, acute acalculous cholecystitis, mesenteric thrombosis, hepatic artery thrombosis, and colonic perforation.[61] Lupus mesenteric vasculitis preferentially affects the superior mesenteric artery; ileum and jejunum are most frequently affected (80–85%), and rectum less often (14%).[62]

The ischemic change differ depending upon the sensitivity of the vessels in four different bowel layers; mucosal damage leads to ulceration and hemorrhage, submucosal involvement cause edema, pseudo-obstruction occurs due to muscular damage, and ascites due to serosal damage.[56] Clinical features of LMV are listed in Table 21.3. Gastrointestinal vasculitis in SLE indicates severe disease and is mostly accompanied by active disease elsewhere in the body. However, LMV can present as the initial manifestation of SLE.

Leukopenia, hypoalbuminemia, and elevated serum amylase are associated with serious complications. Ascites can be present in 55–78% of patients with SLE.[61,64] Acute peritoneal effusion can be due to mesenteric vasculitis or peritonitis. Peritonitis may be due to SLE activity, infection, bowel infarction, perforated viscera, or pancreatitis. Chronic peritoneal effusion can be caused by lupus peritonitis, hypoalbuminemia (nephrotic syndrome, protein-losing enteropathy, and liver cirrhosis), right heart failure, constrictive pericarditis, hepatic venous thrombosis, malignancy, or chronic infections like tuberculosis.

Endoscopy and Histopathology

Though histopathological diagnosis of LMV can be obtained, most endoscopic superficial biopsies do not yield a definitive diagnosis because the affected vessels are usually located in an inaccessible area.[56] Colonoscopy and endoscopy may show mucosal congestion, mucosal edema, erosions, and ulcers (superficial or deep, variable sizes, occasionally punched-out ulcers). Vasculitic changes are rarely reported in endoscopic biopsies and are more frequently picked up in resected specimens.

Radiological Investigation

Abdominal X-ray may reveal pneumoperitoneum, pneumatosis cystoides intestinalis, ileus, etc. Barium enema may show "thumbprinting" suggestive of ischemic bowel. CT abdomen is becoming increasingly popular as gold standard investigation. The imaging characteristics are given in Table 21.4, Figures 21.5 and 21.6.

There are conflicting reports about hepatic involvement with lupus vasculitis. In an autopsy study from Japan, evidence of hepatic arteritis was found in 21% patients with SLE and liver disease. In contrast, in another series of 33 patients with histologically proven liver disease, none had vasculitis. Rarely, hepatic vasculitis can result in hepatic hematoma, abscess formation, and spontaneous rupture of liver.

The reported annual incidence of acute pancreatitis in SLE patients is 2.3/1,000.[65] In SLE patients, acute pancreatitis

Table 21.3 Clinical characteristics of lupus mesenteric vasculitis (n = 97)[63]

Clinical features	Frequency (%)
Abdominal pain	90.7
Abdominal distension	70.1
Diarrhea	58.8
Nausea and vomiting	72.2
Fever	29.9
Abdominal tenderness	67.0
Bladder irritations symptoms/dysuria	9.3
Elevated serum amylase	30.9
Alimentary tract hemorrhage	33.0
Intestinal obstruction	40.2
Intestinal perforation	2.1
Lupus urinary tract involvement	22.7
Other organ involvement	
Polyserositis	22.7
Arthralgia	30.9
Renal involvement	67.0
Cardiac involvement	33.0
Pulmonary involvement	15.5
Central nervous system involvement	10.3

Table 21.4 Imaging findings in lupus mesenteric vasculitis (n = 97)[63]

Imaging finding	Frequency (%)
Bowel wall thickening	94.8
Target sign	83.5
Dilatation of intestinal segments	86.6
Engorgement of mesenteric vessels	100
Increased attenuation of mesenteric fat	96.9
Small bowel wall thickening	81.4
Large bowel wall thickening	69.1
Gastric wall thickening	6.2
Bowel wall thickness	
Slight (4–5 mm)	37.1
Moderate (6–8 mm)	42.3
Severe (>8 mm)	20.6
Ascites	55.7
Lymphadenopathy	15.5
Pancreas enlargement	3.1
Thickened bladder wall and/or reduced bladder size	6.2
Hydronephrosis	12.4
Stenosis/dilatation of the ureters	15.5

can occur by a variety of mechanisms, one of them being vasculitis.

Treatment

All lupus enteritis patients require corticosteroid and/or immunosuppressive therapy in view of severe systemic vasculitis. More than two-thirds of them require immunosuppression with cyclophosphamide. In a series of 97 patients, 84.5% patients achieved remission after appropriate treatment. In fact, 51.5% were on steroid treatment before the onset of LMV, and additional immunosuppressive

agents (hydroxychloroquine, azathioprine, methotrexate, or cyclophosphamide) were also administered in 43.3% patients.[63] Remission was obtained in 84.5% with medical treatment alone and surgical intervention was rarely required. Mortality of 13.2% was noted in this study, mostly related to infections, heart failure and multiorgan dysfunction. Relapse of LMV occurs in about approximately 25% of patients. Bowel wall thickness of more than 8 mm is a risk factor for relapse, whereas high-dose cyclophosphamide (≥ 1 g/m^2 per month) seems to be a protective factor.

Rheumatoid Vasculitis

Rheumatoid vasculitis (RV) involves the small- and medium-sized vessels and occurs in a small percentage of patients with established rheumatoid arthritis (RA). Although autopsy data have reported a high incidence of 15–30% in different series, clinically apparent vasculitis is much less common with frequency ranging between 1 and 5%.[66] Rheumatoid vasculitis occurs predominantly after long-standing RA. It is more frequent in the presence of rheumatoid nodules, hypocomplementemia, and high titers of rheumatoid factor. It most commonly affects skin followed by peripheral nervous system. In a large cohort of 86 patients of RV, the median age at presentation was 63 years and the median duration of RA was 10.8 years.[67]

Intestinal involvement occurs in 10–38% of cases of RV. Small bowel involvement results in ulceration, perforation, and necrosis of the small bowel. Vasculitis of the colon may manifest as pancolitis, clinically similar to ulcerative colitis. Rectal biopsies can be positive for vasculitis in up to 40% of cases.[68]

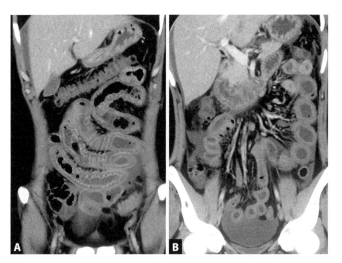

Figs 21.5A and B CT scan of abdomen of a male patient with lupus enteritis showing thickening and layering of bowel wall, more prominent in small bowel

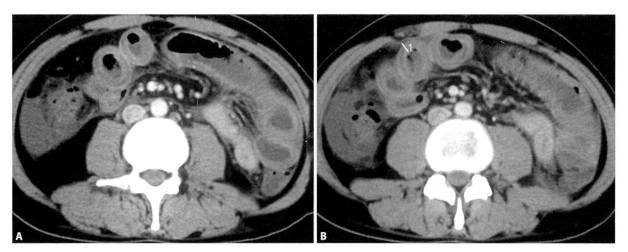

Figs 21.6A and B CT scan of abdomen in a case of small-vessel vasculitis of GIT showing mural thickening of small and large bowel with multilayered appearance

BEHÇET'S DISEASE VASCULITIS

- Gastrointestinal tract involvement in Behçet's disease is seen in approximately 7% patients.
- Oral ulcers are presenting manifestation in 70% patients, occurring later in nearly all patients.
- Behçet's disease can virtually involve any part of GIT.
- The most common site of involvement is small intestine, particularly the terminal ileum. There may be aphthous ulcerations or deep punched-out lesions which may lead to perforation or fistula formation.
- Clinically, Behçet's disease needs to be differentiated from Crohn's disease (CD). Deep ulceration and bowel perforation are more common in Behçet's disease, lack granulomas, and do not form abscesses like CD.
- Intestinal BD often requires surgical intervention and is usually followed by a high recurrence rate.

Behçet's disease is characterized by recurrent oral and/or genital aphthous ulcers along with cutaneous, ocular, gastrointestinal, articular, and/or CNS inflammatory lesions. Small-vessel vasculitis, arterial aneurysms, and thrombosis may occur.[1] Behçet's disease is a disease of young people, seen in second (26.6%), third (39.1%), and the fourth decade (20%) of life.[69] Among BD patients requiring laparotomy, the presenting manifestations include abdominal pain in 92%, mass in 21%, and melena in 17%.[70] In literature, the frequency of GI involvement has varied between 4 and 34%, with a large series from Iran reporting GI involvement in 7.4%.[69] Behçet's disease can cause ulceration throughout the digestive tract which is similar to the aphthous lesions seen in the mouth and genital area.

Oral ulcers are presenting manifestation in 70% patients, occurring later in all patients. The oral lesions are punched-out ulcers with a necrotic base, surrounded by an erythematous rim. They are generally multiple and painful, and heal with little scarring. Esophageal involvement is quite infrequent and is commoner in male patients. The most common site is middle third of esophagus. Symptoms include substernal pain, dysphagia, and hematemesis. Several morphological forms of esophageal lesions including erosions, perforated ulcers, widely spreading esophagitis, and severe stenosis can be seen.[71] Endoscopic biopsy and culture are required to differentiate this condition from viral and candidial esophagitis, as it is important in view of treatment perspective. Esophageal involvement is accompanied by involvement of other part of GI tract in more than 50% cases.

The most common site of involvement in the small intestine is the terminal ileum. Small-vessel involvement results in mucosal inflammation and ulceration, whereas large-vessel involvement causes ischemia and infarction of the bowel wall. Ileocecal involvement is frequent and tends to affect the antimesenteric aspect of the wall. The ulcers may be aphthous or may have a punched-out appearance. The ulcers can complicate into perforation, fistula formation, or hemorrhage. They may heal with medical therapy but usually relapse later. Anastomotic site ulcers are known to occur in patients undergoing surgery and usually tend to occur along ileal side of ileocolic anastomoses. Typical colonoscopic findings in intestinal BD include single or a few deep ulcers with discrete margins in the ileocecal area or anastomotic site.

There are some common features between CD and BD. Behçet's disease manifests as discrete ulcers and skip lesions involving the intestines with relative sparing of the rectum similar to that seen in CD. Uveitis and arthritis can be seen in both CD and BD. However, deep ulcerations and intestinal perforation are more common in BD. Intestinal wall thickness is normal in BD and generally it lacks granulomas and do not complicate into abscess formation like CD (Table 21.5).

Superficial and deep vein thrombophlebitis are common in BD. Arterial manifestation includes pseudoaneurysm as most common finding though large abdominal arterial involvement is rare. Large-vessel thrombosis can be seen in 11% of cases. Of these, approximately 26% have hepatic vein thrombosis leading on to Budd–Chiari syndrome.[72]

Various hepatobiliary complications include fatty liver, acute hepatitis, cholelithiasis, cholecystitis, primary biliary cirrhosis, and hepatic abscesses. Alkaline phosphatase is elevated in 11% of BD patients. Serum alkaline phosphatase level correlates with disease activity.[73]

Characteristic radiographic findings on barium study include single or multiple discrete ulcers with mucosal fold thickening. CT shows concentric bowel wall thickening that enhances after giving contrast material (Table 21.6).

Table 21.5 Clinical manifestations of Behçet's disease (n = 167)[76]

Clinical features	Frequency
Age at diagnosis of BD	38.5 ± 12.2 years
Age at diagnosis of intestinal BD	41.4 ± 12.3 years
Systemic symptoms and signs of BD	
Recurrent oral ulcer	95.2%
Recurrent genital ulcer	46.7%
Ocular lesion	6.0%
Skin lesion	49.1%
Positive pathergy test	2.4%
Arthritis or arthralgia	39.5%
Neurologic lesion	0%
Vascular lesion	1.2%
Symptoms and signs of intestinal involvement	
Abdominal pain	71.8%
Diarrhea	85.0%
Abdominal mass	2.4%
Tenderness	71.2%
Nausea/vomiting	2.4%
Melena/hematochezia	18.6%

A recent study showed that patients <25 years of age with intestinal BD, those with history of surgery or volcano-shaped intestinal ulcers, have an increased risk of bowel perforation.[74] Intestinal BD often requires surgical treatment and there is tendency for recurrent disease. The patients achieving a complete remission (Table 21.7 assessment of activity in Behçets disease) with medical treatment and those without previous intestinal perforation have better outcomes.[75] Details of medical treatment of BD has been discussed in other sections of the book.

LOCALIZED VASCULITIS OF GASTROINTESTINAL TRACT

Vasculitis of the GIT may occur as a form of single-organ vasculitis (SOV). Single-organ vasculitis is the vasculitis in arteries or veins in a single organ, with no features of systemic involvement. It may involve organs in a multifocal fashion or may be confined to focal sites. Focal SOV tends to have a good prognosis and excision of the vasculitic lesion can be curative. However, SOV can also progress to a systemic illness, and systemic therapy is almost always required for diffuse forms of SOV.[78]

Localized vasculitis of gastrointestinal tract (LVGT) usually occurs in the fifth decade with female predominance. The clinical presentation includes abdominal pain in 94%, weight loss in 72%, nausea or vomiting in 66%, diarrhea in 44%, gastroduodenal ulcers in 33%, and GI bleeding in 13% cases (Table 21.8 showing manifestation of LVGT). In a large series of LVGT, most common presentation was acute abdomen, two-thirds of patients requiring surgical intervention.[14]

Endoscopic biopsies are not helpful in making the diagnosis of LVGT. Histopathology can establish the diagnosis in surgically resected specimens. Abdominal angiography is

Table 21.6 Colonoscopy findings in intestinal Behçet's disease (n = 167)[76]

Colonoscopic findings	Frequency (%)
Location of intestinal lesion	
Ileal area	2.4%
Ileocecal area	93.4%
Ascending colon	15.0%
Other colonic segment	10.8%
Distribution of intestinal lesion	
Localized involvement	85.0%
Diffuse involvement 25	15.0%
Number of intestinal ulcer	
Solitary 86	51.5%
2–5	31.7%
≥5	16.8%
Depth of intestinal ulcer	
Aphthous	7.2%
Shallow	27.5%
Deep	65.3%
Shape of intestinal ulcer	
Oval	47.3
Geographic 52	31.1
Volcano 36	21.6
Size of intestinal ulcer (mm)	
<5	6.6%
5–10	17.4%
10–20	26.9 %
≥20	49.1%
Margin of intestinal ulcer	
Discrete	44.9%
Elevation	7.8%
Nodular elevation	19.2%
Marginal erythema	28.1%

Table 21.7 Disease activity index for intestinal Behçet's disease[77]

Parameter	Score
General well-being for 1 week	
Well	0
Fair	10
Poor	20
Very poor	30
Terrible	40
Fever	
<38°C	0
>38°C	10
*Extraintestinal manifestations**	5 per item
Abdominal pain in 1 week	
None	0
Mild	20
Moderate	40
Severe	80
Abdominal mass	
None	0
Palpable mass	10
Abdominal tenderness	
None	0
Mildly tender	10
Moderately or severely tender	20
Intestinal complications†	10 per item
No. of liquid stools in 1 week	
0	0
1–7	10
8–21	20
22–35	30
>36	40

*Score 5 for oral ulcer, genital ulcer, eye lesion, skin lesion, or arthralgia; score 15 for vascular involvement or central nervous system involvement.
†Fistula, perforation, abscess, or intestinal obstruction.

Table 21.8 Demographical, GI symptoms, and findings in patients with isolated GI vasculitis (n = 18)[14]

Demography and GI symptoms	
Male/female	1:2
Age at diagnosis, years	53.5 (17.4–83.3)
Months from symptom onset to diagnosis	10 (0.5–45)
Abdominal pain	94.4%
Abdominal angina	44.4%
Nausea or vomiting	66.7%
Diarrhea	44.4%
Weight loss	72.2%
Hematochezia or melena	16.7%
Gastroduodenal ulcers	33.3%
Gastroduodenal mucosal hemorrhage/active bleeding	13.4%
Colorectal ulcers	25%
Colorectal mucosal hemorrhage/active bleeding	8.3%
Acute abdomen	66.6%
Cholecystitis	27.7%
Appendicitis	5.5%
Pancreatitis	5.5%
Peritonitis	5.5%
Bowel perforation	5.5%
Intestinal occlusion	22.2%
GI ischemia/infarction	38.8%
Splenic infarction	22.2%
Liver infarction	16.6

the investigation of choice for demonstrating involvement of mesenteric vessels. Stenosis is the most common lesion (seen in 86% patients), followed by dilatation in 53%, aneurysm in 33%, obstruction in 26%, and wall thickening in 13%. Blood vessels involved in the decreasing order of frequency are the superior mesenteric artery in 73%, celiac artery in 60%, hepatic artery in 53%, inferior mesenteric artery in 46%, and splenic artery in 40% cases. Raised ESR is seen in 50% cases.

An important concern in such patients is whether a single-organ vasculitis of the GI tract is actually a localized GI vasculitis or simply an initial manifestation of a more severe systemic vasculitis. Hence, in patients presenting with LGVT, laboratory determinations including ANCAs, antinuclear antibodies, rheumatoid factor, cryoglobulins, C3 and C4 serum complement levels, HIV, and hepatitis B and C serology should be performed. Moreover, close follow-up, in particular during the first 5 years after the diagnosis of LGVT, is required to confirm that the vasculitis is strictly restricted to the GIT and there is no progression to a more threatening systemic vasculitis in the following years after the diagnosis of this condition.[79]

The outcome of LVGT depends upon the extent and site of involvement. In general, patients with SOV involving the gall bladder, pancreas, and appendix are cured by surgical intervention only and the prognosis is excellent. However, those with intestinal involvement have more variable outcome, depending on disease extent and immunosuppressive treatment.

KEY POINTS

- Systemic vasculitides are multisystem diseases, with wide spectrum of manifestations and variable presentation.
- Gastrointestinal is uncommon or rare in large-vessel vasculitis but involvement is rather common in medium- and small-vessel vasculitis. It is essential for internists, gastroenterologists, GI surgeons, and rheumatologists to be aware of various GI manifestations of vasculitis, as it can be life threatening at times.
- Gastrointestinal complications generally indicate a severe disease and they adversely affect the prognosis.
- Medical treatment with steroid, immunosuppressants, or biologics is indicated in most cases of systemic vasculitis with GI involvement.
- Endoscopic evaluation and treatment are required in those presenting with GI ulceration and bleeding but endoscopic findings including endoscopic biopsies rarely clinch the diagnosis.
- Surgical treatment is required in a small subset of patients presenting with bowel gangrene, perforation peritonitis, strictures, or severe GI bleeding not responding to medical and endoscopic measures.
- Localized vasculitis of GIT is a rather rare condition and surgical intervention is commonly required in this condition.

REFERENCES

1. Jennette JC, Falk RJ, Bacon PA, et al. 2012 revised International Chapel Hill Consensus Conference Nomenclature of Vasculitides. Arthritis Rheum. 2013;65:1-11.
2. Ha HK, Lee SH, Rha SE, et al. Radiologic features of vasculitis involving the gastrointestinal tract. Radiographics. 2000;20:779-94.
3. Gayraud M, Guillevin L, le Toumelin P, et al. Long-term followup of polyarteritis nodosa, microscopic polyangiitis, and Churg–Strauss syndrome: analysis of four prospective trials including 278 patients. Arthritis Rheum. 2001;44:666-75.
4. Sharma BK, Sagar S, Singh AP, et al. Takayasu arteritis in India. Heart Vessels Suppl. 1992;7:37-43.
5. Rits Y, Oderich GS, Bower TC, et al. Interventions for mesenteric vasculitis. J Vasc Surg. 2010;51:392-400, e2.

6. Hokama A, Kinjo F, Arakaki T, et al. Pulseless hematochezia: Takayasu's arteritis associated with ulcerative colitis. Intern Med. 2003;42:897-8.

7. Reny JL, Paul JF, Lefebvre C, et al. Association of Takayasu's arteritis and Crohn's disease. Results of a study on 44 Takayasu patients and review of the literature. Ann Med Interne (Paris). 2003;154:85-90.

8. Annamalai A, Francis ML, Ranatunga SK, et al. Giant cell arteritis presenting as small bowel infarction. J Gen Intern Med. 2007;22:140-4.

9. Kyle V. Laboratory investigations including liver in polymyalgia rheumatica/giant cell arteritis. Baillieres Clin Rheumatol. 1991;5:475-84.

10. Pagnoux C, Seror R, Henegar C, et al. Clinical features and outcomes in 348 patients with polyarteritis nodosa: a systematic retrospective study of patients diagnosed between 1963 and 2005 and entered into the French Vasculitis Study Group Database. Arthritis Rheum. 2010;62:616-26.

11. Nuzum JW Jr. Polyarteritis nodosa; statistical review of one hundred seventy-five cases from the literature and report of a typical case. AMA Arch Intern Med. 1954;94:942-55.

12. Levine SM, Hellmann DB, Stone JH. Gastrointestinal involvement in polyarteritis nodosa (1986–2000): presentation and outcomes in 24 patients. Am J Med. 2002;112:386-91.

13. Burke AP, Sobin LH, Virmani R. Localized vasculitis of the gastrointestinal tract. Am J Surg Pathol. 1995;19:338-49.

14. Salvarani C, Calamia KT, Crowson CS, et al. Localized vasculitis of the gastrointestinal tract: a case series. Rheumatology (Oxford). 2010;49:1326-35.

15. Guillevin L, Lhote F, Gallais V, et al. Gastrointestinal tract involvement in polyarteritis nodosa and Churg–Strauss syndrome. Ann Med Interne (Paris). 1995;146:260-7.

16. Pagnoux C, Mahr A, Cohen P, et al. Presentation and outcome of gastrointestinal involvement in systemic necrotizing vasculitides: analysis of 62 patients with polyarteritis nodosa, microscopic polyangiitis, Wegener granulomatosis, Churg–Strauss syndrome, or rheumatoid arthritis-associated vasculitis. Medicine (Baltimore). 2005;84:115-28.

17. Kojima H, Uemura M, Sakurai S, et al. Clinical features of liver disturbance in rheumatoid diseases clinicopathological study with special reference to the cause of liver disturbance. J Gastroenterol. 2002;37:617-25.

18. Ebert EC, Hagspiel KD, Nagar M, et al. Gastrointestinal involvement in polyarteritis nodosa. Clin Gastroenterol Hepatol. 2008;6:960-6.

19. Guillevin L, Mahr A, Callard P, et al. Hepatitis B virus-associated polyarteritis nodosa: clinical characteristics, outcome, and impact of treatment in 115 patients. Medicine (Baltimore). 2005;84:313-22.

20. Shusterman N, London WT. Hepatitis B and immune-complex disease. N Engl J Med. 1984;310:43-6.

21. Guillevin L, Lhote F, Cohen P, et al. Polyarteritis nodosa related to hepatitis B virus. A prospective study with long-term observation of 41 patients. Medicine (Baltimore). 1995;74:238-53.

22. Guillevin L, Lhote F, Jarrousse B, et al. Polyarteritis nodosa related to hepatitis B virus. A retrospective study of 66 patients. Ann Med Interne (Paris). 1992;143:63-74.

23. Guillevin L, Lhote F, Gayraud M, et al. Prognostic factors in polyarteritis nodosa and Churg–Strauss syndrome. A prospective study in 342 patients. Medicine (Baltimore). 1996;75:17-28.

24. Zizic TM, Classen JN, Stevens MB. Acute abdominal complications of systemic lupus erythematosus and polyarteritis nodosa. Am J Med. 1982;73:525-31.

25. Fortin PR, Larson MG, Watters AK, et al. Prognostic factors in systemic necrotizing vasculitis of the polyarteritis nodosa group—a review of 45 cases. J Rheumatol. 1995;22:78-84.

26. Flaherty J, Bradley EL 3rd. Acute pancreatitis as a complication of polyarteritis nodosa. Int J Pancreatol. 1999;25:53-7.

27. Hernandez-Rodriguez J, Alba MA, Prieto-Gonzalez S, et al. Diagnosis and classification of polyarteritis nodosa. J Autoimmun. 2014;48-9,84-9.

28. Zulian F, Falcini F, Zancan L, et al. Acute surgical abdomen as presenting manifestation of Kawasaki disease. J Pediatr. 2003;142:731-5.

29. Yim D, Curtis N, Cheung M, et al. An update on Kawasaki disease II: clinical features, diagnosis, treatment and outcomes. J Paediatr Child Health. 2013;49:614-23.

30. Morgan MD, Savage CO. Vasculitis in the gastrointestinal tract. Best Pract Res Clin Gastroenterol. 2005;19:215-33.

31. Guillevin L, Cohen P, Gayraud M, et al. Churg–Strauss syndrome. Clinical study and long-term follow-up of 96 patients. Medicine (Baltimore). 1999;78:26-37.

32. Cojocaru M, Cojocaru IM, Silosi I, et al. Gastrointestinal manifestations in systemic autoimmune diseases. Maedica (Buchar). 2011;6:45-51.

33. Pavone L, Grasselli C, Chierici E, et al. Outcome and prognostic factors during the course of primary small-vessel vasculitides. J Rheumatol. 2006;33:1299-306.

34. Lanham JG, Elkon KB, Pusey CD, et al. Systemic vasculitis with asthma and eosinophilia: a clinical approach to the Churg–Strauss syndrome. Medicine (Baltimore). 1984;63:65-81.

35. Mir O, Nazal EM, Cohen P, et al. Esophageal involvement as an initial manifestation of Churg–Strauss syndrome. Presse Med. 2007;36:57-60.

36. Ahn E, Luk A, Chetty R, et al. Vasculitides of the gastrointestinal tract. Semin Diagn Pathol. 2009;26:77-88.

37. Guillevin L, Durand-Gasselin B, Cevallos R, et al. Microscopic polyangiitis: clinical and laboratory findings in eighty-five patients. Arthritis Rheum. 1999;42:421-30.

38. Calvo-Rio V, Loricera J, Mata C, et al. Henoch–Schönlein purpura in northern Spain: clinical spectrum of the disease in 417 patients from a single center. Medicine (Baltimore). 2014;93:106-13.

39. Zhang Y, Huang X. Gastrointestinal involvement in Henoch–Schönlein purpura. Scand J Gastroenterol. 2008;43:1038-43.

40. Chen SY, Kong MS. Gastrointestinal manifestations and complications of Henoch–Schönlein purpura. Chang Gung Med J. 2004;27:175-81.

41. Blanco R, Martinez-Taboada VM, Rodriguez-Valverde V, et al. Henoch–Schönlein purpura in adulthood and childhood: two different expressions of the same syndrome. Arthritis Rheum. 1997;40:859-64.

42. Cull DL, Rosario V, Lally KP, et al. Surgical implications of Henoch–Schönlein purpura. J Pediatr Surg. 1990;25:741-3.

43. Choong CK, Kimble RM, Pease P, et al. Colo-colic intussusception in Henoch–Schönlein purpura. Pediatr Surg Int. 1998;14:173-4.

44. Choong CK, Beasley SW. Intra-abdominal manifestations of Henoch–Schönlein purpura. J Paediatr Child Health. 1998;34:405-9.

45. Yavuz H, Arslan A. Henoch–Schönlein purpura-related intestinal perforation: a steroid complication? Pediatr Int. 2001;43:423-5.

46. Bilici S, Akgun C, Melek M, et al. Acute appendicitis in two children with Henoch–Schönlein purpura. Paediatr Int Child Health. 2012;32:244-5.

47. Connolly B, O'Halpin D. Sonographic evaluation of the abdomen in Henoch–Schönlein purpura. Clin Radiol. 1994;49:320-3.

48. Jeong YK, Ha HK, Yoon CH, et al. Gastrointestinal involvement in Henoch–Schönlein syndrome: CT findings. AJR Am J Roentgenol. 1997;168:965-8.

49. Esaki M, Matsumoto T, Nakamura S, et al. GI involvement in Henoch–Schönlein purpura. Gastrointest Endosc. 2002;56:920-3.

50. Weiss PF, Feinstein JA, Luan X, et al. Effects of corticosteroid on Henoch–Schönlein purpura: a systematic review. Pediatrics. 2007;120:1079-87.

51. Lin SJ, Huang JL. Henoch–Schönlein purpura in Chinese children and adults. Asian Pac J Allergy Immunol. 1998;16:21-5.

52. Uppal SS, Hussain MA, Al-Raqum HA, et al. Henoch–Schönlein's purpura in adults versus children/adolescents: a comparative study. Clin Exp Rheumatol. 2006;24:S26-30.

53. Hung SP, Yang YH, Lin YT, et al. Clinical manifestations and outcomes of Henoch–Schönlein purpura: comparison between adults and children. Pediatr Neonatol. 2009;50:162-8.

54. Sultan SM, Ioannou Y, Isenberg DA. A review of gastrointestinal manifestations of systemic lupus erythematosus. Rheumatology (Oxford). 1999;38:917-32.

55. Barile-Fabris L, Hernandez-Cabrera MF, Barragan-Garfias JA. Vasculitis in systemic lupus erythematosus. Curr Rheumatol Rep. 2014;16:440.

56. Ju JH, Min JK, Jung CK, et al. Lupus mesenteric vasculitis can cause acute abdominal pain in patients with SLE. Nature Rev Rheumatol. 2009;5:273-81.

57. Tian XP, Zhang X. Gastrointestinal involvement in systemic lupus erythematosus: insight into pathogenesis, diagnosis and treatment. World J Gastroenterol. 2010;16:2971-7.

58. Ramos-Casals M, Nardi N, Lagrutta M, et al. Vasculitis in systemic lupus erythematosus: prevalence and clinical characteristics in 670 patients. Medicine (Baltimore). 2006;85:95-104.

59. Lee CK, Ahn MS, Lee EY, et al. Acute abdominal pain in systemic lupus erythematosus: focus on lupus enteritis (gastrointestinal vasculitis). Ann Rheum Dis. 2002;61:547-50.

60. Yuan S, Lian F, Chen D, et al. Clinical features and associated factors of abdominal pain in systemic lupus erythematosus. J Rheumatol. 2013;40:2015-22.

61. Janssens P, Arnaud L, Galicier L, et al. Lupus enteritis: from clinical findings to therapeutic management. Orphanet J Rare Dis. 2013;8:67.

62. Drenkard C, Villa AR, Reyes E, et al. Vasculitis in systemic lupus erythematosus. Lupus. 1997;6:235-42.

63. Yuan S, Ye Y, Chen D, et al. Lupus mesenteric vasculitis: clinical features and associated factors for the recurrence and prognosis of disease. Semin Arthritis Rheum. 2014;43:759-66.

64. Yuan S, Ye Y, Chen D, et al. Lupus mesenteric vasculitis: clinical features and associated factors for the recurrence and prognosis of disease. Semin Arthritis Rheum. 2013.

65. Pascual-Ramos V, Duarte-Rojo A, Villa AR, et al. Systemic lupus erythematosus as a cause and prognostic factor of acute pancreatitis. J Rheumatol. 2004;31:707-12.

66. Genta MS, Genta RM, Gabay C. Systemic rheumatoid vasculitis: a review. Semin Arthritis Rheum. 2006;36:88-98.

67. Makol A, Crowson CS, Wetter DA, et al. Vasculitis associated with rheumatoid arthritis: a case–control study. Rheumatology (Oxford). 2014;53:890-9.

68. Ebert EC, Hagspiel KD. Gastrointestinal and hepatic manifestations of rheumatoid arthritis. Dig Dis Sci. 2011;56:295-302.

69. Davatchi F, Shahram F, Chams-Davatchi C, et al. Behçet's disease in Iran: analysis of 6500 cases. Int J Rheum Dis. 2010;13:367-73.

70. Kasahara Y, Tanaka S, Nishino M, et al. Intestinal involvement in Behçet's disease: review of 136 surgical cases in the Japanese literature. Dis Colon Rectum. 1981;24:103-6.

71. Mori S, Yoshihira A, Kawamura H, et al. Esophageal involvement in Behçet's disease. Am J Gastroenterol. 1983;78:548-53.

72. Bismuth E, Hadengue A, Hammel P, et al. Hepatic vein thrombosis in Behçet's disease. Hepatology. 1990;11:969-74.

73. Ebert EC. Gastrointestinal manifestations of Behçet's disease. Dig Dis Sci. 2009;54:201-7.

74. Moon CM, Cheon JH, Shin JK, et al. Prediction of free bowel perforation in patients with intestinal Behçet's disease using clinical and colonoscopic findings. Dig Dis Sci. 2010;55:2904-11.

75. Choi IJ, Kim JS, Cha SD, et al. Long-term clinical course and prognostic factors in intestinal Behçet's disease. Dis Colon Rectum. 2000;43:692-700.

76. Lee HJ, Kim YN, Jang HW, et al. Correlations between endoscopic and clinical disease activity indices in intestinal Behçet's disease. World J Gastroenterol. 2012;18:5771-8.

77. Cheon JH, Han DS, Park JY, et al. Development, validation, and responsiveness of a novel disease activity index for intestinal Behçet's disease. Inflamm Bowel Dis. 2011;17:605-13.

78. Hernandez-Rodriguez J, Hoffman GS. Updating single-organ vasculitis. Curr Opin Rheumatol. 2012;24:38-45.

79. Gonzalez-Gay MA, Vazquez-Rodriguez TR, Miranda-Filloy JA, et al. Localized vasculitis of the gastrointestinal tract: a case report and literature review. Clin Exp Rheumatol. 2008;26:S101-4.

CHAPTER 22

Head and Neck Manifestations

Naresh K Panda, Roshan K Verma

INTRODUCTION

Vasculitides are a heterogeneous group of disorders characterized by inflammation and necrosis of the vessel wall leading to thrombosis of the vessel and tissue ischemia. Vasculitis may be localized or systemic, and hence may present with wide variety of signs and symptoms. The classification of systemic vasculitis is commonly based on the size of the vessels involved.[1] Broadly, these are classified as small-sized vessel disease that includes granulomatosis with polyangiitis [GPA, previously Wegener's granulomatosis (WG)], eosinophilic granulomatosis with polyangiitis (EGPA, previously Churg–Strauss vasculitis) and microscopic polyangiitis (MPA), medium-sized vessel disease that includes Kawasaki disease and polyarteritis nodosa (PAN) and large-sized vessel disease giant cell arteritis and Takayasu arteritis. GPA and EGPA, PAN and GCA are associated with significant head and neck manifestation and are important to the otolaryngologist.

Granulomatosis with polyangiitis, formerly known as WG named after Friedrich Wegener, who described it in 1936.[2]

Granulomatosis with polyangiitis is characterized by necrotizing granulomatous inflammation of the upper and lower respiratory tracts in combination with vasculities of medium and small arteries and focal glomerulonephritis.[3] Freidrich Wegener's (1936) original report describes a small group of patients who presented with upper respiratory disease and who died of renal failure.[2] He described the clinical and histopathological features of the disease. It was Goldmann and Churg (1954) who are credited for defining the three criteria required for the diagnosis of GPA: presence of necrotizing granulomatous inflammation of respiratory tract, vasculitis, and glomerulonephritis.[4] Granulomatosis with polyangiitis was thought to be multisystem disease with presence of classic triad considered essential for diagnosis until the concept of limited disease was introduced by Fienberg (1951) and expanded by Carrington and Liebow (1966).[5,6] Limited disease is anatomically restricted form of disease being restricted to one organ involvement. ELK (E stands for ear, nose, throat, L for lung involvement, and K for kidney involvement) system of classification proposed by De Remee et al. (1976) classifies according to the extent of an organ involvement observed during course of disease.[7] It is now believed that GPA is a continuous disease, starts with limited involvement and progresses with unpredictable speed to multisystem disease with features of classic triad of upper airway, lung, and kidney involvement (Table 22.1).

In 1990, the American College of Rheumatology accepted classification criteria for GPA. These criteria were not intended for diagnosis, but for inclusion in randomized controlled trials. Two or more positive criteria have a sensitivity of 88.2% and a specificity of 92.0% of describing WG.[8]

OTOLARYNGOLOGIST PERSPECTIVE

As head and neck involvement is common in GPA, the role of otolaryngologist is very critical. Initially these patients may

Table 22.1 The frequency of involvement of various sites in systemic vasculitis

Organ site	Frequency at presentation, %	Frequency during disease course, %
Upper airway	73	92
Lower airway	48	85
Kidney	20	80
Joint	32	67
Eye	15	52
Skin	13	46
Nerve	1	20

Source: Kornblut AD, Wolff SM, deFries HO, et al. Wegener's granulomatosis. Laryngoscope. 1980;90:1453-65.

have limited GPA, the symptoms may be limited to head and neck, and frank systemic involvement may occur later on. In one study of 22 patients with GPA, head and neck symptoms were seen in 100% of patients at the time of presentation, while lung, orbital, and joint involvement were seen in 75% while only 27% had renal involvement.[9] A high index of suspicion along with good communication between the clinicians and pathologist is essential for making a diagnosis of GPA.

HEAD AND NECK MANIFESTATIONS IN GPA

Granulomatosis with polyangiitis is a rare disease with incidence of 1–3 cases/million.[10] It usually occurs in the age group of 20-40 years without any sexual predilection.[11] It classically presents as triad with involvement of lung, renal parenchyma, and head and neck. Not all patients show involvement of all three regions at presentation. It may or may not present with constitutional symptoms like malaise, fever, weight loss, night sweats, and arthralgias.

Head and Neck involvement is the most common and is present in all most all patients at the time of presentation. In the head and neck, sites of involvement will dictate the characteristic clinical presentation.

OTOLOGIC MANIFESTATION

Otologic involvement is seen in 20–61% of the cases of GPA and rarely might be the only presenting feature.[12] Ear involvement in GPA may involve all the components of ear but most commonly involves the middle ear presenting as otits media with effusion.

External Ear

Granulomatosis with polyangiitis may rarely involve the external ear and present with auricular pain, edema, and erythema of the pinna. Erythema of the auricle may occur in approximately 15-20% of patients with otological signs and symptoms.[13] Involvement of pinna closely resembles relapsing polychondritis. The condition responds to treatment with glucocorticoids or cytotoxic agents.

Middle Ear

Granulomatosis with polyangiitis most commonly involves the middle ear. Otits media with effusion is the most common otological finding occurring secondary to eustachian tube dysfunction. It may be unilateral or involves both ears. Eustachian tube dysfunction may be granulation tissue within the lumen of eustachian tube or nasopharyngeal

inflammation causing obstruction of the tube.[14] Otitis media with effusion of GPA responds poorly to drug therapy.

Chronic suppurative otitis media is seen in 24% of patients of GPA.[12] It occurs due to direct involvement of middle ear and mastoid by necrotizing granulomatous inflammation and lead to effusion, otomastoiditis, and facial nerve palsy.[13] It typically presents as severe post auricular pain, profuse ear discharge not responding to topical medication, and deafness typically conductive hearing loss. Otomastoiditis with facial nerve palsy is presenting feature in 10% of GPA.[15,16]

Inner Ear

Sensorineural deafness occurs in 8% of patients of GPA and usually develops gradually within days to weeks.[17] Tinnitus may be associated with sensorineural deafness. The cause of sensorineural deafness is postulated to be due to vasculitis affecting the vasa nervosa and cochlear vessels and also thought to be due to deposition of immune complexes within labyrinth.[12,18,19] Vertigo and nystagmus may very rarely be the presenting feature of GPA. It is thought to be due to deposition of immune complex within the vestibule.[20]

RHINOLOGIC MANIFESTATIONS

Nose and the paranasal sinuses is the most common sub site of involvement in GPA, seen in up to 60% patients.[21] Nasal symptoms consist of nasal congestion, nasal obstruction, and profuse foul smelling rhinorrhea, pain over the dorsum of nose and anosmia.[22] Patient may also complain of recurrent epistaxis and epiphora. Chronic sinusitis is very common and may sometimes be the initial presenting symptom.[23] Patient may present with headache, postnasal drip, chronic cough, and sinus tenderness. Typically the symptoms of chronic sinusitis do not respond to medical treatment. The patient may also complain of nasal collapse, saddle nose deformity, and nasal airway stenosis.[24] Saddle nose deformity may be seen in 10-25% of patients with sinonasal involvement.[25]

Nasal examination in GPA may show congested mucosa, superficial ulcerations of nasal mucosa, nasal crusting, and septal perforation and sinus tenderness (Fig. 22.1). Nasal endoscopy may show purulent discharge in the middle meatus, crusting over the septum and turbinates, friable nasal mucosa, and rarely nasal polyps[26] (Figs 22.2 and 22.3).

Radiology in GPA shows characteristic features. Computed tomography of nose and paranasal sinuses typically show bone destruction in background of generalized mucosal thickening (Fig. 22.4). The bone destruction is typically in midline affecting nasal septum and turbinate's

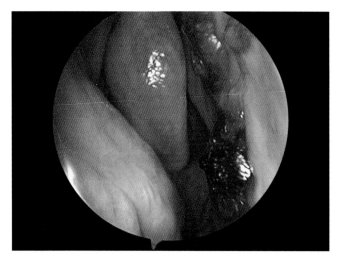

Fig. 22.1 Nasal endoscopy showing extensive crusting and septal destruction in a patient with GPA

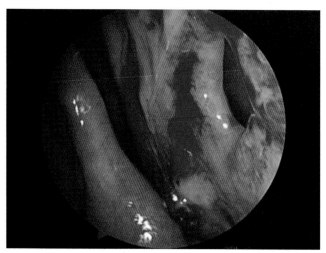

Fig. 22.2 Nasal endoscopy showing septal perforation in a patient with GPA

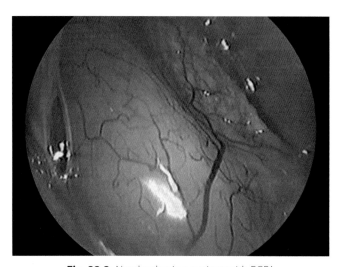

Fig. 22.3 Nasal polyp in a patient with EGPA

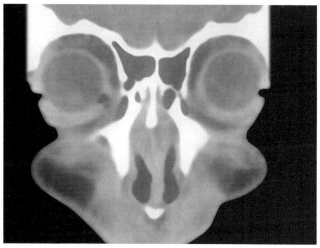

Fig. 22.4 NCCT PNS coronal view showing destruction of nasal septum

initially and symmetrically extends laterally to involve the maxillary antrum and other sinuses with sclerotic changes of walls of sinus.[27] The end result is single large cavity with loss of nasal septum, turbinates, and lateral walls of maxillary antrum.[28] Magnetic resonance imaging shows high signal intensity of T1 weighted sequence and evidence of fat signal from the sclerotic walls of the sinus.[29]

OTOLARYNGOLOGIST'S ROLE

A patient of GPA might present initially to otolaryngologist with features of recurrent sinusitis, epistaxis, and recurrent nasal obstruction. Chronic sinusitis not responding to medical treatment with extensive crusting seen in the nasal cavity should arouse a suspicion of WG. Nasal mucosal biopsy may be needed to confirm the diagnosis on histopathology. It is important to remove all visible nasal crusts followed by liberal removal of tissue from the septum, nasal floor, and turbinates in order to provide ample tissue for histopathology. However, the results of nasal biopsy are highly unpredictable. Jennings in his study has reported that nasal biopsy has positive predictive value of 100% and negative predictive value of 74%.[30] Thus, a significant number of specimens are reported as false positive for GPA on nasal biopsy.

Functional endoscopic sinus surgery may be required in refractory cases of chronic sinusitis. Management of recurrent epistaxis may be required in the initial stages. Septal perforation repair and correction of saddle nose deformity may be required when the disease is in remission phase.

LARYNGEAL AND TRACHEAL MANIFESTATION

Involvement of larynx and trachea is common and in 25% of cases airway involvement may be the sole presenting symptom.[31] Airway involvement is more common in the younger patients <30 years of age and in females.[32] Ulceration, granuloma formation, pseudomembranes, and cobble stone appearance of the mucosa of larynx and trachea may be seen. They usually present with recurrent cough, change in voice, respiratory difficulty, and hemoptysis. Subglottic stenosis is a rare complication and occurs in 8–10% cases.[33] It is more commonly seen in association with generalized GPA. Patients with subglottic stenosis usually present with hoarseness and stridor. Fiberoptic bronchoscopy shows concentric narrowing of the subglottis with congestion, erythema, and discrete granuloma formation. Biopsy from the subglottic area may confirm the diagnosis of GPA but the positive result is usually infrequent.[34]

Patients with laryngotracheal involvement may present in stridor and may require emergency tracheostomy. Fibrotic scarring of subglottoic stenosis rarely responds to immunosuppressive therapy. The options for management of subglottic stenosis include repeated endoscopic dilations with intralesional injection of corticosteroids, balloon dilation, use of laryngeal stents like M Tube, laser excision of the stenosis, surgical resection of subglottic segment, and reanastomosis.[35]

ORAL MANIFESTATIONS

Oral cavity involvement is uncommon and usually occurs in advanced stages of GPA. Less than 6% of patients present with oral manifestation and oral symptoms rarely are the initial indicator of GPA.[36] In oral cavity the classical lesion is strawberry gingivitis: reddish-to-pinkish hyperplastic gingivitis with numerous petechiae with associated pain and bleeding gums are pathognomonic of WG.[37] Other oral cavity lesion include either mucosal ulcers on the tongue, buccal mucosa, gums or palate, cobblestone-like lesion over the palate, nonhealing extraction socket, and oroantral fistula.

Salivary Gland Involvement

This is rare in GPA (WG) but may occur during the course of the disease. Submandibular or parotid gland of one or both sides may become enlarged and rarely may be the presenting feature in WG.[38] Involvement of the salivary glands may simulate Sjögren syndrome.[39]

DIFFERENTIAL DIAGNOSIS

- Gingival hyperplasia secondary to drugs like phenytoin or some calcium channel blockers, cyclosporine, or conjugated estrogens
- Sarcoidosis
- Churg-Strauss syndrome
- Tuberculosis
- Polyarteritis nodosa
- Scurvy
- Some neoplastic diseases like leukemia, Kaposis's sarcoma, or squamous cell carcinoma of oral cavity.

EOSINOPHILIC GRANULOMATOSIS WITH POLYANGIITIS (CHURG-STRAUSS VASCULITIS)

Eosinophilic granulomatosis with polyangiitis is a complex multisystem disease characterized by upper and lower respiratory tract involvement, blood and tissue eosinophilia, and vasculitis.[40] It is a rare disease with incidence of 0.5–6.8/per million per year.[41] Histology is characterized by eosinophilic core of necrosis with fibrinoid collagen degeneration and surrounded by granulomatous infiltrate consisting of histiocytes, lymphocytes, and giant cells.[42,43] The most accepted criteria for diagnosis of EGPA is given by the American College of Rheumatology (1990) that includes history of asthma, eosinophilia > 10%, mononeuropathy or polyneuropathy, nonfixed pulmonary infiltrates, paranasal sinus abnormalities, and biopsy showing extravascular eosinophils. Presence of four out of the six criteria is essential for diagnosis of Churg–Strauss vasculitis.[44]

Head and Neck Manifestations

Otolaryngologists may play an important role in diagnosing this disease.

Otologic Manifestations

Involvement of ear is extremely rare in EGPA and occurs in advanced stage of disease. It may present with profuse aural discharge, chronic suppurative otitis media due to eosinophilic granulomatous infiltration of middle ear, and mastoid without any response to and not responding to conventional medication. The patient may also present with progressive sensorineural hearing loss that may be unilateral or bilateral.[45] SNHL is believed to be the result of arteritis of the internal auditory artery producing ischemia of the eighth cranial nerve.[45] Facial nerve palsy can also be one of the presenting manifestations.

Nasal Manifestations

Seventy percent of patients of EGPA have nasal symptoms at presentation.[46] Allergic rhinitis, chronic rhinosinusitis, pan sinusitis, nasal polyps, thick nasal crust, and septal perforation have been associated with Churg-Strauss vasculitis. Rhinitis is present in 70% of cases of Churg-Strauss vasculitis and do not respond to conventional medication.[47] Nasal polyps are seen in 50% of patients and may require functional endoscopic sinus surgery for relief of nasal obstruction.[48] Nasal biopsies are usually inconclusive and do not reliably show features of vasculitis as compared to biopsy from other organ.[46] Nasal symptoms favorably respond to corticosteroid medication.

Laryngeal Involvement

Laryngeal involvement is extremely rare in EGPA. Mazzantini et al. have reported an isolated case of laryngeal involvement; the patient presented with dysphonia and had superior laryngeal nerve palsy.[49] Eosinophilic granulomatosis with polyangiitis poses a diagnostic challenge to the otolaryngologists. The otolaryngologist should consider the entity in a patient with adult onset asthma with chronic rhinosinusitis with fever, malaise, and paresthesia of limbs. The additional predicting indicators are increased ESR, CRP, ANCA positivity, and parenchyma changes in the X-ray chest.

KAWASAKI DISEASE

Introduction

Kawasaki disease is also known as an acute febrile mucocutaneous lymph node syndrome that most commonly affects infants and children. It was first described by Dr. Tomisaku Kawasaki (1967).[50] It is a multisystemic vasculitis affecting medium-sized vessels and most commonly involves coronary arteries.[51,52] It is the disease of young children and 80% cases occur in children below 5 years, with male-to-female ratio of 1.62:1 and overall incidence of 62 per 100,000 children.[53] The clinical findings in Kawasaki disease are usually nonspecific, and hence high index of suspicion is required to clinch the diagnosis. Clinical criteria for diagnosis of Kawasaki disease require the presence of fever for at least 5 days and at least four of the following five signs: (1) a bilateral nonpurulent bulbar conjunctival injection; (2) changes in the mucosa of the oropharynx, including an injected pharynx, injected and/or dry fissured lips, and a strawberry tongue;

(3) changes in the peripheral extremities, such as edema and/or erythema of the hands or feet in the acute phase, or periungual desquamation; (4) a rash polymorphous nonvesicular, primarily truncal; and (5) cervical adenopathy, 1.5 cm, usually unilateral.[54,55]

Head and Neck Manifestation of Kawasaki Disease

Neck

Cervical lymphadenopathy is the most common and occurs in 75% of cases of Kawasaki disease.[56] It may be presenting symptom in 12% of cases of Kawasaki disease.[57] Lymphadenopathy is usually unilateral and appears to involve commonly single node. However, there are case reports of Kawasaki disease presenting with bilateral multiple nodes in the neck.[58] Deep neck space infection and retropharyngeal abscess may also be presenting features of Kawasaki disease.[59] There are reports in literature when Kawasaki disease was initially misdiagnosed as retropharyngeal abscess on CT neck of febrile child with cervical lymphadenopathy.[60] In such cases the possibility of Kawasaki disease was considered when the fever was refractory to antibiotic treatment.

Oral Manifestations

Lips may become erythematous and swollen and later on fissuring, cracking, and bleeding may occur. Tongue may be erythematous and appear like strawberry tongue.[61] Oral and oropharyngeal mucosa may become erythematous with mucosal ulcerations. Patients may present to clinician with sore throat, acute tonsillitis, and pharyngitis.[62]

Ear Manifestations

It may present with features of mastoiditis, sensorineural hearing loss, and facial palsy.[61]

Nasal Manifestations

Patient may present to otolaryngologist with nasal bleed due to thrombocytopenia.

POLYARTERITIS NODOSA

Introduction

It is a systemic vasculitic disease characterized by inflammation and necrosis of small- and medium- sized-muscular arteries affecting mainly renal, cardiovascular, and gastrointestinal tract.[1] Hepatitis B infection and hepatitis B antigenemia are strongly associated with polyarteritis and seen in 7–22% of cases.[63] Initial presenting symptoms may include constitutional symptoms like low-grade fever, myalgia, weight loss, weakness, and fatigue.[64,65] Renal, cardiovascular, neurological, and gastrointestinal involvement is most common.[64] Visceral angiography showing microaneurysm, stenosis, ectasia, and irregularities in vessel walls of renal and mesenteric beds clinches the diagnosis of PAN.[65] Histopathology shows focal segmental granulomatous vasculitis with mixed cell infiltrate affecting medium-sized vessels.[66]

Head and Neck Involvement

Head and neck involvement is not very common in PAN.

Ear Involvement

Bilateral progressive sensorineural hearing loss has been reported in patients with PAN.[67] Sudden onset of sensorineural hearing loss has also been reported as the initial presenting symptom of PAN.[67] Experimental studies on temporal bones and PAN have reported fibrosis and ossification of the basal turn of cochlea thus making cochlear implantation difficult in such cases.[68] Vasculitis of stylomastoid and labyrinthine artery were also seen. Temporal bone studies have also shown endolymphatic hydrops of the basal turn of the cochlea and chronic perforation of the free wall of the saccule.[69] Polyarteritis nodosa can also present with initial symptom of facial paralysis.

Nasal Manifestations

Ployateritis nodosa may present with features of sinusitis, nasal crusting, nasal vestibulitis, and septal perforation.[70]

GIANT CELL ARTERITIS

Giant cell arteritis, temporal arteritis, or Hourton's arteritis is multisystemic vasculitis of elderly people primarily involving large- and medium-sized blood vessels especially involving extra cranial branches of external carotid artery.[71] Giant cell arteritis is a disease of elderly and occurs exclusively in persons older than > 50 years.[72] It is more common in females than males. Histology of involved vessel shows granulomatous arteritis with lymphocytic infiltration of tunica adventitia and disruption of tunica media and destruction of elastic lamina by giant cell granuloma with prominence of Langerhans giant cells. Inflammatory process results in loss of elastic properties of tunica media of vessel wall leading to dilatation and aneurysm formation.[73]

Classical presentation of giant cell arteritis includes severe pain in the head, fever, decreased vision, diplopia, and rapidly progressive blindness of one or both eyes. Sometimes, patient might present with severe unbearable neuralgic pain of occiput, jaw, face, and head with edema of face and neck. Classically, there is tenderness over the course of temporal and occipital arteries and they are thickened, reddened, and nonpulsatile. It may also present with myocardial infarction and aortic aneurysm.[74]

ESR is raised in all cases of giant cell arteritis, hypochromic anemia, and leukocytosis. Arterial biopsy of accessible vessels clinches diagnosis. Features of intimal thickening, cellular infiltration with presence of giant cells, and thrombus formation clinches the diagnosis.[75]

HEAD AND NECK MANIFESTATIONS

Otology

High-frequency sensorineural hearing loss has been reported in patients with giant cell arteritis that recovers partially with steroid therapy.[76] Vestibular dysfunction is common in patients with giant cell arteritis and high incidence of BPPV has been reported in these groups of patients.[77] Sometimes giant cell arteritis may present with Meniere's syndrome.[78]

Oral Manifestations

Jaw claudication is one of the common initial presenting symptoms of giant cell arteritis.[79] Difficulty in opening jaw, masticatory claudication, painful tongue, painful swallowing, necrosis of tongue, and toothache may also be one of the presenting symptoms.[80,81]

Neck and Face

Severe pain over the face, neck, and occiput is common presenting symptom of giant cell arteritis. Carotidynia (pain and tenderness over the course of carotid vessels) may be present.[82] Facial edema and swelling over the neck is common in giant cell arteritis. The most common picture is the presence of bilateral, painful, slightly pink, nonpitting swelling of the cheeks, and maxilla region in elderly person, should raise suspicion of giant cell arteritis.[83]

KEY POINTS

- Various ENT manifestations can occur.
- These manifestations can give a clue of the underlying systemic disease.

REFERENCES

1. Jennette JC, Falk RJ, Andrassy K, et al. Nomenclature of systemic vasculitides. Proposal of an international consensus conference. Arthritis Rheum. 1994;37:187-92.
2. Wegener's F. Uber eine eigenartige rhinogene granulomatose mit besonderer Beteiligung des arteriensystems und der Nieren. Beitr Pathol. 1939;102;36-58.
3. Kornblut AD, Wolff SM, deFries HO, et al. Wegener's granulomatosis. Laryngoscope. 1980;90:1453-65.
4. Godman GC, Churg J. Wegener's granulomatosis: pathology and review of the literature. Arch Pathol 1954;58:533-53.
5. Fienberg R. Necrotizing granulomatosis and angiitis of the lungs. Am J Clin Pathol. 1953;23:413-28.
6. Carrington CB, Liebow M. Limited forms of angiitis and granulomatosis of Wegener's type. Am J Med. 1966;41:497-527.
7. DeRemee RA, McDonald TJ, Harrison EG Jr, et al. Wegener's granulomatosis. Anatomic correlates, a proposed classification. Mayo Clin Proc. 1976; 51:777-81.
8. Leavitt RY, Fauci AS, Bloch DA, et al. "The American College of Rheumatology 1990 criteria for the classification of Wegener's granulomatosis." Arthritis Rheum. 1990;33:1101-7.
9. D'Cruz DP, Baguley E, Asherson RA, et al. Ear, nose, and throat symptoms in ear, nose, and throat symptoms in subacute Wegener's granulomatosis. BMJ. 1989;299:419-22.
10. Cotch MF, Hoffmann GS, Yerg DE, et al. The epidemiology of Wegener's granulomatosis. Estimates of 5 years prevalence annual mortality and geographic distribution from population based data sources. Arthritis Rheuma. 1996;39:87-92.
11. Hoffmann GS, Kerr GS, Levitt RY, et al. Wegener's granulomatosis: analysis of 158 cases. Ann intern Med. 1992;116:488-98.
12. Takagi D, Nakamaru Y, Maguchi S, et al. Otologic manifestations of Wegener's granulomatosis. Laryngoscope. 2002;112:1684-90.
13. McCaffrey TV, McDonald TJ, Facer GW, et al. Otologic manifestations of Wegener's granulomatosis. Otolaryngol Head Neck Surg. 1980;88:586-93.
14. Fauci AS, Haynes BF, Katz P, et al. Wegener's granulomatosis: prospective clinical and therapeutic experience with 85 patients for 21 years. Ann Intern Med. 1983;98:76-85.
15. Bradley PJ. Wegener's granulomatosis of the ear. J Laryngol Otol. 1983;97:623-6.
16. Dagum P, Roberson JB Jr. Otologic Wegener's granulomatosis with facial nerve palsy. Ann Otol Rhinol Laryngol. 1998;107:555-9.
17. Erickson VR, Hwang PH. Wegener's granulomatosis: current trends in diagnosis and management. Curr Opin Otolaryngol Head Neck Surg. 2007;15:170-6.
18. Shivaprasad BN, Balasubramaniam R. Chronic otitis media and facial paralysis presenting feature of Wegener's granulomatosis. Singapore Med J. 2009;50:e155.
19. Illum P, Thorling K. Otological manifestations of Wegener's granulomatosis. Laryngoscope. 1982;92:801-4.
20. Dagum P, Roberson JB Jr. Otologic Wegener's granulomatosis with facial nerve palsy. Ann Otol Rhinol Laryngol. 1998;107:555-9.
21. Rasmussen N. Management of the ear, nose, and throat manifestations of Wegener granulomatosis: an otorhinolaryngologist's perspective. Curr Opin Rheumatol. 2001;13:3-11.
22. McDonald T, DeRemee RA. Wegener's granulomatosis. Laryngoscope. 1983;93:220-31.
23. Thomas V. Mccaffrey. Nasal manifestation of systemic disease. Otolaryngol Pol. 2009;63:228-35.
24. Rijuneeta, Panda N, Bambery P, et al. Nasal polyposis in Wegener's granulomatosis: a rare presentation. Internet J Otorhinolaryngol. 2005;4:28.
25. Martinez Del Pero M, Walsh M, Luqmani R, et al. Long-term damage to the ENT system in Wegener's granulomatosis. Eur Arch Otorhinolaryngol. 2011;268:733.
26. McDonald TJ, DeRemee RA, Kern EB, et al. Nasal manifestations of Wegener's granulomatosis. Laryngoscope. 1974;84:2101-12.
27. Lloyd G, Lund VJ, Beale T, et al. Rhinologic changes in Wegener's granulomatosis. J Laryngology Otol. 2002;116:565-9.
28. Simmons JT, Leavitt R, Kornblut AD, et al. CT of the paranasal sinuses and orbits in patients with Wegener's granulomatosis. Ear Nose Throat J. 1987;66:134-40.
29. Provenzale JM, Allen NB. Wegener's granulomatosis: CT and MR findings. Am J Neuroradiol. 1996;17:785-92.
30. Jennings CR, Jones NS, Dugar J, et al. Wegener's granulomatosis–a review of diagnosis and treatment in 53 subjects. Rhinology. 1998;36:188-91.
31. Lebovics RS, Hoffman GS, Leavitt RY, et al. The management of subglottic stenosis in patients with Wegener's granulomatosis. Laryngoscope. 1992;102:1341-5.
32. Alaani A, Hogg RP, Drake Lee AB. Wegener's granulomatosis and subglottic stenosis: management of the airway. J Laryngol Otol. 2004;118:786-90.
33. Langford CA, Sneller MC, Hallahan CW, et al. Clinical features and therapeutic management of subglottic stenosis in patients with Wegener's granulomatosis. Arthritis Rheum. 1996;39:1754-60.
34. Devaney KO, Travis WD, Hoffman G, et al. Interpretation of head and neck biopsies in Wegener's granulomatosis. A pathologic study of 126 biopsies in 70 patients. Am J Surg Pathol. 1990;14:555-64.
35. Eliachar I, Chan J, Akst L. New approaches to the management of subglottic stenosis in Wegener's granulomatosis. Cleve Clin J Med. 2002;69:SII149-51.
36. Eufinger H, Machtens E, Akuoma-Boetang E. Oral manifestations in Wegener's granulomatosis. Review of literature and report of case. J Oral Maxillofac Surg. 1992;21:50-3.
37. Stewart C, Cohen D, Bhattacharya L, et al. Oral manifestations of Wegener's granulomatosis. Report of three cases and literature review. J Am Dent Assoc. 2007;138:338-48.

38. Ah-See KW, McLaren K, Maran AG. Wegener's granulomatosis presenting as major salivary gland enlargement. J Laryngol Otol. 1996;110:691-3.

39. Specks U, Colby TV, Olsen KD, et al. Salivary gland involvement in Wegener's granulomatosis. Arch Otolaryngol Head Neck Surg. 1991;117:218-23.

40. Abril A, Clamia KT, Cohen MD. The Churg–Strauss syndrome (allergic granulomatous angiitis): review update. Semin Arthritis Rheum. 2003;33:106-14.

41. Watts RA, Lane SE, Bentham G, et al. Epidemiology of systemic vasculitis: a ten-year study in the United Kingdom. Arthritis Rheum. 2000;43:414.

42. Jennette JC, Falk RJ. Small-vessel vasculitis. N Engl J Med. 1997;337:1512-23.

43. Guillevin L, Cohen P, Gayraud M, et al. Churg–Strauss syndrome. Clinical study and long-term follow-up of 96 patients. Medicine (Baltimore). 1999;78:26-37.

44. Masi AT, Hunder GG, Lie JT, et al. The American College of Rheumatology 1990. Criteria for the classification of Churg–Strauss syndrome (allergic granulomatosis and angiitis). Arthritis Rheum.1990;33:1094-100.

45. Ishiyama A, Canalis RF. Otological manifestations of Churg–Strauss syndrome. Laryngoscope. 2001;111:1619-24.

46. Bacciu A, Bacciu S, Mercante G, et al. Ear, nose, and throat manifestations of Churg–Strauss syndrome. Acta Otolaryngol. 2006;126:503-9.

47. Olsen KD, Neel HB 3rd, Deremee RA, et al. Nasal manifestations of allergic granulomatosis and angiitis (Churg-Strauss syndrome). Otolaryngol Head Neck Surg. 1980;88:85-9.

48. Chumbley LC, Harrison EG, DeRemee RA. Allergic granulomatosis and angiitis (Churg–Strauss Syndrome): report and analysis of 30 cases. Mayo Clin Proc. 1977;52:477-84.

49. Mazzantini M, Fattori B, Matteucci F, et al. Neurolaryngeal involvement in Churg–Strauss syndrome. Eur Arch Otorhinolaryngol. 1998;255:302-6.

50. Kawasaki T. Acute febrile mucocutaneous syndrome with lymphoid involvement with specific desquamation of fingers and toes in children (Japanese). Arerugi. 1967;16:178-222.

51. Jennete JC. Ronald JF. Small vessel vasculitis. New Eng J Med. 2006;337:1512-21.

52. Naoe S, Shibuya K, Takahashi K, et al. Pathologic observations concerning the cardiovascular lesions in Kawasaki disease. Cardiol Young. 1991;1:212-20.

53. Kawasaki T. General review and problems in Kawasaki disease. Jpn Heart J. 1995;36:1-12.

54. Yanagawa H, Yashiro M, Nakamura Y, et al. Results of 12 nationwide epidemiological incidence surveys of Kawasaki disease in Japan. Arch Pediatr Adolesc Med. 1995;149:779-83.

55. Surjit S, Kawasaki T. Kawasaki disease-an Indian perspective. Indian Pediatr. 2009;46:563-71.

56. April MM, Burns JC, Newburger JW, et al. Kawasaki disease cervical lymphadenopathy. Arch Otolaryngol Head Neck Surg. 1989;115:512-4.

57. Stamos JK, Corydon K, Donaldson J, et al. Lymphadenitis as the dominant manifestation of Kawasaki disease. Pediatrics. 1994;93:525-8.

58. Falcini F, Simonini G, Calabri GB, et al. Multifocal lymphadenopathy associated with severe Kawasaki disease: a difficult diagnosis. Ann Rheum Dis. 2003;62:688-9.

59. Hung MC, Wu KG, Hwang B, et al. Kawasaki disease resembling a retropharyngeal abscess case report and literature review. Int J Cardiol. 2007;115:e94-6.

60. Homicz MR, Carvalho D, Kearns DB, et al. An atypical presentation of Kawasaki disease resembling a retropharyngeal abscess. Int J Pediatr Otorhinolaryngol. 2000;54:45-9.

61. Yoskovitch A, Tewfik TL, Duffy CM, e al. Head and Neck manifestations of Kawasaki disease. Int J Pediatr Otorhinolaryngol. 2000;52:123-9.

62. Hathursinghe HR, Patel S, Uppal HS, et al. Acute tonsillitis: an unusual presentation of Kawasaki syndrome: a case report and review of the literature. Eur Arch Otorhinolaryngol. 2006;263:336-8.

63. Guillevin L, Lhote F, Sauvaget F, et al. Treatment of polyarteritis nodosa related to hepatitis B virus with interferon-alpha and plasma exchanges. Ann Rheum Dis. 1994;53:334-7.

64. Guillevin L, Le Thi Huong Du, Godeau P, et al. "Clinical findings and prognosis of polyarteritis nodosa and Churg–Strauss angiitis: a study in 165 patients." Rheumatology. 1988;27:258-64.

65. Ewald EA, Griffin D, McCune WJ. Correlation of angiographic abnormalities with disease manifestations and disease severity in polyarteritis nodosa. J Rheumatol. 1987;14:952-6.

66. Waldherr R, Eberlein-Gonska M, Noronha IL. Histopathological differentiation of systemic necrotizing vasculitides. APMIS. 1990;98:17-28.

67. Rowe-Jones JM, Macallan DC, Sorooshian M. Polyarteritis nodosa presenting as bilateral sudden onset cochleo-vestibular failure in a young woman. J Laryngol Otology. 1990; 104:562-4.

68. Peitersen E, Carlsen BH. Hearing impairment as the initial sign of polyarteritis nodosa. Acta Otolaryngol. 1966;61:189-95.

69. Gussen P. Polyarteritis nodosa and deafness. A human temporal bone study. Arch Otorhinolaryngol. 1977;217:263-71.

70. Oristrell Salva J, Bosch Gil JA, Valdés Oliveras M, et al. [Polyarteritis nodosa and perforation of the nasal septum]. Med Clin (Brac). 1985;84:673-4.

71. Liozon E, Ouattara B, Portal MF, et al. Head-and-neck swelling: an under-recognized feature of giant cell arteritis. A report of 37 patients. Clin Exp Rheumatol. 2006;24:S20-5.

72. Paulley JW, Hughes JP. Giant-cell arteritis, or arteritis of the aged. Br Med J. 1960;26:1562-7.

73. Salvarani Carlo, Fabrizio Cantini, Luigi Boicardi, et al. Polymyalgia rheumatica and giant-cell arteritis. Eng J Med. 2002;37:261-71.

74. Calvo-Romero JM. Giant cell arteritis. Postgrad Med J. 2003;79:511-5.

75. Lie JT. Illustrated histopathologic classification criteria for selected vasculitis syndromes. Arthritis Rheum. 1990;33(8):1074-87.

76. Amor-Dorado JC, Llorca J, Garcia-Porrua C, et al. Audiovestibular manifestations in giant cell arteritis: a prospective study. Medicine (Baltimore). 2003;82:13-26.

77. Amor-Dorado JC, Llorca J, Costa-Ribas C, et al. Giant cell arteritis: a new association with benign paroxysmal positional vertigo. Laryngoscope. 2004;114:1420-5.

78. Mckennan KX, Nielsen SL, Watson C, et al. Meniere's syndrome: an atypical presentation of giant cell arteritis (temporal arteritis). Laryngoscope. 1993;103:1103-7.

79. Brodmann M, Dorr A, Hafner F, et al. Tongue necrosis as first symptom of giant cell arteritis (GCA). Clin Rheum. 2009;28:47-9.

80. Hellmann DB. Temporal arteritis: a cough, toothache, and tongue infarction. JAMA. 2002;287:2996-3000.

81. Healey LA, Wilske KR. Presentation of occult giant cell arteritis. Arthritis Rheum. 1980;23:641-3.

82. García-Porrua C, González-Gay MA. Carotid tenderness: an ominous sign of giant cell arteritis. Scand J Rheumatol. 1998;27:154-6.

83. Turner RG, Henry J, Friedmann AI, et al. Giant cell arteritis. Postgrad Med J. 1974;50:265-9.

Principles of Management

CHAPTER 23

Approach to Childhood Vasculitis

Amita Aggarwal, Anuj Shukla

INTRODUCTION

Though vasculitis is less common in children as compared to adults, there are some forms of vasculitis that occur exclusively in children like Kawasaki disease (KD). In addition some forms of vasculitis are more common in children like Henoch-Schönlein purpura (HSP). Common vasculitis in adults like ANCA associated vasculitis, polyarteritis nodosa (PAN) are rare, and giant cell arteritis does not occur in children. In view of infections being more common in children, the diagnosis of vasculitis is often delayed in a child.

PREVALENCE

The data on prevalence of childhood vasculitis is mainly derived from registries, US registry with 434 patients found HSP to be the commonest childhood vasculitis constituting 49.1% of cases whereas Canadian registry with 252 patients reported KD to be the commonest constituting 65.3% of cases (Table 23.1).[1,2]

The data on incidence of vasculitis is very limited and it is reported to be 20.4 per 100,000 children in United Kingdom[3] and in Czech Republic[4] it was 10.2 per 100,000 children.

Table 23.1 Prevalence of different vasculitis among children

	US registry[1] (434)		Canadian registry[2] (225)	
	Number	%	Number	%
Kawasaki	97	22.4	147	65.3
HSP	213	49.1	38	16.9
WG	6	1.4	5	2.2
PAN	14	3.2	4	1.8
Behçet's	–	–	2	0.9
Takayasu's arteritis	8	1.8	2	0.9
Miscellaneous	96	22.1	27	12.0

Disease specific surveys have revealed incidence of HSP in Dutch population to be 6.1 per 100,000 children.[5]

Though no large prevalence data are available from India, probably HSP and KD are the common vasculitis followed by Takayasu's arteritis.

CLINICAL FEATURES

Clinical features in vasculitis can occur either because of vessel occlusion leading to ischemia that manifests as gangrene, stroke, gastrointestinal bleed and claudication or due to injury to the vessel wall presenting as palpable purpura, livedo reticularis, aneurysms or aortic regurgitation. Capillary involvement in glomerulus leads to glomerulonephritis while in pulmonary circulation it leads to pulmonary hemorrhage. The systemic inflammatory response leads to fever, malaise, myalgias, arthralgias, anemia and weight loss.

The onset can be acute as in HSP and KD or subacute/chronic as in PAN, TA, etc. In the initial phase, the patient may have only systemic features and present as fever of unknown origin. At this stage abnormal urine analysis, pulse deficit or presence of anti-neutrophil cytoplasmic antibody may raise a suspicion. Once patient develops features suggesting vascular involvement approach depends on size of suspected vessel involved (Table 23.2). Thought there can be some overlap in the symptoms.

The common forms of vasculitis in children based on vessel size are listed in Table 23.3.

Once the diagnosis of vasculitis is suspected a detailed history to exclude secondary causes like infections, drugs, other connective tissue diseases and travel needs to be elicited. A thorough examination to look for pulse inequality or bruit, hypertension or blood pressure inequality in limbs, skin rash in hidden areas like buttocks, scrotal ulcers, cardiac murmurs, sensory loss or mild motor weakness suggestive of

Table 23.2 Clinical features depending on size of blood vessel involved

Size of vessel	Common symptoms
Small	Skin rash (palpable purpura, skin infarct), glomerulonephritis, abdominal pain, GI bleed, pulmonary hemorrhage
Medium	Digital gangrene, livedo reticularis, nodules along vessels, hypertension, mononeuritis multiplex, myocardial infarction
Large	Claudication, hypertension, stroke, aortic incompetence, syncope

Table 23.3 Classification of vasculitis based on size of vessel

- Small vessel vasculitis
  - Henoch-Schönlein purpura
  - Granulomatosis with polyangiitis
  - Leukocytoclastic vasculitis
  - Eosinophilic granulomatosis with polyangiitis
- Medium vessel vasculitis
  - Polyarteritis nodosa
  - Kawasaki disease
- Large vessel vasculitis
  - Takayasu's arteritis

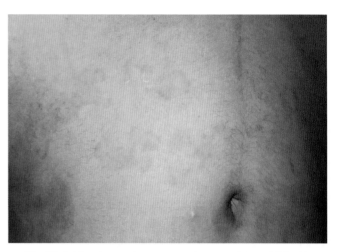

Fig. 23.1 Macular erythematous rash on trunk in a child with Kawasaki disease

Table 23.4 EULAR/PRES classification criteria for Kawasaki's disease

Fever lasting for more than 5 days plus 4 of the 5 following criteria
1. Bilateral conjunctival injection
2. Polymorphous rash
3. Cervical adenopathy
4. Changes in oral mucosa
5. Changes in the peripheral extremities and perineal area

mononeuritis, fundus examination for hypertensive changes or ischemic changes of TA should be done.

Laboratory evaluation includes complete blood count, serum creatinine, urine analysis, chest radiograph and acute phase reactants like ESR and CRP. If small vessel vasculitis is suspected ANA and ANCA should be done to exclude lupus and ANCA-associated vasculitis. Further investigations depend upon the type of vasculitis being considered and the pattern of organ involvement.

CASE VIGNETTE

A 5-year-old child presents with high-grade fever for 7 days associated with redness of eyes and skin rash. In addition, there is history of abdominal pain for 3 days. On examination the child was toxic looking, irritable, had polymorphous erythematous rash on the trunk, oral mucosal congestion, suffused conjunctiva, and right cervical tender lymphadenopathy. Investigation revealed leukocytosis and high CRP.

In view of short history differential diagnosis would include viral, bacterial or rickettsial infection, drug reaction and Kawasaki disease. However presence of abdominal symptoms, irritability, unilateral cervical nodes along with other features makes KD a more likely possibility though infections always need to be excluded by appropriate tests.

Kawasaki disease is predominantly a medium vessel vasculitis that usually presents below 5 years of age. Though it has been described from all parts of the world, it is much more common in South Asia with an incidence of 66.5 per 100,000 in Taiwan.[6] In India reported incidence from Chandigarh in children below 15 years of age is 4.54 per100,000.[7]

It has an acute onset with high fever, skin rash, mucosal inflammation and unilateral cervical adenopathy due to which it was also called mucocutaneous lymph node syndrome. The skin rash is typically erythematous, macular, nonpruritic and polymorphous (Fig. 23.1). Strawberry tongue and ulceration of lips occurs as a consequence of mucosal inflammation. Bilateral nonexudative conjunctivitis is seen in majority of children. Hands and feet may show edema and diffuse redness which is followed by sheet-like peeling of skin on palms and soles starting from periungual area. Presence of rash in the perineal area, erythema in BCG scar is also suggestive of KD. The proposed diagnostic criteria for KD are as follows (Table 23.4).[8]

Other features include abdominal pain, nausea, vomiting, paralytic ileus, irritability, uveitis and keratitis. Resolution of fever heralds the second phase of KD characterized by peeling of skin, thrombocytosis and development of coronary artery changes in some children.

The differential diagnosis includes toxic shock syndrome, scarlet fever, viral exanthema, severe drug reaction, systemic onset juvenile arthritis and rarely SLE. Laboratory investigations suggest acute inflammation (leukocytosis, high ESR and CRP). Echocardiography to look for coronary artery dilatation and aneurysm is the most important investigation. Echo may also reveal myocarditis or pericarditis. Besides this liver and renal function tests, urine analysis and infection screen is a must. Time is the key as IVIG given within 10 days of illness markedly reduces the risk of coronary artery aneurysms the major cause of long-term cardiac morbidity.[9]

CASE VIGNETTE

An 8-year-old girl presents with rash on legs for 4 days. In addition, she has episodic abdominal pain and pain in both knees for 1 day. She denies any vomiting, diarrhea, fever, pedal edema, hematuria, or any other systemic features. On examination, she has palpable purpura over both legs and buttocks along with mild swelling and tenderness in both knees. Rest of the examination is normal. Investigations revealed mild leukocytosis, normal renal function and microscopic hematuria. Her ANA was negative but serum IgA was elevated. The diagnosis is HSP in view of short history of palpable purpura, arthritis, abdominal pain and microscopic hematuria.

Henoch-Schönlein purpura: The HSP is a small vessel vasculitis that occurs 2–3 times more commonly in children than adults and presents with dependent purpura mainly over legs and buttocks (Fig. 23.2). Arthralgia or arthritis of large joints occur in half the children. Gastrointestinal vasculitis presents as colicky abdominal pain, melena or hematochezia, abdominal distension and in severe cases as intussusception. Abdominal symptoms can precede purpura by up to 14 days and in such situation diagnosis is difficult. Glomerulonephritis is usually asymptomatic and microscopic hematuria and/or mild proteinuria is its hallmark. Severe renal disease may present with nephrotic syndrome, nephritic illness, renal insufficiency or hypertension. Few patients can have angioedema like picture with swelling of lips, eyelid, scrotum, etc. The illness usually follows an upper respiratory tract infection.

Diagnosis is mainly clinical (Table 23.5) and can be confirmed by skin biopsy showing leukocytoclastic vasculitis with IgA and C3 deposits.

Other laboratory abnormalities include neutrophilic leukocytosis, increased CRP, urinary abnormalities. Kidney biopsy is indicated only in patients presenting with marked proteinuria or renal insufficiency. As compared to adults children have a higher frequency of arthralgia but upper limb purpura, severe renal involvement is seen more often in adults.[11]

It is a self-limiting illness, though relapses can occur in about one-fourth patients and may occur up to few years. Most children can be managed with reassurance or NSAIDs. Corticosteroids are indicated for GI vasculitis and nephritis. Routine use of corticosteroids does not affect the long-term outcome.[12] Severity of renal involvement determines the need of other immunosuppressive agents like azathioprine or cyclophosphamide.

Other Forms of Leukocytoclastic Vasculitis

Hypersensitivity vasculitis: It presents mainly with palpable purpura and is associated with drugs, infections and rarely no cause is discernible. It is also self-limiting or may require a short course of corticosteroids. Absence of internal organ involvement and complete recovery helps in making a diagnosis.[13]

Vasculitis-associated with other connective tissue diseases: Systemic lupus erythematosus, mixed connective tissue

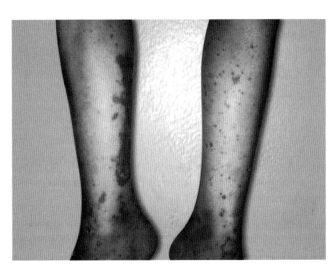

Fig. 23.2 Palpable purpura in a child with HSP

Table 23.5 EULAR/PRINTO/PRES Ankara 2008 classification criteria for HSP[10]

Purpura or petechiae (mandatory) with lower limb predominance with at least one of the following
- Abdominal pain
- Histopathology showing leukocytoclastic vasculitis with predominant IgA deposits or glomerulonephritis
- Arthritis or arthralgia
- Renal disease

disease or dermatomyositis may rarely have leukocytoclastic vasculitis. Presence of other associated features and autoantibodies helps in clinching the diagnosis.

Hypocomplementemic urticarial vasculitis: Though the pathology is small vessel vasculitis, it presents as urticarial lesion that last for a few days. The cause is not known but children have consistently low C4 but normal or low C3. The other abnormalities include anemia, high ESR and CRP. It may be associated with SLE thus ANA needs to be done.

CASE VIGNETTE

A 10-year-old boy presented with blurring of vision in right eye for 5 days along with mild pain. He also had history of recurrent oral ulcers for last 2 years. In addition, he had on episode of scrotal ulcers. There was no history of any skin lesions or fever. Eye examination revealed posterior uveitis. Presence of recurrent oral ulcers, genital ulcer and posterior uveitis suggests a diagnosis of Behçet's syndrome.

Behçet's syndrome: It is more common in adults but can be seen in adolescents. It is a syndrome characterized by neutrophilic vasculitis of both arteries and veins and is seen more often in Mediterranean. Clinically, it presents as recurrent oral ulcers that are deep, large, painful and heal in 1–3 weeks. Other skin manifestations include pseudofolliculitis, pathergy, genital ulcers, palpable purpura, erythema nodosum. Eye involvement is common and can involve any part of eye like anterior uveitis, posterior uveitis and retinal vasculitis. Other symptoms include venous thrombosis, thrombophlebitis, arteritis with aneurysm formation. There is a need to develop criteria for pediatric onset Behçet's disease as children have more GI involvement.[14]

There is no diagnostic test. Due to inflammation there is anemia, high ESR, CRP and mild leukocytosis. Other investigations are mainly to exclude other causes of disease manifestation like infection, malignancy or autoimmune disease.

CASE VIGNETTE

A 9-year-old boy presented with fever for 6 months associated with malaise and weight loss of 8 kg. He has episodic abdominal pain for last 2 months and developed weakness of left hand 5 days ago. On examination, he was sick looking thin built boy with BP of 140/95 mm Hg and left wrist drop and sensory loss in right sural nerve distribution. In view of systemic feature, hypertension, weight loss and mononeuritis multiplex, a diagnosis of classical PAN was made.

Classical polyarteritis nodosa (cPAN): It is a medium vessel vasculitis characterized by transmural neutrophilic infiltration. It is a monophasic illness and occurs mainly in older children.

Systemic features are common, occur early and include fever, myalgias, arthralgias, weight loss. Any system can get be affected however kidney, gut and peripheral nerves are often involved resulting in bland proteinuria, hypertension, abdominal pain, gastrointestinal bleed and mononeuritis multiplex (Fig. 23.3). The skin lesions include subcutaneous nodules along vessel wall, livedo reticularis and gangrene.[15] The diagnosis is confirmed by biopsy of the involved tissue or CT angiogram/conventional angiogram showing narrowing, irregularity and microaneurysms (Table 23.6).

Cutaneous PAN is a localized variant of PAN that presents with skin lesions and may in addition have fever, arthritis, myalgias and rarely neuropathy. Cutaneous PAN rarely progresses to involve internal organ.[16] In a child with recurrent cutaneous PAN streptococcal infection should be considered and treated.

Recently children with PAN-like disease have been described to have mutations in adenosine deaminase 2 gene and its deficiency may alter endothelial function or cause increased inflammation.[17]

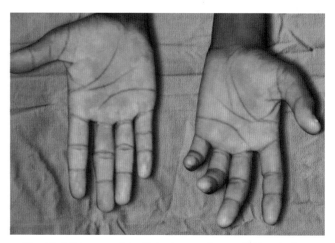

Fig. 23.3 Mononeuritis of left ulnar nerve in a child with cPAN

Table 23.6 EULAR/PRINTO/PRES Ankara 2008 classification criteria for diagnosis of cPAN[10]
Histological or angiographic confirmation of medium vessel vasculitis along one out of the following 5 criteria
1. Skin involvement
2. Hypertension
3. Myalgias or muscle tenderness
4. Kidney involvement
5. Peripheral neuropathy

CASE VIGNETTE

A 9-year-old girl presented with headache for last 2 months. On examination, she had hypertension and feeble left radial and brachial artery. In addition, she had a left subclavian and renal bruit. Investigation revealed anemia, high ESR, normal renal functions. Ultrasound revealed small sized left kidney and CT angiogram showed 70% stenosis of left subclavian artery, abdominal aorta irregularity and left renal artery stenosis. In view of pulse inequality, bruit, hypertension and stenotic lesions on angiogram the diagnosis is TA.

Takayasu's arteritis (TA): It is a large vessel vasculitis seen more commonly in Asians. It generally presents in adolescents with hypertension, headache or it could be detected asymptomatically when a pulse is found to be absent during examination.[18] The other important features are intermittent claudication, thinning of limb, syncope and abdominal angina. A small proportion of patients however can present with PUO associated with nonspecific symptoms, like fever, arthralgia, myalgia, fatigue, weight loss and anemia. A meticulous examination can provide the first clue by finding a difference in blood pressure between extremities or a loss of pulse or vascular bruit (Table 23.7).[19]

The long-term complications of TA include aortic incompetence, aneurysm formation, end-stage renal disease and stroke.

The diagnosis is based on demonstration of arterial narrowing near the origin of vessels from the aorta, as well as of the aorta itself by angiogram (Fig. 23.4). As it can be asymptomatic, some patients have extensive collaterals at diagnosis. MR, CT or conventional digital subtraction angiograms can be used with MR angiogram avoiding radiation exposure. Doppler US is also being used for follow-up and diagnosis. It can be also picked up on FDG PET done to evaluate PUO when it shows increased uptake in aorta or its main branches.

Treatment is mainly aimed at controlling inflammation in a hope to prevent further pulse loss. Corticosteroids and immunosuppressive drugs are used and in resistant cases biologicals have also been tried.[20] Endovascular interventions

Table 23.7 EULAR/PRINTO/PRES classification criteria for diagnosis of TA[10]
Angiographic abnormalities of aorta and its branches along with 1 of the 5 following features
• Pulse deficit or claudication
• BP unequality
• Vascular bruit
• Hypertension
• Elevated acute phase proteins

also are useful in control of hypertension and in improving claudication.[21]

ANCA-associated Vasculitis

Though granulomatosis with polyangiitis is the most common of the ANCA-associated vasculitis in children, microscopic polyangiitis and eosinophilic. Granulomatosis with polyangiitis (Churg-Strauss syndrome) are also described in children. The clinical presentation is very similar to that seen in adults and most cases are described in adolescent age group.[22]

Majority of the children with GPA have systemic features, glomerulonephritis, lower and upper airway diseases (Fig. 23.5). Antibodies to PR-3 and presence of pauci-immune

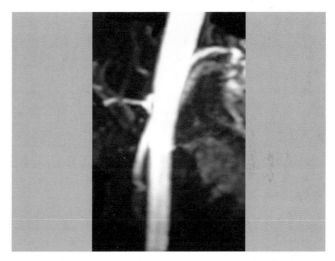

Fig. 23.4 MR angiogram showing complete stenosis of right renal artery and near complete stenosis of left renal artery in a patient with TA

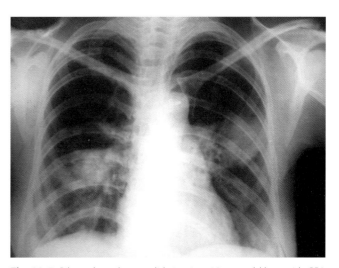

Fig. 23.5 Bilateral patch consolidation in a 18-year-old boy with GPA

Flow chart 23.1 Algorithm for approaching a child with vasculitis

Table 23.8 EULAR/PRINTO/PRES Ankara 2008 classification definition of WG in children[10]

At least 3 of the 6 following criteria should be present
1. Histopathology—vascular or extravascular granulomas
2. Upper airway involvement
3. Subglottic, tracheal or bronchial stenosis
4. Pulmonary involvement
5. Presence of ANCA
6. Renal disease—proteinuria, hematuria, RBC casts or pauci-immune glomerulonephritis

glomerulonephritis on kidney biopsy helps in establishing the diagnosis (Table 23.8).

Children with MPA also have an acute onset with systemic features associated with lung and kidney disease (almost 50% presenting with renal failure). Upper airway disease does not occur in MPA.[23] The EGPA is rare in children and has insidious onset with palpable purpura. Children have higher prevalence of cardiopulmonary features and a lower prevalence of peripheral neuropathy.[24]

Other uncommon vasculitis is primary CNS angiitis that presents with focal neurological deficit or alteration of sensorium.[25]

Though most vasculitis in children present similar to adults, their relative prevalence and outcome is different. In some vasculitis, the diagnosis is obvious like in HSP or in most cases of TA but in other systemic vasculitis a high index of suspicion is required for early diagnosis. Recording of blood pressure, good urine analysis can provide clues to a diagnosis of vasculitis. A simple algorithm for approach to childhood vasculitis is given in Flow chart 23.1.

KEY POINTS

- Childhood vasculitis can have variable clinical manifestations.
- HSP and KD are the most common forms of childhood vasculitis.
- Diagnosis requires high index of suspicion.

REFERENCES

1. Malleson PN, Fung MY, Rosenberg AM. The incidence of pediatric rheumatic diseases from the Canadian Rheumatology Association disease registry. J Rheumatol. 1996;23:1981-7.
2. Bowyer S, Roettcher P. Pediatric rheumatology clinic populations in the United States: result of a 3 year survey. Pediatric rheumatology database research group. J Rheumatol 1996;23:1968-74.
3. Gardner-Medwin JM, Dolezalova P, Cumminis C, et al. Incidence of Henoch-Schönlein pupura, Kawasaki Disease and rare vasculitides in children of different ethnic origin. Lancet. 2002;360:1197-202.
4. Dolezalova P, Telekesova P, Nemcova D, et al. Incidence of vasculitis in children in the Czech Republic: 2 year prospective epidemiologic survey. J Rheumatol 2004;31:2295-9.
5. Yang YH, Hung CF, Hsu CR, et al. A nationwide survey on epidemiological characteristics of childhood Henoch-Schönlein purpura in Taiwan. Rheumatology. 2005;44:618-22.
6. Lue HC, Chen LR, Lin MT, et al. Epidemiological features of kawasaki disease in Taiwan, 1976–2007: Results of five nationwide questionnaire hospital surveys. Pediatr Neonatol. 2014;55:92-6.
7. Singh S, Aulakh R, Kawasaki T. Kawasaki disease and the emerging coronary artery disease epidemic in India: is there a correlation? Indian J Pediatr. 2014;81:328-32
8. Ozen S, Ruperto N, Dillon MU, et al. EULAR/PRES endorsed consensus criteria for the classification of childhood vasculitides. Ann Rheum Dis. 2006;65:936-41.
9. Newburger JW, Takahashi M, Burns JC, et al. The treatment of Kawasaki syndrome with intravenous gamma globulin. N Engl J Med. 1986;315:341-7.
10. Ozen S, Pistorio A, Lusan SM, et al. EULAR/PRINTO/ PReS criteria for Henoch-Schönlein purpura, childhood polyarteritis nodosa, childhood Wegener's granulomatosis and childhood Takayasu's arteritis Ankara 2008: Part II: Final classification criteria. Ann Rheum Dis. 2010;69:798-806.
11. Kang Y, Park JS, Ha YJ, et al. Differences in clinical manifestations and outcomes between adult and child patients with Henoch-Schönlein purpura. J Korean Med Sci. 2014;29:198-203.
12. Jauhola O, Ronkainen J, Koskimies O, et al. Outcome of Henoch-Schönlein purpura 8 years after treatment with a placebo or prednisone at disease onset. Pediatr Nephrol. 2012;27:933-9.
13. Calvo-Río V, Loricera J, Ortiz-Sanjuán F, et al. Revisiting clinical differences between hypersensitivity vasculitis and Henoch-Schönlein purpura in adults from a defined population. Clin Exp Rheumatol. 2014 Feb 11. [Epub ahead of print].
14. Ozen S, Eroglu FK. Pediatric-onset Behçet disease. Curr Opin Rheumatol. 2013;25:636-42.
15. Dhillon MJ, Elfeitheriou D, Brogan P. Medium vessel vasculitis. Ped Nephrol. 2010;25:1641-52.
16. Furukawa F. Cutaneous polyarteritis nodosa: an update. Ann Vasc Dis. 2012;5:282-8.
17. Navon Elkan P, Pierce SB, Segel R, et al. Mutant adenosine deaminase 2 in a polyarteritis nodosa vasculopathy. N Engl J Med. 2014;370:921-31.
18. Kumar S, Goel R, Danda D, et al. A103: childhood onset Takayasu arteritis-experience from a tertiary care centre in South India. Arthritis Rheumatol. 2014;66:S139.
19. Forsey J, Dhandayuthapani G, Hamilton M, et al. Takayasu arteritis: key clinical factors for early diagnosis. Arch Dis Child Educ Pract Ed. 2011;96:176-82.

20. Brunner J, Feldman BM, Tyrrell PN, et al. Takayasu arteritis in children and adolescents. Rheumatology (Oxford). 2010;49:1806-14.

21. Gulati A, Bagga A. Large vessel vasculitis. Pediatr Nephrol. 2010;25:1037-48.

22. Cabral DA, Uribe AG, Benseler S, et al. Classification, presentation and initial treatment of Wegener's granulomatosis in childhood. Arthritis Rheum. 2009;60:3413-34.

23. Peco-Antic A, Bonaci-Nikolic B, Basta-Jovanovic G, et al. Childhood microscopic polyangiitis associated with MPO-ANCA. Pediatric Nephrology. 2006;21:46-53.

24. Zwerina J, Eger G, Engelbrecht M, et al. Churg-Strauss syndrome in childhood: A systematic literature review and clinical comparison with adult patients.Semin Arthritis Rheum. 2009;39:108-15.

25. Cellucci T, Benseler S. Central nervous system vasculitis in children. Curr Opin Rheumatol. 2010;22:590-7.

CHAPTER 24

Approach to Adult with Systemic Vasculitis

Pradeep Bambery, Vinay Sagar, Aman Sharma

INTRODUCTION

Vasculitides are a heterogeneous group of uncommon inflammatory autoimmune disorders represented by inflammation and necrosis of vessel wall, eventually culminating in loss of vascular integrity. Damaged walls either result in compromised lumen with downstream ischemia or weakening of vessel wall with rupture and aneurysm formation. The estimated incidence of primary systemic vasculitis is ≥ 100 cases per million.[1] These disorders have a wide spectrum of clinical presentations, dependent upon size, type and location of the involved vessel.

These patients may present with nonspecific symptoms in the beginning of illness and symptoms pertaining to inflicted organ systems might develop later. The diagnosis of systemic vasculitis must be considered among the differential diagnosis when the patient presents with multisystem involvement. A detailed and comprehensive history along with physical examination, usually suggests the diagnosis of systemic vasculitis, which can be further substantiated by laboratory investigations, radiologic imaging such as computed tomography, angiogram and tissue biopsy of the involved organ. The most important key to the diagnosis is to keep systemic vasculitis amongst the differential diagnosis. The pattern of organ involvement often provides valuable clue to a given vasculitic disorder, however, significant overlaps have been observed.

The vasculitis syndromes have variable course, and can often have a relentless downhill course. Thus, these require prompt recognition and institution of appropriate and often aggressive treatment with immunosuppressive therapy to prevent irreversible organ damage or death. Current immunosuppressive treatments have significantly reduced mortality; however, most patients still have poor quality of life due to permanent organ damage, multiple relapses, and drug toxicity.[2-4] Outcome in vasculitis patients is dependent upon the type of vasculitic syndrome, organ involvement, treatment regimen administered, presence of antineutrophilic cytoplasmic antibodies (ANCA), older age group and male gender.[5] The approach to an adult is shown in Figure 24.1.

Clinical Features

The diagnosis of vasculitis is often delayed because of the presence of nonspecific symptoms, which are usually mimicked by various other disorders. A detailed history and physical examination is essential part of work-up to arrive a particular diagnosis and to exclude secondary causes of vasculitis, such as inflammatory disorders (rheumatoid arthritis, systemic lupus erythematosus, Sjögren's syndrome, inflammatory bowel disease and sarcoidosis), infections (hepatitis B and C virus, human immunodeficiency virus, mycobacterium tuberculosis, syphilis and infective endocarditis), neoplasias (myelo- and lymphoproliferative disorder and solid tumors), drugs (hydralazine, propyl-thiouracil, and montelukast). Infection endocarditis can present with fever and multisystem involvement and should be excluded. Age and gender have important bearing, as the ANCA associated vasculitis (AAV) and polyarteritis nodosa (PAN) predominantly affect middle age population (45–50 years), whereas IgA vasculitis [Henoch–Schönlein purpura (HSP)] and Takayasu arteritis (TA) affect younger population (17–26 years) and giant cell arteritis (GCA) affects the older population (>50 years). The TA and GCA are more prevalent in female gender.[6] The signs common to all vasculitides are constitutional features like fatigue, weakness,

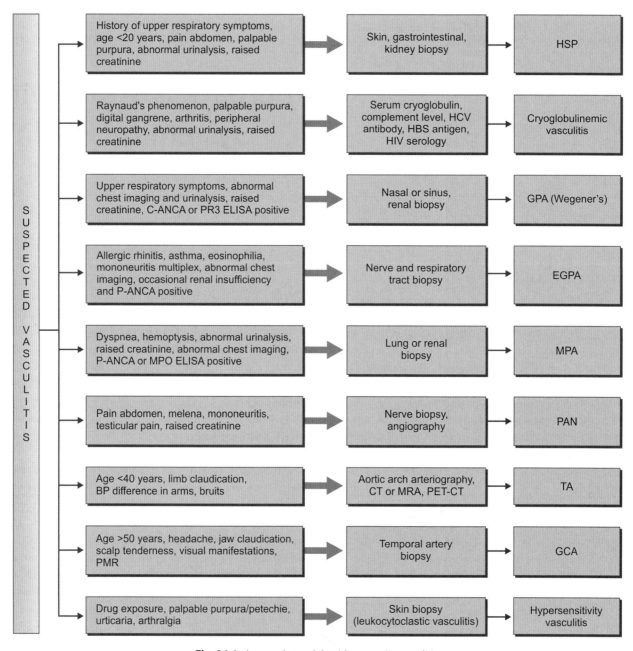

Fig. 24.1 Approach to adult with systemic vasculitis

low grade fever, joints or muscle aches, anorexia and weight loss.[7] Systemic vasculitides such as GCA, Behçet's disease (BD), PAN, hypersensitivity vasculitis, TA, granulomatosis with polyangiitis (GPA) are frequently considered as a differential diagnosis for pyrexia of unknown origin.[8] However, other causes of unexplained fever should also be explored and excluded, which include, infections, neoplastic, non-infectious inflammatory disorders, drugs, inherited and metabolic diseases.

The presence of certain characteristic features that strongly indicate diagnosis of systemic vasculitis are mononeuritis multiplex, palpable purpura and pulmonary renal syndrome. Mononeuritis multiplex or asymmetric polyneuropathy, which typically manifested with both sensory and motor deficit, occurs in up to 70% patients with PAN and up to 75% patients with eosinophilic granulomatosis with polyangiitis (EGPA).[9-12] It usually manifests as initial picture of dysesthesias and pain, which later progresses to weakness in the distribution of the affected peripheral nerves, like foot and wrist drop. Patients with isolated palpable purpura most likely have cutaneous leukocytoclastic vasculitis (hypersensitivity vasculitis), whereas, in patients with purpura along with systemic symptoms, IgA vasculitis or microscopic polyangiitis (MPA) should be suspected. Patients with pulmonary renal syndrome, manifesting in the form of hemoptysis and renal failure due to glomerulonephritis suggests the diagnosis of GPA, MPA, and antiglomerular basement membrane disease (anti-GBM).

Upper airway involvement occurs in patients of both GPA and EGPA. However, it is estimated to present in up to 90% of patients with GPA, as compared to 30–35% patients with EGPA.[13,14] Upper respiratory tract symptoms usually manifest in the form of nasal crusting, persistent rhinorrhea, purulent or bloody nasal discharge, chronic sinusitis, otitis media, nasal bridge destruction leading to saddle nose deformity and subglottic stenosis. Patients may also complaint of earache, conductive and sensorineural hearing loss and ear discharge. There are varieties of other skin lesions that are associated with vasculitis, such as, ulcerations, digital infarcts, urticaria, livedo reticularis, bullous or vesicular eruptions, and subcutaneous nodules.

Polyarteritis nodosa (PAN) and TA are the most likely diagnosis in the patients with recently detected hypertension, along with presence of constitutional symptoms and other clinical pictures consistent with vasculitis. The hypertension in PAN and TA is due to involvement of renal artery, leading to renal artery stenosis. The PAN patients may also complaint of abdominal pain and lower gastrointestinal bleeding, due to mesenteric ischemia. The discomfort is most prominent after taking meals (abdominal angina), leading to decreased food intake. The etiologies for secondary PAN should also be explored such as hepatitis B virus (HBV), and hairy cell leukemia.[15,16] Orchitis with testicular pain and tenderness occurs in almost 10% of patients of PAN. Pulmonary involvement is typically absent in PAN, pulmonary capillaritis, and parenchymal involvement strongly suggest other systemic vasculitis, such as GPA, MPA, or EGPA.[17] Discrepancy in blood pressure recordings in any limb or absent peripheral pulses, raise the possibility of TA or GCA with large artery involvement. In addition, GCA patients may have characteristic findings such as constitutional symptoms, headache, jaw claudication, and sometimes visual manifestations. Bronchial asthma is the foremost important clinical manifestation of EGPA and present in ≥ 90% of patients.[18] The EGPA should always be suspected in patients with poorly controlled asthma, despite being on treatment along with a skin rash with other manifestations like mononeuritis multiplex. Asthma usually precedes the other clinical features by approximately 8–10 years.[19]

Laboratory Investigations

Hematological Parameters

Normocytic normochromic anemia due to chronic inflammatory process, leukocytosis, and thrombocytosis may be seen. Peripheral blood eosinophilia is a characteristic finding in patients with EGPA. Erythrocyte sedimentation rate (ESR) and C-reactive protein (CRP) are nonspecific acute phase reactants, which are usually elevated during acute phase of disease and relapse. These parameters may not be differentiated between acute flare of vasculitis or superimposed infections. However, ESR as well as CRP plays a significant role in diagnosing and following-up GCA patients. The ESR often reaches ≥ 100 mm in first hour and CRP levels tend to parallel with ESR. A meta-analysis has demonstrated normal ESR level in only 4% of patients in biopsy proven GCA.[20]

Antineutrophil Cytoplasmic Antibodies

Antineutrophil cytoplasmic antibodies (ANCA) is a serological marker for some primary vasculitic syndromes, which predominantly involve small to medium sized vessels. These vasculitis are collectively known as ANCA associated vasculitis (AAV), and comprise of GPA, MPA, EGPA and renal limited vasculitis.[21] Currently, two types of assays are available to detect circulating ANCA. First one is, indirect immunofluorescence assay (IIF) and this technique is performed by using normal human ethanol fixed neutrophils, and second assay is, enzyme linked immunosorbent assay (ELISA), which use purified vasculitis-specific antigens.[22] Out of these two assays, IIF is more sensitive and ELISA is more specific. Thus, it is recommended that ANCA testing should be carried out by both IIF and ELISA.[22]

The two major fluoroscopic staining pattern observed are the C-ANCA with diffuse, granular cytoplasmic staining, in which the antibody in the patients serum is directed against proteinase 3 (PR3); however, the perinuclear or P-ANCA pattern results from a staining pattern around the nucleus and the antibody responsible for this pattern is directed against myeloperoxidase (MPO).[23-25] ANCA serology is positive in up to 90% of patients with active generalized GPA, whereas it is positive in only up to 40% of patients with limited GPA, and hence, the sensitivity of PR3-ANCA depends on extent, severity and activity of disease.[26] However, among GPA patients with ANCA, 80–90% have PR3-ANCA and rest have MPO-ANCA positive. The MPA patients have ANCA association up to 70% and most of them are directed against MPO. ANCA both PR3 and MPO are detected with variable frequency in patients with EGPA.[26] The P-ANCA is not as specific as C-ANCA for ANCA associated vasculitis and may be found in association with other inflammatory diseases such as inflammatory bowel diseases and other connective tissue disorders such as rheumatoid arthritis and systemic lupus erythematosus.[27] The details about ANCA are discussed in Chapter 5.

Other Laboratory Tests

Hepatitis B virus (HBV) infection has been observed in up to 36% of PAN patients and PAN is also reported occasionally with HCV patients.[9,15,28] However, HCV infection is often observed concomitantly with other viral infections like HBV.[29-32]

Similarly, hepatitis C antibody testing needs to be done in patients with mixed cryoglobulinemia.[33-35] Hypocomplementemia may be detected in patients with cryoglobulinemic and hypersensitive vasculitis.

Urinalysis detects hematuria and proteinuria, and further assessment is essential for red blood cell casts and dysmorphic red blood cells indicating glomerular inflammation, and quantification of 24 hours urinary protein excretion along with serum creatinine to estimate extent of glomerular damage in small vessel vasculitis. Electromyography or nerve conduction studies should be performed to confirm the clinically established diagnosis of mononeuritis multiplex in patients with PAN, EGPA and rarely GPA.

Biopsy from Affected Organs

Biopsy examination is essential part of investigations and it helps to arrive at definitive diagnosis. Whenever possible it should be obtained from the involved tissue. Now, the biopsy can be performed more accurately under ultrasound or computed tomographic guidance. Biopsy has a role to define the extent, severity and phase (acute vs chronic) of vasculitis. Thus, accordingly clinicians can formulate intensity of immunosuppression and prognosticate.

Skin Biopsy

In patients with skin involvement in the form of palpable purpura, urticaria, cutaneous infarcts, nonhealing ulcers, nodular lesions, it is logical to perform skin biopsy from the edge of the lesion. A deep punch or incisional biopsy is taken from a fresh lesion, usually within 18–36 hours of onset of lesion. The biopsy specimen should be sent for histopathology and immunofluorescence study. Histopathology study usually demonstrates small vessel involvement with leukocytoclasia. However, in drug-induced vasculitis, additional some degree of tissue eosinophilia may also be seen. In direct immunofluorescence study, the most common immune deposits found in blood vessels are IgM, C3, and fibrin.[36] Prominent IgA deposits within blood vessel wall helps to differentiate IgA vasculitis from other small vessel cutaneous vasculitis.[37]

Nasal or Sinus Biopsy

In suspected patients of GPA with nasal or sinus symptoms, a nasal or sinus biopsy should be done. Although it is relatively less invasive, it has high false-negative rates due to small amount of tissue obtained. The typical histopathological finding is granulomatous inflammation that in the presence of clinical picture consistent with GPA and C-ANCA positivity, is sufficient to establish the diagnosis of GPA.

Lung Biopsy

Patients with clinical and radiological evidence consistent with pulmonary involvement in GPA and MPA, without involvement of other easily accessible sites should be planned to undergo a lung biopsy, which is most often performed through open or thoracoscopic approach. The characteristic histopathologic picture of pulmonary capillaritis is seen in MPA; however, necrotizing granulomatous inflammation may be seen in GPA.

Nerve Biopsy

Nerve biopsy is considered in patients with clinical features compatible with vasculitic neuropathy. The nerve biopsy is mostly done from sural sensory nerve or the superficial peroneal sensory nerve in the lower limbs. Sometimes superficial peroneal sensory nerve biopsy is combined with biopsy of peroneus brevis muscle and is shown to increase the diagnostic yield.[38] Superficial radial nerve is biopsied whenever there is predominant upper limb involvement. It has been demonstrated that addition of muscle biopsy improves the yield of definitive vasculitic neuropathy.[39] Histopathological findings include perivascular and transmural mononuclear cell infiltration of the epineural blood vessels, with resulting fibrinoid necrosis of vessel wall and axonal loss.

Kidney Biopsy

Renal biopsy is indicated in patients with ANCA associated vasculitis with overt renal dysfunction such as reduced estimated glomerular filtration rate or evidence of active urinary sediments. Some experts preclude the need of renal biopsy if the diagnosis is already established in the presence of consistent clinical feature with compatible histopathology report from more easily accessible site and positive ANCA report. Renal biopsy typically demonstrates segmental necrotizing glomerulonephritis, often with crescents and pauci-immune on immunofluorescence and electron microscopy.

Temporal Artery Biopsy

The temporal artery biopsy should be performed in patients with suspected GCA. It is a reasonably safe procedure, and generally obtained in out patient setting under local anesthesia. Biopsy should be obtained from the clinically involved side. The GCA affects temporal artery focally and segmentally; thus, the sample length needs to be adequate to include pathologic site. There is no unanimous opinion regarding optimal length of the sample.[40-42] Different studies have recommended different length of sample, which ranges from 1.5 to 5 cm.[40-42] In patients with strong clinical suspicion of GCA and negative temporal artery, biopsy from most symptomatic side, should undergo temporal artery biopsy from the contralateral side.[43]

Radiologic Imaging

Ultrasound Doppler Study

Ultrasound has a role mainly in large vessel vasculitis, particularly in GCA, TA and idiopathic aortitis. Findings that are observed are stenosis, occlusion or hypoechoic swollen (halo sign) temporal artery wall. A prospective study in biopsy proven GCA patients had demonstrated sensitivity of halo sign of only 40%.[44] A meta-analysis published has illustrated sensitivity and specificity of 87% and 96%, respectively, of temporal artery duplex ultrasound with respect to the clinical diagnosis.[45]

Angiogram

Arteriogram is useful in identifying and characterizing a vasculitis into large or medium vessel vasculitis. Arteriographic findings are very nonspecific and helpful in establishing diagnosis only in association with compatible clinical data and other supportive laboratory reports. The typical features of angiography that are observed in vasculitis patients include narrowing, aneurysm formation, or vascular wall irregularities.

Mesenteric and renal arteriography is an alternative to biopsy for diagnosis, especially in situations where obvious site for biopsy is absent in patients with PAN.[46] The arteriographic findings suggestive of PAN include multiple aneurysms and irregular constrictions of larger vessels with occlusion of smaller penetrating arteries. Computed tomography (CT) and magnetic resonance (MR) angiogram are less invasive techniques and can also be used. These modalities can also show renal infarcts.

Arteriography of aorta and its major branches is a viable option to diagnose suspected TA and large vessel GCA. Primary abnormalities which may be observed include smooth walled, tapered, or narrowed areas with some areas of dilatation along with collateral circulation. It has both diagnostic and therapeutic value with interventions such as angioplasty and stent placement can be performed in single arterial puncture. Although, arteriography can clearly delineate the luminal outline, it does not allow the assessment of vessel wall thickening. The CT and MR angiography has shown promising results with demonstration of arterial abnormalities as well as thickening of the vessel wall.[47-49]

Positron emission tomography has a role in identifying the site of inflammation and treatment response in large vessel vasculitis.[50,51] However, it has no additional benefit over routine imaging modality for identifying extent of involvement in small vessel vasculitis.[52]

Hence to conclude, it is important to note that most of the systemic vasculitides have a multisystem involvement. Detailed clinical history, physical examination along with relevant investigations can help in arriving at the correct diagnosis.

KEY POINTS

- Systemic vasculitides are systemic multisystem disorders.
- The key to the diagnosis is keeping vasculitides among the differential diagnosis.
- Detailed history, clinical examination and relevant investigations can help in achieving the correct diagnosis.
- The biopsy is generally the gold standard but may have different sensitivity at different sites and moreover, it may not show the complete picture due to small biopsy sample size.

REFERENCES

1. Watts RA, Scott DGI. Epidemiology of vasculitis. In: Ball GV, Bridges SL Jr (Eds). Vasculitis, 2nd edn. Oxford: Oxford University Press; 2008.pp.7-21.
2. Gordon M, Luqmani RA, Adu D, et al. Relapses in patients with a systemic vasculitis. Q J Med. 1993;86:779-89.
3. Exley AR, Carruthers DM, Luqmani RA, et al. Damage occurs early in systemic vasculitis and is an index of outcome. Q J Med. 1997;90:391-9.
4. Seo P, Luqmani RA, Flossmann O, et al. The future of damage assessment in vasculitis. J Rheumatol. 2007;34:1357-71.
5. Mukhtyar C, Flossmann O, Hellmich B, et al. Outcomes from studies of antineutrophil cytoplasm antibody associated vasculitis: a systematic review by the European League against rheumatism systemic vasculitis task force. Ann Rheum Dis. 2008;67:1004-10.
6. Hunder GG, Arend WP, Bloch DA, et al. The American College of Rheumatology 1990 criteria for the classification of vasculitis. Introduction. Arthritis Rheum 1990;33:1065-7.
7. Conn DL. Update on systemic necrotizing vasculitis. Mayo Clin Proc. 1989;64:535-43.
8. Hayakawa K, Ramasamy B, Chandrasekar PH. Fever of unknown origin: an evidence-based review. Am J Med Sci. 2012;344:307-16.
9. Pagnoux C, Seror R, Henegar C, et al. French Vasculitis Study Group. Clinical features and outcomes in 348 patients with polyarteritis nodosa: a systematic retrospective study of patients diagnosed between 1963 and 2005 and entered into the French Vasculitis Study Group Database. Arthritis Rheum. 2010;62:616-26.
10. Tervaert JW, Kallenberg C. Neurologic manifestations of systemic vasculitides. Rheum Dis Clin North Am. 1993;19:913-40.
11. Sinico RA, Bottero P. Churg-Strauss angiitis. Best Pract Res Clin Rheumatol. 2009;23:355-66.
12. Guillevin L, Cohen P, Gayraud M, et al. Churg-Strauss syndrome. Clinical study and long-term follow-up of 96 patients. Medicine (Baltimore). 1999;78:26-37.
13. Seo P, Stone JH. The antineutrophil cytoplasmic antibody-associated vasculitides. Am J Med. 2004;117:39-50.
14. Hoffman GS, Kerr GS, Leavitt RY, et al. Wegener granulomatosis: an analysis of 158 patients. Ann Intern Med. 1992;116:488-98.
15. Guillevin L, Mahr A, Callard P, et al. French Vasculitis Study Group. Hepatitis B virus-associated polyarteritis nodosa: clinical characteristics, outcome, and impact of treatment in 115 patients. Medicine (Baltimore). 2005;84:313-22.
16. Hasler P, Kistler H, Gerber H. Vasculitides in hairy cell leukemia. Semin Arthritis Rheum. 1995;25:134-42.
17. Boki KA, Dafni U, Karpouzas GA, et al. Necrotizing vasculitis in Greece: clinical, immunological and immunogenetic aspects. A study of 66 patients. Br J Rheumatol. 1997;36:1059-66.
18. Comarmond C, Pagnoux C, Khellaf M, et al. French Vasculitis Study Group. Eosinophilic granulomatosis with polyangiitis (Churg-Strauss): clinical characteristics and long-term follow-up of the 383 patients enrolled in the French Vasculitis Study Group cohort. Arthritis Rheum. 2013;65:270-81.
19. Cottin V, Khouatra C, Dubost R, et al. Persistent airflow obstruction in asthma of patients with Churg-Strauss syndrome and long-term follow-up. Allergy. 2009;64:589-95.
20. Smetana GW, Shmerling RH. Does this patient have temporal arteritis? JAMA. 2002;287:92-101.
21. Savige J, Davies D, Falk RJ, et al. Antineutrophil cytoplasmic antibodies and associated diseases: a review of the clinical and laboratory features. Kidney Int. 2000;57:846-62.
22. Savige J, Gillis D, Benson E, et al. International Consensus Statement on Testing and Reporting of Antineutrophil Cytoplasmic Antibodies (ANCA). Am J Clin Pathol. 1999;111:507-13.
23. Jennette JC, Wilkman AS, Falk RJ. Diagnostic predictive value of ANCA serology. Kidney Int. 1998;53:796-8.
24. Niles JL, Pan GL, Collins AB, et al. Antigen-specific radioimmunoassays for anti-neutrophil cytoplasmic antibodies in the diagnosis of rapidly progressive glomerulonephritis. J Am Soc Nephrol. 1991;2:27-36.
25. Falk RJ, Jennette JC. Anti-neutrophil cytoplasmic autoantibodies with specificity for myeloperoxidase in patients with systemic vasculitis and idiopathic necrotizing and crescentic glomerulonephritis. N Engl J Med. 1988;318:1651-7.
26. Hoffman GS, Specks U. Antineutrophil cytoplasmic antibodies. Arthritis Rheum. 1998;41:1521-37.
27. Merkel PA, Polisson RP, Chang Y, et al. Prevalence of antineutrophil cytoplasmic antibodies in a large inception cohort of patients with connective tissue disease. Ann Intern Med. 1997;126:866-73.
28. Carson CW, Conn DL, Czaja AJ, et al. Frequency and significance of antibodies to hepatitis C virus in polyarteritis nodosa. J Rheumatol. 1993;20:304-9.
29. Sharma A, Sharma K. Hepatotropic viral infection associated systemic vasculitides—HBV associated polyarteritis nodosa and HCV associated cryoglobulinemic vasculitis. J Clin Exp Hepatol. 2013;3:204-12.
30. Pagnoux C, Cohen P, Guillevin L. Vasculitides secondary to infections. Clin Exp Rheumatol. 2006;24(Suppl. 41):S71-S81.
31. Cacoub P, Lunel-fabiani F, Le Thi Huong D. Polyarteritis nodosa and hepatitis C virus infection. Ann Intern Med. 1992;116:605-6.
32. Servant A, Bogard M, Delaugerre C, et al. GB virus C in systemic medium- and small-vessel necrotizing vasculitides. Br J Rheumatol. 1998;37:1292-4.
33. Monti G, Galli M, Invernizzi F, et al. Cryoglobulinaemias: a multi-centre study of the early clinical and laboratory manifestations of primary and secondary disease. GISC. Italian Group for the Study of Cryoglobulinaemias. QJM. 1995;88:115-26.
34. Kawakami T, Ooka S, Mizoguchi M, et al. Remission of hepatitis B virus-related cryoglobulinemic vasculitis with entecavir. Ann Intern Med. 2008;149:911-2.
35. Dimitrakopoulos AN, Kordossis T, Hatzakis A, et al. Mixed cryoglobulinemia in HIV-1 infection: the role of HIV-1. Ann Intern Med 1999;13:226-30.
36. Russell JP, Gibson LE. Primary cutaneous small vessel vasculitis: approach to diagnosis and treatment. Int J Dermatol. 2006;45:3-13.

37. Jennette JC, Falk RJ. Small-vessel vasculitis. N Engl J Med. 1997;337:1512-23.
38. Said G, Lacroix C. Primary and secondary vasculitic neuropathy. J Neurol. 2005;252:633-41.
39. Vital C, Vital A, Canron M-H, et al. Combined nerve and muscle biopsy in the diagnosis of vasculitic neuropathy. A 16-year retrospective study of 202 cases. J Periph Nerv Syst. 2006;11:20-9.
40. Klein RG, Campbell RJ, Hunder GG, et al. Skip lesions in temporal arteritis. Mayo Clin Proc. 1976;51:504-10.
41. Kent RB 3rd, Thomas L. Temporal artery biopsy. Am Surg. 1990;56:16-21.
42. Taylor-Gjevre R, Vo M, Shukla D, et al. Temporal artery biopsy for giant cell arteritis. J Rheumatol. 2005;32:1279-82.
43. Gonzalez-Gay MA. The diagnosis and management of patients with giant cell arteritis. J Rheumatol. 2005;32:1186-8.
44. Salvarani C, Silingardi M, Ghirarduzzi A, et al. Is duplex ultrasonography useful for the diagnosis of giant-cell arteritis? Ann Intern Med. 2002;137:232-8.
45. Karassa FB, Matsagas MI, Schmidt WA, et al. Meta-analysis: test performance of ultrasonography for giant-cell arteritis. Ann Intern Med. 2005;142:359-69.
46. Ewald EA, Griffin D, McCune WJ. Correlation of angiographic abnormalities with disease manifestations and disease severity in polyarteritis nodosa. J Rheumatol. 1987;14:952-6.
47. Yamada I, Numano F, Suzuki S. Takayasu arteritis: evaluation with MR imaging. Radiology. 1993;188:89-94.
48. Yamada I, Nakagawa T, Himeno Y, et al. Takayasu arteritis: evaluation of the thoracic aorta with CT angiography. Radiology. 1998;209:103-9.
49. Keenan NG, Mason JC, Maceira A, et al. Integrated cardiac and vascular assessment in Takayasu arteritis by cardiovascular magnetic resonance. Arthritis Rheum. 2009;60:3501-9.
50. Prieto-González S, Depetris M, García-Martínez A, et al. Positron emission tomography assessment of large vessel inflammation in patients with newly diagnosed, biopsy-proven giant cell arteritis: a prospective, case-control study. Ann Rheum Dis. 2014;73:1388-92.
51. Santhosh S, Mittal BR, Gayana S, et al. F-18 FDG PET/CT in the evaluation of Takayasu arteritis: An experience from the tropics. J Nucl Cardiol. 2014.
52. Soussan M, Abisror N, Abad S, et al. FDG-PET/CT in patients with ANCA-associated vasculitis: case-series and literature review. Autoimmun Rev. 2014;13:125-31.

CHAPTER 25

Assessment of Disease Activity and Damage

Aman Sharma, Ram Nath Misra

INTRODUCTION

The systemic vasculitides are heterogeneous group of uncommon autoimmune diseases characterized by the inflammation of the vessel wall.[1-3] There has been a change in the perception of these disease over the last fifty years, from acute life-threatening conditions to chronic manageable disorders. This has resulted from the significant advancement in the available treatment options for these disorders converting these previously invariably fatal diseases to chronically manageable disorders. These treatment options, however, have their own safety concerns. Thus there is a need to have objective measures of assessing disease activity. Since the spectrum of clinical presentations may vary from mild to severe life-threatening, it is pertinent to have objective tools for assessment of disease activity. These tools should not only be responsive but should also be discriminant.

The clinical manifestations in these disorders are not only because of disease activity but also because of accrual damage, either due to disease or therapy. As the irreversible damage may be due to healed disease or drug toxicity, this damage should be differentiated from disease activity to prevent undue immunosuppression. Multisystem nature of these disorders, and variability in disease activity in different organ systems makes the assessment difficult. Closely mimicking presentations of drug toxicity and infection compound the matters further. For example, hematuria in a patient with GPA could be due to relapse of the basic disease, hemorrhagic cystitis due to cyclophosphamide toxicity or urinary tract infection. Thus, the assessment of the current disease activity depends both upon clinical evaluation and investigations. There are various validated tools for measuring disease activity and damage, which have been used in various multicenter randomized controlled therapeutic trials. In the absence of a validated biomarker of disease activity, the structured assessment tools for a qualitative and quantitative assessment of systemic vasculitis are surrogate markers of disease activity. The future goal of therapy in vasculitis should be tailored treatment regimens for different clinical and these assessment tools should play an important role in achieving this goal.

TOOLS FOR ASSESSMENT

Histopathology

Histopathology not only provides the definitive evidence of organ involvement but also gives information on the extent of activity, damage and possible outcomes in patients with vasculitis.[4]

The biopsy should be done from the organ involved. The common sites for biopsy are sinuses, kidney and lungs in GPA; kidney and nerves in microscopic polyangiitis (MPA), nerves in eosinophilic granulomatosis with polyantiitis (EGPA) and polyarteritis nodosa (PAN) and temporal artery in giant cell arteritis (GCA). The yield of biopsy also varies considerably, e.g. from almost 100% yield in renal biopsy in patient with renal involvement to around 60% from nasal biopsy.[5,6] Although, histologic demonstration and grading of vasculitic injury would appear to be a gold standard, the patchy nature of involvement and the impracticality of repetitive biopsy, makes this unviable.

RADIOLOGICAL ASSESSMENT

Radiological investigations have a vital role in the diagnosis and assessment of the vasculitides. Chest X-ray and X-ray of the paranasal sinuses can help in making the initial diagnosis and monitoring of ANCA-associated vasculitis. Conventional arteriography can demonstrate aneurysms, occlusion and stenosis. However, this method has a limitation of being invasive and carries a substantial radiation exposure besides posing technical difficulties in patients with lengthy stenotic lesions. It is also unable to image the vessel wall.

COMPUTERIZED TOMOGRAPHY

Computerized tomography is not only helpful in assessing structural lesions but also monitoring the response to therapy. Most patients with GPA have paranasal sinus or lung involvement. The CT scan of nose and paranasal sinuses typically shows bone destruction in background of generalized mucosal thickening. The bone destruction is typically in midline affecting nasal septum and turbinate's initially and symmetrically extends laterally to involve the maxillary antrum and other sinuses with sclerotic changes of walls of sinus.[7] The end result is single large cavity with loss of nasal septum, turbinates and lateral walls of maxillary antrum.[8] The various CT findings in GPA can be lung nodules or masses. Nodules are usually multiple, bilateral, and subpleural. Bronchial wall thickening, large airways abnormality, patchy consolidation, and ground-glass shadowing can be the other findings. Pleural effusion is uncommon. Infiltrative lesions are more common in MPA and EGPA. Severely abnormal chest CT scans with involvement of $\geq 80\%$ of the lung parenchyma is an independent predictor of mortality.[9] The CT scanning of the chest is of value in the monitoring of disease in GPA. While the nodular infiltrates respond very well to treatment and often resolve completely, atelectasis, fibrotic bands and areas of bronchiectasis represent the damage/scars.

The CT angiography is superior to conventional angiography because both mural as well as luminal changes can be studied. Thus, it has a role in diagnosis and monitoring of Takayasu's arteritis (TA). The CT angiography can demonstrate stenosis, occlusions, aneurysms, concentric arterial wall thickening and heavy transmural calcification (differentiating from atherosclerosis) in chronic disease. CT angiography can also demonstrate microaneurysms or end organ changes in polyarteritis nodosa.

Magnetic resonance imaging and angiography provides information regarding the state of the vessel wall like vessel wall edema and progressive vessel wall thickening in large vessel vasculitis. The major limitations of MRA are an over estimation of the degree of stenosis; and poor correlation between gadolinium enhancement of the vessel wall and disease activity.[10]

ULTRASONOGRAPHY

Ultrasonography (USG) is useful modality with high sensitivity and specificity for diagnosis of temporal arteritis. There is a 'halo' around the temporal artery, which can be shown to resolve with institution of glucocorticoids. The USG has a sensitivity and specificity of 95% and 93% respectively when compared to histology.[11] It may play an important role in management, as the histological involvement of temporal arteries is patchy and can result in low sensitivity of temporal artery biopsy. A color Doppler ultrasound scoring system (CDUS) has been shown to have good correlation with Indian Takayasu clinical activity score (ITAS 2010) in patients of Takayasu's arteritis recently.[12]

POSITRON EMISSION TOMOGRAPHY

Positron emission tomography (PET) can be used to assess vessels with a caliber of ≥ 4 mm. It can demonstrate widespread, often clinically silent involvement of other areas in temporal arteritis like the involvement of subclavian arteries and the aorta.[13] It is not suitable for imaging temporal arteries due to the intense background signal from the brain. Diagnosis of large vessel vasculitis, particularly in the abdominal aorta should not be solely based on PET as inflammatory atherosclerotic plaques may exhibit isotope uptake. The PET is also useful in assessment of Takayasu arteritis.[14] A recent meta-analysis of six studies on the role of PET in assessing disease activity in Takayasu arteritis showed the pooled sensitivity, and specificity of 70.1% (95% CI, 58.6-80.0) and 77.2% respectively. The positive likelihood ratio and negative likelihood ratio were 2.313 and 0.341 respectively.[15]

SEROLOGICAL MARKERS IN DISEASE ASSESSMENT

Anti-neutrophil cytoplasmic antibodies (ANCA) are directed against primary granules of neutrophils and monocytes. Discovery of ANCA has been a major advancement in the diagnosis and understanding of the immunopathogenesis of small vessel vasculitis.[16,17] Two patterns are identified using an indirect immunofluorescence technique namely, C-ANCA (diffuse cytoplasmic uptake), and P-ANCA (perinuclear uptake). These antibodies are specifically targeted against antigens in the primary granules of neutrophils.

Proteinase 3 (PR3) and myeloperoxidase (MPO) are the two most relevant antigens and the ANCA to those antigens can be measured using an ELISA technique. The international consensus statement on reporting of ANCA recommends that both IIF and ELISA testing should be done when seeking to identify ANCA.[18] Role of ANCA in monitoring disease activity is controversial. Although it has been shown that PR 3 ANCA levels rise in patients with reactivation of GPA, upto one-third of patients may have a rise in these titers without any clinical consequence.[19] A recent study on relevance of monitoring PR3-ANCA titers in predicting relapse in GPA patients showed that no strict clinical-immunological correspondence was observed for 25% of the patients. It was concluded that GPA management cannot be based on ANCA levels alone.[20]

Erythrocyte sedimentation rate (ESR) and C-reactive protein (CRP) cannot differentiate between disease activity and infection. While normal ESR and CRP cannot exclude systemic vasculitis, their levels can be used for following up the therapeutic response.

CLINICAL INDICES OF DISEASE ASSESSMENT

The development of clinical assessment tools has been necessitated by the failure to develop any serological biomarker. The three domains of clinical assessment are: (1) disease activity (2) disease damage and (3) functional status. These indices help in bringing the objectivity to the outcomes of various treatment interventions.

DISEASE ACTIVITY

The cornerstone of disease activity assessment remains to be the clinical assessment. The clinical assessment tools take into account the clinical and laboratory data. The advantages of these assessment tool are reproducibility, a numeric score for future comparison, and a standardized way of data collection

INSTRUMENTS FOR ASSESSING DISEASE ACTIVITY

Various disease activity assessment tools have been developed and the ones that have been used commonly are as follows:
- Five-factor score (FFS)
- Groningen index
- Disease extent index (DEI)
- Birmingham vasculitis activity score (BVAS)
- Indian Takayasu clinical activity score (ITAS2010)

Five-Factor Score

Five-factor score (FFS) is a simple yet effective tool proposed in 1988.[21] The five-factors taken into account were proteinuria of > 1 g/day, renal insufficiency, gastrointestinal, cardiac and CNS involvement, with each component getting a score of one. This tool is a simple measure of disease activity that helps in prognostication. When FFS = 0, mortality at five years was 12%, when FFS = 1, mortality was 26% and when FFS was >2, mortality was 46%. Although, it has not been an established basis for treatment decisions, it seems logical to consider it during risk stratification. This score has been used for measuring disease activity in polyarteritis nodosa and EGPA.

Groningen Index

This is a GPA specific disease activity assessment tool. As both clinical and histological features are taken into consideration while determining the disease activity, its requirement of biopsy limits its value in serial assessment of disease activity.[22]

Disease Extent Index

The disease extent index (DEI) is again a GPA specific tool.[23] This is an extension of old ELK (ear/nose-throat, lung, kidney) system for GPA, first hinted at by Godman et al in 1954, but that was established by De Remee's group in 1976. A score is given to active disease in various organ systems namely ENT and upper airways, inflammatory eye lesions, heart, lung and lower airways, kidney, gastrointestinal tract, peripheral nervous system, central nervous system, skin, arthralgia/arthritis and also constitutional symptoms. Each organ system involvement is given a score of two irrespective of whether one or more than one manifestation are there in a system. The maximum score is 21. The most important thing is to ensure that all symptoms in an organ system are due to active vasculitis and other causes like infection/malignancy and damage have been excluded. DEI was developed for long term outcome studies to include full extent of GPA.

Vasculitis Activity Index

This score was introduced by a group in Baltimore .There are nine rating scales for the amount of disease activity in each organ system.[24] The laboratory abnormalities are also taken into account. Despite the possibility of an observer bias, it is a useful tool for experienced observers.

Birmingham Vasculitis Activity Score

This is the most widely used tool to quantify disease activity in systemic vasculitis presently in use. The original version (version 1) was developed by consensus expert opinion in 1994.[25] It consisted of 59 items grouped into nine organ systems. The BVAS was subsequently modified (version 2) for use in the European Vasculitis Study Group (EUVAS) trials and has been modified again, to its current version (version3; BVAS v.3).[26,27] The main difference between BVAS v. 3 and v. 2 is that the persistent boxes for each variable in version 2 have been replaced by a single box for the whole form, which is only ticked if all the items are due to persistent disease. Though there has been a reduction in the number of items from 64 to 56, the overall maximum score has been maintained. The weighting of items in the original version has remained relatively unchanged between the three versions. The maximum score is 63. The BVAS v. 3, which was initially validated in a cohort of 313 patients with mixed primary and secondary vasculitis from the UK, has also been revalidated in other cohorts.[28] The BVAS is an attempt to produce a tool with a strong emphasis on items determined clinically. A simplified disease specific version of BVAS was also developed for GPA (previously known as Wegener's granulomatosis). The BVAS calculator can be accessed online at http://www.epsnetwork.co.uk/BVAS/bvas_flow.html.

Indian Takayasu Clinical Activity Score

As the standard tools, BVAS and vasculitis damage index (VDI), did not perform well for the different disease patterns in Takayasu arteritis (TA), and MR and PET are expensive and lack established correlation with active inflammation, The Indian Rheumatology Association's Vasculitis (IRAVAS) group devised and validated a clinical index to capture the activity and damage of TA.[29,30] The Indian Takayasu Clinical Activity Score (ITAS) was initially derived from disease manifestations scored in the Disease Extent Index (DEI.Tak). The final ITAS2010 has 44 items with 33 features arising from the cardiovascular system. Seven key items are weighted to score 2 and all others score 1 only. This score has been used in various clinical studies, a few drug trials and as a comparator for validation of an ultrasound scoring system in takayasu arteritis.[12, 31-35]

DAMAGE

It is very important to understand that during the course of illness, the multisystem organ involvement will result in accrual damage in various organs and may result in some clinical manifestations. These manifestations may not only be due to the disease damage per se but also because of the detrimental effects of the drugs, procedures or therapeutic interventions.

The other important aspect of measuring the damage is its irreversibility and hence the damage score can either remain same or worsen over a period of time but can never improve.

VASCULITIS DAMAGE INDEX

The most comprehensive damage index available, and the most widely used instrument for assessing damage is VDI.[36] The 64 damage items grouped into 11 organ systems are represented in this index. In order to avoid scoring for disease activity, the damage has to be present for at least 3 months before it is scored. The measurement of damage may be for single time events like myocardial infarction and stroke, or even for chronic ongoing damage like persistent skin ulcers. This index has been widely used in trials of vasculitis and carries a prognostic value with a 6-month VDI score ≥4 associated with increased mortality. The regular use of VDI has shown that damage occurs early in the course of vasculitis.[37]

QUALITY OF LIFE ASSESSMENT

The outcomes of patients with vasculitides have improved significantly, and once fatal conditions have been converted in chronic disease states. The morbidity in these diseases however is still very significant, due to disease relapses and immunosuppressive treatment. Thus despite being in remission, there may be significant impairment in the quality of life and improvement in survival rates without improvement in functional status is not the most desirable outcome. There are disease specific tool for assess quality of life in vasculitides. The clinical instrument used is the Medical Outcomes Study 36 item Short-form General Health Survey (SF-36).[38] It has been translated and validated into several other languages. Since it is of a generic nature, it might fail to capture items more specific for patients with systemic vasculitis. There is no significant correlation between the VDI and any of the SF36 domains.

PATIENT REPORTED OUTCOMES

The outcomes are always measured in terms of the presentations considered important and most relevant by the physicians. These are dependent upon the type of different organ involvements in vasculitis. While these might be important to the physicians, the patient subjective experiences may represent key domains of illness that differ from physicians. In a study of 264 patients from three countries, fatigue (75%), followed by pain (31%), musculoskeletal symptoms (24%), difficult breathing (19%), financial aspects (13%), nasal discharge/crusting (14%) were the most common items reported from the free text sections. Severe manifestations like dialysis, seizures and oxygen dependency were ranked lower.[39] This study suggested that there are various manifestations, which are important to the patients but are not measured in the present outcome measures used in various clinical trials. This highlights the need for development and validation of patient reported outcome instrument in vasculitis.

KEY POINTS

- The primary systemic vasculitides have now become more chronic, manageable, diseases due to advancement in treatment options.
- In the absence of a biomarker of disease activity, proper assessment of vasculitides is important to differentiate damage from disease activity.
- These tools not only serve as an objective outcome measure in various clinical trials but also can help in day to day management of these patients.
- The BVAS (version 3) is the clinical tool of choice for assessment of disease activity in GPA.
- The ITAS2010 is a validated tool for assessing disease activity in TA.
- The VDI is the most commonly used tool for assessment of damage in vasculitis and also has a role in assessing prognosis.

REFERENCES

1. Bambery P, Sakhuja V, Bhusnurmath SR, et al. Wegener's granulomatosis: Clinical experience with eighteen patients. J Assosc Physicians India. 1992;40:597-600.
2. Malaviya AN, Kumar A, Singh YN, et al. Wegener's granulomatosis in India: not so rare. Br J Rheumatol. 1990;29:499-500.
3. Kumar A,Pandhi A, Menon A, et al. Wegener's granulomatosis in India: clinical features, treatment and outcome of twenty-five patients. Ind J Chest Dis Allied Sci. 2001;43:197-204.
4. Naidu GS, Sharma A, Nada R, et al. Histopathological classification of pauci-immune glomerulonephritis and its impact on outcome. Rheumatol Int. 2014 May 18. [Epub ahead of print]
5. Aasarod K, Bostad L, Hammerstrom J, et al. Renal histopathology and clinical course in 94 patients with Wegener's granulomatosis. Nephrol Dial Transplant. 2001;16: 953-60.
6. Devaney KO, Travis WD, Hoffman G, et al. Interpretation of head and neck biopsies in Wegener's granulomatosis. A pathologic study of 126 biopsies in 70 patients. Am J Surg Pathol. 1990;14: 555-64.
7. Lloyd G, Lund VJ, Beale T, et al. Rhinologic changes in Wegener's granulomatosis. J Laryngol Otol. 2002;116: 565-9.
8. Simmons JT, Leavitt R, Kornblut AD, et al. CT of the paranasal sinuses and orbits in patients with Wegener's granulomatosis. Ear Nose Throat J. 1987;66:134-40.
9. Lohrmann C, Uhl M, Kotter E, et al. Pulmonary manifestations of Wegener granulomatosis: CT findings in 57 patients and a review of the literature. Eur J Radiol. 2005;53:471-7.
10. Andrews J, Al-Nahhas A, Pennell D, et al. Non-invasive imaging in the diagnosis and management of Takayasu's arteritis. Ann Rheum Dis. 2004;63:995-1000.
11. Schmidt WA, Gromnica E. Incidence of temporal arteritis in patients with polymyalgia rheumatica: a prospective study using colour Doppler ultrasonography of the temporal arteries. Rheumatology (Oxford) 2002;41:46-52.
12. Sinha D, Mondal S, Nag A, Ghosh A. Development of a colour Doppler ultrasound scoring system in patients of Takayasu's arteritis and its correlation with clinical activity score (ITAS 2010). Rheumatology. 2013;52:196-202.
13. Blockmans D, Stroobants S, Maes A, et al. Positron emission tomography in giant cell arteritis and polymyalgia rheumatica: evidence for inflammation of the aortic arch. Am J Med 2000;108:246-9.
14. Santhosh S, Mittal BR, Gayana S, Bhattacharya A, Sharma A, Jain S. F-18 FDG PET/CT in the evaluation of Takayasu arteritis: an experience from the tropics. J Nucl Cardiol. 2014 May 30. [Epub ahead of print].
15. Cheng Y, Lv N, Wang Z, et al. 18-FDG-PET in assessing disease activity in Takayasu arteritis: a meta-analysis. Clin Exp Rheumatol. 2013;31:S22-7.
16. van der Woude FJ, Rasmussen N, Lobatto S, et al. Autoantibodies against neutrophils and monocytes: tool for diagnosis and marker of disease activity in Wegener's granulomatosis. Lancet 1985;1:425-9.
17. Davies DJ, Moran JE, Niall J, et al. Segmental necrotising glomerulonephritis with antineutrophil antibody: possible arbovirus aetiology. Br Med J (Clin Res Ed). 1982;285:606.
18. Savige J, Paspaliaris B, Silvestrini R, et al. A review of immunofluorescent pattern associated with anti neutrophil cytoplasmic antibodies (ANCA) and their differentiation from other autoantibodies. J Clin Pathol. 1998;51:568-75.
19. Boosma MM, Stegeman CA, van der Leij MJ, et al. Prediction of relapse in Wegener's granulomatosis by measurement of anti

neutrophil cytoplasmic antibody levels: a prospective study. Arthritis Rheum 2000;43:2025-33.

20. Thai LH, Charles P, Resche-Rigon M, et al. Are anti-proteinase-3 ANCA a useful marker of granulomatosis with polyangiitis (Wegener's) relapses? Results of a retrospective study on 126 patients. Autoimmun Rev. 2014;13:313-8.

21. Guillevin L, Lhote F, Gayraud M, et al. Prognostic factors in polyarteritis nodosa and Churg-Strauss syndrome. A prospective study in 342 patients, Medicine (Baltimore) 1996;75:17-28.

22. Kallenberg CG, Tervaert JW, Stageman CA, et al. Criteria for disease activity in Wegener's granulomatosis: a requirement for longitudinal studies. APMIS Suppl. 1990;19:37-9.

23. de Groot K, Gross WL, Herlyn K, et al. Development and validation of disease extent index for Wegener's granulomatosis. Clin Nephrol. 2001;55:31-8.

24. Whiting-O'Keefe QE, Stone JH, Hellman DB, et al Validity of vasculitis activity index for systemic necrotizing vasculitis. Arthritis Rheum. 1999;42:2365-71.

25. Luqmani RA, Bacon PA Moots RJ, et al. Birmingham vasculitis activity score (BVAS) in systemic necrotizing vasculitis. Quart J Med. 1994;87:671-8.

26. Luqmani RA, Exley AR, Kitas GD, et al. Disease assessment and management of the vasculitides. Baillieres Clin Rheumatol. 1997;11:423-46.

27. Mukhtyar C, Lee R, Brown D, et al. Modification and validation of the Birmingham vasculitis activity score (version 3). Ann Rheum Dis. 2009;68:1827-32.

28. Suppiah R, Mukhtyar C, Flossman O, et al. A cross-sectional study of the Birmingham Vasculitis Activity Score version 3 in systemic vasculitis. Rheumatology (Oxford). 2011;50: 899-905.

29. Sivakumar MR, Misra RN, Bacon PA, et al. The Indian perspective of Takayasu arteritis and development of a disease extent index (DEI.TAK) to assess Takayasu arteritis. Rheumatology 2005;44, iii6-iii7.

30. Misra R, Danda D, Rajappa SM, et al. Indian Rheumatology Vasculitis (IRAVAS) group. Development and initial validation of the Indian Takayasu Clinical Activity Score (ITAS2010). Rheumatology (Oxford). 2013;52:1795-801.

31. Goel R, Kumar TS, Danda D, et al. Childhood-onset Takayasu arteritis-Experience from a tertiary care center in South India. J Rheumatol. 2014;41:1183-9

32. Kumar S, Goel R, Danda D, et al. A103: childhood onset Takayasu arteritis-experience from a tertiary care centre in South India. Arthritis Rheumatol. 2014;66:S139.

33. Goel R, Danda D, Kumar S, et al. Rapid control of disease activity by tocilizumab in 10 'difficult-to-treat' cases of Takayasu arteritis. Int J Rheum Dis. 2013;16:754-61.

34. Salvarani C, Magnani L, Catanoso M, et al. Tocilizumab: a novel therapy for patients with large-vessel vasculitis. Rheumatology (Oxford). 2012;51:151-6.

35. Goel R, Danda D, Mathew J, et al. Mycophenolate mofetil in Takayasu's arteritis. Clin Rheumatol. 2010;29:329-32.

36. Exley AR, Bacon PA, Luqmani R, et al. Development and initial validation of the vasculitis damage index (VDI) for standardized clinical assessment of damage in systemic vasculitides. Arthritis Rheum. 1997;40:371-80.

37. Exley A, Carruthers DM, Luqmani RA, et al. Damage occurs early in systemic vascultis and is an index of outcome. Quart J Med. 1997;90:391-9.

38. Ware JE, Scherbourne CD. The MOS 36-item short-form health survey(SF-36).1.Conceptual framework and item selection. Med Care. 1992;30:473-83.

39. HerlynK, Hellmich B, Seo P, et al. Patient reported outcome assessment in vasculitis may provide important data and a unique perspective. Arthritis Care Res. 2010;62:1639-45.

CHAPTER **26**

Newer and Future Treatment of Vasculitis

David Jayne

INTRODUCTION

Glucocorticoids were first used in granulomatosis with polyangiitis (GPA, previously known as Wegener's granulomatosis) and polyarteritis in the late 1940s and a randomized trial of ACTH performed by the Medical Research Council (UK) reported better survival of polyarteritis at one year.[1] In a retrospective survey of polyarteritis, mortality was lower with combination azathioprine/glucocorticoid therapy than glucocorticoids alone or no therapy. Cyclophosphamide was first used in GPA by Novack and Pearson in 1967 and subsequently by Fauci and colleagues at the National Institutes of Health (USA).[2] It became apparent that the combination of cyclophosphamide and glucocorticoids resulted in stable remissions in GPA and polyarteritis and permitted reduction or withdrawal of glucocorticoids. The toxicity of cyclophosphamide, especially the risks of infertility and malignancy has subsequently encouraged the development of alternative therapies.

Rituximab is established as an alternative to cyclophosphamide for remission induction in ANCA vasculitis.[3] It represents the first drug that has achieved a license for the treatment of ANCA vasculitis. High-dose glucocorticoids are now the major cause of early adverse events in vasculitis therapy and a target for future drug development. Improved understanding of the biology of vasculitis has offered up a range of further targets for future therapy.

CURRENT OUTCOMES

Vasculitis patients continue to have a higher mortality than a matched background population as shown by a recent study of long-term outcomes of patients recruited to the European Vasculitis Study Group (EUVAS) studies (EUVAS, European Vasculitis Society). The mortality rate ratio was 2.6 compared to a control population, with advanced renal failure, increasing age and a high disease activity at diagnosis being the main adverse predicators.[4] Several other studies have identified increasing age and worsening renal function as poor prognostic markers. The MPO-ANCA subtype appears to predict both worse renal and patient survival. The increase in mortality is highest in the first year with one, two and five years survival being 88%, 85% and 78%. Disease and therapy-related deaths, particularly infection, account for the majority of deaths in the first year. While infection remains an important cause beyond the first year, malignancy and cardiovascular becomes more common with longer follow-up.

The majority of vasculitis patients develop at least one item of irreversible damage as a result of vasculitis or its therapy.[5] Damage of the upper respiratory tract is common in GPA with deafness, and chronic nasal and sinus symptomatology. Twenty percent of patients develop end-stage renal disease (ESRD) by five years with more having chronic kidney disease of less severity. Renal survival is associated with serum creatinine at diagnosis and the percentage of normal glomeruli in the renal biopsy. However even in those presenting with severe histological findings and low numbers of normal glomeruli, treatment should be given as the chance of renal recovery is greater than for therapy-related death. A renal histology score has been developed with four categories associating with a progressively worse renal survival, focal, crescentic, mixed and fibrotic.

Relapse occurs in around 50% by five years.[6] Many factors are associated with an increased relapse risk including treatment reduction or withdrawal, diagnosis of GPA, PR3-ANCA subtype, persisting ANCA positivity after induction therapy, respiratory involvement, younger age, nasal carriage of *Staphylococcus aureus* and absence of severe renal involvement. Relapses are categorized as minor/non-severe or major/severe if vasculitic activity threatens vital organ function. Relapse is not a mortality predictor suggesting that the majority of relapses do not contribute to vital organ dysfunction. However, therapy must be prolonged to prevent relapse and appropriate monitoring instituted to detect relapse at an early stage. A CD8+ T-cell transcription signature, using microarray analysis of purified T cells, has been identified that can predict patients at risk of relapse. The subset of genes defining the poor prognostic group were enriched for genes involved in the IL-7 receptor pathway, T cell receptor signaling and genes expressed by memory T cells.[7]

NEWER THERAPIES

Rituximab

B-cell depletion with rituximab is as effective as cyclophosphamide for the induction of remission of in GPA or microscopic polyangiitis (MPA). The RITUXVAS trial employed two cyclophosphamide pulses with rituximab 375 mg/m^2/week x 4, but the results in the RAVE trial, with the same rituximab dose but no cyclophosphamide, were similar.[8,9] No early benefits of cyclophosphamide avoidance were observed in either trial. The relapse risk after rituximab in the RAVE trial when no remission therapy was employed was the same as for cyclophosphamide followed by azathioprine.[10] Rituximab can be recommended as an alternative to cyclophosphamide for remission induction and is preferred when cyclophosphamide is contraindicated, for example, by infection, cytopenia, intolerance, malignancy or fertility protection. A simpler regimen of rituximab 1 g repeated after 14 days appears to be similar in efficacy to the four dose regimen.[11] Rituximab is now the favored treatment for refractory vasculitis and has delivered to most benefit to patients in this subgroup where there are few alternatives.

Relapse rates after rituximab are particularly high when treating relapsing disease with rituximab.[12] Controversy exists as to the best relapse prevention management with alternatives including conventional immunosuppressives, azathioprine or methotrexate, further rituximab at time of relapse, or at time of B cell or ANCA return, or fixed interval repeat dose rituximab as maintenance therapy.[13] The latter approach has been successful in the MAINRITSAN trial, where after cyclophosphamide induction 1 g of rituximab at 6 months followed by 500 mg every 6 months was more effective than azathioprine. The RITAZAREM trial is comparing a regimen of fixed interval repeat dose rituximab to azathioprine for patients receiving rituximab as treatment of relapsing GPA or MPA.

The use of rituximab is increasing in patients with AAV. No change in infection rates was observed when rituximab was substituted for cyclophosphamide in two induction trials. Whether this reflects an infection risk with rituximab similar to cyclophosphamide or the role of concomitant high-dose steroid is unclear. *Progressive multifocal leukoencephalopathy*, caused by the JC virus, has occurred in AAV patients treated with rituximab but it is unclear whether the prevalence of PML is actually increased by rituximab.[14] Patients should be counseled that such a risk might exist. Infusion reactions to rituximab occur in 20% but have been mild without sequelae and have not prevented repeat treatment. Hypogammaglobulinemia occurs after rituximab in a minority and is related to the use of previous immunosuppressives, cumulative exposure to rituximab and length of follow-up.[15] While mild reductions of IgG do not appear to influence infective risk, severe deficiency to below 3 g/L has occurred and led to recurrent infection and need for immunoglobulin replacement. Rituximab impairs the humoral response to immunizations, and, where possible, these should be administered at least two weeks before, or four months after, rituximab.

Methotrexate

Cyclophosphamide substitution by methotrexate, dosed at 20–25 mg/week, for non-severe AAV presentations was found to be effective in the NORAM trial with similar remission rates at six months.[16] Enthusiasm for this approach has waned with a higher relapse rate following methotrexate induction and higher subsequent glucocorticoid and cyclophosphamide requirement in a five year follow-up report of this study.[17] Also, non-severe patients accrue high frequencies of organ damage and chronic morbidity, so more aggressive strategies are justified. As a remission maintenance agent after cyclophosphamide induction, methotrexate was equivalent to azathioprine in the WEGENT trial.[18]

Mycophenolate Mofetil

In a recent trial comparing mycophenolate mofetil (MMF) to cyclophosphamide for remission induction of new patients with early or generalized AAV, the MMF group had similar response at six months but more relapses by 18 months. The increased relapse risk with MMF occurred in PR3-ANCA positive patients and MMF may be a more appropriate treatment for the MPO-ANCA subgroup.[19] The MMF was shown not to be superior to azathioprine for the prevention of relapse in the IMPROVE trial and is now only recommended after azathioprine has failed in patients in whom methotrexate is contraindicated.[20]

Plasma Exchange

Plasma exchange improves the chances of renal recovery in those presenting in renal failure, creatinine> 500 μmol, but it is uncertain whether it also has a role in renal vasculitis with deteriorating, renal function below this level, or in severe non-renal presentations, such as, diffuse alveolar hemorrhage.[21] A meta-analysis failed to confirm a significant benefit of plasma exchange on the composite outcome of death and end stage renal disease.[22] The increasing evidence for the pathogenicity of ANCA in renal vasculitis provides a rationale for its use, but removal of coagulation factors, cytokines or other substances may also be important. Plasma filtration or centrifugation appear equally effective and, on average, seven daily or alternate day exchanges of 1–1.5 plasma volumes are used. Double filtration apheresis, selective IgG and MPO-ANCA selective immunoabsorption have also been employed but until there is better understanding of the mechanisms of plasma exchange, non-selective procedures are preferred. The procedure usually requires central vascular access, and may be complicated by hemorrhage and thrombocytopenia. Volume replacement with albumin is recommended but plasma or coagulation factor rich plasma fractions are used in the setting of increased bleeding risk, such as, after a renal biopsy or in the presence of alveolar hemorrhage. The ongoing PEXIVAS trial is assessing the benefit of plasma exchange in prevention death and end stage renal disease in patients with renal AAV or alveolar hemorrhage.[23]

Intravenous Immunoglobulin

Intravenous immunoglobulin reduces disease activity in refractory AAV but the effect lasts ≤ 3 months.[24] This option can be considered if conventional therapy is contraindicated, for example, by infection or in pregnancy. A potential mechanism of immunoglobulin, as proposed in Kawasaki disease, is the neutralization of microbial toxins. Blockade of tumor necrosis alpha with infliximab or etanercept has led to remission when used also as an additional agent but prolonged use appears ineffective and it may increase the risks of infection.[25]

Other Newer Agents

Patients failing to achieve remission by six months, or possibly before, should have their non-glucocorticoid treatment reassessed as for progressive disease. Deoxyspergualin (gusperimus) is an immunosuppressive with a range of activity on the innate and cognate immune systems that has demonstrated high response levels in refractory GPA.[26] Leukopenia is common but rapidly reversible and not accompanied by increased infection frequency. There does not appear to be a sustained effect after deoxyspergualin withdrawal when relapses are common. Lymphocyte, eosinophil and macrophage depletion with the anti-CD52 therapeutic antibody alemtuzumab has led to sustained treatment free remissions.[27] The profound, transient lymphopenia induced by alemtuzumab is poorly tolerated in those over 60 or with impaired renal function. Those relapsing are treated as described above with multiple minor relapses or at least one major relapse requiring a change of immunosuppressive. Changing the non-cyclophosphamide immunosuppressive, for example, from azathioprine to methotrexate, or vice versa, or switching to mycophenolic acid preparations or leflunomide, can be considered.[28]

OTHER FORMS OF VASCULITIS

Eosinophilic Granulomatosis with Polyangiitis (EGPA, Churg Strauss Syndrome)

A similar approach to GPA and MPA is adopted with cyclophosphamide and high dose glucocorticoids for severe EGPA. Non-severe disease has been treated with glucocorticoids alone but this has led to a high relapse frequency and glucocorticoid exposure, which is probably reduced by using azathioprine or other immunosuppressive. Rituximab has been used in small case series with similar levels of success to GPA.[29] The interleukin 5 inhibitor, mepolizumab is under evaluation for EGPA and has shown promise in two small non-randomized trials.[30]

Large Vessel Vasculitis

Glucocorticoids remain the standard therapy for giant cell arteritis and Takayasu's disease but are associated with considerable toxicity. Tumor necrosis factor inhibitors, such as infliximab have been used for refractory or relapsing disease but did not have efficacy in a double blind induction trial.[31] Tocilizumab, an anti-interleukin 6 receptor antibody, is also used as a treatment for refractory disease and is being evaluated as a routine induction agent for giant cell arteritis in the GIACTA trial (Giant Cell Arteritis Clinical Research Study).

FUTURE THERAPIES FOR VASCULITIS

Depleting B-cells

Other anti-CD20 and anti-CD19 antibodies have been developed, with increased affinity, reduced immunogenicity, improved antibody-dependent cellular cytotoxicity (ADCC) or complement-dependent cytotoxicity: humanized ocrelizumab has been tested-but abandoned because of high infectious complications rate-in lupus nephritis and fully humanized ofatuzumab, has not yet been used in nephrology.

Other depleting monoclonal antibodies targeting multiple cell populations, including B-cells, are actually evaluated in autoimmune glomerulonephritides. Alemtuzumab (or Campath-1), an anti-CD52 antibody targeting B-cells, activated T-cells and monocytes has been used in to treat refractory renal transplant rejection and is being evaluated in relapsing ANCA-vasculitis (NCT01405807). Milatuzumab, a depleting antibody that binds to CD74, a marker expressed by cells of both T and B lymphocyte lineages, is tested in B-cell malignancy and lupus nephritis (NCT01845740).

Blocking B-cell Activation

Belimumab is a monoclonal antibody that inhibits the B-cell activating factor (BAFF), also known as B-lymphocyte stimulator (BLyS). This agent has been approved for treatment of SLE but the major phase III trials of belimumab did not include patients with severe renal involvement.[32] Belimumab is now being evaluated in ANCA vasculitis (BREVAS study, NCT01663623). Of interest, two other anti-BAFF agents, tabalumab and blisibimod, are also being tested in SLE (NCT01196091) and IgA nephropathy (NCT02062684 and NCT02052219). Finally, atacicept, a soluble recombinant fusion protein that inhibits both BAFF and APRIL, another B-cell stimulating factor, is being evaluated in SLE.[33]

Epratuzumab is a new monoclonal antibody targeting B-cells. The target of epratuzumab is CD22, a transmembrane sialoglycoprotein expressed on mature B-cell lineage, involved in activation and migration of these lymphocytes. Administration of this molecule induces mild B-cell depletion but marked B-cell anergy, via a mechanism called trogocytosis. Although not yet tested in lupus nephritis,

preliminary studies have shown interesting results in moderate-to-severe forms of SLE.[34]

A new potential way to interfere with B-cell activation is targeting of the spleen tyrosine kinase (Syk). This tyrosine kinase is recruited and activated after B-cell receptor (BCR) signaling and is crucial for several downstream events amplifying the B-cell response. Fostamatinib is a selective inhibitor of Syk. Importantly, Syk is also involved in the activation of mesangial cells after IgA1 binding, leading to production of proinflammatory cytokines in the glomerulus and cell proliferation. Although its development in rheumatoid arthritis has been stopped due to lack of efficacy, preclinical data have shown efficacy in experimental vasculitis.[35]

Inhibiting Complement Activation

Eculizumab is the first-in-class agent that binds and inhibits the complement compound C5, interrupting the final steps of the complement cascade. By inhibiting the cleavage of C5 by C5 convertase, it prevents the production of C5a (a potent proinflammatory anaphylatoxin) and the formation of the membrane-attack complex (terminal complement complex C5b-9) responsible for cell destruction. Eculizumab has been approved in atypical hemolytic uremic syndrome (aHUS), even if some uncertainties remain concerning the exact indications and the duration of this expensive treatment. Nevertheless, eculizumab may also have efficacy in other glomerular diseases involving alternative pathway activation such as membranoproliferative glomerulonephritis and C3 glomerulopathy or endothelial dysfunction - such as catastrophic antiphospholipid syndrome or antibody-mediated acute rejection in kidney transplantation. Other complement inhibitors are under development, including CCX168, which is a small molecule, targeting the C5a receptor. C5a is released when the C5 convertase cleaves C5 and has a role in chemotaxis and inflammatory response activation. Based on the observation that complement activation is crucial in ANCA-associated renal vasculitis and that C5a receptor mediates neutrophil activation, this drug is being tested in human disease, in association with a cyclophosphamide-based immunosuppressive regimen (NCT01363388). In the animal model of anti-MPO associated nephropathy using a transgenic mouse expressing the human C5a receptor, CCX168 significantly improved the glomerular lesions and reduced both hematuria and proteinuria.[36] Of interest, a soluble complement receptor 1 (CR1), named CDX-1135 has been used in dense-deposit disease (NCT01791686). This molecule blocks the complement cascade by regulating both C3 and C5-convertase by a process known as decay-acceleration. Nevertheless, this phase 1 trial was prematurely discontinued, due to lack of efficacy of CDX-1135 in this type of nephropathy. One of the most promising molecules in this field is TT30, which is a novel therapeutic fusion protein combining the C3-binding domain of complement receptor 2 (CR2) with the inhibitory region of factor H. This biologic agent targeting specifically the complement alternative pathway is effective in different animal models and is actually in evaluation in a phase 1 safety study. Recombinant C1 inhibitor is given in hereditary angioedema, a disease characterized by a genetic deficiency of this enzyme, but it is also actually under evaluation for the treatment of antibody-mediated acute rejection in renal transplantation.

Blocking Systemic Inflammation

Biologic agents targeting the major cytokines involved in systemic inflammation, such as tumor necrosis factor alpha (TNF-α), interleukin 1 (IL-1) or interleukin 6 (IL-6) have been used in rheumatology or gastroenterology for many years, showing good results in diseases such as rheumatoid arthritis, ankylosing spondylitis or inflammatory bowel disease.

As concerning the direct anti-inflammatory action of these drugs, an open-label clinical trial was published 10 years ago, suggesting that infliximab was effective at inducing remission in patients refractory ANCA vasculitis, when combined with standard immunosuppressive drugs. However, a controlled randomized trial evaluating etanercept in granulomatous forms of ANCA vasculitis, showed no beneficial effects on the rate of disease relapse.[37]

Several studies have demonstrated a pivotal role of a newer cytokine, called (TNF)-like weak inducer of apoptosis (TWEAK) in the physiopathology of lupus nephritis. This soluble cytokine is released by inflammatory cells that infiltrate the kidney, such as neutrophils or macrophages, and promote renal cell activation, proliferation and apoptosis, endothelial cell activation and fibrosis.[38] Urinary levels or TWEAK correlate with disease activity in human LN and blockade or deficiency of the TWEAK pathway in animal models of LN results in improvement of renal damage. BIIB023, is a monoclonal antibody against TWEAK in clinical development for the treatment of LN. The ATLAS study (NCT01499355)—Anti-T weak in lupus nephritis patient study—is an ongoing randomized double-blind placebo-controlled, proof of concept study evaluating this new biologic in patients with active lupus nephritis.

Interfering with Lymphocyte Costimulation and Activation Pathways

Abatacept, is a fusion protein composed of the extracellular domain of CTLA-4 and the Fc fragment of IgG1. Binding to CD80 (B7-1) on antigen-presenting cells (APC), abatacept inhibits the costimulation of T-cells. This molecule, actually used in anti-TNF-resistant rheumatoid arthritis, has been evaluated in a small study in patients with non-severe GPA where it appeared effective.[39] Inhibition of the CD40-CD40L costimulatory pathway by a monoclonal anti-CD40L antibody was also tested in autoimmunity. Although preliminary studies showed an impact both on immunological and urinary markers (hematuria and proteinuria), it had to be stopped prematurely because of an increased risk of thromboembolic complications. Alternatives agents that inhibit CD40:CD4 ligand interactions have been developed.

Complications and Barriers of Future Therapies

Some of the main complications of biologics are due to their specific effects. For instance, inhibition of B-cells can lead to hypogammaglobulinemia and subsequent increase in infectious complication rate.[15] Allergic or hypersensitivity reactions can sometimes be observed, even if newer, fully humanized biological agents tend to be safer. Antidrug antibodies such as human antichimeric antibodies (HACA) can sometimes be detected, not always neutralizing the effects of the drug but leading sometimes to decrease of its efficacy or to clinical adverse events, such as infusion reactions. Finally, vasculitis patients may require specific tailoring of the therapeutic regimen, with reduced doses of drugs in cases of renal dysfunction, or increased doses in cases of nephrotic syndrome, where part of the drug can be eliminated in the urine due to excessive glomerular permeability. For instance, it has been reported that nephrotic patients with membranous nephritis treated with rituximab have shorter duration of B-cell depletion when compared with patients with other autoimmune diseases and no kidney involvement.

CONCLUSION

Major stages in the evolution of vasculitis therapy have been the introduction of glucocorticoids, the combination of cyclophosphamide with glucocorticoids, the use of alternative immunosuppressives to maintain remission, and the introduction of rituximab. As a result, the outlook for patients with vasculitis has been slowly improving. However, many problems with current therapies remain and there are uncertainties as to how to dose rituximab. None of the current approaches are curative and vasculitis patients continue to require prolonged medical follow-up. Newer agents have allowed reduced glucocorticoid and cyclophosphamide exposure, which is reducing some of the irreversible drug associated toxicity that occurred in the past. The development of international collaborative networks, such as the European Vasculitis Society (EUVAS) and Vasculitis Clinical research Consortium (VCRC) have enabled trials to be performed and provide a platform for the testing of future therapies.

ACKNOWLEDGMENT

David Jayne is supported by the Cambridge Biomedical Research Centre.

DISCLOSURES

David Jayne has received research grants from Roche/Genentech and Sanofi/Genzyme. He has received consultancy fees from BIOGEN, Chemocentryx, GSK, Merck Serono, and Roche/Genentech.

KEY POINTS

- The traditional treatment of ANCA vasculitis with high dose glucocorticoids and cyclophosphamide is effective in the majority of patients but associated with early and late treatment related morbidity and mortality.
- Rituximab is an alternative to cyclophosphamide now licensed for the treatment of ANCA vasculitis in many countries. It is especially useful in the management of refractory and relapsing disease.
- Relapse after rituximab is common and there is uncertainty as to how to reduce relapse risk. Fixed interval repeat dose rituximab is an option under evaluation.
- Although well tolerated rituximab is associated with a risk of low immunoglobulin levels in vasculitis patients that lead to an increased rate of infections and, occasionally, the need for supplemental immunoglobulins.
- Many newer immunotherapeutic agents are potential future treatments for vasculitis, including complement and cytokine inhibitors and blockade of co-stimulatory interactions.

REFERENCES

1. Moore PM, Beard EC, Thoburn TW, et al. Idiopathic (lethal) granuloma of the midline facial tissues treated with cortisone: Report of a case. Trans Am Laryngol Rhinol Otol Soc. 1951;57:154-65.
2. Fauci AS, Katz P, Haynes BF, et al. Cyclophosphamide therapy of severe systemic necrotizing vasculitis. N Engl J Med. 1979;301:235-8.
3. Guerry MJ, Brogan P, Bruce IN, et al. Recommendations for the use of rituximab in anti-neutrophil cytoplasm antibody-associated vasculitis. Rheumatology (Oxford) 2012;51:634-43.
4. Flossmann O, Berden A, de Groot K, et al. Long-term patient survival in ANCA-associated vasculitis. Ann Rheum Dis. 2011;70:488-94.
5. Robson J, Doll H, Suppiah R, et al. Damage in the ANCA-associated vasculitides: Long-term data from the European Vasculitis Study Group (EUVAS) therapeutic trials. Ann Rheum Dis. 2013;doi: 10.1136/annrheumdis-2013-203927.
6. Walsh M, Flossmann O, Berden A, et al. Risk factors for relapse of antineutrophil cytoplasmic antibody-associated vasculitis. Arthritis Rheum. 2012;64:542-8.
7. McKinney EF, Lyons PA, Carr EJ, et al. A CD8+ T-cell transcription signature predicts prognosis in autoimmune disease. Nat Med. 2010;16:586-91.
8. Jones RB, Tervaert JW, Hauser T, et al. Rituximab versus cyclophosphamide in ANCA-associated renal vasculitis. N Engl J Med. 2010;363:211-20.
9. Stone JH, Merkel PA, Spiera R, et al. Rituximab versus cyclophosphamide for ANCA-associated vasculitis. N Engl J Med. 2010;363:221-32.
10. Specks U, Merkel PA, Seo P, et al. Efficacy of remission-induction regimens for ANCA-associated vasculitis. N Engl J Med. 2013;369:417-27.
11. Jones RB, Ferraro AJ, Chaudhry AN, et al. A multicenter survey of rituximab therapy for refractory antineutrophil cytoplasmic antibody-associated vasculitis. Arthritis Rheum. 2009;60:2156-68.
12. Smith RM, Jones RB, Guerry MJ, et al. Rituximab for remission maintenance in relapsing antineutrophil cytoplasmic antibody-associated vasculitis. Arthritis Rheum. 2012;64:3760-9.
13. Cartin-Ceba R, Golbin JM, Keogh KA, et al. Rituximab for remission induction and maintenance in refractory granulomatosis with polyangiitis (Wegener's): Ten-year experience at a single center. Arthritis Rheum. 2012;64:3770-8.
14. Pugnet G, Pagnoux C, Bezanahary H, et al. Progressive multifocal encephalopathy after cyclophosphamide in granulomatosis with polyangiitis (Wegener) patients: Case report and review of literature. Clin Exp Rheumatol. 2013;31:S62-4.
15. Marco H, Smith RM, Jones RB, et al. The effect of rituximab therapy on immunoglobulin levels in patients with multisystem autoimmune disease. BMC Musculoskelet Disord. 2014;15:178.
16. De Groot K, Rasmussen N, Bacon PA, et al. Randomized trial of cyclophosphamide versus methotrexate for induction of remission in early systemic antineutrophil cytoplasmic antibody-associated vasculitis. Arthritis Rheum. 2005;52:2461-9.

17. Faurschou M, Westman K, Rasmussen N, et al. Brief report: Long-term outcome of a randomized clinical trial comparing methotrexate to cyclophosphamide for remission induction in early systemic antineutrophil cytoplasmic antibody-associated vasculitis. Arthritis Rheum. 2012;64:3472-7.

18. Pagnoux C, Mahr A, Hamidou MA, et al. Azathioprine or methotrexate maintenance for ANCA-associated vasculitis. N Engl J Med. 2008;359:2790-803.

19. Hu W, Liu C, Xie H, et al. Mycophenolate mofetil versus cyclophosphamide for inducing remission of ANCA vasculitis with moderate renal involvement. Nephrol Dial Transplant. 2008;23:1307-12.

20. Hiemstra TF, Walsh M, Mahr A, et al. Mycophenolate mofetil vs azathioprine for remission maintenance in antineutrophil cytoplasmic antibody-associated vasculitis: A randomized controlled trial. JAMA. 2010;304:2381-8.

21. Jayne DR, Gaskin G, Rasmussen N, et al. Randomized trial of plasma exchange or high-dosage methylprednisolone as adjunctive therapy for severe renal vasculitis. J Am Soc Nephrol. 2007;18:2180-8.

22. Walsh M, Catapano F, Szpirt W, et al. Plasma exchange for renal vasculitis and idiopathic rapidly progressive glomerulonephritis: A meta-analysis. Am J Kidney Dis. 2011;57:566-74.

23. Walsh M, Merkel PA, Peh CA, et al. Plasma exchange and glucocorticoid dosing in the treatment of anti-neutrophil cytoplasm antibody associated vasculitis (pexivas): Protocol for a randomized controlled trial. Trials. 2013;14:73.

24. Jayne DR, Chapel H, Adu D, et al. Intravenous immunoglobulin for anca-associated systemic vasculitis with persistent disease activity. QJM. 2000;93:433-9.

25. Booth A, Harper L, Hammad T, et al. Prospective study of TNF-alpha blockade with infliximab in anti-neutrophil cytoplasmic antibody-associated systemic vasculitis. J Am Soc Nephrol. 2004;15:717-21.

26. Perenyei M, Jayne DR, Flossmann O. Gusperimus: Immunological mechanism and clinical applications. Rheumatology (Oxford) 2014;doi: 10.1093/rheumatology/ket451.

27. Walsh M, Chaudhry A, Jayne D. Long-term follow-up of relapsing/refractory anti-neutrophil cytoplasm antibody associated vasculitis treated with the lymphocyte depleting antibody alemtuzumab (campath-1h). Ann Rheum Dis. 2008;67:1322-7.

28. Metzler C, Miehle N, Manger K, et al. Elevated relapse rate under oral methotrexate versus leflunomide for maintenance of remission in Wegener's granulomatosis. Rheumatology (Oxford). 2007;46:1087-91.

29. Koukoulaki M, Smith KG, Jayne DR. Rituximab in Churg-Strauss syndrome. Ann Rheum Dis. 2006;65:557-9.

30. Kim S, Marigowda G, Oren E, et al. Mepolizumab as a steroid-sparing treatment option in patients with Churg-Strauss syndrome. J Allergy Clin Immunol. 2010;125:1336-43.

31. Langford CA. L41. Perspectives on the treatment of giant cell arteritis. Presse Med. 2013;42:609-12.

32. Furuta S, Jayne D. Emerging therapies in antineutrophil cytoplasm antibody-associated vasculitis. Curr Opin Rheumatol. 2014;26:1-6.

33. Isenberg D, Gordon C, Licu D, et al. Efficacy and safety of atacicept for prevention of flares in patients with moderate-to-severe systemic lupus erythematosus (SLE): 52-week data (april-SLE randomised trial). Ann Rheum Dis. 2014; doi:10.1136/annrheumdis-2013-205067.

34. Rossi EA, Chang CH, Goldenberg DM. Anti-cd22/cd20 bispecific antibody with enhanced trogocytosis for treatment of lupus. PLoS One. 2014;9:e98315.

35. McAdoo SP, Reynolds J, Bhangal G, et al. Spleen tyrosine kinase inhibition attenuates autoantibody production and reverses experimental autoimmune GN. J Am Soc Nephrol. 2014;doi: 10.1681/ASN.2013090978.

36. Xiao H, Dairaghi DJ, Powers JP, et al. C5a receptor (cd88) blockade protects against MPO-ANCA GN. J Am Soc Nephrol. 2014;25:225-31.

37. The Wegener's granulomatosis etanercept trial (WGET) research group. Etanercept plus standard therapy for Wegener's granulomatosis. N Engl J Med. 2005;352:351-61.

38. Schwartz N, Rubinstein T, Burkly LC, et al. Urinary tweak as a biomarker of lupus nephritis: A multicenter cohort study. Arthritis Res Ther. 2009;11:R143.

39. Langford CA, Monach PA, Specks U, et al. An open-label trial of abatacept (CTLA4-IG) in non-severe relapsing granulomatosis with polyangiitis (Wegener's). Ann Rheum Dis. 2014;73:1376-9.

Individual Vasculitis Syndromes

- Giant Cell Arteritis and Polymyalgia Rheumatica
- Takayasu's Arteritis
- Kawasaki Disease
- Polyarteritis Nodosa
- Granulomatosis with Polyangiitis (Wegener's Granulomatosis)
- Microscopic Polyangiitis
- Eosinophilic Granulomatosis with Polyangiitis (Churg-Strauss Syndrome)
- Immunoglobulin A Vasculitis
- Primary Angiitis of Central Nervous System
- Behçet's Disease
- Cryoglobulinemic Vasculitis
- Relapsing Polychondritis
- IgG4 Disease
- Infection-associated Vasculitis
- Vasculitis Mimics
- Secondary Vasculitis
- Cogan's Syndrome
- Malignancy-associated Vasculitis
- Pregnancy and Vasculitis
- Prevention and Management of Infections

CHAPTER 27

Giant Cell Arteritis and Polymyalgia Rheumatica

Tanaz A Kermani

INTRODUCTION

Polymyalgia Rheumatica

Polymyalgia rheumatica (PMR) is a chronic, inflammatory condition in individuals over the age of 50 years. Polymyalgia rheumatica has most commonly been reported in individuals of Northern European descent.[1] The diagnosis of PMR is based on clinical symptoms consistent with this diagnosis and evidence of systemic inflammation. There are many conditions that may mimic PMR, particularly late-onset spondyloarthritis (SpA) and rheumatoid arthritis (RA).[2] Evidence of bursitis and tendonitis on ultrasound of the shoulder and hips is common in patients with PMR and may add to the specificity of the diagnosis.[3,4] There is a well-known association between PMR and giant cell arteritis (GCA). Temporal artery evaluation in asymptomatic patients with PMR suggests that PMR may be a forme fruste.[5] An estimated 16–21% of patients with PMR may develop GCA.[6]

Giant Cell Arteritis

Giant cell arteritis is the most common form of systemic vasculitis in people over the age of 50 years. Like PMR, GCA is most common in people of Northern European descent.[1] While GCA preferentially involves the extracranial branches of the carotid artery, involvement of the aorta, and its primary and secondary branches also occurs.[7] Temporal artery biopsy remain the diagnostic test of choice. However, in the subset with predominantly large-vessel involvement, imaging of the aorta and its branches with computed tomography angiography (CTA), magnetic resonance angiography (MRA), or ultrasonography (USG) is helpful.

CASE VIGNETTE

A 69-year-old woman who was previously in excellent health presents to her physician for increased joint pain for the past month. She denies any inciting events. Symptoms initially started in both shoulders and now also affect the proximal thighs. She feels stiff in the morning and has difficulty getting out of bed. As the day progresses, she can move better and has less pain. She has minimal relief with ibuprofen. She also reports an unexplained 5 pound weight loss around the same time but no other constitutional symptoms. She denies any joint swelling, chest pain, pulmonary symptoms, gastrointestinal symptoms, headaches, jaw pain, visual changes, paresthesias, or weakness. On examination, she appears well. She is afebrile. Blood pressure is 90/60 in the left arm. Heart rate is 70 beats per minute and regular. Cardiopulmonary examination is normal. Joint examination reveals limited active range of motion in both shoulders. Passive range of motion is intact. There is no swelling of the shoulders or any of the joints. No skin changes. Strength is normal in the upper and lower extremities proximally and distally.

Laboratory testing includes a complete blood count (CBC) with hemoglobin 10.2 g/dL, normal white cell count but elevated platelet count at 480,000. Chemistry panel is normal. Creatine kinase, thyroid stimulating hormone TSH is normal. Sedimentation rate (Westergren method) is abnormal at 70 mm/hour with a C-reactive protein of 7.9 mg/dL. She was diagnosed with PMR and started on prednisone 15 mg daily with resolution of her symptoms. Markers of inflammation normalized with treatment.

She did well until 8 months later when prednisone was at 5 mg daily. She reported new onset cyanotic changes in the hands suggestive of Raynaud's-like phenomenon. She also developed a new pain in both arms although more prominent on the left side. She noted "fatiguing" of the arms with any exertion. The pain was more prominent in the muscles and not the joints. She said the muscle cramping would start within a few minutes of activity and resolve with rest. She otherwise felt well, and she denied any joint pain, constitutional symptoms, headaches, jaw claudication, scalp tenderness, visual

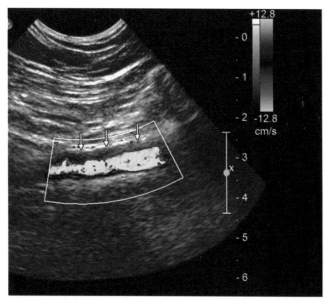

Fig. 27.1 Color duplex ultrasound of the right subclavian artery in longitudinal axis showing circumferential wall thickening, so called "halo sign" (increased intimal medial complex) in the patient described in the vignette. The white arrows outline the medial wall of the artery and the halo is the portion between the arrows and the color Doppler flow in the lumen of the artery (increased intimal medial wall thickening).

changes, cardiopulmonary, or gastrointestinal symptoms. On examination, blood pressure was not obtainable in the left arm, 90/60 in the right arm. Left radial pulse was absent. She had bilateral subclavian artery bruits and carotid bruits. Range of motion in all joints was normal without synovitis. No cardiac murmurs. Pulmonary examination was normal. Remainder of her physical examination was normal. Laboratory testing revealed an elevated sedimentation rate of 46 mm/hour with a C-reactive protein of 2.5 mg/dL. Upper extremity arterial ultrasound showed wall thickening (Fig. 27.1) and stenosis of bilateral subclavian and axillary arteries. Computed tomography angiography of the chest showed mural thickening of the thoracic (Fig. 27.2A) and abdominal aorta with thickening and narrowing of the left proximal subclavian artery (Fig. 27.2B), and high-grade stenosis of the right axillary artery consistent with vasculitis.

A diagnosis of GCA was made. Prednisone was increased to 60 mg daily with gradual improvement of symptoms 1 month later and normalization of markers of inflammation. This was gradually tapered.

EPIDEMIOLOGY

Polymyalgia Rheumatica

The estimated annual incidence of PMR is 58.7 per 100,000 people ≥50 years of age.[8-10] The incidence increases with age and mean age at diagnosis is approximately 73 years.[9,10] Polymyalgia rheumatica most commonly affects Caucasian individuals.[1] The highest incidences of PMR have been reported in Norway while lowest incidences have been reported in Southern European countries.[11-13] Very little is known about the incidence and prevalence of PMR in

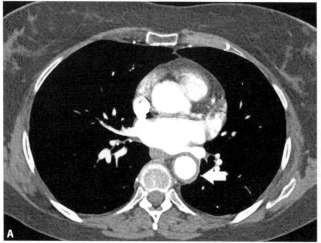

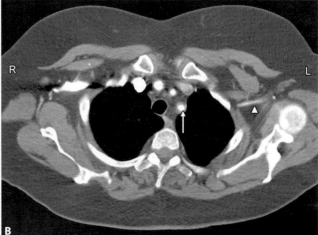

Figs 27.2A and B CTA of the chest showing circumferential thickening of the wall of the descending thoracic aorta (A, arrow). Thickening (white arrow) with stenosis (arrowhead) of the left subclavian artery noted on CTA chest consistent with giant cell arteritis (B).

non-Caucasian populations. In a population-based study from Japan, the estimated prevalence was 1.47 per 100,000 people ≥50 years.[14] The etiology of PMR is unknown. While infectious and environmental agents have been suspected, no causative agent has been identified to date.[2]

Giant Cell Arteritis

Giant cell arteritis is the most common form of vasculitis in people over the age of 50 years. As in the case of PMR, the incidence of GCA increases with age, with the highest rates reported for those individuals in the seventh decade of life.[1] Additionally, GCA is also most commonly observed in Caucasian individuals with the highest incidence rates reported among individuals in Scandinavian countries and North American populations of Northern European ancestry.[1] It is extremely rare in African Americans and Asians.[1] In a study from Tennessee in the United States of America, the incidence of GCA in African Americans was 0.4 per 100,000 people over the age of 50 years.[15] Likewise, in a population-based study from Japan, the prevalence of GCA was estimated at 1.47 per 100,000 people ≥ 50 years old.[14]

Women are affected two to three times more often than the men.[1] The causative agent in GCA has not been identified to date.

DIAGNOSIS

Polymyalgia Rheumatica

There are no diagnostic tests that are specific for PMR. Multiple conditions can mimic present with polymyalgia-like symptoms and the diagnosis requires exclusion of other conditions. Markers of inflammation are often elevated. Several diagnostic criteria for PMR have been proposed based on retrospective clinical series.[16-19] Most of these include an age cut-off, presence of bilateral shoulder girdle and hip girdle pain, morning stiffness, and elevated markers of inflammation. An international collaborative initiative is currently underway to develop classification criteria for PMR.[3,4] Ultrasonography of the shoulders and hips may add to the specificity of a diagnosis of PMR.[3,4] However, ultrasound cannot distinguish inflammatory changes from PMR from other inflammatory arthritis like RA or SpA.

Giant Cell Arteritis

Temporal artery biopsy is still considered the "gold standard" for diagnosis of GCA.[6] The hallmark histopathological feature of GCA is transmural inflammation. However, temporal artery biopsy is insensitive in the subset of patients with GCA who present with upper extremity arterial involvement (limb claudication, large-vessel bruits). In one study, 42% of GCA patients with subclavian, axillary, or brachial artery involvement had a negative temporal artery biopsy.[20] In this subset, large-vessel imaging with CTA, MRA, or ultrasound may be helpful in establishing a diagnosis.[21]

CLINICAL FEATURES

Polymyalgia Rheumatica

Patients with PMR present with pain and stiffness affecting the neck, shoulder, low back, and hip or proximal thighs. The absence of shoulder involvement is unusual in patients with this diagnosis.[22] Stiffness lasting half an hour or longer, generally occurring in the morning or after periods of inactivity is common. In contrast to osteoarthritis or rotator cuff tendinopathy, the stiffness and pain in PMR is worse with inactivity and improves with activity. Constitutional symptoms such as fatigue, malaise, anorexia, weight loss, and fever are also common.[17] Pain and swelling of distal joints like wrists, hands, and feet should raise concern for an inflammatory arthritis like RA or SpA.[2] A subset of patients with PMR may present with swelling and pitting edema (RS3PE) of the hands and feet due to tenosynovitis, so called remitting seronegative symmetrical synovitis with RS3PE syndrome.[23] However, this variant can also be a presenting feature of other inflammatory forms of arthritis including SpA and RA.

Musculoskeletal examination in patients with PMR often reveals painful and limited active range of motion of the shoulders and hips. Swelling of the wrists and knees has been reported in up to one-third of patients with PMR.[24-28] While synovitis of the wrist, metacarpophalangeal or proximal interphalangeal joints has been reported in patients with PMR, these findings are more consistent with RA.[29] Patients may have give-way muscle weakness due to pain, but true muscle weakness is not a feature of PMR. Given the close association of PMR with GCA and the fact that other conditions like GCA may present with PMR-like symptoms, examination should also include evaluation of the temporal arteries, peripheral pulses, and auscultation for bruits. If vascular abnormalities are present, evaluation for GCA should be undertaken.

Giant Cell Arteritis

Patients with GCA often present with new temporal or occipital headaches. Scalp tenderness may be present.[6] Abnormalities of the temporal artery on inspection and palpation such as thickening and nodularity of the temporal arteries may be observed, and, if present, are specific for the diagnosis.[30] Jaw claudication from the involvement of the facial and internal maxillary arteries supplying the muscles of mastication, while only present in one-third of the patients, is also very specific for this diagnosis.[30] Symptoms of PMR with aching and prolonged morning stiffness of the shoulder and hip-girdle are present in 40–60% of patients with GCA. Constitutional symptoms such as fatigue, fever, or weight loss are also often present at diagnosis.[6]

Approximately 20% of patients experience partial or complete vision loss from acute arteritic anterior ischemic optic neuropathy (AAION).[6] Other visual symptoms related to ischemia may include amaurosis fugax and diplopia. Fundoscopic examination of patients with AAION shows pallor and edema of the optic disc in contrast to nonarteritic anterior ischemic optic neuropathy, a more common cause of sudden vision loss.[31] Any patient with GCA and visual symptoms should be evaluated by an ophthalmologist.

A subset of GCA patients present with constitutional symptoms in the absence of more typical cranial symptoms. Therefore, GCA should be in the differential diagnosis for an elderly person who presents with fever of unknown origin or unexplained constitutional symptoms. Another less recognized manifestation of GCA is vascular insufficiency affecting the extremities, especially the arms.[20,32] These patients present with cyanosis of the digits, limb claudication as in the patient presented above.

While uncommon, case series of patients with GCA from India report similar presentation as those observed in individuals from Western countries with the exception of fever being a prominent clinical manifestations in these patients.[33-35]

On physical examination for anyone suspected of having GCA, special attention should be given to the vascular examination. The presence or absence of temporal artery abnormalities (diminished pulses, nodularity, thrombosis) should be noted. Peripheral pulses, including radial, carotid, femoral, and pedal pulses, should be assessed. Auscultation over the major vessels, including carotid, subclavian, abdominal, and femoral arteries, may disclose vascular bruits. The presence of diminished or absent peripheral pulses, bruits, and/or asymmetric blood pressures in the upper extremities suggests large-artery involvement due to vasculitis and should prompt large-vessel imaging. Aortic insufficiency murmur may indicate aortic root involvement and should also be evaluated with echocardiogram or imaging since patients with GCA have increased risk of aneurysms, particularly thoracic aortic aneurysms.[36]

INVESTIGATIONS

Polymyalgia Rheumatica

Laboratory Findings

Laboratory findings in PMR are nonspecific and may include anemia, leukocytosis, and elevated markers of inflammation.[16,17] Erythrocyte sedimentation rate (ESR) and C-reactive protein (CRP) are often elevated, although low (≤30 mm/hour) or normal ESR has been reported in 6–20% of patients with PMR.[2] Autoantibodies including rheumatoid factor (RF) and anti-cyclic citrullinated peptide are negative in PMR and if present are consistent with RA.[17,37-40] Thyroid stimulating hormone, muscle enzymes (creatine phosphokinase), calcium, electrolytes, renal function, serum protein electrophoresis, and urinalysis are also recommended tests to exclude PMR mimics.[41,42]

Imaging Studies

Plain radiographs are helpful in excluding other conditions that can present with symptoms of PMR (Flow chart 27.1) but there are no diagnostic findings in patients with PMR. The presence of bony erosions on radiographs of the wrist, hands, or feet is more consistent with RA.[29]

Ultrasonography may aid in distinguishing PMR from other noninflammatory causes of shoulder and hip pain.[3,4] The predominant finding on in patients with PMR is inflammation of periarticular structures particularly tendons and bursae. Bicipital tendonitis, subacromial bursitis, subdeltoid bursitis, and trochanteric bursitis are commonly observed on MRI or ultrasound in patients with PMR.[43-46] Glenohumeral and hip joint effusions and synovitis have also been reported.[3,4,45-49] These abnormalities, however, are not specific to PMR and are also seen in other inflammatory forms of arthritis like RA or SpA. In general, the presence of subacromial/subdeltoid bursitis or tenosynovitis of the long head of the biceps appears to be more prevalent in patients with PMR than other forms of inflammatory arthritis.[43,45,48] Patients with PMR also often report neck and back pain. Detailed imaging of these areas shows inflammatory changes, particularly, interspinous bursitis.[50-54]

Biopsy

Tissue biopsies are not necessary in patients with PMR. Muscle biopsy would only be indicated in those suspected of having an inflammatory myositis. Temporal artery biopsy should be pursued in patients with PMR who have cranial symptoms or vascular abnormalities that may suggest GCA.[6]

Flow chart 27.1 Suggested algorithm for evaluation of a patient with suspected giant cell arteritis

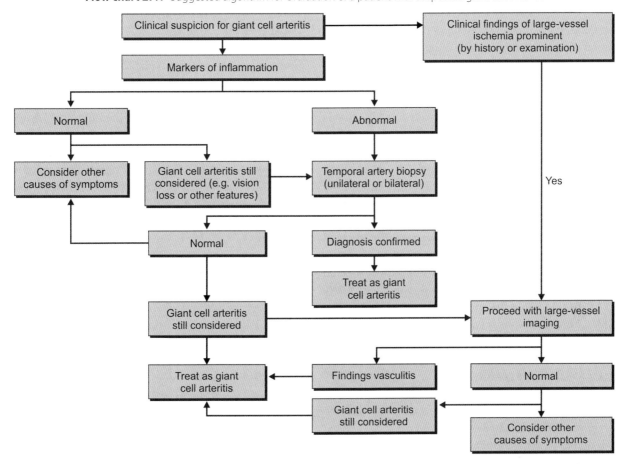

Giant Cell Arteritis

Laboratory Findings

Patients with GCA often have evidence of systemic inflammation on laboratory evaluation with anemia, thrombocytosis, or elevated ESR and CRP. While elevated ESR is considered a hallmark of this diagnosis, approximately 4% patients with GCA can have normal markers of inflammation at diagnosis.[30,55] Therefore, in cases where clinical suspicion is high, a biopsy and/or imaging studies should be pursued even in the absence of a systemic inflammatory response.

Biopsy

Given the need for prolonged corticosteroid therapy and the morbidity associated with treatment in GCA, confirmation of the diagnosis should be pursued with a temporal artery biopsy. Temporal artery biopsy shows transmural inflammation. Macrophages concentrate near the internal elastic lamina with fragmentation of this layer by Verhoeff-Van Gieson stain.

Macrophages coalesce to form multinucleated giant cells but absence of giant cells does not exclude the diagnosis. Necrotizing arteritis is not a feature of GCA and is more consistent with other forms of vasculitis such as polyarteritis nodosa or antineutrophil cytoplasmic antibody vasculitis that can rarely affect the temporal artery.[56]

The overall sensitivity of a temporal artery biopsy is estimated at 87%.[57,58] Since the vasculitis can be segmental and the presence of "skip lesions" may result in false negative results, the biopsy needs to be of sufficient length. A length of approximately 1 cm postfixation is recommended based on observations of decreased sensitivity in specimens less than 0.5–0.7 cm in length.[59,60] In general, unilateral temporal artery biopsy is sufficient. However, discordance (positive biopsy on one side but negative findings on the contralateral side) has been reported in 1.4–12.7% cases.[61-66]

In patients with GCA with primarily large-artery involvement (e.g. upper extremity arterial involvement), temporal artery biopsy is insensitive and can be negative in up to 42% of cases.[20] Therefore, in this subset of patients, imaging should be pursued to confirm the diagnosis of GCA.

Imaging

Several noninvasive imaging modalities that are useful in the evaluation of patients with GCA are discussed in this section. Ultrasound, CTA, and MRA allow evaluation of the vessel wall and the lumen.[67] Positron emission tomography (PET) scan can also be useful in the diagnosis of large-vessel vasculitis. It is the only functional test but this is a costly modality that is not widely available and is not necessary in most cases.

Duplex USG can evaluate the vessel wall and the lumen and is helpful in evaluation of subjects with GCA. In addition to being noninvasive, USG has no radiation and allows the evaluation of multiple arteries.[68] Arteries affected by vasculitis have a "dark halo", a hypoechoic area surrounding the vessel walls that may represent edema of the arterial wall.[69] In a meta-analysis of 23 studies with 2,036 patients who had USG evaluation of temporal arteries for suspected GCA, the sensitivity of the halo sign was estimated at 69% (95% CI: 57–79%) while the specificity was high (82%; 95% CI 75–87%) when compared with temporal artery biopsy.[70] When evaluating the sensitivity of any USG abnormality (halo, stenosis, and/or occlusion), the sensitivity of USG improved to 87% with a specificity of 96%.[70] Ultrasonography can also be a valuable modality in the evaluation of proximal upper extremity arteries, particularly the subclavian, axillary, and brachial arteries that may be involved in GCA.[71-73] As in the case of biopsy, other forms of vasculitis that can affect the temporal artery (e.g. polyarteritis nodosa) can also cause the "halo" sign so these diagnostic tests must be interpreted in the context of the clinical findings.[74,75] This modality is also very operator-dependent and therefore, should not be a substitute for biopsy unless performed by someone with expertise.

Magnetic resonance imaging and MRA allows evaluation of both the vessel wall as well as the lumen. Magnetic resonance imaging findings that correlate with vasculitis include the vessel wall thickening, edema on T2-weighted images, and postgadolinium enhancement of the vessel wall. Bley and colleagues have evaluated the diagnostic value of T2-weighted imaging of the superficial temporal arteries.[76] However, the findings have not been reproduced in other studies and sensitivity of this modality dramatically decreases with initiation of glucocorticoids. Magnetic resonance imaging is a useful modality for the evaluation of large-vessel (extracranial) involvement from GCA and can visualize the aorta and its branches. The sensitivity of this modality in the diagnosis of GCA has not been studied.

Computed tomography angiography can evaluate the aorta and its branches in patients suspected of having GCA. Findings of vasculitis on CTA may include wall thickening, delayed wall enhancement, or long segments of tapered stenoses.[77,78] The performance of CTA as a diagnostic tool in patients suspected of having GCA is unknown.

Patients with large-vessel vasculitis, such as GCA often have increased fluorodeoxyglucose (FDG) uptake in the aorta and major branches (subclavian, carotid, and femoral arteries) on PET. In a prospective study of patients with GCA who underwent PET imaging at diagnosis, vascular FDG uptake was seen in 76% of patients.[79] However, this expensive modality may not be widely available and has not been well studied. It is a reasonable study in patients with fever unknown origin, those with negative imaging where vasculitis is considered or in cases where there is concern for malignancy. However, FDG uptake has also been reported in atherosclerosis.

DIAGNOSTIC APPROACH

The demographic characteristics of these two conditions should be kept in mind when evaluating patients suspected of having PMR or GCA. These diagnoses are not seen in people under the age of 50 years. Additionally, they are most common in individuals of Caucasian ancestry.

Polymyalgia Rheumatica

Evaluation begins with a careful history and physical examination. When evaluating any patient suspected of having PMR, a broad differential should be considered (Table 27.1). Laboratory testing in those suspected of having PMR should include acute phase reactants (ESR and CRP), CBC, chemistries, thyroid testing, muscle enzymes, RF, cyclic citrullinated peptide, and if appropriate, testing for hepatitis, infections. X-ray imaging can be helpful in evaluating other causes of shoulder or hip pain. If available, ultrasound can also be used to evaluate the presence of inflammatory findings as those reported in patients with PMR. In patients with cranial findings suspicious for GCA or vascular bruits, additional evaluation with biopsy and/or imaging as appropriate should be pursued. Once other causes have been excluded and a diagnosis has been made, it is very important to follow these patients closely with serial evaluation over time. Between 2–30% of patients initially thought to have PMR may later be reclassified as RA.[2]

Giant Cell Arteritis

Patients with suspected GCA should undergo a careful history and physical examination. A suggested approach is in Flow chart 27.1. Laboratory testing should include ESR and CRP. While normal ESR and CRP make the diagnosis of GCA

Table 27.1 Clinical findings and useful diagnostic evaluations in other conditions that may present with symptoms of polymyalgia rheumatica

Diagnosis	Clinical findings	Evaluations
Rheumatoid arthritis	Polyarthritis, peripheral joint involvement	Markers of inflammation elevated, rheumatoid factor, cyclic citrullinated peptide may be positive or negative. X-rays may show erosions
Spondyloarthropathy	Inflammatory back pain	Markers of inflammation often elevated, consider imaging (X-ray or MRI) of the sacroiliac joint
Calcium pyrophosphate disease and calcium hydroxyapatite disorders	Large shoulder effusion	Chondrocalcinosis, calcium deposits on imaging. Consider joint aspiration
Giant cell arteritis	Cranial symptoms, symptoms of vascular insufficiency or abnormal vascular examination	Biopsy or large-vessel imaging to evaluate
Inflammatory myopathies (dermatomyositis, polymyositis)	Muscle weakness on examination, skin findings of myositis	Muscle enzymes elevated, skin biopsy if appropriate, normal thyroid stimulating hormone
Rotator-cuff disease	Unilateral involvement	Normal markers of inflammation, imaging to evaluate for tears or other findings if diagnostic uncertainty
Degenerative joint disease	Bony hypertrophy, history of trauma, unilateral involvement	Normal markers of inflammation, X-ray with degenerative changes
Fibromyalgia	Diffuse, widespread pain	Normal laboratory tests, exclusion other causes
Thyroid diseases	Symptoms of hypothyroidism	Abnormal thyroid stimulating hormone
Disorders of the parathyroid gland		Abnormal serum calcium, parathyroid hormone
Septic arthritis	Fever, history of trauma, drug use, warmth, erythema, swelling, pain on examination	Elevated white cell count, elevated markers of inflammation, joint aspiration to confirm diagnosis
Parkinsonism	Features of Parkinsonism on examination	Evaluation usually all normal
Drug-induced myopathy, e.g. statins	History of drug exposure	Elevated CK

very unlikely, it does not exclude the diagnosis. All patients suspected of having GCA should undergo a temporal artery biopsy. If biopsy is negative and the clinical suspicion for GCA remains, consideration should be given to large-vessel imaging although the yield of pursuing this in patients with negative biopsy has not been studied. Large-vessel imaging is also recommended in patients suspected of having large-vessel manifestations (limb claudication, stroke, bruits on examination). In patients with aortic insufficiency murmurs, thoracic aortic imaging (echocardiography or CTA/MRA) should be performed given increased risk of aneurysms (particularly thoracic aneurysms) in patients with GCA.

MANAGEMENT

Glucocorticoids are the mainstay for treatment for both diseases.

Polymyalgia Rheumatica

Nonsteroidal anti-inflammatory medications are not recommended for treatment of PMR.[80] Low doses of glucocorticoids (prednisone or equivalent of 10–20 mg daily) are usually effective.[42,80] Higher doses are not needed for isolated PMR and should only be used in patients suspected of having GCA.

Clinical response is usually prompt and other diagnoses should be considered in cases where the response is incomplete or markers of inflammation remain elevated. While there are no standardized protocols for tapering prednisone in PMR, prednisone dose is gradually decreased by 2.5 mg every 2–4 weeks until the patient is at 10 mg daily following which the daily dose of prednisone is tapered by 1 mg a month.[42,80] Relapses in PMR are common and most patients require 1–2 years of therapy.[81-83]

In cases where frequent relapses occur or, in patients with comorbidities or toxicities related to prolonged glucocorticoid treatment, methotrexate may be considered.[80,84,85] A multicenter, randomized, placebo-controlled trial evaluating infliximab in patients with newly diagnosed PMR did not show any steroid-sparing effect.[86]

Giant Cell Arteritis

Given the concern for vision loss, prednisone at daily doses of 40–60 mg should be initiated in all patients suspected of having GCA while awaiting temporal artery biopsy. Temporal artery biopsy can be diagnostic even after several weeks of corticosteroid therapy.[87] In patients with visual symptoms or vision loss, high-dose intravenous methylprednisolone (1 g daily for 3 days) is recommended and may decrease the chances of contralateral eye involvement.[88] It should be noted that vision loss is often irreversible. Escalation of therapy is not recommended based solely on lack of improvement of visual symptoms. Addition of low-dose aspirin may reduce the risk of ischemic complications and should be considered unless there are contraindications. In retrospective studies fewer patients with GCA on aspirin had vision loss compared to patients not on aspirin.[89,90]

The high-doses of prednisone are maintained for approximately 4 weeks followed by a gradual taper of about 10% every 2–4 weeks.[6] Disease relapses are common and typical duration of treatment is 1–2 years.[6]

Methotrexate may be a useful adjunct to glucocorticoid therapy in patients with GCA in whom corticosteroid taper is complicated by frequent relapses or in patients with comorbidities and toxicities related to glucocorticoid use. In a meta-analysis treatment with methotrexate lowered the risk of relapse and reduces corticosteroid exposure.[91]

Patients with GCA need long-term monitoring for complications, particularly aortic aneurysms that are late complications and have been associated with increased mortality.[92,93]

KEY POINTS

- PMR and GCA are common conditions in people ≥50 years and are most often seen in Caucasian individuals.
- Given the absence of any diagnostic tests specific to PMR, careful consideration should be given excluding other mimics.
- Ultrasonography of affected joints may complement the clinical evaluation of patients suspected of having PMR.

- In addition to affecting the superficial temporal artery, GCA also affects the aorta and its branches.
- Glucocorticoid treatment should be promptly initiated in anyone with moderate to high-suspicion of GCA given the dreaded complication of vision loss that is irreversible.
- Temporal artery biopsy should be pursued in all patients suspected of having GCA.
- Large-vessel imaging may be helpful in the evaluation of patients suspected of having GCA.
- Patients with GCA should be monitored long-term for aortic aneurysm formation.

REFERENCES

1. Gonzalez-Gay MA, Vazquez-Rodriguez TR, Lopez-Diaz MJ, et al. Epidemiology of giant cell arteritis and polymyalgia rheumatica. Arthritis Rheum. 2009;61:1454-61.
2. Kermani TA, Warrington KJ. Polymyalgia rheumatica. Lancet. 2013;381:63-72.
3. Dasgupta B, Cimmino MA, Kremers HM, et al. 2012 provisional classification criteria for polymyalgia rheumatica: a European League Against Rheumatism/American College of Rheumatology collaborative initiative. Arthritis Rheum. 2012;64:943-54.
4. Dasgupta B, Cimmino MA, Maradit-Kremers H, et al. 2012 provisional classification criteria for polymyalgia rheumatica: a European League Against Rheumatism/American College of Rheumatology collaborative initiative. Ann Rheum Dis. 2012;71:484-92.
5. Weyand CM, Hicok KC, Hunder GG, et al. Tissue cytokine patterns in patients with polymyalgia rheumatica and giant cell arteritis. Ann Intern Med. 1994;121:484-91.
6. Salvarani C, Cantini F, Hunder GG. Polymyalgia rheumatica and giant-cell arteritis. Lancet. 2008;372:234-45.
7. Muratore F, Pazzola G, Pipitone N, et al. Large-vessel involvement in giant cell arteritis and polymyalgia rheumatica. Clin Exp Rheumatol. 2014;32:S106-11.
8. Crowson CS, Matteson EL, Myasoedova E, et al. The lifetime risk of adult-onset rheumatoid arthritis and other inflammatory autoimmune rheumatic diseases. Arthritis Rheum. 2011;63:633-9.
9. Lawrence RC, Felson DT, Helmick CG, et al. Estimates of the prevalence of arthritis and other rheumatic conditions in the United States. Part II, Arthritis Rheum. 2008;58:26-35.
10. Salvarani C, Gabriel SE, O'Fallon WM, et al. Epidemiology of polymyalgia rheumatica in Olmsted County, Minnesota, 1970-1991. Arthritis Rheum. 1995;38:369-73.
11. Gran JT, Myklebust G. The incidence of polymyalgia rheumatica and temporal arteritis in the county of Aust Agder, south Norway: a prospective study 1987-94. J Rheumatol. 1997;24:1739-43.
12. Salvarani C, Macchioni P, Zizzi F, et al. Epidemiologic and immunogenetic aspects of polymyalgia rheumatica and giant cell arteritis in northern Italy. Arthritis Rheum. 1991;34:351-6.

13. Gonzalez-Gay MA, Garcia-Porrua C, Vazquez-Caruncho M, et al. The spectrum of polymyalgia rheumatica in northwestern Spain: incidence and analysis of variables associated with relapse in a 10 year study. J Rheumatol. 1999;26:1326-32.

14. Kobayashi S, Yano T, Matsumoto Y, et al. Clinical and epidemiologic analysis of giant cell (temporal) arteritis from a nationwide survey in 1998 in Japan: the first government-supported nationwide survey. Arthritis Rheum. 2003;49:594-8.

15. Smith CA, Fidler WJ, Pinals RS. The epidemiology of giant cell arteritis. Report of a ten-year study in Shelby County, Tennessee. Arthritis Rheum. 1983;26:1214-9.

16. Bird HA, Esselinckx W, Dixon AS, et al. An evaluation of criteria for polymyalgia rheumatica. Ann Rheum Dis. 1979;38:434-9.

17. Chuang TY, Hunder GG, Ilstrup DM, et al. Polymyalgia rheumatica: a 10-year epidemiologic and clinical study. Ann Intern Med. 1982;97:672-80.

18. Healey LA. Long-term follow-up of polymyalgia rheumatica: evidence for synovitis. Semin Arthritis Rheum. 1984;13:322-8.

19. Jones JG, Hazleman BL. Prognosis and management of polymyalgia rheumatica. Ann Rheum Dis. 1981;40:1-5.

20. Brack A, Martinez-Taboada V, Stanson A, et al. Disease pattern in cranial and large-vessel giant cell arteritis. Arthritis Rheum. 1999;42:311-7.

21. Kermani TA, Warrington KJ. Recent advances in diagnostic strategies for giant cell arteritis. Curr Neurol Neurosci Rep. 2012;12:138-44.

22. Dasgupta B, Salvarani C, Schirmer M, et al. Developing classification criteria for polymyalgia rheumatica: comparison of views from an expert panel and wider survey. J Rheumatol. 2008;35:270-7.

23. Salvarani C, Cantini F, Olivieri I, et al. Polymyalgia rheumatica: a disorder of extraarticular synovial structures? J Rheumatol. 1999;26:517-21.

24. Myklebust G, Gran JT. A prospective study of 287 patients with polymyalgia rheumatica and temporal arteritis: clinical and laboratory manifestations at onset of disease and at the time of diagnosis. Br J Rheumatol. 1996;35:1161-8.

25. Gran JT, Myklebust G. The incidence and clinical characteristics of peripheral arthritis in polymyalgia rheumatica and temporal arteritis: a prospective study of 231 cases. Rheumatology (Oxford). 2000;39:283-7.

26. Salvarani C, Cantini F, Macchioni P, et al. Distal musculoskeletal manifestations in polymyalgia rheumatica: a prospective followup study. Arthritis Rheum. 1998;41:1221-6.

27. Salvarani C, Cantini F, Olivieri I. Distal musculoskeletal manifestations in polymyalgia rheumatica. Clin Exp Rheumatol. 2000;18:S51-2.

28. Ceccato F, Roverano SG, Papasidero S, et al. Peripheral musculoskeletal manifestations in polymyalgia rheumatica. J Clin Rheumatol. 2006;12:167-71.

29. Pease CT, Haugeberg G, Montague B, et al. Polymyalgia rheumatica can be distinguished from late onset rheumatoid arthritis at baseline: results of a 5-yr prospective study. Rheumatology (Oxford). 2009;48:123-7.

30. Smetana GW, Shmerling RH. Does this patient have temporal arteritis? JAMA. 2002;287:92-101.

31. Hayreh SS. Ischaemic optic neuropathy. Indian J Ophthalmol. 2000;48:171-94.

32. Nuenninghoff DM, Hunder GG, Christianson TJ, et al. Incidence and predictors of large-artery complication (aortic aneurysm, aortic dissection, and/or large-artery stenosis) in patients with giant cell arteritis: a population-based study over 50 years. Arthritis Rheum. 2003;48:3522-31.

33. Desai MC, Vas CJ. Temporal arteritis. The Indian scene. J Assoc Physicians India. 1989;37:609-11.

34. Mathew T, Aroor S, Devasia AJ, et al. Temporal arteritis: a case series from south India and an update of the Indian scenario. Ann Indian Acad Neurol. 2012;15:27-30.

35. Singh S, Balakrishnan C, Mangat G, et al. Giant cell arteritis in Mumbai. J Assoc Physicians India. 2010;58:372-4.

36. Evans JM, O'Fallon WM, Hunder GG. Increased incidence of aortic aneurysm and dissection in giant cell (temporal) arteritis. A population-based study. Ann Intern Med. 1995;122:502-7.

37. Dasgupta B, Hutchings A, Hollywood J, et al. Autoantibodies to cyclic citrullinated peptide in a PMR inception cohort from The PMR Outcomes Study. Ann Rheum Dis. 2008;67:903-4.

38. Lopez-Hoyos M, Ruiz de Alegria C, Blanco R, et al. Clinical utility of anti-CCP antibodies in the differential diagnosis of elderly-onset rheumatoid arthritis and polymyalgia rheumatica. Rheumatology (Oxford). 2004;43:655-7.

39. Pease CT, Haugeberg G, Morgan AW, et al. Diagnosing late onset rheumatoid arthritis, polymyalgia rheumatica, and temporal arteritis in patients presenting with polymyalgic symptoms. A prospective longterm evaluation. J Rheumatol. 2005;32:1043-6.

40. Ceccato F, Roverano S, Barrionuevo A, et al. The role of anticyclic citrullinated peptide antibodies in the differential diagnosis of elderly-onset rheumatoid arthritis and polymyalgia rheumatica. Clin Rheumatol. 2006;25:854-7.

41. Michet CJ, Matteson EL. Polymyalgia rheumatica. BMJ. 2008;336:765-9.

42. Dasgupta B, Borg FA, Hassan N, et al. BSR and BHPR guidelines for the management of polymyalgia rheumatica. Rheumatology (Oxford). 2010;49:186-90.

43. Salvarani C, Cantini F, Olivieri I, et al. Proximal bursitis in active polymyalgia rheumatica. Ann Intern Med. 1997;127:27-31.

44. McGonagle D, Pease C, Marzo-Ortega H, et al. Comparison of extracapsular changes by magnetic resonance imaging in patients with rheumatoid arthritis and polymyalgia rheumatica. J Rheumatol. 2001;28:1837-41.

45. Cantini F, Salvarani C, Olivieri I, et al. Shoulder ultrasonography in the diagnosis of polymyalgia rheumatica: a case-control study. J Rheumatol. 2001;28:1049-55.

46. Cantini F, Niccoli L, Nannini C, et al. Inflammatory changes of hip synovial structures in polymyalgia rheumatica. Clin Exp Rheumatol. 2005;23:462-8.

47. Koski JM. Ultrasonographic evidence of synovitis in axial joints in patients with polymyalgia rheumatica. Br J Rheumatol. 1992;31:201-3.

48. Frediani B, Falsetti P, Storri L, et al. Evidence for synovitis in active polymyalgia rheumatica: sonographic study in a large series of patients. J Rheumatol. 2002;29:123-30.

49. Falsetti P, Acciai C, Volpe A, et al. Ultrasonography in early assessment of elderly patients with polymyalgic symptoms: a role in predicting diagnostic outcome? Scand J Rheumatol. 2011;40:57-63.

50. Salvarani C, Barozzi L, Boiardi L, et al. Lumbar interspinous bursitis in active polymyalgia rheumatica. Clin Exp Rheumatol. 2013;31:526-31.

51. Salvarani C, Barozzi L, Cantini F, et al. Cervical interspinous bursitis in active polymyalgia rheumatica. Ann Rheum Dis. 2008;67:758-61.

52. Blockmans D, De Ceuninck L, Vanderschueren S, et al. Repetitive 18-fluorodeoxyglucose positron emission tomography in isolated polymyalgia rheumatica: a prospective study in 35 patients. Rheumatology (Oxford). 2007;46:672-7.

53. Yamashita H, Kubota K, Takahashi Y, et al. Whole-body fluorodeoxyglucose positron emission tomography/computed tomography in patients with active polymyalgia rheumatica: evidence for distinctive bursitis and large-vessel vasculitis. Mod Rheumatol. 2012;22:705-11.

54. Adams H, Raijmakers P, Smulders Y. Polymyalgia rheumatica and interspinous FDG uptake on PET/CT. Clin Nucl Med. 2012;37:502-5.

55. Kermani TA, Schmidt J, Crowson CS, et al. Utility of erythrocyte sedimentation rate and C-reactive protein for the diagnosis of giant cell arteritis. Semin Arthritis Rheum. 2012;41:866-71.

56. Hamidou MA, Moreau A, Toquet C, et al. Temporal arteritis associated with systemic necrotizing vasculitis. J Rheumatol. 2003;30:2165-9.

57. Salvarani C, Crowson CS, O'Fallon WM, et al. Reappraisal of the epidemiology of giant cell arteritis in Olmsted County, Minnesota, over a fifty-year period. Arthritis Rheum. 2004;51:264-8.

58. Niederkohr RD, Levin LA. A Bayesian analysis of the true sensitivity of a temporal artery biopsy. Invest Ophthalmol Vis Sci. 2007;48:675-80.

59. Mahr A, Saba M, Kambouchner M, et al. Temporal artery biopsy for diagnosing giant cell arteritis: the longer, the better? Ann Rheum Dis. 2006;65:826-8.

60. Ypsilantis E, Courtney ED, Chopra N, et al. Importance of specimen length during temporal artery biopsy. Br J Surg. 2011;98:1556-60.

61. Durling B, Toren A, Patel V, et al. Incidence of discordant temporal artery biopsy in the diagnosis of giant cell arteritis. Can J Ophthalmol. 2014;49:157-61.

62. Ponge T, Barrier JH, Grolleau JY, et al. The efficacy of selective unilateral temporal artery biopsy versus bilateral biopsies for diagnosis of giant cell arteritis. J Rheumatol. 1988;15:997-1000.

63. Boyev LR, Miller NR, Green WR. Efficacy of unilateral versus bilateral temporal artery biopsies for the diagnosis of giant cell arteritis. Am J Ophthalmol. 1999;128:211-5.

64. Danesh-Meyer HV, Savino PJ, Eagle RC Jr, et al. Low diagnostic yield with second biopsies in suspected giant cell arteritis. J Neuroophthalmol. 2000;20:213-5.

65. Pless M, Rizzo JF 3rd, Lamkin JC, et al. Concordance of bilateral temporal artery biopsy in giant cell arteritis. J Neuroophthalmol. 2000;20:216-8.

66. Breuer GS, Nesher G, Nesher R. Rate of discordant findings in bilateral temporal artery biopsy to diagnose giant cell arteritis. J Rheumatol. 2009;36:794-6.

67. Pipitone N, Versari A, Salvarani C. Role of imaging studies in the diagnosis and follow-up of large-vessel vasculitis: an update. Rheumatology (Oxford). 2008;47:403-8.

68. Blockmans D, Bley T, Schmidt W. Imaging for large-vessel vasculitis. Curr Opin Rheumatol. 2009;21:19-28.

69. Schmidt WA, Kraft HE, Vorpahl K, et al. Color duplex ultrasonography in the diagnosis of temporal arteritis. N Engl J Med. 1997;337:1336-42.

70. Karassa FB, Matsagas MI, Schmidt WA, et al. Meta-analysis: test performance of ultrasonography for giant-cell arteritis. Ann Intern Med. 2005;142:359-69.

71. Schmidt WA, Natusch A, Moller DE, et al. Involvement of peripheral arteries in giant cell arteritis: a color Doppler sonography study. Clin Exp Rheumatol. 2002;20:309-18.

72. Schmidt WA, Seifert A, Gromnica-Ihle E, et al. Ultrasound of proximal upper extremity arteries to increase the diagnostic yield in large-vessel giant cell arteritis. Rheumatology (Oxford). 2008;47:96-101.

73. Diamantopoulos AP, Haugeberg G, Hetland H, et al. Diagnostic value of color Doppler ultrasonography of temporal arteries and large vessels in giant cell arteritis: a consecutive case series. Arthritis Care Res. 2014;66:113-9.

74. Karahaliou M, Vaiopoulos G, Papaspyrou S, et al. Colour duplex sonography of temporal arteries before decision for biopsy: a prospective study in 55 patients with suspected giant cell arteritis. Arthritis Res Ther. 2006;8:R116.

75. Schmidt WA. Doppler ultrasonography in the diagnosis of giant cell arteritis. Clin Exp Rheumatol. 2000;18:S40-2.

76. Bley TA, Uhl M, Carew J, et al. Diagnostic value of high-resolution MR imaging in giant cell arteritis. AJNR Am J Neuroradiol. 2007;28:1722-7.

77. Lefebvre C, Rance A, Paul JF, et al. The role of B-mode ultrasonography and electron beam computed tomography in evaluation of Takayasu's arteritis: a study of 43 patients. Semin Arthritis Rheum. 2000;30:25-32.

78. Chung JW, Kim HC, Choi YH, et al. Patterns of aortic involvement in Takayasu arteritis and its clinical implications: evaluation with spiral computed tomography angiography. J Vasc Surg. 2007;45:906-14.

79. Blockmans D, Stroobants S, Maes A, et al. Positron emission tomography in giant cell arteritis and polymyalgia rheumatica: evidence for inflammation of the aortic arch. Am J Med. 2000;108:246-9.

80. Hernandez-Rodriguez J, Cid MC, Lopez-Soto A, et al. Treatment of polymyalgia rheumatica: a systematic review. Arch Intern Med. 2009;169:1839-50.

81. Gabriel SE, Sunku J, Salvarani C, et al. Adverse outcomes of antiinflammatory therapy among patients with polymyalgia rheumatica. Arthritis Rheum. 1997;40:1873-8.

82. Maradit Kremers H, Reinalda MS, Crowson CS, et al. Glucocorticoids and cardiovascular and cerebrovascular events in polymyalgia rheumatica. Arthritis Rheum. 2007;57: 279-86.

83. Barraclough K, Liddell WG, du Toit J, et al. Polymyalgia rheumatica in primary care: a cohort study of the diagnostic criteria and outcome. Fam Pract. 2008;25:328-33.

84. Dasgupta B, Matteson EL, Maradit-Kremers H. Management guidelines and outcome measures in polymyalgia rheumatica (PMR). Clin Exp Rheumatol. 2007;25:130-6.

85. Spies CM, Burmester GR, Buttgereit F. Methotrexate treatment in large vessel vasculitis and polymyalgia rheumatica. Clin Exp Rheumatol. 2010;28:S172-7.

86. Salvarani C, Macchioni P, Manzini C, et al. Infliximab plus prednisone or placebo plus prednisone for the initial treatment of polymyalgia rheumatica: a randomized trial. Ann Intern Med. 2007;146:631-9.

87. Achkar AA, Lie JT, Hunder GG, et al. How does previous corticosteroid treatment affect the biopsy findings in giant cell (temporal) arteritis? Ann Intern Med. 1994;120:987-92.

88. Liu GT, Glaser JS, Schatz NJ, et al. Visual morbidity in giant cell arteritis. Clinical characteristics and prognosis for vision. Ophthalmology. 1994;101:1779-85.

89. Nesher G, Berkun Y, Mates M, et al. Low-dose aspirin and prevention of cranial ischemic complications in giant cell arteritis. Arthritis Rheum. 2004;50:1332-7.

90. Mackie SL, Hensor EM, Haugeberg G, et al. Can the prognosis of polymyalgia rheumatica be predicted at disease onset? Results from a 5-year prospective study. Rheumatology (Oxford). 2010;49:716-22.

91. Mahr AD, Jover JA, Spiera RF, et al. Adjunctive methotrexate for treatment of giant cell arteritis: an individual patient data meta-analysis. Arthritis Rheum. 2007;56:2789-97.

92. Kermani TA, Warrington KJ, Crowson CS, et al. Large-vessel involvement in giant cell arteritis: a population-based cohort study of the incidence-trends and prognosis. Ann Rheum Dis. 2013;72:1989-94.

93. Mackie SL, Hensor EM, Morgan AW, et al. Should I send my patient with previous giant cell arteritis for imaging of the thoracic aorta? A systematic literature review and meta-analysis. Ann Rheum Dis. 2014;73:143-8.

CHAPTER 28

Takayasu's Arteritis

Aravind G Hegde, Ruchika Goel, George Joseph, Debashish Danda

INTRODUCTION

Takayasu's arteritis (TA) is a prototype large-vessel vasculitis (LVV) of unknown etiology affecting the aorta, its main branches, and pulmonary arteries. This chronic granulomatous vasculitis predominantly affects young women. It is characterized by stenosis, occlusion, dilatation, and aneurysm formation in the affected arteries. Takayasu's arteritis is also famously known as the "pulseless disease," albeit its misleading connotation in view of other prevalent illnesses with weak or absent arterial pulse.[1]

CASE VIGNETTE

A 26-year-old lady presented with exertional dyspnea (NYHA class III), anginal symptoms (CCS class III), and claudication of both upper limbs for 3 years. Her first coronary and peripheral angiogram performed in June 2012 had shown 90% stenosis of left main ostium, 80% stenosis of bilateral subclavian arteries, and 90% stenosis of right vertebral artery (RVA) ostium and bilateral renal artery stenosis. She had undergone percutaneous transluminal angioplasty with renal angioplasty in June 2012. Further re-evaluation at another center in July 2012 diagnosed her disease as aortoarteritis.

In view of cardiac involvement, she was given pulse methylprednisolone IV 15 mg/kg for 3 days, followed by 1 mg/kg per day of oral steroids and azathioprine in 2 mg/kg per day dosage along with statins, aspirin, nitrates, beta blockers, and angiotensin converting enzyme (ACE) inhibitors.

In December 2012, she underwent coronary angiography (CAG) and percutaneous transluminal coronary angioplasty of left main artery; she was continued on medical management with tapering doses of steroid.

She continued to have angina in March 2013, and a possibility of in-stent restenosis (ISR)/right coronary artery (RCA) involvement was considered. She underwent CAG that showed patent left main artery stent and mild ISR. She was continued on medical management with prednisolone 5 mg daily, azathioprine 100 mg once daily, and an escalation of antianginal measures was done. She did not consult her rheumatologist or cardiologist after December 2013.

She presented to Christian Medical College Vellore in May 2014 with exertional dyspnea, a recent progression to NYHA Class IV over the preceding 2 months along with rest angina, claudication of all four limbs and acute onset gradually progressive weakness of left half of the body with giddiness over the preceding 3 days.

On examination, she was found to have bilateral carotid and subclavian bruits with weak left carotid and subclavian pulses; no pulse was felt beyond subclavians in both upper limbs, and pulses in both lower limb arteries were weak. Blood pressure was not recordable in both upper limbs, and it was markedly low (70 mm systolic) in both lower limbs. She also had left-sided hemiparesis; other systemic examinations were normal.

Her erythrocyte sedimentation rate (ESR) and C-reactive protein (CRP) were 68 mm/h and 85.5 mg/L, respectively. Her MRI brain showed acute infarct in the perforator branches of right middle cerebral artery and anterior cerebral artery.

She was pulsed with Inj methylprednisolone 15 mg/kg IV for 3 days in view of recent onset stroke followed by introduction of daily oral corticosteroids (CS) at 1 mg/kg dose and mycophenolate mofetil at 1 g twice daily dose along with antiplatelet agents.

Cardiology consultation was taken and her CAG, peripheral angiography, and pulmonary angiography revealed significant ostial disease in the dominant RCA, diffuse significant disease of right subclavian artery with 60–70% stenosis, 80% ostial stenosis in RVA, occlusion of right common carotid artery (RCCA), diffuse disease with 50–60% stenosis of left common carotid artery (LCCA), ostioproximal diffuse disease with 70% narrowing of left subclavian artery (LSCA), occlusion of left vertebral artery (LVA), minor disease of celiac arteries and diffusely narrowed infrarenal aorta.

She was advised interventions in a staged manner after a month of medical management to control the disease activity. She underwent percutaneous transluminal angioplasty with stenting of the RCA, RVA, and percutaneous balloon angioplasty of RCCA and LSCA in June 2014. PTA with stenting of RCCA, reassessment of LSCA and visceral aorta for stenting was advised after another 1 month. She has been symptomatically better with relief from angina, and left hemiparesis got markedly resolved. She maintained the improvements with continued mycophenolate therapy even after steroid tapering.

HISTORY

The earliest report of a patient presenting with manifestations suggestive of TA dates back to 1830 in Japanese literature describing patients with fever and absent pulses. It was a latency of another 75 years when Mikito Takayasu, an ophthalmologist presented the case of a 21-year-old woman with arteriovenous anastomosis in the retina at the 12th Annual Meeting of the Japan Ophthalmology Society in 1905.[2] He, however, did not describe absent pulses in his patient. Nevertheless, the research committee of the Department of Health and Welfare in Japan recognized the case as the first description of TA and attributed the term "Takayasu arteritis" in his memory in 1975.[2,3]

Originally classified by Ishikawa in 1988 and American College of Rheumatology (ACR) in 1990, TA continues to be categorized as a LVV by the 1994 Chapel Hill Consensus Conference (CHCC) as well as the subsequent 2012 revised CHCC.

EPIDEMIOLOGY

Takayasu's arteritis has been a rare disease, and it affects mostly young Asian women.[3,4] The highest prevalence rate of TA has been described in Japan (40 cases per million), while in other countries, it ranges from 4.7 to 8.0 cases per million.[5-7] According to most case series, females comprise between 82.9% and 97.0% of all cases of TA;[5-8] male: female ratio, however, is less skewed in India, Kuwait and Israel with reports ranging it from 1.6:1 to 2 :1.[5,9,10]

Takayasu's arteritis is usually diagnosed in young individuals in the second or third decade,[4] but it can also occur in early childhood. In India, mean age of onset of symptoms was 24.0 (± 8.8) years in a series (9). It is the third most common cause of vasculitis in the pediatric age group.[11] In our recent report of 40 patients with childhood onset TA from south India, the median age of onset was 12.5 years (range: 1–16 years) and the median delay in diagnosis was 11.3 months (range: 1–60 months).[12] American College of Rheumatology defines age of onset below 40 years as one of the criteria for classification of TA,[13] although 13.0–17.5% of patients fulfilling adequate classification criteria for TA have disease onset after the age of 40 years.[14,15] Delay in diagnosis by months to years from the onset of the first symptoms is a commonplace. Younger patients with TA, in particular, have up to four times higher diagnostic delay than their adult counterparts.[14,16]

It has been speculated by some believers that TA and giant cell arteritis (GCA) form a spectrum within the same disease because of the similarities in terms of nature and distribution of arterial involvement and gender bias.[17,18] However, the 2012 revised CHCC has categorically classified both these large-vessel vasculitides as separate entities in view of their differences in age of disease onset, with most TA patients having onset before the age of 50 years in contrast to GCA heralding itself in vast majority only after their 50th birthday.[19]

The mortality rate in TA ranges from 3%to 27%, as cited in various studies from across the world.[18,20-22] The 5- and 10-year survival rates reported are in the 81–95% and 73–90% range, respectively.[10,21] Congestive heart failure, reportedly, seems to be the leading cause of death in TA.[10,23-25]

CLASSIFICATION CRITERIA AND DIAGNOSIS

No diagnostic or classification criteria for TA existed until 1988 when the first set of criteria were described by Ishikawa.[26] It comprised of an obligatory criterion, two major criteria and nine minor criteria (Table 28.1). In the presence of the obligatory criterion, either (i) two major criteria or (ii) one major criterion and ≥two minor criteria or (iii) ≥ four minor criteria led to a highly probable diagnosis of TA. While the sensitivity of this criterion was 84%, TA patients with predominantly aortic disease were missed out by Ishikawa's criteria.

In 1990, ACR came out with its classification criteria for TA (Table 28.2).[13] The presence of three or more criteria yielded a sensitivity of 90.5% and a specificity of 97.8% for classifying a patient as TA.

Table 28.1 Ishikawa's proposed set of diagnostic criteria for TA[26]

Obligatory criterion	Age less than or equal to 40 years with characteristic symptoms and signs of TA
Major criteria	Lesion of the left mid subclavian artery
	Lesion of the right mid subclavian artery
Minor criteria	High ESR
	Common carotid artery tenderness
	Hypertension
	Aortic regurgitation or annuloaortic ectasia
	Lesions of the pulmonary artery
	Lesions of the left mid common carotid artery
	Lesions of the distal brachiocephalic trunk
	Lesions of the thoracic aorta
	Lesions of the abdominal aorta

Table 28.2 ACR 1990 classification criteria for TA[13]

Age at disease onset <40 years	Development of symptoms or findings related to TA at age <40 years
Claudication of extremities	Development and worsening of fatigue and discomfort in muscles of one or more extremity while in use, especially the upper extremities
Decreased brachial artery pulse	Decreased pulsation of one or both brachial arteries
Blood pressure difference >10 mm Hg	Systolic BP difference greater than 10 mm Hg between arms
Bruit over subclavian arteries or aorta	Bruit audible on auscultation over one or both subclavian arteries or abdominal aorta
Arteriogram abnormality	Arteriographic narrowing or occlusion of the entire aorta, its primary branches, or large arteries in the proximal upper or lower extremities, not due to arteriosclerosis, fibromuscular dysplasia, or similar causes; changes usually focal or segmental

As in Ishikawa's diagnostic criteria, ACR classification criteria for TA too face the similar criticisms, namely the age restriction imposed for disease onset (<40 years); both criteria also have limitation in diagnosing TA in patients with predominantly aortic disease without involvement of branches, which is prevalent amongst Indian patients. When Ishikawa's diagnostic criteria and the 1990 ACR classification criteria for TA were applied to Indian patients with angiographically proven TA, the sensitivity decreased to 60.4 and 77.4%, respectively. Nonetheless, the specificity of both criteria remains higher than 95%.[27]

Sharma et al., in 1995, had proposed a modification of Ishikawa's diagnostic criteria for TA. The modifications in major criteria included (a) removal of the obligatory criterion, namely age of onset <40 years and (b) addition of characteristic signs and symptoms of TA as a major criterion. Minor criteria were also modified by (a) removal of age in the definition of hypertension, (b) nonexclusion of aortoiliac lesions in defining abdominal aortic lesions, and (c) inclusion of coronary artery lesions in patients younger than 30 years of age in the absence of risk factors. A high probability of TA is considered when (i) two major criteria are present or (ii) one major and two minor criteria or (iii) four minor criteria are present. The sensitivity and specificity of Sharma's diagnostic criteria for TA is 92.5 and 95.0%, respectively.[27,28]

In children, another classification criterion for the more common childhood vasculitides was proposed by the European League Against Rheumatism (EULAR), the Pediatric Rheumatology European Society (PRES), and the Pediatric Rheumatology International Trials Organization (PRINTO) in 2005, which was subsequently validated in 2008. The EULAR/PRINTO/PRES criteria for c-TA had a 100% sensitivity and 99.9% specificity due to inclusion of angiographic abnormality as its mandatory criterion.[29]

While none of these are formal diagnostic tools, such criteria help differentiate TA from other forms of vasculitides in clinical practice.

PATHOLOGY

Since biopsy specimens are seldom available in TA, pathological features are mostly based on autopsy findings or segments excised during bypass surgery. On histology, the lesions may be active, chronic, or healed.

Gross histopathology is characterized by thickening and fibrosis of all three layers of large vessels with patchy areas of focal luminal narrowing. In rapidly progressive cases where fibrosis is not extensive, aneurysms may be seen. Intima is thickened with ridging, classically described as tree bark appearance.[30] One or more patterns of disease are noted on gross appearance : (a) involvement of a localized aortic segment for a length of 2–7 cm, (b) multiple short-segment disease with normal or "skip" areas in between, or (c) diffuse aortic disease with or without small stretch of normal segments in between.

Microscopically, TA is usually characterized by skip lesions in aortic wall. Autopsy studies have revealed three types of lesions in biopsy, viz. active lesions with inflammatory infiltrate, chronic lesions with fibrosis, or more commonly a combination of active and chronic lesions.[31] Active lesions are characterized by inflammatory infiltrate, predominantly consisting of lymphoplasmacytic cells in the aortic tissue with granulomas and giant cell formation. In chronic cases, there is evidence of degeneration of internal elastic lamina of tunica media, neovascularization, and adventitial fibrosis.

PATHOGENESIS

Etiopathogenesis of TA is not fully elucidated mainly due to unavailability of biopsy from large vessels and lack of any animal model for TA. Most of the evidence is indirect from in vitro studies on blood and peripheral blood mononuclear cells.

Similar to other autoimmune conditions, TA is also suggested to be an outcome of interplay between genetic susceptibility, environmental trigger like infectious agents, and possible epigenetic changes.

HLA: Human leukocyte antigen (HLA) B region polymorphisms, especially in HLA-B*52 allele, have been shown to be associated with disease susceptibility in most of the candidate gene-based studies from India, Japan, and Turkey; it was further replicated in two separate genome-wide association studies (GWASs), namely the one involving Japanese patients and the other on combined Turkish/American patient population.[32-37] Both these recent GWASs have implicated polymorphism in interleukin-12B (IL-12B) region encoding for p40 subunit of IL-12 in imparting disease susceptibility synergistically with HLAB*52.[38,39] Amino acid residues at positions 67 and 171 in peptide-binding groove of this HLA-B molecule are specifically shown to be associated with TA, thus suggesting the role of antigen binding in causation of this disease.[36] Genes associated with TA in various studies have been listed in Table 28.3.

Mycobacterial theory: Even though immunological studies suggest oligoclonality of T cells and thus a role of limited antigens in TA, the exact nature of antigen is not known.[40] Role of *Mycobacterium tuberculosis* in TA is controversial. Studies have shown coexistence of TA and tuberculosis as well as common genetic associations and cross reactivity of antiendothelial cell antibodies (AECAs) in serum of TA patients to mycobacterial antigen Hsp-65.[46-49] However, the presence of the mycobacterial antigen in TA has not been shown as yet, although a recent study has identified presence of IS6110 and HupB gene sequences of *Mycobacterium bovis* and *M. tuberculosis*, respectively in aortic tissues of 70% of TA patients.[50] Possibilities of *Mycobacterium leprae* and viral agents as potential antigenic triggers have also been postulated.

T cells: Initial lesion in TA is mostly restricted to vasa vasoritis in tunica adventitia of large arteries followed by immune cell infiltration in adventitia-media region. Direct histological studies and indirect evidences suggest a role of cell-mediated immunity predominantly involving Th1 cells in the

Table 28.3 List of genetic studies with genes implicated in TA

Implicated genes	Geographic population	Reference
Results from GWASs		
IL12B, HLA-B/MICA, HLA-DRB1/HLA-DQB1, FCGR2A/3A,	Turkey/ US	40
IL12B, MLX, HLA-B	Japan	35
Results from candidate gene studies		
HLA B 52/ HLA B*52:01	India, Japan, Mexico	33–39
HLA B*51	India	33
HLA B39.2	Japan	36, 41
HLA B* 67	Japan	34, 35
MICA/C12-A	Japan	42
HLA B 44	Japan	39
HLA DPB1*09, HLA DQB1*1701	China	43
IL12, IL2, IL6	Turkey	44
IL12B, HLA-B (GWAS)	Japan, Turkey and N. America	38, 40
FCGR2A/3A	Turkey/ N. America	40
NFKBIL1	Japan	45

pathogenesis. Inflammatory infiltrates in TA consist of mainly Th1 cells, γδ T cells, NK cells, monocyte, and macrophages. γδ T cells in TA are observed to have a restricted repertoire with reactivity to heat shock protein-60 (hsp-60).[31,51,52] These cells were shown to exhibit cytotoxicity to endothelial cells.[40] Cytokine gene expression analysis has shown increased mRNA expression of tumor necrosis factor alpha (TNF-α) and IL-4 in patients with TA.[53]

Humoral immunity: Although the possible role of humoral immunity has long been thought to be limited and a remote possibility, it is currently a contentious issue. Antiendothelial cell antibodies, antiannexin V antibodies (AA5A), and anticardiolipin antibodies (ACLAs) have all been reported in serum of 54, 36, and 12% of TA patients, respectively.[54-56] AECA and AA5A, also shown to be abundant in circulation of patients with several other vasculitides, are thought to act by mediating adhesion of leukocytes to inflamed vascular endothelial cells and by enhancing apoptosis of endothelial cells.[54,56,57] Higher frequency of circulating plasmablast have also been observed in a subset of patients with active TA.[58]

A simplified flow chart of proposed hypothesis for etiopathogenesis of TA incorporating the results for various genetic, histopathological, and immunological studies is shown in Flow chart 28.1.

Flow chart 28.1 Proposed pathogenesis of TA

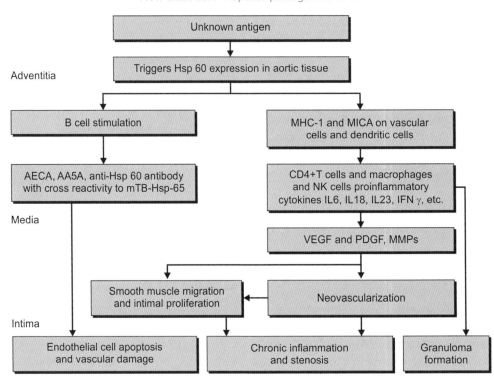

CLINICAL FEATURES

Clinical manifestations of TA include nonspecific symptoms associated with inflammation such as fever, fatigue, malaise, arthralgias, night sweats, weight loss, headache, carotid artery tenderness (carotidodynia), and symptoms related to organ hypoperfusion such as claudication, angina, abdominal angina, and renovascular hypertension. Carotidynia, a pathognomonic physical finding reflecting inflammation of the carotid arteries, is found in 29% of patients with TA.[1] Clinical features may be divided into three stages.

1. Prepulseless stage—characterized by nonspecific constitutional symptoms and signs
2. Stage of vessel wall inflammation—manifested by characteristic sign such as carotidodynia
3. Stage of burnt out or fibrotic process—characterized by ischemic symptoms due to arterial stenosis

Difficulty in diagnosing TA during prepulseless phase and the stage of vessel wall inflammation due to nonspecific constitutional symptoms accounts for commonly encountered delays in TA diagnosis. As a result, a precious therapeutic window of opportunity during this potentially reversible phase of the disease is lost. Pyrexia of unknown origin (PUO) is a well-known presentation of LVV; and

LVVs account for 17 % of cases with PUO.[45] However, newer noninvasive investigational modality such as PET imaging is able to detect subclinical vessel wall inflammation in early TA presenting as PUO and other nonspecific manifestations. A high degree of suspicion in combination with PET may help clinicians diagnose and treat TA in its early reversible stages, thus salvaging patients from disease progression, damage, and expensive as well as risky interventions.

Subclavian artery is involved in up to 90% patients (left more common than right) (Table 28.4), leading to upper extremity claudication and occasional Raynaud's phenomenon. Carotids and vertebral arteries are also commonly involved leading to visual changes, syncope, transient ischemic attacks, and stroke.

Aorta is significantly involved in > 50% patients, leading to aortic insufficiency, hypertension, congestive heart failure, abdominal pain, nausea, and vomiting. When it causes profound aortic narrowing in the descending thoracic aorta, abdominal aorta, or both, it can present as midaortic syndrome. However, there are many other differentials including fibromuscular dysplasia, a number of genetic diseases such as neurofibromatosis, mucopolysaccharidosis, Williams syndrome, Turner syndrome, Alagille syndrome, and congenital rubella syndrome with similar presentations.

Table 28.4 Frequency of blood vessel involvement in TA [14]

Blood vessel	Involvement in total numbers of patients (%)*
Aorta	65
Aortic arch/root	35
Abdominal	47
Thoracic	17
Subclavian artery	93
Common carotid artery	58
Renal artery	38
Vertebral artery	35
Celiac artery	18
Common iliac artery	17
Pulmonary artery	5

*One or more vessels may be involved in a single patient (hence, total will exceed 100%).

Occlusion of visceral arteries such as renal arteries can give rise to renovascular hypertension. Celiac artery and mesenteric arteries can be involved leading to postprandial abdominal angina and mesenteric ischemia. Occlusion of iliac arteries leads to lower limb claudication.

Coronary involvement may be present in up to one-third of patients with TA. Occlusion of the ostia of the left main coronary artery and proximal segments of the coronary arteries are the most common angiographic findings in the coronary vasculature of patients with TA. Apart from the vasculitic process, enhanced atherosclerosis in TA has significantly unfavorable impact on the disease process. Aortic regurgitation develops in 20% of patients as a result of aortic root dilation. Congestive cardiac failure is common and leading cause of mortality in TA patients. The underlying basis for this complication in most cases is hypertension or ischemia of the hypertrophied myocardium. But, dilated and poorly contractile heart with features similar to dilated cardiomyopathy also can be seen in TA. Myocarditis may be the basis and it is reported.[59]

Involvement of the pulmonary artery may be relatively common though it may not be clinically apparent. According to arteriographic studies, pulmonary artery disease may occur between 50% and 86% of TA patients.[25,60] Most patients do not have symptoms, but few may present with features of pulmonary arterial hypertension or very rarely with hemoptysis.

Cutaneous manifestations in TA vary widely between countries. The frequency of skin lesions is estimated to be between 2.8% and 28% of all cases.[61] Specific skin manifestations in TA include Raynaud phenomenon, pyoderma gangrenosum, erythema nodosum-like lesions, necrotic or ulcerated nodules, livedo reticularis, and purpura.[61,62]

Retinal disease as reported by Takayasu himself occurs in 14% of patients and is a result of compromise in the internal carotid circulation leading to central retinal hypoperfusion.[63]

DIAGNOSIS

Laboratory data may be nonspecific in TA. Anemia of chronic disease, mild-to-moderate thrombocytosis, elevated acute phase reactants, viz. ESR and CRP can be present. Although CRP and ESR can be useful to follow-up patients with TA, worsening of vasculitis without an increase in CRP or ESR is not so uncommon.[18,64]

IMAGING

At least one of the several available modalities is essential for establishing the diagnosis, determining the distribution of lesions and monitoring the activity of disease.

Conventional angiography or digital subtraction angiography (DSA) is considered the "gold standard" for diagnosis of TA.

However, noninvasive imaging methods including magnetic resonance angiography (MRA), color Doppler ultrasound (CDU), computerized tomography angiography (CTA), PET with 18F-fluorodeoxyglucose (18F-FDG), and 18F-FDG PET/CT[65-74] have recently gained ground.

Digital subtraction angiography may miss minor, nonocclusive lesions, as it shows only radiological lesions affecting the vessel lumen without giving any information about the vessel wall. Besides, it is an invasive method causing exposure to contrast media and radioactivity.[70,71]

The MRA, CTA and CDU can simultaneously visualize the characteristic, homogenously thickened vessel walls as well as luminal changes of large arteries. They can demonstrate early inflammatory signs (vessel wall thickening and mural inflammation) as well as late complications (stenoses and aneurysms).[75] MRA and CTA provide a good overview of the involved vessels in different locations.

The highest resolution achieved is with ultrasound, but it fails to depict the thoracic aorta unless performed as a transesophageal examination.[72]

The 18F-FDG PET is a noninvasive imaging method that measures 18F-FDG, which accumulates in hypermetabolic, activated inflammatory cells infiltrating the vessels. 18F-FDG PET/CT combines the functional information from PET and anatomical information from CT. However, vascular uptake on PET is not specific for vasculitis, and differentiating between atherosclerotic and vasculitic lesions may be difficult. Also, PET cannot delineate the structure of vessel wall from luminal flow. Radiation exposure is high in CT, particularly in PET–CT.[65-67] Increased vessel wall thickness, vessel wall edema, and mural contrast enhancement are usually considered evidence of active disease.[70]

With involvement of the branches, the lesions are usually noted around the ostia. The subclavian (especially the left) and renal arteries are commonly affected. Rarely, all arch arteries are involved. The disease may begin at the aortic annulus, but the infrarenal aorta, inferior mesenteric artery, and iliac arteries are usually not affected. Pulmonary arterial involvement, found in about 70% of patients, is usually mild, and may extend into segmental and subsegmental branches.[76] Coronary arterial involvement is usually rare; it can be ostial, and/or proximal.[77] About 40% of patients develop cardiac abnormalities, predominantly as cardiac failure, and this complication is seen more often in children.

In 1996, Hata et al. proposed the angiographic classification of TA[78] (Table 28.5 and Fig. 28.1).

Involvement of coronary arteries is labeled C (+), and involvement of pulmonary arteries is denoted as *P* (+).

Japanese patients have a higher incidence of arch involvement (reverse coarctation), while "mid aortic syndrome" with diffuse involvement of thoracoabdominal aorta and renal arteries is more common in southeast Asia, India, and Africa. In North America, arch vessels and abdominal aorta are more frequently affected.

DIFFERENTIAL DIAGNOSIS

Other diseases that may affect the aorta are considered as differentials of TA including GCA, Cogan's syndrome, relapsing polychrondritis, ankylosing spondylitis, rheumatoid arthritis, lupus aortitis, Buerger's disease, Behçet's disease, syphilis, tuberculosis, atherosclerosis, radiation-induced damage, inflammatory bowel disease, sarcoidosis, neurofibromatosis, congenital coarctation, Marfan's syndrome, Ehlers-Danlos syndrome, and IgG4-related disease (IgG4-RD). IgG4-related disease is a recently recognized systemic inflammatory condition associated with high levels of IgG4 in blood and involved tissue, and this entity may account for a minority of cases with TA.[79]

TREATMENT

It is vital to understand the pattern and extent of arterial involvement and the current disease activity status prior to management of TA. Since there is no completed, placebo-controlled, randomized clinical trial, the evidence-based data

Table 28.5 Angiographic classification of TA proposed by Hata et al.[78]

Type	Vessel involvement
Type I	Branches from the aortic arch
Type IIa	Ascending aorta, aortic arch, and its branches
Type IIb	Ascending aorta, aortic arch and its branches, thoracic descending aorta
Type III	Thoracic descending aorta, abdominal aorta, and/or renal arteries
Type IV	Abdominal aorta and/or renal arteries
Type V	Combined features of type IIb and IV

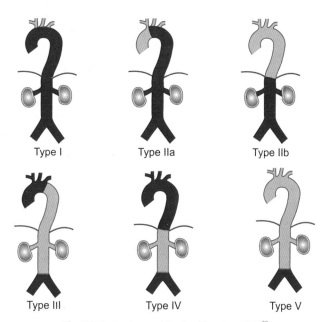

Fig. 28.1 Angiographic classification of TA[78]

for management of TA are negligible. Much of the available data in this regard come from open-label studies, case series, and expert opinion. Management of TA is a collective endeavor of physicians, rheumatologists, interventional cardiologists, radiologists as well as cardiovascular surgeons. Medical treatment with CS and other immunosuppressive agents are used to control ongoing inflammation, whereas endovascular and surgical interventions may be employed to reverse the sequelae of vessel inflammation and damage; together they form the cornerstones in the management of TA.

CORTICOSTEROIDS

In the presence of active disease, standard initial treatment of TA starts with high-dose (0.5–1 mg/kg per day) prednisolone or its equivalents. The response to high-dose prednisolone is generally favorable, but relapse is the rule while tapering. Adverse effects of long-term CS treatment is another limiting factor. This calls for initiation of steroid sparing, conventional immunosuppressants (IS) along with the initial high-dose CS treatment, and continuing IS onto the maintenance phase while tapering the CS dose. Deflazacort, a metabolite of prednisolone produces much less metabolic toxicities in our experience in terms of cushingoid features, glucose impairment, and osteoporosis.

CONVENTIONAL IMMUNOSUPPRESSIVES

The *MTX* is an inexpensive drug, easily available and relatively safe, that has widespread use in rheumatological practice; it is the first choice for many practitioners. Hoffman et al. reported 16 patients with TA who were given standard CS treatment and MTX. 81% went into remission and eight patients (50%) remained in remission for a mean period of 18 months.[80] MTX is initiated at a dose of 0.3 mg/kg per week, with the initial dose not exceeding 15 mg per week; dose is gradually escalated to 25 mg per week.

Azathioprine (AZA) at 2 mg/kg per day is another widely used option of IS agent in the treatment of TA. In an open study from India,[81] 65 IS naive patients with TA were given AZA in 2 mg/kg per day dose in addition to CS treatment for 1 year. Acute phase responses were considerably reduced and follow-up angiography showed no progression of disease without any major adverse events.

Mycophenolate mofetil is a promising agent to be used in TA, at a dose of 2000 mg daily (exceptionally can be escalated up to a maximum of 4000 mg per day). In a study from our center, we have reported outcome of 21 consecutive TA patients treated with MMF for 9.6 ± 6.4 months. Improvement in disease activity was shown using Indian Takayasu activity score (ITAS) and physician global assessment. The CS requirement was also reduced. The only adverse event was skin rash in a single patient. This study shows favorable efficacy and safety profiles of MMF in Indian patients with TA.[82] There are several other reports with similarly high success rate with MMF in TA. With high safety profile, MMF is an excellently efficacious IS in our experience. Those who encounter failure with MMF often failed to instruct the patients to take MMF at least 1–2 hour away from food for optimum absorption. Facilities for estimating 6 hour area under the curve and the trough level of mycophenolic acid (MPA) are useful in deciding dose escalation and documenting any noncompliance by patient. In occasional cases with gastrointestinal adverse effects from mycophenolate mofetil, mycophenolate sodium can be the ideal replacement to achieve the desired efficacy.[83]

Cyclophosphamide (CYC) is used in TA with severe disease having at least one of the following complications: retinal vasculitis, pulmonary artery involvement with or without aneurysm, severe aortic regurgitation, or myocarditis.[84,85] Cyclophosphamide has been given at 2 mg/kg per day dose in some case series.[85] There is also a case report of a resistant TA patient treated successfully with autologous stem cell transplantation following high-dose CYC therapy.[86]

Other IS: Cyclosporine (CSA),[87-89] tacrolimus,[90] and leflunomide[91] have also been tried in select cases with successful results. Cyclosporine may also be effective in some cases for the treatment of pyoderma gangrenosum complicating TA.[87,89]

Similar to cyclophosphamide, in our personal experience, IVIg may also be helpful in certain complicated cases such as TA with myocarditis requiring aggressive and fast-acting immunosuppression, especially when steroids are contraindicated.

DEFINITION OF REFRACTORY DISEASE IN TA

There is no universally accepted consensus definition for refractory disease. Earlier studies had defined refractory disease when disease activity worsened following reduction of CS dose or persisted despite use of at least one conventional IS agent. The Turkish TA Study Group[38] defined refractory disease as (1) angiographic or clinical progression despite treatment or (2) the presence of any of the following characteristics: (i) prednisolone dose >7.5 mg per day after 6 months of treatment, despite administration of conventional IS agents (ii) need for new surgery due to persistent disease activity, (iii) frequent flares (more than three per year), and (iv) death associated with disease activity. Biologic agents are reserved for patients refractory to combination of CS and a conventional IS or rarely to combination of two conventional IS agents.

BIOLOGIC AGENTS

TNF blockers: Serum TNF-α levels are increased in TA. Patients with active TA have a higher TNF-α production compared with those in remission or healthy controls.[92,93]

Therefore, anti-TNF agents, mostly infliximab (IFX), have been tried in refractory adult TA and c-TA patients. The results of long-term follow-up of anti-TNF treatment were reported in a case series of 20 refractory TA patients from a single center.[94] Infliximab was the most frequently used agent for a median duration of 23 months. Remission was achieved in 90% of patients, and CS treatment could be discontinued in

50% patients. However, 33% of patients relapsed. Recently, Comarmond et al.[95] reported five new patients and reviewed the data of 79 patients from literature who were treated with infliximab as an add-on therapy along with IS. While 37% of patients achieved complete remission, 53.5% showed a partial response. Corticosteroids treatment could be discontinued in 40%. Only <10% of patients remained resistant.

Rituximab (RTX), a chimeric monoclonal antibody binding to CD20 expressed on the surface of B cells, has also been tried in TA. Surprisingly, there are case reports showing good clinical response to RTX treatment in refractory TA patients.[96] Rituximab treatment also reduced the expansion of newly generated plasmablasts in TA cases.[58]

Tocilizumab (TCZ): Since IL-6 expression is high within inflamed arteries and serum levels of IL-6 correlate with disease activity, blocking IL-6 seems to be a biologically effective option for TA.[91,92] Tocilizumab is a humanized monoclonal antibody against the IL-6 receptor, and the first report of successful use of TCZ in a patient with refractory TA was published in 2008.[97] Our data of 10 patients showed a good clinical response in 60% of patients while on TCZ infusions. Tocilizumab facilitated rapid reduction in steroid dose from 24 ± 15 to 5.4 ± 4.9 mg per day ($P = 0.003$). However, following discontinuation of TCZ therapy after six infusions, only two patients maintained stable disease state and the majority needed rescue therapy.[98] In spite of these observations, TCZ remains a fast-acting, steroid-sparing stopgap measure in active and refractory disease. Simultaneous institution of IS agents appears to be a must option to sustain the benefit achieved with TCZ in a rapid fashion. While TCZ can be discontinued after four to six infusions at monthly intervals, IS like MMF should be started concurrently with TCZ and continue indefinitely to sustain response including remission.

Abatacept is another upcoming biologic agent inhibiting the costimulation of T cells and is presently being investigated in the first ever randomized, placebo-controlled trial on patients with LVV including TA.[99]

Experimental regime: There is a case report of a TA patient who underwent multitarget therapy with the calcineurin inhibitor tacrolimus and the purine antimetabolic immunosuppressant mizoribine (MZR) after a failed trial with a conventional combination therapy of corticosteroid, MTX, and IFX. Mizoribine is thought to have a mechanism of action identical to that of MMF, with fewer myelosuppressive and hepatotoxic effects.[100]

ENDOVASCULAR AND SURGICAL INTERVENTIONS

Both vascular surgery and percutaneous intervention play important roles in the revascularization of obstructed vessels as well as repair of aneurysms and spontaneous dissection in TA.

In view of relatively higher restenosis rates after percutaneous interventions reported in observational studies over the last several decades, surgery established itself as a more effective technique with wider acceptance.[18,101-106] Surgery is also the only option available for treating severe aortic regurgitation and ascending aortic or complex aneurysmal disease. Surgery, however, has the disadvantage of limited applicability to treat multiple vascular territories (which is often required in TA). In addition, there are complexities of a repeat surgery to treat "not so infrequent" complications of TA such as anastomotic aneurysm, graft occlusion, and progression of disease, besides the inherently associated morbidities of any major surgical intervention.[18,105,107]

Percutaneous intervention is less invasive than surgery, permits treatment of multiple lesions through one vascular access, and can be easily repeated through the same access site if restenosis occurs. Outcomes of both treatment modalities can be compromised by persisting disease activity,[102,105,108-110] a situation made worse by the fact that conventionally adopted medical treatment for TA (like use of methotrexate) is frequently ineffective in controlling disease activity optimally.[18] Waiting for disease activity to subside before intervening may not be possible when risk of complications or significant symptoms are present. A practical approach in patients with active disease is to intervene after a few weeks of aggressive medical treatment that could include newer agents such as TCZ in resistant cases.[98] In recent years, percutaneous intervention in TA has seen significant progress in the areas of chronic occlusion by recanalization using contemporary technique (Figs 28.2A to C), step-wise dilatation of resistant lesions using noncompliant balloons in multiple sittings, treatment of recurrently restenotic lesions by prolonged long-balloon dilatation, prevention of restenosis using covered stents, and repair of aneurysms and spontaneous dissections using aortic stent grafts; these measures have resulted in the ability to treat a much wider range of lesions with better immediate outcomes and improved assisted patency rates in the long run.[111,112] Figure 28.2 illustrates an example of successful endovascular intervention.

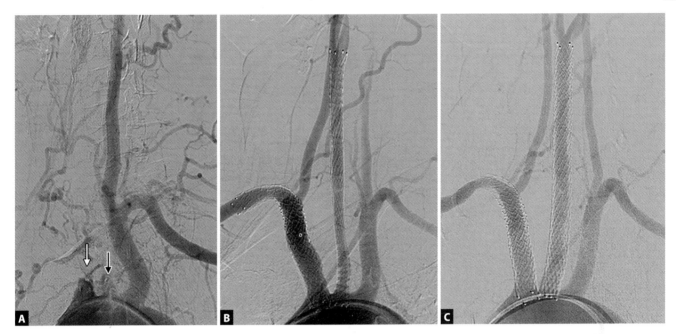

Figs 28.2A to C (A) Aortic arch angiogram in a 31-year-old woman who had sustained multiple cerebral infarctions. The innominate (white arrow) and left common carotid (black arrow) arteries are occluded at their ostia. Left vertebral artery is the sole supply to the brain; (B) Postintervention angiogram showing successful outcome after recanalization and self-expanding stent deployment in the innominate—right subclavian and LCCAs; (C) A 19-month follow-up angiogram showing sustained patency of the recanalized arch vessels with spontaneous positive remodeling of the stented arteries

Supportive treatment: Other aspects of the disease such as dyslipidemia, atherosclerosis, systemic and pulmonary hypertension, ischemic heart disease, cardiac failure, seizures, neurological deficits, and side effects arising out of medications also need to be addressed in order to decrease morbidity and mortality in TA patients. Statins, antiplatelets, antihypertensives, and occasional antifailure drugs as and when needed are adjunct therapeutic agents in TA.

DISEASE ACTIVITY ASSESSMENT AND MONITORING

Unlike other medium- and small-vessel vasculitides, histopathology does not have a major role in diagnosis or monitoring disease activity in TA due to various reasons mentioned above. Conventionally, ESR and CRPs are the only markers available for disease monitoring, in addition to physical examination for new vascular signs. However, discordance between clinical activity using these inflammatory markers and histopathological findings has been observed in 20–40% of cases according to various studies.[18,64] Acute-phase reactant values were normal and misleading in approximately one fifth of patients with active disease, whereas nearly three fourths of patients with active disease had concordant increases in acute phase reactants

in a study.[18] In a recent report from United States, there was discordance between clinical activity and histological findings in 38% of patients.[64]

In an effort to attain uniformity and add sensitivity to clinician's assessment, composite outcome measures have been proposed. Initially in a study from NIH, disease was defined as active in the presence of systemic symptoms, new vascular bruits, elevated acute phase reactants, or angiographic evidence of progression of vascular lesions.[14]

ITAS: Recently, Indian Rheumatology Vasculitis Group has devised a tool, namely the ITAS based on Birmingham Vasculitis Index.[113] Initially, a disease extent score (DEI. TAK)[114] was devised incorporating clinical signs pertaining to large-vessel involvement that was further modified to the current format of ITAS 2010. Indian Takayasu activity score 2010 is a weighted score for vascular items (0–2) related to six organ systems and has been validated in a large cohort of Indian patients with TA.[115]

Biomarkers: Apart from ESR and CRP, pentraxin-3 is another promising biomarker being studied to monitor disease activity with a higher sensitivity.[116] Other molecules in serum explored as disease activity markers are matrix metalloproteinase (MMP)-2, -3, -9, IL-6, regulated upon activation and normal T expressed and secreted, vascular cell adhesion molecules, and unacylated and acylated ghrelin levels.[105,117,118] The leptin/ghrelin ratio was significantly higher in TA patients than controls and had a positive correlation with disease activity.[118]

FUTURE DIRECTIONS

Even though research related to TA has gained momentum in the recent decade, the paucity of data in the understanding of etiopathogenesis of this disease and disease monitoring remains a stumbling block in management. Contribution of genetic susceptibility is modest with a maximum odds ratio of around 4.0, and hence the role of epigenetics in disease causation needs to be studied. Composite disease activity indices need to be refined further with higher sensitivity and specificity. A composite biomarker index in addition to clinical indices would probably help in better assessment of disease. Studies exploring targeted therapies, such as biological agents, are being planned for better management of steroid refractory and steroid-dependent disease. A better classification system too may evolve from the ongoing DCVAS-EULAR study.

KEY POINTS

- TA is a chronic granulomatous vasculitis of aorta and its main branches at origin.
- Angiography remains the gold standard in evaluation.
- Recently validated Indian Takayasu activity score 2010 is the only useful clinical tool in assessing disease. Disease extent index-Takayasu (DEI. TAK) is a validated disease extent score. Takayasu arteritis damage score (TADS) as damage score is under evaluation.

REFERENCES

1. Numano F, Kakuta T. Takayasu arteritis—five doctors in the history of Takayasu arteritis. Int J Cardiol. 1996;54:S1-10.
2. Numano F. The story of Takayasu arteritis. Rheumatology (Oxford). 2002;41:103-6.
3. Maksimowicz-McKinnon K, Clark TM, Hoffman GS. Takayasu arteritis and giant cell arteritis: a spectrum within the same disease? Medicine (Baltimore). 2009;88:221-6.
4. Richards BL, March L, Gabriel SE. Epidemiology of large-vessel vasculidities. Best Pract Res Clin Rheumatol. 2010;24:871-83.
5. Moriwaki R, Noda M, Yajima M, et al. Clinical manifestations of Takayasu arteritis in India and Japan: new classification of angiographic findings. Angiology. 1997;48:369-79.
6. Waern AU, Andersson P, Hemmingsson A. Takayasu's arteritis: a hospital-region based study on occurrence, treatment and prognosis. Angiology. 1983;34:311-20.
7. Watts R, Al-Taiar A, Mooney J, et al. The epidemiology of Takayasu arteritis in the UK. Rheumatology (Oxford). 2009;48:1008-11.
8. Dreyer L, Faurschou M, Baslund B. A population-based study of Takayasu's arteritis in eastern Denmark. Clin Exp Rheumatol. 2011;29:S40-42.
9. Rosenthal T, Morag B, Itzchak Y. Takayasu arteritis in Israel. Heart Vessels Suppl. 1992;7:44-47.
10. Subramanyan R, Joy J, Balakrishnan KG. Natural history of aortoarteritis (Takayasu's disease). Circulation. 1989;80:429-37.
11. Katsicas MM, Pompozi L, Russo R. Takayasu arteritis in pediatric patients. Arch Argent Pediatr. 2012;110:251-5.
12. Goel R, Kumar TS, Danda D, et al. Childhood-onset Takayasu arteritis: experience from a tertiary care center in south India. J Rheumatol. 2014;41:1183-9.
13. Arend WP, Michel BA, Bloch DA, et al. The American college of rheumatology 1990 criteria for the classification of Takayasu arteritis. Arthritis Rheum. 1990;33:1129-34.
14. Kerr GS, Hallahan CW, Giordano J, et al. Takayasu arteritis. Ann Intern Med. 1994;120:919-29.
15. Vanoli M, Daina E, Salvarani C, et al. Takayasu's arteritis: a study of 104 Italian patients. Arthritis Rheum. 2005;53:100-7.
16. Johnston SL, Lock RJ, Gompels MM. Takayasu arteritis: a review. J Clin Pathol. 2002;55:481-6.
17. Grayson PC, Maksimowicz-McKinnon K, Clark TM, et al. Distribution of arterial lesions in Takayasu's arteritis and giant cell arteritis. Ann Rheum Dis. 2012;71:1329-34.
18. Maksimowicz-McKinnon K, Clark TM, Hoffman GS. Limitations of therapy and a guarded prognosis in an American cohort of Takayasu arteritis patients. Arthritis Rheum. 2007;56:1000-9.
19. Jennette JC, Falk RJ, Bacon PA, et al. 2012 revised International Chapel Hill Consensus Conference Nomenclature of Vasculitides. Arthritis Rheum. 2013;65:1-11.
20. Bicakcigil M, Aksu K, Kamali S, et al. Takayasu's arteritis in Turkey: clinical and angiographic features of 248 patients. Clin Exp Rheumatol. 2009;27:S59-64.
21. Soto ME, Espinola N, Flores-Suarez LF, et al. Takayasu arteritis: clinical features in 110 Mexican Mestizo patients and cardiovascular impact on survival and prognosis. Clin Exp Rheumatol. 2008;26:S9-15.
22. Ueda H, Morooka S, Ito I, et al. Clinical observation of 52 cases of aortitis syndrome. Jpn Heart J. 1969;10:277-88.
23. Ishikawa K, Maetani S. Long-term outcome for 120 Japanese patients with Takayasu's disease. Clinical and statistical analyses of related prognostic factors. Circulation. 1994;90:1855-60.
24. Jain S, Kumari S, Ganguly NK, et al. Current status of Takayasu arteritis in India. Int J Cardiol. 1996;54:S111-6.
25. Lupi-Herrera E, Sanchez-Torres G, Marcushamer J, et al. Takayasu's arteritis. Clinical study of 107 cases. Am Heart J. 1977;93:94-103.

26. Ishikawa K. Diagnostic approach and proposed criteria for the clinical diagnosis of Takayasu's arteriopathy. J Am Coll Cardiol. 1988;12:964-72.

27. Sharma BK, Jain S, Suri S, et al. Diagnostic criteria for Takayasu arteritis. Int J Cardiol. 1996;54:S141-7.

28. Sharma BK, Siveski-Iliskovic N, Singal PK. Takayasu arteritis may be underdiagnosed in North America. Can J Cardiol. 1995;11:311-6.

29. Ozen S, Pistorio A, Iusan SM, et al. EULAR/PRINTO/PRES criteria for Henoch-Schönlein purpura, childhood polyarteritis nodosa, childhood Wegener granulomatosis and childhood Takayasu arteritis: Ankara 2008. Part II: final classification criteria. Ann Rheum Dis. 2010;69:798-806.

30. Gravanis MB. Giant cell arteritis and Takayasu aortitis: morphologic, pathogenetic and etiologic factors. Int J Cardiol. 2000;75:S21-33; discussion S35-26.

31. Sharma BK, Jain S, Radotra BD. An autopsy study of Takayasu arteritis in India. Int J Cardiol. 1998;66:S85-90; discussion S91.

32. Mehra NK, Jaini R, Balamurugan A, et al. Immunogenetic analysis of Takayasu arteritis in Indian patients. Int J Cardiol. 1998;66:S127-132; discussion S133.

33. Sahin Z, Bicakcigil M, Aksu K, et al. Takayasu's arteritis is associated with HLA-B*52, but not with HLA-B*51, in Turkey. Arthritis Res Ther. 2012;14:R27.

34. Soto ME, Vargas-Alarcon G, Cicero-Sabido R, et al. Comparison distribution of HLA-B alleles in Mexican patients with Takayasu arteritis and tuberculosis. Hum Immunol. 2007;68:449-53.

35. Takamura C, Ohhigashi H, Ebana Y, et al. New human leukocyte antigen risk allele in Japanese patients with Takayasu arteritis. Circ J. 2012;76:1697-702.

36. Terao C, Yoshifuji H, Ohmura K, et al. Association of Takayasu arteritis with HLA-B 67:01 and two amino acids in HLA-B protein. Rheumatology (Oxford). 2013;52:1769-74.

37. Yoshida M, Kimura A, Katsuragi K, et al. DNA typing of HLA-B gene in Takayasu's arteritis. Tissue Antigens. 1993;42:87-90.

38. Saruhan-Direskeneli G, Hughes T, Aksu K, et al. Identification of multiple genetic susceptibility loci in Takayasu arteritis. Am J Hum Genet. 2013;93:298-305.

39. Terao C, Yoshifuji H, Kimura A, et al. Two susceptibility loci to Takayasu arteritis reveal a synergistic role of the IL12B and HLA-B regions in a Japanese population. Am J Hum Genet. 2013;93:289-97.

40. Chauhan SK, Singh M, Nityanand S. Reactivity of gamma/delta T cells to human 60-kd heat-shock protein and their cytotoxicity to aortic endothelial cells in Takayasu arteritis. Arthritis Rheum. 2007;56:2798-2802.

41. Kimura A, Kobayashi Y, Takahashi M, et al. Mica gene polymorphism in Takayasu's arteritis and Buerger's disease. Int J Cardiol. 1998;66:S107-13; discussion S115.

42. Lv N, Dang A, Wang Z, et al. Association of susceptibility to Takayasu arteritis in Chinese Han patients with HLA-DPB1. Hum Immunol. 2011;72:893-6.

43. Saruhan-Direskeneli G, Bicakcigil M, Yilmaz V, et al. Interleukin (IL)-12, IL-2, and IL-6 gene polymorphisms in Takayasu's arteritis from Turkey. Hum Immunol. 2006;67:735-40.

44. Shibata H, Yasunami M, Obuchi N, et al. Direct determination of single nucleotide polymorphism haplotype of NFKBIL1 promoter polymorphism by DNA conformation analysis and its application to association study of chronic inflammatory diseases. Hum Immunol. 2006;67:363-73.

45. Vanderschueren S, Knockaert D, Adriaenssens T, et al. From prolonged febrile illness to fever of unknown origin: the challenge continues. Arch Intern Med. 2003;163:1033-41.

46. Aggarwal A, Chag M, Sinha N, et al. Takayasu's arteritis: role of *Mycobacterium tuberculosis* and its 65 kDA heat shock protein. Int J Cardiol. 1996;55:49-55.

47. Castillo-Martinez D, Amezcua-Guerra LM. Self-reactivity against stress-induced cell molecules: the missing link between Takayasu's arteritis and tuberculosis? Med Hypotheses. 2012;78:485-8.

48. Duzova A, Turkmen O, Cinar A, et al. Takayasu's arteritis and tuberculosis: a case report. Clin Rheumatol. 2000;19:486-9.

49. Kothari SS. Aetiopathogenesis of Takayasu's arteritis and BCG vaccination: the missing link? Med Hypotheses. 1995;45:227-30.

50. Soto ME, Del Carmen Avila-Casado M, Huesca-Gomez C, et al. Detection of IS6110 and HupB gene sequences of mycobacterium tuberculosis and bovis in the aortic tissue of patients with Takayasu's arteritis. BMC Infect Dis. 2012;12:194.

51. Chauhan SK, Tripathy NK, Sinha N, et al. T-cell receptor repertoire of circulating gamma delta T-cells in Takayasu's arteritis. Clin Immunol. 2006;118:243-9.

52. Seko Y, Minota S, Kawasaki A, et al. Perforin-secreting killer cell infiltration and expression of a 65-kd heat-shock protein in aortic tissue of patients with Takayasu's arteritis. J Clin Invest. 1994;93:750-8.

53. Tripathy NK, Chauhan SK, Nityanand S. Cytokine mRNA repertoire of peripheral blood mononuclear cells in Takayasu's arteritis. Clin Exp Immunol. 2004;138:369-74.

54. Chauhan SK, Tripathy NK, Nityanand S. Antigenic targets and pathogenicity of anti-aortic endothelial cell antibodies in Takayasu arteritis. Arthritis Rheum. 2006;54:2326-33.

55. Tripathy NK, Sinha N, Nityanand S. Anti-annexin v antibodies in Takayasu's arteritis: prevalence and relationship with disease activity. Clin Exp Immunol. 2003;134:360-4.

56. Wang H, Ma J, Wu Q, et al. Circulating B lymphocytes producing autoantibodies to endothelial cells play a role in the pathogenesis of Takayasu arteritis. J Vasc Surg. 2011;53:174-80.

57. Tobon GJ, Alard JE, Youinou P, et al. Are autoantibodies triggering endothelial cell apoptosis really pathogenic? Autoimmun Rev. 2009;8:605-10.

58. Hoyer BF, Mumtaz IM, Loddenkemper K, et al. Takayasu arteritis is characterised by disturbances of B cell homeostasis and responds to B cell depletion therapy with rituximab. Ann Rheum Dis. 2012;71:75-79.

59. Rav-Acha M, Plot L, Peled N, et al. Coronary involvement in Takayasu's arteritis. Autoimmun Rev. 2007;6:566-71.

60. Zheng D, Fan D, Liu L. Takayasu arteritis in China: a report of 530 cases. Heart Vessels Suppl. 1992;7:32-36.

61. Frances C, Boisnic S, Bletry O, et al. Cutaneous manifestations of Takayasu arteritis. A retrospective study of 80 cases. Dermatologica. 1990;181:266-72.

62. Pascual-Lopez M, Hernandez-Nunez A, Aragues-Montanes M, et al. Takayasu's disease with cutaneous involvement. Dermatology. 2004;208:10-15.

63. Chun YS, Park SJ, Park IK, et al. The clinical and ocular manifestations of Takayasu arteritis. Retina. 2001;21:132-40.

64. Schmidt J, Kermani TA, Bacani AK, et al. Diagnostic features, treatment, and outcomes of Takayasu arteritis in a US cohort of 126 patients. Mayo Clin Proc. 2013;88:822-30.

65. Arnaud L, Haroche J, Malek Z, et al. Is (18)F-fluorodeoxyglucose positron emission tomography scanning a reliable way to assess disease activity in Takayasu arteritis? Arthritis Rheum. 2009;60:1193-200.

66. Fuchs M, Briel M, Daikeler T, et al. The impact of 18F-FDG PET on the management of patients with suspected large vessel vasculitis. Eur J Nucl Med Mol Imaging. 2012;39:344-53.

67. Karapolat I, Kalfa M, Keser G, et al. Comparison of F18-FDG PET/CT findings with current clinical disease status in patients with Takayasu's arteritis. Clin Exp Rheumatol. 2013;31:S15-21.

68. Kissin EY, Merkel PA. Diagnostic imaging in Takayasu arteritis. Curr Opin Rheumatol. 2004;16:31-37.

69. Magnoni M, Dagna L, Coli S, et al. Assessment of Takayasu arteritis activity by carotid contrast-enhanced ultrasound. Circ Cardiovasc Imaging. 2011;4:e1-2.

70. Mavrogeni S, Dimitroulas T, Chatziioannou SN, et al. The role of multimodality imaging in the evaluation of Takayasu arteritis. Semin Arthritis Rheum. 2013;42:401-12.

71. Pipitone N, Versari A, Salvarani C. Role of imaging studies in the diagnosis and follow-up of large-vessel vasculitis: an update. Rheumatology (Oxford). 2008;47:403-8.

72. Schmidt WA. Imaging in vasculitis. Best Pract Res Clin Rheumatol. 2013;27:107-18.

73. Tso E, Flamm SD, White RD, et al. Takayasu arteritis: utility and limitations of magnetic resonance imaging in diagnosis and treatment. Arthritis Rheum. 2002;46:1634-42.

74. Yamazaki M, Takano H, Miyauchi H, et al. Detection of Takayasu arteritis in early stage by computed tomography. Int J Cardiol. 2002;85:305-7.

75. Pipitone N, Pazzola G, Muratore F, et al. L30. Assessment of vasculitis extent and severity. Presse Med. 2013;42:588-9.

76. Toledano K, Guralnik L, Lorber A, et al. Pulmonary arteries involvement in Takayasu's arteritis: two cases and literature review. Semin Arthritis Rheum. 2011;41:461-70.

77. Lanjewar C, Kerkar P, Vaideeswar P, et al. Isolated bilateral coronary ostial stenosis—an uncommon presentation of aortoarteritis. Int J Cardiol. 2007;114:e126-8.

78. Hata A, Noda M, Moriwaki R, et al. Angiographic findings of Takayasu arteritis: new classification. Int J Cardiol. 1996;54:S155-63.

79. Stone JR. Aortitis, periaortitis, and retroperitoneal fibrosis, as manifestations of IgG4-related systemic disease. Curr Opin Rheumatol. 2011;23:88-94.

80. Hoffman GS, Leavitt RY, Kerr GS, et al. Treatment of glucocorticoid-resistant or relapsing Takayasu arteritis with methotrexate. Arthritis Rheum. 1994;37:578-82.

81. Valsakumar AK, Valappil UC, Jorapur V, et al. Role of immunosuppressive therapy on clinical, immunological, and angiographic outcome in active Takayasu's arteritis. J Rheumatol. 2003;30:1793-8.

82. Goel R, Danda D, Mathew J, et al. *Mycophenolate mofetil* in Takayasu's arteritis. Clin Rheumatol. 2010;29:329-32.

83. Cofan F, Rosich E, Arias M, et al. Quality of life in renal transplant recipients following conversion from mycophenolate mofetil to enteric-coated mycophenolate sodium. Transplant Proc. 2007;39:2179-81.

84. Cash JM, Engelbrecht JA. Takayasu's arteritis in western South Dakota. S D J Med. 1990;43:5-9.

85. Rodriguez-Hurtado FJ, Sabio JM, Lucena J, et al. Ocular involvement in Takayasu's arteritis: response to cyclophosphamide therapy. Eur J Med Res. 2002;7:128-30.

86. Kotter I, Daikeler T, Amberger C, et al. Autologous stem cell transplantation of treatment-resistant systemic vasculitis—a single center experience and review of the literature. Clin Nephrol. 2005;64:485-9.

87. Fearfield LA, Ross JR, Farrell AM, et al. Pyoderma gangrenosum associated with Takayasu's arteritis responding to cyclosporin. Br J Dermatol. 1999;141:339-43.

88. Horigome H, Kamoda T, Matsui A. Treatment of glucocorticoid-dependent Takayasu's arteritis with cyclosporin. Med J Aust. 1999;170:566.

89. Ujiie H, Sawamura D, Yokota K, et al. Pyoderma gangrenosum associated with Takayasu's arteritis. Clin Exp Dermatol. 2004;29:357-9.

90. Yamazaki H, Nanki T, Harigai M, et al. Successful treatment of refractory Takayasu arteritis with tacrolimus. J Rheumatol. 2012;39:1487-8.

91. Unizony S, Stone JH, Stone JR. New treatment strategies in large-vessel vasculitis. Curr Opin Rheumatol. 2013;25:3-9.

92. Park MC, Lee SW, Park YB, et al. Serum cytokine profiles and their correlations with disease activity in Takayasu's arteritis. Rheumatology (Oxford). 2006;45:545-8.

93. Tripathy NK, Gupta PC, Nityanand S. High TNF-alpha and low IL-2 producing T cells characterize active disease in Takayasu's arteritis. Clin Immunol. 2006;118:154-8.

94. Schmidt J, Kermani TA, Bacani AK, et al. Tumor necrosis factor inhibitors in patients with Takayasu arteritis: experience from a referral center with long-term followup. Arthritis Care Res (Hoboken). 2012;64:1079-83.

95. Comarmond C, Plaisier E, Dahan K, et al. Anti TNF-alpha in refractory Takayasu's arteritis: Cases series and review of the literature. Autoimmun Rev. 2012;11:678-84.

96. Ernst D, Greer M, Stoll M, et al. Remission achieved in refractory advanced Takayasu arteritis using rituximab. Case Rep Rheumatol. 2012;2012:406963.

97. Nishimoto N, Nakahara H, Yoshio-Hoshino N, et al. Successful treatment of a patient with Takayasu arteritis using a humanized anti-interleukin-6 receptor antibody. Arthritis Rheum. 2008;58:1197-1200.

98. Goel R, Danda D, Kumar S, et al. Rapid control of disease activity by tocilizumab in 10 'difficult-to-treat' cases of Takayasu arteritis. Int J Rheum Dis. 2013;16:754-61.

99. Abatacept for Treating Adults With Giant Cell Arteritis and Takayasu's Arteritis - Full Text View - ClinicalTrials.

gov [Internet]. [cited 2014 Jun 8]. Available from: http://clinicaltrials.gov/show/NCT00556439

100. Shimizu M, Ueno K, Ishikawa S, et al. Successful multitarget therapy using mizoribine and tacrolimus for refractory Takayasu arteritis. Rheumatology (Oxford). 2014;53:1530-2.

101. Cong XL, Dai SM, Feng X, Wang ZW, et al. Takayasu's arteritis: clinical features and outcomes of 125 patients in china. Clin Rheumatol. 2010;29:973-81.

102. Ham SW, Kumar SR, Wang BR, et al. Late outcomes of endovascular and open revascularization for nonatherosclerotic renal artery disease. Arch Surg. 2010;145:832-9.

103. Kim YW, Kim DI, Park YJ, et al. Surgical bypass vs endovascular treatment for patients with supra-aortic arterial occlusive disease due to Takayasu arteritis. J Vasc Surg. 2012;55:693-700.

104. Mukhtyar C, Guillevin L, Cid MC, et al. EULAR recommendations for the management of large vessel vasculitis. Ann Rheum Dis. 2009;68:318-23.

105. Saadoun D, Lambert M, Mirault T, et al. Retrospective analysis of surgery versus endovascular intervention in Takayasu arteritis: A multicenter experience. Circulation. 2012;125:813-9.

106. Wu X, Duan HY, Gu YQ, et al. Surgical treatment of brachiocephalic vessel involvement in Takayasu's arteritis. Chin Med J (Engl). 2010;123:1122-6.

107. Miyata T, Sato O, Koyama H, et al. Long-term survival after surgical treatment of patients with Takayasu's arteritis. Circulation. 2003;108:1474-80.

108. Fields CE, Bower TC, Cooper LT, et al. Takayasu's arteritis: operative results and influence of disease activity. J Vasc Surg. 2006;43:64-71.

109. Matsuura K, Ogino H, Kobayashi J, et al. Surgical treatment of aortic regurgitation due to Takayasu arteritis: long-term morbidity and mortality. Circulation. 2005;112:3707-12.

110. Park MC, Lee SW, Park YB, et al. Post-interventional immunosuppressive treatment and vascular restenosis in Takayasu's arteritis. Rheumatology (Oxford). 2006;45:600-5.

111. Joseph G. L49. Percutaneous interventions in Takayasu arteritis. Presse Med. 2013;42:635-7.

112. Joseph G, Danda D. Outcome of 1516 percutaneous interventions in 401 patients with Takayasu arteritis a single-center experience from south India. Presse Med. 2013;42:721.

113. Mukhtyar C, Lee R, Brown D, et al. Modification and validation of the Birmingham vasculitis activity score (version 3). Ann Rheum Dis. 2009;68:1827-32.

114. Sivakumar MR, Misra RN, Bacon PA. OP14. The Indian perspective of Takayasu arteritis and development of a disease extent index (DEI.TAK) to assess Takayasu arteritis. Rheumatology. 2005;44:iii6-iii7.

115. Misra R, Danda D, Rajappa SM, et al. Development and initial validation of the Indian Takayasu clinical activity score (ITAS2010). Rheumatology (Oxford). 2013;52:1795-801.

116. Noris M, Daina E, Gamba S, et al. Interleukin-6 and RANTES in Takayasu arteritis: a guide for therapeutic decisions? Circulation. 1999;100:55-60.

117. Matsuyama A, Sakai N, Ishigami M, et al. Matrix metalloproteinases as novel disease markers in Takayasu arteritis. Circulation. 2003;108:1469-73.

118. Yilmaz H, Gerdan V, Kozaci D, et al. Ghrelin and adipokines as circulating markers of disease activity in patients with Takayasu arteritis. Arthritis Res Ther. 2012;14:R272.

CHAPTER 29

Kawasaki Disease

S Madhusudan, Surjit Singh

INTRODUCTION

If one were to be given the task of creating a disease that could vex the most astute of clinicians, what would its attributes be?

- Clinical features that mimic other common illnesses.
- Fleeting clinical signs that are already passive by the time the child comes to medical attention or are yet to appear.
- The more atypical the presentation, more sinister the complications.
- Few clues in laboratory investigations with none being diagnostic.
- Devastating short-term and long-term complications if the diagnosis is missed.
- The absence of specific guidelines for diagnosis or treatment, and, fortunately, the availability of an expensive drug that dramatically alters the prognosis, but unfortunately with no specific guidelines for its use.

Few diseases in medicine possibly have all these attributes. In the 1960s, a Japanese pediatrician stumbled upon one such disease when he came across several febrile children with characteristic skin and mucosal findings and published a detailed account of them, calling the disease mucocutaneous lymph node syndrome.[1] Over the next few decades, similar children were seen all over the world. Today, we know it as Kawasaki disease (KD), the commonest childhood vasculitis and the most common cause of acquired heart disease in children of the developed world.[2]

CASE VIGNETTE

A 4-year-old girl-child was brought to the hospital with high-grade fever for three days and marked irritability. Initial work-up for fever carried out at the referring hospital was noncontributory. On examination, she was found to have conjunctival edema, erythematous maculopapular rash, strawberry tongue, and bilateral cervical lymphadenopathy. There was reactivation of the Bacillus Calmette-Guerin (BCG) vaccination site. Her hemoglobin was 89 g/L; total leucocyte count 18,200/cumm; 80% polymorphs, as differential count showed; erythrocyte sedimentation rate (ESR) 86 mm/h; and C-reactive protein (CRP) 120 mg/L. Urine examination showed traces of albumin and 40 pus cells per high-power field. Blood and urine cultures were sterile. A diagnosis of KD was made, and she was started on intravenous immunoglobulin 2 g/kg as a single bolus. There was prompt resolution of fever and the irritability subsided within a few hours. Two-dimensional echocardiography done a week after admission did not show any evidence of coronary artery abnormalities (CAA).

EPIDEMIOLOGY

Kawasaki disease has been reported worldwide but the maximum incidence is seen in Japan, followed by Korea and Taiwan.[3] Incidence rates over the years, in several countries, are increasing. Japan reported an incidence of 239.6 per 100,000 children 0-4 years old, the highest ever till date.[3] The Japanese incidence rates are several times those of China (60.7), Canada (25.1), Northern European countries (5-10), and Australia (3.5).[3] A hospital-based analysis in our own institute showed an increasing incidence from 0.51 in 1994 to 4.54 in 2007 per 100,000 children under 15 years of age.[4]

Though more common in childhood, KD has been described in almost all age groups including neonates and the elderly. The maximum incidence of KD is seen under the age of 5 years.[5] It has been seen to be more common in boys than in girls.[5,6]

An intriguing feature of KD is its characteristic seasonal variation that has been seen all over the world. The Kawasaki Disease Global Climate Consortium reported statistically significant and consistent seasonal fluctuations in KD. In the Northern Hemisphere, high numbers were found in winter and low numbers in late summer and fall, but no such pattern was seen in the tropics or the Southern Hemisphere.[7] In a study from our institute, we demonstrated two peaks, with most children presenting in October and May, and least in February.[4]

ETIOPATHOGENESIS

The exact pathogenetic mechanisms underlying KD are obscure and a matter of intense investigation all over the world. From microbial organisms to changing wind patterns in the stratosphere, the theories postulated over the years have been as diverse as the clinical manifestations. Data demonstrating higher risk of KD among siblings of children with KD and higher probability of parents having had KD as children suggest a genetic basis.[8] Another pointer toward a genetic basis is the striking difference between the average annual incidence rates seen in Hawaiian children, with Japanese American children having rates as high as those in the Japanese mainland, whereas white children had rates similar to those in the US mainland.[9] Three areas identified in this regard include single nucleotide polymorphisms (SNP) in calcineurin nuclear pathway of activated T cells, TGF-beta signaling pathway, and the FCGR2A pathways.[10] Recent studies have shown that SNP in the inositol 1,4,5-triphosphate receptor type 3 (ITPR3) gene is associated with the risk of developing CAA in children with KD.[11]

The occurrence of KD in epidemics, the seasonal variation, increased risk in siblings and the presence of IgA plasma cells, monocytes/macrophages, and CD8 lymphocytes in autopsy cases, all point to an infective agent at the root of KD, probably, a virus that enters through the respiratory or the gastrointestinal route.[12] Recently, studies have also suggested the possibility that the elusive agent may be wind borne and may be carried by the wind currents originating in Central Asia, and that studying the microbiology of aerosols might help.[13]

CLINICAL FEATURES

As no laboratory parameter is pathognomonic and the diagnosis is primarily clinical, sound knowledge of the clinical features and the natural course of the disease are essential.

The natural course of KD can be divided into three phases: the acute phase constituting the first 10 days of the illness, the subacute phase from day 10 to day 28, and the convalescent phase that lasts up to 6–8 weeks after the onset of illness.

The disease starts like any other infective illness with high grade, remittent fever that should last at least five days to satisfy the diagnostic criteria. However, in the presence of four or more principal criteria, the diagnosis can be made as early as day 4 of the illness. Fever lasts for a mean of 11 days in the absence of appropriate treatment but can continue for 3–4 weeks.[14] Continuing fever with no response to antibiotics is a key feature that differentiates KD from common infections, including its closest mimic, streptococcal infection. Conversely, the resolution of fever with appropriate therapy within two days is a retrospective clue. Fever is accompanied by one or more of the following features at different times during its course.

Bilateral, nonexudative conjunctival injection typically involving the bulbar conjunctiva, with limbal sparing appears shortly after the onset of fever. Conjunctival edema, corneal ulceration, pain, and photophobia are unusual. Acute anterior uveitis is well known but is usually asymptomatic and self-limited.

The rash of KD is highly variable, but is usually an erythematous maculopapular rash. Less commonly, it can be an urticarial exanthem, a scarlatiniform rash, an erythroderma, an erythema-multiforme-like rash, or, rarely, a fine micropustular eruption. Vesicles and bullae are extremely rare.

Cervical lymphadenopathy is the least common feature that figures in the diagnostic criteria. It is usually unilateral, involves one or more nodes that are at least 1.5 cm in size, firm, and nontender. Like fever, lymphadenopathy also lures the unsuspecting clinician to continue treating the child on the lines of an infection. Unilateral cervical lymphadenopathy unresponsive to antibiotics in a febrile child should always remind one of KD.

Characteristic changes occur in the extremities in each phase of the disease. In the acute phase, there is bilateral, symmetrical, occasionally painful swelling of the hands and feet that may be associated with erythema of the palms and soles. This gradually disappears by the end of the second week when the characteristic periungual desquamation starts. In the convalescent phase, transverse ridging at the base of the nails called "Beau's lines" may be seen.

Some of the most characteristic features of KD are the typical changes that occur in the lips, tongue, and the oral mucosa. Red, swollen, and cracked lips with peeling and occasional bleeding, occur in few other diseases and again differentiate KD from streptococcal infection. The tongue is also red and the fungiform papillae stand out giving rise to the characteristic "strawberry tongue." Oropharyngeal mucosa is diffusely erythematous.

Perianal desquamation is characteristic of KD and occurs in the first week of the illness as compared to periungual desquamation that occurs after 10 days in the convalescent phase. Desquamation, especially perianal, occurs in few other conditions and is virtually pathognomonic of KD.

Children with KD, especially infants, have been seen to be extremely irritable, and this irritability, which is out of proportion to fever, can again be a clue to KD.

Another typical feature that can be a valuable clue in countries where the BCG vaccine is commonly used is reactivation at the site of BCG vaccination that may appear as erythema, induration, and rarely necrosis and ulceration. Virtually, any organ system can be involved and the diversity of symptoms that have been described, including arthritis, arthralgia, vomiting, pain abdomen, diarrhea, hepatomegaly, jaundice, transient unilateral facial nerve palsy, and transient sensorineural hearing loss, testify to this fact.[15]

The dreaded complication of KD is the development of CAA that can occur in up to 15–25% of untreated cases but in < 5% in children treated with intravenous immunoglobulin (IVIg).[14] In fact, some of the young adults with CAA and myocardial infarction without the traditional risk factors may have had KD that went unrecognized in their childhood.

The following section lists the diagnostic criteria of KD.[15]

CLINICAL CRITERIA FOR THE DIAGNOSIS OF KD

Fever persisting at least 5 days and presence of at least four principal features:

1. *Changes in extremities:*
   - *Acute:* Erythema of palms and soles; edema of hands and feet.
   - *Subacute:* Periungual peeling of fingers and toes in weeks 2 and 3.
2. Polymorphous exanthema.
3. Bilateral bulbar conjunctival injection without exudates.
4. *Changes in lips and oral cavity:* Erythema, lips cracking, strawberry tongue, and diffuse injection of oral and pharyngeal mucosae.
5. Cervical lymphadenopathy (≥ 1.5 cm diameter), usually unilateral.

INVESTIGATIONS

Laboratory investigations that aid in the diagnosis of KD are nonspecific and include raised inflammatory markers such as ESR and CRP. Polymorphonuclear leukocytosis and normocytic anemia are common in the acute phase. Platelet counts are characteristically normal in the first week and start rising by the seventh day of illness. Thrombocytopenia has also been described in this setting.[16] Dengue fever can be a close imitator, given the seasonal predilection that it shares with KD and the simultaneous occurrence of both has also been described.[17]

Needless to say, a comprehensive search for an infective focus should be undertaken that if positive may mean either an alternative diagnosis or a coexisting illness, which in fact may have been the inciting agent of KD in the first place. This includes a blood culture, urine analysis and culture, chest X-ray, and ultrasound of abdomen. The presence of sterile pyuria and that of hydrops of the gall bladder are soft markers of KD.

INCOMPLETE AND ATYPICAL KD

Incomplete KD refers to those cases who fail to "completely" satisfy the diagnostic criteria of KD, whereas atypical KD refers to those cases that do not show the "typical" features of KD. Atypical manifestations can be significant hypertension, renal failure, stroke or acute "surgical" abdomen, urethritis, orchitis, and pleural effusion, none of which are commonly seen in KD.

DIFFERENTIAL DIAGNOSIS

Not surprisingly, the differential diagnosis is wide and encompasses varied conditions such as scarlet fever, Stevens-Johnson syndrome, measles and other viral exanthemata, toxic shock syndrome, staphylococcal scalded skin syndrome, and systemic onset juvenile idiopathic arthritis. Clinical features that are typical of KD and seldom seen in other conditions include persistent fever unresponsive to antibiotics, extreme irritability, changes in the lips and tongue, and perianal and periungual desquamation.

The single most worrisome aspect of KD is the failure to make a diagnosis and this worry stems from the numerous red herrings that one encounters in the history, examination, and laboratory investigations, the important ones being listed below:

Feature	Possible misdiagnosis
Fever, rash	Viral fever
Rash	Drug reaction
Cervical lymphadenopathy, pharyngeal erythema	Acute streptococcal pharyngitis
Sterile pyuria	UTI
Fever, extreme irritability	Meningitis
Thrombocytopenia with fever and rash	Dengue fever

As highlighted all along, KD is a clinical dilemma.

It would be useful for clinicians caring for children with suspected KD to remember the following practical aspects.

- It is always a good idea to manage a child with suspected KD as an inpatient rather than an outpatient, as it makes the following points easier.
- Given the flitting and fleeting nature of the symptoms and signs, a complete first-hand history taken from the primary caretaker of the child, often more than once, is crucial.
- Due to high-grade fever persisting despite conventional antibiotics, the child is often evaluated by several physicians who could have documented clinical signs at different times as the disease evolves. Communication with these physicians might help in assembling pieces together to solve the jigsaw that KD is.
- A complete, meticulous physical examination should be performed daily to avoid missing new clinical signs. Periungual and perianal desquamation and reactivation at the BCG site can be extremely subtle initially and are likely to be missed unless specifically looked for.
- Isolated laboratory parameters do not carry as much significance as monitoring their trends does. In conjunction with the presence or absence of fever, they help the clinician in deciding the need for therapy.
- The ultimate decision of treating a child with KD should be based not on any single clinical or laboratory parameter but on the child's risk profile and the family in Toto, which in developing countries means considering the financial constraints as well.

TREATMENT

The availability of a drug that dramatically decreases the incidence of CAA from 25 to 2% is a boon for these children and the role of IVIg is well established in this regard.[18] Several dose and infusion regimens have been compared and 2 g/kg as a single infusion around over 10 hours has been seen to be most effective and is followed in our unit.[14] The rate of infusion should be low initially and gradually increased every 15–30 min, to a maximum of 4 mL/kg/h.

Adverse events following IVIg infusions can be immediate (occurring during the infusion itself) or delayed (occurring after the infusion is complete). Commonly, adverse effects occur immediately after infusion and include headache, flushing, chills, myalgia, wheezing, tachycardia, lower back pain, nausea, and hypotension.

Treatment failure, seen in approximately 10–15% of cases, is defined as persistence or recurrence of fever ≥ 36 hours after the completion of the initial IVIg infusion.[14] Retreatment

with IVIg is recommended in such cases, other options being intravenous methylprednisolone and more recently the tumor necrosis factor alpha antagonist, infliximab.

Infliximab has also been tried as an addition to the primary therapy in KD but has not been seen to reduce treatment resistence.[19]

Aspirin is used at an anti-inflammatory dose of 30–50 mg/kg per day during the acute phase of the illness. Compared to the higher dose of 80–120 mg/kg per day, it may be better tolerated in terms of gastrointestinal and other side effects. The dose is then reduced to an antiplatelet dose of 3–5 mg/kg once fever and inflammation subside and continued till the child shows no evidence of coronary changes in the echocardiogram done at 6–8 weeks. In case the child has coronary changes, aspirin is continued indefinitely.[14]

CONCLUSION

Kawasaki disease is increasingly being recognized in our country and is no longer uncommon. Optimal management demands a timely diagnosis that, being entirely clinical, requires a strong clinical acumen and awareness with repeated reinforcement is the key.

KEY POINTS

- Kawasaki disease is a medium-vessel vasculitis seen predominantly in childhood.
- It should be considered in the differential diagnosis of all children with high-grade fever persisting beyond 5 days and, especially, when it is accompanied by conjunctival injection, rash, oral cavity changes, and cervical lymphadenopathy.
- Coronary artery abnormalities are the dreaded complication.
- Intravenous immunoglobulin is the standard treatment.

REFERENCES

1. Kawasaki T. Pediatric acute febrile mucocutaneous lymph node syndrome with characteristic desquamation of fingers and toes: my clinical observation of fifty cases. Pediatr Infect Dis. J 2002;21:1-38.
2. Taubert KA, Rowley AH, Shulman ST. Nationwide survey of Kawasaki disease and acute rheumatic fever. J Pediatr. 1991;119:279-82.
3. Abstracts of the 10th International Kawasaki Disease Symposium. February 7-10, 2012. Kyoto, Japan. Pediatr Int. 2012;54:38-142.

4. Singh S, Aulakh R, Bhalla AK, et al. Is Kawasaki disease incidence rising in Chandigarh, North India? Arch Dis Child. 2011;96:137-40.
5. Uehara R, Belay ED. Epidemiology of Kawasaki disease in Asia, Europe, and the United States. J Epidemiol. 2012;22:79-85.
6. Singh S, Aulakh R. Kawasaki disease and Henoch-Schönlein purpura: changing trends at a tertiary care hospital in north India (1993–2008). Rheumatol Int. 2010;30:771-4.
7. Burns JC, Herzog L, Fabri O, et al. Seasonality of Kawasaki disease: a global perspective. Kawasaki Disease Global Climate Consortium. PLoS One. 2013;8:e74529.
8. Uehara R, Yashiro M, Nakamura Y, et al. Kawasaki disease in parents and children. Acta Paediatr. 2003;92:694-7.
9. Holman RC, Christensen KY, Belay ED, et al. Racial/ethnic differences in the incidence of Kawasaki syndrome among children in Hawaii. Hawaii Med J. 2010;69:194-7.
10. Burns JC, Newburger JW. Genetics insights into the pathogenesis of Kawasaki disease. Circ Cardiovasc Genet. 2012;5:277-8.
11. Onouchi Y, Gunji T, Burns JC, et al. ITPKC functional polymorphism associated with Kawasaki disease susceptibility and formation of coronary artery aneurysms. Nat Genet. 2008;40:35-42.
12. Takahashi K, Oharaseki T, Yokouchi Y. Pathogenesis of Kawasaki disease. Clin Exp Immunol. 2011;164:20-2.
13. Rodó X, Ballester J, Cayan D, et al. Association of Kawasaki disease with tropospheric wind patterns. Sci Rep. 2011;1:152.
14. Newburger JW, Takahashi M, Gerber MA, et al. Diagnosis, treatment, and long-term management of Kawasaki disease: a statement for health professionals from the Committee on Rheumatic Fever, Endocarditis, and Kawasaki Disease, Council on Cardiovascular Disease in the Young, American Heart Association. Pediatrics. 2004;114:1708-33.
15. Sundel RP, Petty RE, Kawasaki disease. In: Cassidy JT, Petty RE, Laxer R, et al. (Eds). Textbook of Pediatric Rheumatology, 6th edition. Philadelphia: Elsevier; 2011. pp. 505-20.
16. Singh S, Gupta D, Suri D, et al. Thrombocytopenia as a presenting feature of Kawasaki disease: a case series from North India. Rheumatol Int. 2009;30:245-8.
17. Singh S, Jat KR, Suri D, et al. Dengue fever and Kawasaki disease: a clinical dilemma. Rheumatol Int. 2009;29:717-9.
18. Newburger JW, Takahashi M, Burns JC, et al. The treatment of Kawasaki syndrome with intravenous gamma globulin. N Engl J Med. 1986;315:341-7.
19. Tremoulet AH, Jain S, Jaggi P, et al. Infliximab for intensification of primary therapy for Kawasaki disease: a phase 3 randomised, double-blind, placebo-controlled trial. Lancet. 2014;383:1731-8.

CHAPTER 30

Polyarteritis Nodosa

Loïc Guillevin

INTRODUCTION

Polyarteritis nodosa (PAN) is a necrotizing angiitis that predominantly affects medium-sized arteries and can involve the majority of organs. Considering the etiologies of PAN, primary and secondary forms can be distinguished, because PAN can be the consequence of hepatitis B virus (HBV) infection[1] and, sometimes, other etiological pathogens.[2] Among vasculitides, PAN has now become even rarer in developed countries since the advent of vaccination against HBV, hygiene measures and specific prophylaxis against infectious diseases.[3] Herein, we review classification criteria for PAN, and characteristics of the disease, its outcome and treatments.

CASE VIGNETTE

A 40-year-old lady complained of the pain in the right shin after a long walk. The pain was persistent, and 2 months later, she developed ankle edema, and skin nodules mimicking erythema nodosum. Ultrasonography was normal. There were no symptoms suggestive of peripheral nerve involvement. Hemogram was normal; CRP was 25 mg/L. No autoantibodies and viral infections were detected (especially HBV). X-ray of the right leg showed a periosteal thickening of right fibula (Fig. 30.1A). Scintigraphy also showed evidence of periostitis and muscle inflammation (Fig. 30.1B) and magnetic resonance imaging (MRI) of the lower limbs showed contrast enhancement of the legs muscles (Fig. 30.1C). Skin biopsy showed necrotizing vasculitis of a medium-sized artery. A diagnosis of PAN was made, and the patient was started on prednisolone 40 mg/day, which was progressively tapered and eventually stopped 2 years later. She had four relapses, and complete

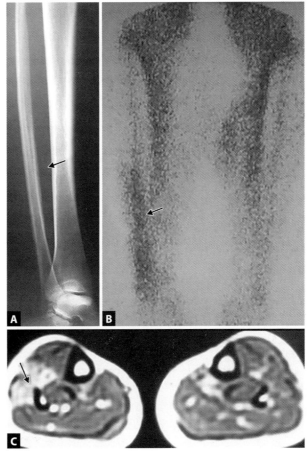

Figs 30.1A to C (A) X-ray of the right leg showing periosteal thickening of right fibula; (B) Scintigraphy showing evidence of periostitis and muscle inflammation; (C) MRI showing contrast enhancement of the legs muscles

remission was achieved with low-dose corticosteroids and methotrexate (7.5 mg/week), which were prescribed for 3 years.

CLASSIFICATION CRITERIA AND DIAGNOSIS

Several classifications of vasculitides have been established. In 1990, the American College of Rheumatology (ACR)[4] (Table 30.1) established criteria for PAN classification, which, unfortunately, did not distinguish between PAN and microscopic polyangiitis (MPA), which had wrongly been considered a different form of the same entity. Antineutrophil cytoplasm antibody (ANCA) testing, histological findings, and the presence of glomerulonephritis and/or alveolar hemorrhage have clearly established that MPA is a disease distinct from PAN. The Chapel Hill Nomenclature[5] (Table 30.2) describes the different vasculitides much more precisely. Polyarteritis nodosa is defined as a necrotizing arteritis of medium- or small-sized arteries, very rarely with vasculitis in arterioles, capillaries or venules, without glomerulonephritis and not associated with ANCA.

Diagnostic criteria based on clinical manifestations and biological or immunological signs could guide clinicians. Because most MPA patients are ANCA positive, these autoantibodies might be a major classification indicator and their presence should exclude the diagnosis of PAN (Table 30.3).[6] Our group established diagnostic criteria and we describe herein the clinical and immunological characteristics able to help diagnose PAN.[6]

EPIDEMIOLOGY

Polyarteritis nodosa is a rare disease that affects all racial groups. Estimates of the annual incidence of PAN-type systemic vasculitides in the general population range from 4.6/1,000,000 inhabitants in England,[7] and 9.0/1,000,000 inhabitants in Olmsted County, Minnesota, to 77/1,000,000 inhabitants in a hepatitis B-hyperendemic Alaskan Eskimo population.[8] In a German study,[9] the PAN incidence was extremely low (0.3–0.4/1,000,000 inhabitants according to the year and part of the country). A comparison of the PAN incidences in two European areas (Lugo, Spain and Norwich, UK) found no significant differences: respectively, 6.2 and 9.7/1,000,000 inhabitants.[10] In France, PAN prevalence was 34/1,000,000 inhabitants in Seine–Saint–Denis, a northern suburb of the Paris.[11]

ETIOLOGY AND PRECIPITATING FACTORS

Infections, mainly viral, have been identified as being responsible for PAN in many patients, with HBV being the most frequent etiological agent.

HBV-related PAN

Although viral antigens or immune complexes have rarely been found in the vessel walls of PAN patients, a close relationship has been demonstrated between PAN and HBV infection. In France, HBV infection transmitted by contaminated blood transfusion has now disappeared, the last proven case occurred in 1987. Meanwhile, intravenous drug abuse has rapidly become a major cause of HBV-related PAN, as is sexual transmission of HBV to nonvaccinated individuals at risk.[12] The development of anti-HBV vaccines and their administration to people at risk also explain the dramatically decreased numbers of new cases since 1989.

Table 30.1 1990 ACR criteria for the classification of polyarteritis nodosa[4]

Criterion	Definition
• Weight loss > 4 kg	Loss of 4 kg or more of body weight since illness began, not due to dieting or other factors
• Livedo reticularis	Mottled reticular pattern over the skin of portions of the extremities or torso
• Testicular pain or tenderness	Pain or tenderness of the testicles, not due to infection, trauma, or other causes
• Myalgias, weakness, or polyneuropathy	Diffuse myalgias (excluding shoulder and hip girdle) or weakness of muscles or tenderness of leg muscles
• Mononeuropathy or polyneuropathy	Development of mononeuropathy, multiple mononeuropathies or polyneuropathy
• Diastolic BP > 90 mm Hg	Development of hypertension with the diastolic BP higher than 90 mm Hg
• Elevated BUN or creatinine	Elevation of BUN >40 mg/dL (14.3 μmol/L) or creatinine >1.5 mg/dL (132 μmol/L), not due to dehydration or obstruction
• Hepatitis B virus	Presence of hepatitis B surface antigen or antibody in serum
• Arteriographic abnormality	Arteriogram showing aneurysms or occlusions of the visceral arteries, not due to arteriosclerosis, fibromuscular dysplasia, or noninflammatory causes
• Biopsy of small- or medium-sized artery containing neutrophils	Histologic changes showing the presence of granulocytes or granulocytes and mononuclear leukocytes in the artery wall

Table 30.2 Definitions adopted by the 2011–2012 International Chapel Hill Consensus Conference nomenclature of vasculitides {Jennette, 2013 #86601; Jennette, 2013 #86115}

CHCC 2012 Names	CHCC 2012 Definitions
Large vessel vasculitis (LVV)	Vasculitis affecting large arteries more often than other vasculitides. Large arteries are the aorta and its major branches. Any size artery may be affected.
Takayasu arteritis (TAK)	Arteritis, often granulomatous, predominantly affecting the aorta and/or its major branches. Onset usually in patients younger than 50.
Giant cell arteritis (GCA)	Arteritis, often granulomatous, usually affecting the aorta and/or its major branches, with a predilection for the branches of the carotid and vertebral arteries. Often involves the temporal artery. Onset usually in patients older than 50 and often associated with polymyalgia rheumatica.
Medium vessel vasculitis (MVV)	Vasculitis predominantly affecting medium arteries defined as the main visceral arteries and their branches. Any size artery may be affected. Inflammatory aneurysms and stenoses are common.
Polyarteritis nodosa (PAN)	Necrotizing arteritis of medium or small arteries without glomerulonephritis or vasculitis in arterioles, capillaries, or venules; and not associated with ANCA.
Kawasaki disease (KD)	Arteritis associated with the mucocutaneous lymph node syndrome and predominantly affecting medium and small arteries. Coronary arteries are often involved. Aorta and large arteries may be involved. Usually occurs in infants and young children.
Small vessel vasculitis (SVV)	Vasculitis predominantly affecting small vessels, defined as small intraparenchymal arteries, arterioles, capillaries and venules. Medium arteries and veins may be affected.
ANCA-associated vasculitis (AAV)	Necrotizing vasculitis, with few or no immune deposits, predominantly affecting small vessels (i.e., capillaries, venules, arterioles, and small arteries), associated with MPO-ANCA or PR3-ANCA. Not all patients have ANCA. Add a prefix indicating ANCA reactivity, e.g. PR3-ANCA, MPO-ANCA, ANCA-negative.
Microscopic polyangiitis (MPA)	Necrotizing vasculitis, with few or no immune deposits, predominantly affecting small vessels (i.e., capillaries, venules, or arterioles). Necrotizing arteritis involving small and medium arteries may be present. Necrotizing glomerulonephritis is very common. Pulmonary capillaritis often occurs. Granulomatous inflammation is absent.
Granulomatosis with polyangiitis (Wegener's) (GPA)	Necrotizing granulomatous inflammation usually involving the upper and lower respiratory tract, and necrotizing vasculitis affecting predominantly small-to-medium vessels (e.g., capillaries, venules, arterioles, arteries, and veins). Necrotizing glomerulonephritis is common.
Eosinophilic granulomatosis with polyangiitis (Churg–Strauss) (EGPA)	Eosinophil-rich and necrotizing granulomatous inflammation often involving the respiratory tract, and necrotizing vasculitis predominantly affecting small-to-medium vessels, and associated with asthma and eosinophilia. ANCA is more frequent when glomerulonephritis is present.
Immune-complex vasculitis	Vasculitis with moderate-to-marked vessel wall deposits of immunoglobulin and/or complement components predominantly affecting small vessels (i.e., capillaries, venules, arterioles and small arteries). Glomerulonephritis is frequent.
Anti-glomerular basement embrane (GBM) disease	Vasculitis affecting glomerular capillaries, pulmonary capillaries, or both, with basement membrane deposition of anti-basement membrane autoantibodies. Lung involvement causes pulmonary hemorrhage, and renal involvement causes glomerulonephritis with necrosis and crescents.
Cryoglobulinemic vasculitis (CV)	Vasculitis with cryoglobulin immune deposits affecting small vessels (predominantly capillaries, venules, or arterioles) and associated with cryoglobulins in serum. Skin, glomeruli and peripheral nerves are often involved.
IgA vasculitis (IgAV) (Henoch–Schönlein)	Vasculitis, with IgA1-dominant immune deposits, affecting small vessels (predominantly capillaries, venules, or arterioles). Often involves skin and gut, and frequently causes arthritis. Glomerulonephritis indistinguishable from IgA nephropathy may occur.
Hypocomplementemic urticarial vasculitis (HUV; Anti-C1q Vasculitis)	Vasculitis accompanied by urticaria and hypocomplementemia affecting small vessels (i.e., capillaries, venules, or arterioles), and associated with anti-C1q antibodies. Glomerulonephritis, arthritis, obstructive pulmonary disease, and ocular inflammation are common.
Variable vessel vasculitis (VVV)	Vasculitis with no predominant type of vessel involved that can affect vessels of any size (small, medium, and large) and type (arteries, veins, and capillaries).
Behçet's disease (BD)	Vasculitis occurring in patients with Behçet's disease that can affect arteries or veins. Behçet's disease is characterized by recurrent oral and/or genital aphthous ulcers accompanied by cutaneous, ocular, articular, gastrointestinal, and/or central nervous system inflammatory lesions. Small vessel vasculitis, thromboangiitis, thrombosis, arteritis and arterial aneurysms may occur.

Contd...

Contd...

CHCC 2012 Names	CHCC 2012 Definitions
Cogan's syndrome	Vasculitis occurring in patients with Cogan's syndrome. Cogan's syndrome is characterized by ocular inflammatory lesions, including interstitial keratitis, uveitis, and episcleritis, and inner ear disease, including sensorineural hearing loss and vestibular dysfunction. Vasculitic manifestations may include arteritis (affecting small, medium or large arteries), aortitis, aortic aneurysms, and aortic and mitral valvulitis.
Single organ vasculitis (SOV)	Vasculitis in arteries or veins of any size in a single organ that has no features that indicate that it is a limited expression of a systemic vasculitis. The involved organ and vessel type should be included in the name (e.g. cutaneous small vessel vasculitis, testicular arteritis, central nervous system vasculitis). Vasculitis distribution may be unifocal or multifocal (diffuse) within an organ. Some patients originally diagnosed with SOV will develop additional disease manifestations that warrant re-defining the case as one of the systemic vasculitides (e.g., cutaneous arteritis later becoming systemic polyarteritis nodosa).
Vasculitis associated with systemic disease	Vasculitis that is associated with and may be secondary to (caused by) a systemic disease. The name (diagnosis) should have a prefix term specifying the systemic disease (e.g., rheumatoid vasculitis, lupus vasculitis).
Vasculitis associated with probable etiology	Vasculitis that is associated with a probable specific etiology. The name (diagnosis) should have a prefix term specifying the association (e.g., hydralazine-associated microscopic polyangiitis, hepatitis B virus-associated vasculitis, and hepatitis C virus-associated cryoglobulinemic vasculitis).

Table 30.3 Proposed diagnostic criteria for PAN*[6]

Criteria	Odds ratio	95% CI	R^2
Positive for PAN			
HBV infection	16.85	6.30–45.08	0.320
Myalgias	1.93	1.06–3.53	0.517
Mononeuropathy or polyneuropathy	3.36	1.93–5.86	0.619
Arteriographic abnormalities	20.40	7.30–56.99	0.640
Testicular pain or tenderness	5.27	1.98–28.26	0.661
Negative (exclusion) for PAN			
ANCA-positivity	0.11	0.05–0.23	0.668
Glomerulonephritis	0.07	0.02–0.29	0.674
Recent asthma onset	0.01	0.01–0.06	0.433

*Based on the analysis of 582 systemic vasculitis patients with all data available in the French Vasculitis Study Group's database: 194 PAN (among whom 117 had HBV-related PAN) and 388 other systemic vasculitides (GPA, n = 144; EGPA, n = 115; MPA, n = 101; cryoglobulinemia, n = 28).

Moreover, the frequency of PAN, due to HBV infection or not, has also decreased in parallel.

Other Etiologies

Some other viruses have also been associated with PAN but could only explain a few cases: hepatitis C virus,[13] parvovirus B19[2] or human immunodeficiency virus infections.[14,15] In addition to infectious causes, PAN has been described in association with cancers and hematological diseases, mainly malignant hemopathies. The closest relationship has been established with hairy-cell leukemia.[16] Malignancies are, for the most part, associated with small-sized vessel vasculitides and very few associated with PAN have been reported.[17]

HISTOLOGY

The histological lesion defining PAN is focal segmental necrotizing vasculitis of medium-sized arteries, much less often arterioles, and only extremely rarely capillaries and venules. The acute phase of arterial wall inflammation is characterized by fibrinoid necrosis of the media and an intense pleomorphic cellular infiltration, predominantly comprised of neutrophils and variable numbers of lymphocytes and eosinophils. The completely destroyed normal architecture of the vessel wall is replaced by a band of amorphous eosinophilic material that resembles fibrin when stained. Arterial aneurysms and thromboses can occur at the site of the lesion. Arterial healing is characterized by fibrotic endarteritis that may lead to aneurysm regression or, when too abundant, to vessel occlusion. Necrotizing vasculitis and healed lesion(s) or normal arteries can coexist in different parts of the same tissues.

Biopsies from several sites can be diagnostic for PAN. In patients complaining of myalgias, with or without concomitant mononeuropathy multiplex, or exhibiting general symptoms, muscle biopsy is useful for diagnosis. The diagnostic sensitivity of biopsies obtained from proximal muscles (deltoid or quadriceps) is lower than that of those taken from distal muscles. Nerve biopsy of a sensory branch of the sciatic or peroneal nerve is an alternative option for patient suffering from distal sensory or sensorimotor mononeuropathy multiplex. A deep skin biopsy is easy to obtain and can show medium-sized vessel involvement in patients with infiltrated necrotic purpura. In patients with visceral involvement, surgical specimens, e.g. small intestine, can also provide the diagnosis. Because renal involvement results from ischemia, renal biopsy is not relevant and strongly contraindicated.

CLINICAL FEATURES

Polyarteritis nodosa can develop at all ages, including children and the elderly, but most patients are between 40 and 60 years old, with no sex predominance (Table 30.4).

Patients with PAN are usually in poor general condition, with two thirds having lost weight and fever. Half of the patients suffer from myalgias. Amyotrophy can be severe, but mostly reflects weight loss, sometimes more than 20 kg. Some patients are bedridden due to the intensity of pain and amyotrophy. Forms of necrotizing vasculitis limited to one muscle or group of muscles with histological features of PAN but no other organ involvement are being described with increasing frequency.[18] Arthralgias predominate in knees, ankles, elbows, and wrists.

Neurological Manifestations

Peripheral neurological symptoms are frequent, while central nervous system (CNS) involvement is rare.

Peripheral Neuropathy

Peripheral neuropathy is the most frequent finding in PAN patients (50–75%)[3,19] and is the earliest symptom for 23–33% of the patients.[19] Rarely, peripheral neuropathy is present without systemic symptoms.[20,21] Its onset is usually acute but may be more indolent. Sensory signs are responsible for hypo- or hyperesthesia, dysesthesia, or frank pain as the prominent and earliest features. Usually, motor deficits start later, also with sudden onset, but may sometimes, precede the sensory sign(s). The first manifestations often affect the lower limbs, with one particular nerve involved. Later, other nerves become affected, with this pattern being referred to

as mononeuritis (or mononeuropathy) multiplex. The main localizations are distal and asymmetric. The following nerves are preferentially involved, superficial peroneal, sural, radial, cubital, and/or median. In its late stage, so many nerves can be involved that mononeuropathy multiplex can be mistaken for a symmetrical process. Segmental edema may precede the development of palsies. The extent of the axonal neuropathy on electromyography may be greater than expected based on clinical manifestations. Mononeuropathy (simplex) is seen less frequently. Very few cases of brachial plexus neuropathy have been reported.[22] Conduction block, suggestive of demyelination, such as in Guillain–Barré syndrome, nerve entrapment, or other acquired demyelinating neuropathies, has been described rarely.

Under treatment, the mononeuropathy multiplex of PAN regresses slowly and patients may recover without sequelae, although 12–18 months are often necessary to obtain and evaluate maximum recovery. The degree of recovery is variable and unpredictable. Sensory symptoms, usually paresthesias, persist longer and, sometimes, indefinitely, and peripheral neuropathy flares cannot be predicted. Electromyography can be used during follow-up to evaluate neuropathy regression or progression, but its reliability remains debatable.

Central nervous system involvement: Central nervous system involvement, much less common than peripheral neuropathy, occurs in around 5% of PAN patients.[3,19] Its common presentations include encephalopathy, affecting cognitive function and characterized by disorientation, psychosis and hallucinations, delusion or diminished consciousness, and focal or multifocal disturbances of the brain and spinal cord, with seizures, strokes and/or subarachnoid hemorrhages, resulting either from vasculitis of a cerebral artery (i.e., arteritis, rupture of cerebral artery aneurysm, and hematoma) or as a consequence of malignant hypertension.

Magnetic resonance imaging may show T2-weighted hyperintensities, localized to the white matter in various brain territories that are suggestive but not specific.

Table 30.4 Percentages of main organ/system involvements or manifestation of PAN according to main published series

Reference	Patients (n)	Mean age	Organ/system involved or manifestation (%)						
			Heart	Hypertension	Skin	CNS	PNS	Kidney	GI
Pagnoux et al., 2010[3]	348	51	22	35	50	5	74	51	38
Cohen et al., 1980*[37]	53	54	4	14	58	—	60	66	25
Leib et al., 1979*[39]	64	47	30	25	28	25	72	63	42
Frohnert & Sheps 1967*[19]	130	—	10	—	58	3	52	8	14

*These older studies may have included PAN patients who would now be diagnosed as having MPA.
CNS, central nervous system; GI, gastrointestinal; PNS, peripheral nervous system.

Magnetic resonance angiography and conventional cerebral angiography (which is performed less frequently than in the past) are often normal, but nonspecific focal or diffuse segmental narrowing of the intracranial vessels may be seen.

Cranial nerve involvement: Cranial nerve palsies, found in approximately 1% of PAN patients,[23] most often affect oculomotor (III), trochlear (IV), abducens (VI), facial (VII), and/or acoustic (VIII) nerves.

Ocular involvement: The eye can be affected in PAN, sometimes severely, e.g. with uni- or bilateral choroiditis, iritis, iridocyclitis, retinal detachment, and/or retinal vasculitis. Blurred vision or visual loss may result from choroiditis, retinitis, or brain parenchymal arteritis.[24] However, the cerebrospinal fluid is usually normal.

Skin Manifestations

Cutaneous lesions have been reported in around half of the patients with systemic PAN, but less frequently in those over 65-year-old. It must be remembered that, in the majority of series, PAN and MPA were not differentiated, and that, today, most cutaneous manifestations would probably to be attributed to MPA. Theoretically, cutaneous or subcutaneous nodules are hallmarks of PAN. They occur along the trajectories of superficial arteries and often disappear spontaneously within a few days. The most common cutaneous finding is palpable purpura, often necrotic, corresponding to subcutaneous small-sized vessel vasculitis, associated with medium-sized vessel involvement. Ulcerations and livedo are less frequent.[3] Livedo reticularis in PAN is typically localized on the lower limbs, the back of the arms, and, sometimes, on the trunk. A biopsy of infiltrated and/or central lesion zones can show vasculitis. Painful ulcerations may develop, frequently associated with indurated plaques resulting from the coalescence of nodules. Peripheral embolization of thrombi may cause infarction of toes and/or fingers or some cutaneous areas. Cholesterol emboli are a possible differential diagnosis.

Polyarteritis nodosa may initially be limited to the skin in a few patients, with systemic disease developing later at some variable time after the first cutaneous sign. Conversely, PAN may remain strictly confined to the skin, as a chronic disease, often associated with multiple cutaneous relapses.[25]

Renal Manifestations

Renal artery involvement can cause mild-to-severe and malignant hypertension and/or vascular ischemic nephropathy with renal insufficiency, which has been identified as a poor-prognosis factor.[26] Angiography (when performed despite renal involvement) may show renal parenchymal infarcts, and characteristic multiple stenoses and microaneurysms of branches of celiac, mesenteric and renal arteries, with or without gastrointestinal (GI) symptoms.[3] Microaneurysms, sometimes, rupture spontaneously or after renal biopsy, which is strongly contraindicated when they are present. Acute renal insufficiency usually occurs early during disease progression or a flare. Renal function outcome remains unpredictable. Hypertension, usually mild, is present in a mean of 40% of PAN patients. When severe, it is the consequence of vascular nephropathy. Hypertension can be attenuated with angiotensin-converting enzyme inhibitors, which have been proven beneficial in this context.

Cardiac Manifestations

Cardiac involvement was mentioned in the first publication on PAN,[27] which described "nodular coronaritis." Congestive heart failure is the main clinical feature, occurring in a few of PAN patients,[3] but usually less frequently than in eosinophilic granulomatosis with polyangiitis (Churg–Strauss) (EGPA). It is specifically due to vasculitis of the coronary arteries or their branches, with myocardial arteriolar infarcts. Specific cardiomyopathy can occur as early as 3–4 months after PAN onset. Angiography can prove coronary involvement in 85% of the patients with clinical signs of infarction. In the remaining 15%, infarction may be due to arteritis of small coronary vessels or spasms. Coronary aneurysms were found but their presence suggests Kawasaki disease rather than PAN. Cardiac MRI seems to be a promising investigative tool to evaluate heart involvement. Valvular involvement is rarely observed in PAN. The pericardium is implicated even more rarely. About half of the first reported cases of pericardial effusion were secondary to renal failure, which is much less frequent now that the diagnosis and overall therapeutic management of patients have improved.

Arrhythmias and conduction disorders, mainly supra-ventricular, result from arteritis of the sinus node or neighboring nerve fibers.

Peripheral Vascular Manifestations

Peripheral arterial occlusions may be responsible for distal gangrene of the toes or fingers.[28] Stenoses and/or microaneurysms can be visualized by angiography.[29] Raynaud's phenomenon, when present, can remain isolated or be complicated by necrosis. In some patients, type II or III cryoglobulins can be found.

Gastrointestinal Manifestations

Gastrointestinal tract involvement is one of the most severe manifestations of PAN, reportedly affecting one third of the patients, more often those with HBV-related PAN (50%).[3] Gastrointestinal manifestations are usually associated with other systemic signs of PAN, but can be the first symptoms of the disease.[30] They are the major cause of deaths within the first year after PAN onset and thereafter the third just after infections and heart disease.[31]

The spectrum of GI symptoms is broad and usually nonspecific, with abdominal pain being the most frequent. Gastrointestinal hemorrhages and small intestine perforations are the most feared manifestations that can occur. When present, ischemic vasculitis mainly affects the small bowel then, more rarely, the colon or stomach. Vasculitis of the gallbladder or the appendix is rare but can be the first sign of PAN, sometimes isolated, hence representing another possible localized form of PAN. However, it was reported that, for the 25% of the patients with isolated and histologically proven vasculitic appendicitis, PAN evolved within the next 5 years to systemic disease. Nonetheless, the prognosis of such limited forms remains good, owing to prompt combined medical treatments and surgery. Likewise, acute necrotizing or, less commonly, chronic pancreatitis, sometimes with pseudocysts, has been diagnosed in approximately 2–3% of the patients,[30] whose prognoses are extremely dismal because of the regular association with severe small intestine ischemia and/or perforations. Liver and/or spleen infarct(s) can occur, even in the absence of HBV infection.

Angiography is the most valuable investigation. It can detect infarcts, hematomas or more suggestive arterial stenoses and microaneurysms, 1–5 mm in diameter or more, in most of the patients with GI symptoms, mainly in renal, celiac, mesenteric, then hepatic or, more rarely, splenic arteries. Intraperitoneal ruptures of these aneurysms have been reported. Severe GI manifestations, like bowel perforations and/or ischemia, peritonitis, intestinal occlusion (and pancreatitis because of its frequent association with bowel perforations) have poor prognoses. Treatment is to combine prompt surgery along with corticosteroids (CS) and immunosuppressants. Indeed, the 5-year survival rate of the patients with these severe GI manifestations was only 56%, compared to 82% for those with less severe GI involvement.[3,30]

Orchitis

While rare, orchitis is one of the most characteristic manifestations of PAN and was retained as one of the ACR classification criteria.[4] Caused by testicular artery ischemia, it is rarely the first disease manifestation and is unilateral. When treated immediately, orchitis may regress under CS. Although no infectious etiology has ever been found, we have observed that orchitis often developed in HBV-related PAN.[32]

Pulmonary Manifestations

The lungs are spared in PAN, unlike MPA, granulomatosis with polyangiitis (Wegener's) (GPA) or EGPA. Although vasculitis of bronchial arteries was found in autopsy studies, it had been clinically asymptomatic.

Miscellaneous

Very rarely, periosteal modifications of the legs can be seen. Localized edema and pain are common symptoms.

Specific Manifestations of HBV-PAN

The immunological process leading to PAN occurs early during the course of HBV infection. When it was possible to date the HBV contamination, most PAN cases developed within less than 6 months thereafter. Hepatitis usually remains silent before PAN onset, which can be the first manifestation of HBV infection. Hepatic cytolysis is usually moderate and cholestasis is minor or absent. When liver biopsies were taken, they frequently showed signs of chronic hepatitis, even when PAN became manifest only a few months after HBV infection. For the group of patients with HBV-related PAN, clinical data were roughly the same as those commonly observed for PAN (Table 30.5),[12] but some differences were found: patients were usually under 40 years old; and malignant hypertension (5%), renal infarction and orchiepididymitis (25%) were more frequent.[12] Other symptoms frequently observed included abdominal manifestations (53%), especially surgical emergencies. In the study by Sergent et al[33] two of the three deaths (among nine patients) were attributed to colon vasculitis. Among the Eskimo patients described by McMahon et al.[8] 31% died and one of the four early deaths was the consequence of small-bowel perforation. Digestive and renal manifestations resulted from ischemia and angiography visualized microaneurysms and infarctions. HBV-related PAN is acute and initially severe but the outcome is excellent for most patients when adequate treatment is prescribed. Seroconversion usually leads to recovery. Sequelae are the consequence of vascular nephropathy but, even in patients with renal insufficiency, it is possible to obtain recovery with little residual impairment of renal function.

Table 30.5 Relevant clinical and biological symptoms in 115 patients with HBV-related PAN[12]

Clinical symptoms	Values*
Age, mean ± SD (years)	51.1 ± 17
Sex ratio, M/F	74/41
General symptoms	97
Fever	69
Weight loss	87
Arthralgias	56
Myalgias	47
Mononeuritis multiplex	84
GI-tract involvement	53
Abdominal pain	51
Bleeding	3
Appendicitis	2
Small intestine perforation	6
Cholecystitis	5
Pancreatitis	6
Renal and/or urogenital involvement	38
Creatininemia, mean ± SD (mg/dL)	1.52 ± 1.39
Orchitis	25
Microaneurysms[†]	69
Renal infarcts[†,‡]	28
Skin involvement	31
Purpura	17
Infiltrated purpura	11
Livedo	10
Nodules	9
Edema (ankles)	16
Vascular manifestations	18
Hypertension	31
Malignant hypertension	5
Cardiac insufficiency	12
Raynaud's phenomenon	3
Pericarditis	5
Digital ischemia	4
Myocardial infarction	1
CNS involvement	10
Retinal vasculitis	2
Erythrocyte sedimentation rate >30 mm/1st h	78
ANCA[§]	0

*Values are %, unless otherwise indicated.
[†] 66 angiographies.
[‡] Not related to vasculitis.
[§] ANCAs were sought in the sera of 66 patients.

Localized Forms of PAN

Localized PAN is rare except for the limited cutaneous forms that represent 10% of all PAN cases. Isolated involvement of one skeletal muscle or a muscle group and isolated neuropathy (mononeuritis multiplex or simplex), without systemic symptoms, have been described,[34] like exceptional cases involving only one organ, in order of decreasing frequency: appendix, gallbladder,[30] or uterus.[35] These forms usually carry good prognoses, often remitting spontaneously, with local therapy (like topical CS for skin lesions) or after surgery (cholecystectomy or appendectomy).

LABORATORY TESTS

Markers of inflammation are found in the majority of patients. An erythrocyte sedimentation rate > 60 mm 1st hour (most of the patients), elevated C-reactive protein, alpha-2 globulin levels and white blood cell counts, sometimes eosinophilia > 1,500/mm³, and normochromic anemia are common laboratory findings. HBsAg should be sought systematically. The frequency of HBV infection fell from 38.5% during 1972–1976 to 17.4% in 1997–2002, with a peak of 48.8% between 1982 and 1986. HBV is now rarely found because of vaccination campaigns and increased safety of blood transfusions.[12] We hypothesize that all PAN are the consequence of infection, even if a micro-organism has not been isolated from all the patients. The general measures to improve transfusion safety and patient care could explain the declining overall frequency of PAN. We also observed that the majority of HBV-infected patients come from northern or sub-Saharan African countries that have no vaccination policies, are IV drug addicts or patients at risk for sexually transmitted infections.

Antineutrophil cytoplasm antibody is not found in PAN, unlike MPA, GPA, and EGPA. In the context of systemic vasculitides, ANCA giving an immunofluorescent perinuclear-labeling pattern (P-), which are primarily directed against myeloperoxidase (anti-MPO) in enzyme-linked immunosorbent assay, should be considered exclusionary for PAN and viewed as an argument in favor of MPA.[6]

ANGIOGRAPHY

Although microaneurysms are not pathognomonic, they are commonly present in PAN and rare in GPA, EGPA, and MPA. Arterial saccular or fusiform aneurysms range in size from 1 to 5 mm and are predominantly seen in the kidneys, mesentery, and liver. The lesions may disappear under effective vasculitis therapy. Angiography is a useful tool when other diagnostic examinations are negative, especially when abdominal pain and nephropathy are present.

OUTCOME AND PROGNOSIS OF PAN

In its systemic form, PAN is an acute disease that can be severe and even fatal, if not treated adequately. Since the introduction of CS, and their later combination with immunosuppressant(s), antiviral therapy for HBV-related PAN and plasma exchanges when appropriate, PAN prognosis has improved and 5-year overall survival rates increased to more than 60%.[3]

A systematic retrospective study was conducted on 348 patients diagnosed with PAN, registered in the French Vasculitis Study Group database and satisfying ACR criteria and Chapel Hill nomenclature.[3] During a mean follow-up of 68.3 months, 76 (21.8%) patients relapsed (63 [28%] with non-HBV-related PAN versus 13 [10.6%] with HBV-related PAN; P < 0.001); 86 (24.7%) patients died (44 [19.6%] with non-HBV-related PAN versus 42 [34.1%] with HBV-related PAN; P = 0.003). Their respective 5-year relapse-free survival rates were 59.4% (95% confidence interval [95% CI] 52.6–67.0) versus 67.0% (95% CI 58.5–76.8). Once remission has been obtained, PAN recurs less frequently than GPA, MPA, or EGPA. In HBV-PAN, relapses occur in those who have persistent, active virus replication after vasculitis treatment. The clinical pattern of relapse does not necessarily repeat the original presentation, in that entirely new organs can be involved at relapse. Although the severity of relapses cannot be predicted, the most patients' clinical features at relapse are rash and arthralgias, and are generally less severe than during the initial presentation.

Deaths

Lethal complications of any form of vasculitis that involve major organs are possible. A few patients die during the first months of the disease from multivisceral involvement unresponsive to treatment.[31]

While fatalities occurring during the first few months of the disease are often caused by uncontrolled vasculitis, those occurring during the following years may be the consequence of treatment side effects and are not rare.

The primary cause of early death from PAN is severe GI involvement, with perforations or hemorrhage, included in the five-factor score (FFS).[26] Notably, HBV infection was not identified as a factor of severity.

TREATMENT OF PAN

Vasculitis Severity

The FFS has significant prognostic value and can guide physicians' choices of therapeutic agents and avoid overtreatment.[26] An earlier FFS version[36] retained the following parameters as being associated with higher mortality: proteinuria >1 g/day, renal insufficiency (creatininemia >140 µmol/L or 1.6 mg/dL), specific cardiomyopathy, GI

manifestations and CNS involvement. When FFS equaled 0, 1, or 2 respective 5-year mortality rates were 12%, 26%, or 46%. Although it has not yet been demonstrated that treatment should be chosen as a function of these criteria, they should probably be considered in deciding the therapeutic strategy. For PAN forms without poor-prognosis symptoms (FFS = 0), we treat patients with CS alone to limit the number of side effects. This strategy is effective, with a few minor relapses necessitating transient intensification of the CS dose or addition of an immunosuppressant (personal observations).

The revisited FFS[26] retained the following factors were significantly associated with higher 5-year mortality: age > 65 years, cardiac symptoms, GI involvement and renal insufficiency (stabilized peak creatinine ≥ 150 µmol/L or 1.7 mg/dL). The presence of each was accorded +1 point. Because ear, nose, and throat symptoms are associated with a better prognosis, their absence is scored +1 point. Respective 5-year mortality rates for FFS of 0, 1, or ≥2 were 9%, 21%, or 40%. The same therapeutic strategy as that previously described for the initial FFS is now applied to PAN patients.

HOW SHOULD PAN BE TREATED?

Since CS were first used to treat PAN in 1950, their use has prolonged the 5-year survival rate from 10% for untreated patients to about 55% in the mid-to-late 1970s.[19,37] Survival was further extended by adding an immunosuppressant, either azathioprine or cyclophosphamide (CYC),[38] to the treatment regimen, attaining a 5-year survival rate of 82% for patients given CS and CYC.[39]

Corticosteroids

The CS are given to all PAN patients. For the specific context of HBV-related PAN, CS should be administered for only a few days (see below). For the other PAN forms, CS use lasts around 12 months. Initial high doses may be useful. Infusion of methylprednisolone pulses (usually 7.5–15 mg/kg IV over 60 min, repeated at 24-h intervals for 1–3 days) has become widely used at treatment onset for severe systemic vasculitis, especially when life-threatening organ involvement is present or during the extension phase of mononeuropathy multiplex. This regimen acts rapidly and is relatively safe. Oral CS (prednisone or its equivalent of methylprednisolone) are given at the starting dose of 1 mg/kg/day. As the patient's clinical status improves and the biological markers of inflammation (C-reactive protein, erythrocyte sedimentation rate) return to normal, usually within 3 weeks, prednisone-dose tapering can begin.

Cyclophosphamide

Oral CYC is prescribed at a dose of 2 mg/kg/day or less for 1 year and, in combination with CS, represents the conventional treatment of systemic necrotizing vasculitides. Although this regimen is effective, it has a low therapeutic/toxic index. Major side effects associated with daily CYC intake include hemorrhagic cystitis, bladder fibrosis, bone-marrow suppression, ovarian failure, and cancer (mainly bladder cancer and hematological malignancies).[40] Severe infections are a major cause of mortality of patients with systemic necrotizing vasculitis, especially while they are receiving high CS doses with adjunctive immunosuppressive drugs.[31,41]

Pulse CYC is now being used increasingly to treat systemic necrotizing vasculitides and is preferred to oral CYC. The CYC content of each pulse, and both the total number and frequency of the pulses, has to be adjusted to the patient's condition: renal function, hematological data, and the disease's response to previous therapies, including previous CYC pulses. Lower dose IV CYC has been evaluated in patients over 65 years. Results showed that the lower dose was as effective as the higher one and caused fewer side effects.[42]

The French Vasculitis Study Group recommends 6 CYC pulses, each at 0.6 g/m², given on days 0, 14, 28, then every 3 weeks for 3 additional pulses. In our opinion, CYC should not be prescribed systematically as first-line treatment for all PAN patients and the management decision must consider the anatomical location of the vasculitis and its severity. When patients fail to respond to pulse CYC, oral CYC has been successfully used to control disease activity or when relapse occurred within the first 6 months of treatment.[43]

Other Cytotoxic Agents

Azathioprine, methotrexate, and several other cytotoxic agents have been tried in PAN patients. They are reserved for patients with contraindications to CYC or as maintenance therapy for a recommended duration of 12–18 months.

The French Vasculitis Study Group trials defined the therapeutic strategy according to the FFS. For patients with poor-prognosis factors (FFS>0), CYC followed by azathioprine maintenance is recommended.[44] However, CS alone can suffice when FFS = 0. But outcomes showed that patients with mononeuritis multiplex without poor-prognosis factors relapsed more frequently than those without this neuropathy. In this subgroup, cytotoxic agents could contribute to preventing relapses.[45]

Plasma Exchanges

To date, no argument supports the systematic use of plasma exchanges at the time of diagnosis of PAN without HBV infection.

Therapeutic Specificities of HBV-related PAN

For HBV-related PAN,[12] conventional CS-and-CYC induction therapy allows the virus to replicate, thereby facilitating evolution towards chronic hepatitis and liver cirrhosis. Thus, CYC and prolonged CS are contraindicated. The preferred initial treatment approach is to combine plasma exchanges and an antiviral drug with CS to rapidly control the most severe life-threatening PAN manifestations, which are common during the first weeks of the disease. CS are then abruptly discontinued to enhance immunological clearance of HBV-infected hepatocytes and favor seroconversion from HBeAg-positivity to anti-HBeAb–positivity.

The combination of antiviral agents gave excellent overall therapeutic results and should be preferred to conventional regimens that jeopardize the final outcome, by allowing continued virus replication and, hence, the long-term risk of cirrhosis or liver failure. Indeed, the benefits of adjunctive antiviral therapy, by eradicating the virus, are probably most evident only after prolonged follow-up by the absence of those severe liver complications.

KEY POINTS

- PAN is a medium vessel vasculitis, commonly presenting with a multisystem involvement
- Hepatitis B viral infection plays a causative role in many of these patients, though the incidence of HBV associated PAN has come down over a period of time.
- Treatment of PAN depends upon the presence or absence of HBV infection
- Antiviral therapy is the cornerstone of therapy for HBV associated PAN.
- Steroids and cytotoxic therapy is the cornerstone of therapy for non-HBV associated PAN.

REFERENCES

1. Trepo C, Thivolet J. Hepatitis associated antigen and periarteritis nodosa (PAN). Vox Sang. 1970;19:410-1.
2. Corman LC, Dolson DJ. Polyarteritis nodosa and parvovirus B19 infection. Lancet. 1992;339:491.

3. Pagnoux C, Seror R, Henegar C, et al. Clinical features and outcomes in 348 patients with polyarteritis nodosa: a systematic retrospective study of patients diagnosed between 1963 and 2005 and entered into the French Vasculitis Study Group Database. Arthritis Rheum. 2010;62:616-26.

4. Lightfoot RW Jr, Michel BA, Bloch DA, et al. The American College of Rheumatology 1990 criteria for the classification of polyarteritis nodosa. Arthritis Rheum. 1990;33:1088-93.

5. Jennette JC, Falk RJ, Bacon PA, et al. 2012 revised International Chapel Hill Consensus Conference Nomenclature of Vasculitides. Arthritis Rheum. 2013;65:1-11.

6. Henegar C, Pagnoux C, Puechal X, et al. A paradigm of diagnostic criteria for polyarteritis nodosa: analysis of a series of 949 patients with vasculitides. Arthritis Rheum. 2008;58:1528-38.

7. Scott DG, Bacon PA, Elliott PJ, et al. Systemic vasculitis in a district general hospital 1972–1980: clinical and laboratory features, classification and prognosis of 80 cases. QJ Med. 1982;51:292-311.

8. McMahon BJ, Heyward WL, Templin DW, et al. Hepatitis B-associated polyarteritis nodosa in Alaskan Eskimos: clinical and epidemiologic features and long-term follow-up. Hepatology. 1989;9:97-101.

9. Reinhold-Keller E, Herlyn K, Wagner-Bastmeyer R, et al. No difference in the incidences of vasculitides between north and south Germany: first results of the German vasculitis register. Rheumatology (Oxford). 2002;41:540-9.

10. Watts RA, Gonzalez-Gay MA, Lane SE, et al. Geoepidemiology of systemic vasculitis: comparison of the incidence in two regions of Europe. Ann Rheum Dis. 2001;60:170-2.

11. Mahr A, Guillevin L, Poissonnet M, et al. Prevalences of polyarteritis nodosa, microscopic polyangiitis, Wegener's granulomatosis, and Churg–Strauss syndrome in a French urban multiethnic population in 2000: a capture-recapture estimate. Arthritis Rheum. 2004;51:92-9.

12. Guillevin L, Mahr A, Callard P, et al. Hepatitis B virus-associated polyarteritis nodosa: clinical characteristics, outcome, and impact of treatment in 115 patients. Medicine (Baltimore). 2005;84:313-22.

13. Cacoub P, Lunel-Fabiani F, Du LT. Polyarteritis nodosa and hepatitis C virus infection. Ann Intern Med. 1992;116:605-6.

14. Calabrese LH. Vasculitis and infection with the human immunodeficiency virus. Rheum Dis Clin North Am. 1991;17:131-47.

15. Gisselbrecht M, Cohen P, Lortholary O, et al. HIV-related vasculitis: clinical presentation and therapeutic approach on six patients. AIDS. 1997;11:121-3.

16. Elkon KB, Hughes GR, Catovsky D, et al. Hairy-cell leukaemia with polyarteritis nodosa. Lancet. 1979;2:280-2.

17. Fain O, Hamidou M, Cacoub P, et al. Vasculitides associated with malignancies: analysis of sixty patients. Arthritis Rheum. 2007;57:1473-80.

18. Nakamura T, Tomoda K, Yamamura Y, et al. Polyarteritis nodosa limited to calf muscles: a case report and review of the literature. Clin Rheumatol. 2003;22:149-53.

19. Frohnert PP, Sheps SG. Long-term follow-up study of periarteritis nodosa. Am J Med. 1967;43:8-14.

20. Abgrall S, Mouthon L, Cohen P, et al. Localized neurological necrotizing vasculitides. Three cases with isolated mononeuritis multiplex. J Rheumatol. 2001;28:631-3.

21. Jennette J, Falk R, Bacon P, et al. Revised International Chapel Hill Consensus Conference Nomenclature of the Vasculitides. Arthritis rheum. 2012; doi: 10.1002/art.37715.

22. Jamieson PW, Giuliani MJ, Martinez AJ. Necrotizing angiopathy presenting with multifocal conduction blocks. Neurology. 1991;41:442-4.

23. Guillevin L, Le Thi Huong D, Godeau P, et al. Clinical findings and prognosis of polyarteritis nodosa and Churg–Strauss angiitis: a study in 165 patients. Br J Rheumatol. 1988;27:258-64.

24. Moore PM. Vasculitis of the central nervous system. Semin Neurol. 1994;14:307-12.

25. Sunderkotter C, Sindrilaru A. Clinical classification of vasculitis. Eur J Dermatol. 2006;16:114-24.

26. Guillevin L, Pagnoux C, Seror R, et al. The five-factor score revisited: assessment of prognoses of systemic necrotizing vasculitides based on the French Vasculitis Study Group (FVSG) cohort. Medicine (Baltimore). 2011;90:19-27.

27. Küssmaul A, Maier R. Ueber eine bischer nicht beschreibene eigenthumliche Arterienerkrankung (Periarteritis nodosa), die mit Morbus Brightii und rapid fortschreitender allgemeiner Muskellhamung einhergeht. Dtsch Arch Klin Med. 1866;1:484-518.

28. Lega JC, Seror R, Fassier T, et al. Characteristics, prognosis, and outcomes of cutaneous ischemia and gangrene in systemic necrotizing vasculitides: a retrospective multicenter study. Semin Arthritis Rheum. 2014;43:681-8.

29. Heron E, Fiessinger JN, Guillevin L. Polyarteritis nodosa presenting as acute leg ischemia. J Rheumatol. 2003;30:1344-6.

30. Pagnoux C, Mahr A, Cohen P, et al. Presentation and outcome of gastrointestinal involvement in systemic necrotizing vasculitides: analysis of 62 patients with polyarteritis nodosa, microscopic polyangiitis, Wegener granulomatosis, Churg–Strauss syndrome, or rheumatoid arthritis-associated vasculitis. Medicine (Baltimore). 2005;84:115-28.

31. Bourgarit A, Le Toumelin P, Pagnoux C, et al. Deaths occurring during the first year after treatment onset for polyarteritis nodosa, microscopic polyangiitis, and Churg–Strauss syndrome: a retrospective analysis of causes and factors predictive of mortality based on 595 patients. Medicine (Baltimore). 2005;84:323-30.

32. Guillevin L, Lhote F, Cohen P, et al. Polyarteritis nodosa related to hepatitis B virus. A prospective study with long-term observation of 41 patients. Medicine (Baltimore). 1995;74:238-53.

33. Sergent JS, Lockshin MD, Christian CL, et al. Vasculitis with hepatitis B antigenemia: long-term observation in nine patients. Medicine (Baltimore). 1976;55:1-18.

34. Gallien S, Mahr A, Rety F, et al. Magnetic resonance imaging of skeletal muscle involvement in limb restricted vasculitis. Ann Rheum Dis. 2002;61:1107-9.

35. Piette JC, Bourgault I, Legrain S, et al. Systemic polyarteritis nodosa diagnosed at hysterectomy. Am J Med. 1987;82:836-8.

36. Guillevin L, Lhote F, Gayraud M, et al. Prognostic factors in polyarteritis nodosa and Churg–Strauss syndrome.

A prospective study in 342 patients. Medicine (Baltimore). 1996;75:17-28.

37. Cohen RD, Conn DL, Ilstrup DM. Clinical features, prognosis, and response to treatment in polyarteritis. Mayo Clin Proc. 1980;55:146-55.

38. Fauci AS, Katz P, Haynes BF, et al. Cyclophosphamide therapy of severe systemic necrotizing vasculitis. N Engl J Med. 1979;301:235-8.

39. Leib ES, Restivo C, Paulus HE. Immunosuppressive and corticosteroid therapy of polyarteritis nodosa. Am J Med. 1979;67:941-7.

40. Le Guenno G, Mahr A, Pagnoux C, et al. Incidence and predictors of urotoxic adverse events in cyclophosphamide-treated patients with systemic necrotizing vasculitides. Arthritis Rheum. 2011;63:1435-45.

41. Gayraud M, Guillevin L, Le Toumelin P, et al. Long-term follow-up of polyarteritis nodosa, microscopic polyangiitis, and Churg–Strauss syndrome: analysis of four prospective trials including 278 patients. Arthritis Rheum. 2001;44:666-75.

42. Pagnoux C, Quéméneur T, Ninet J, et al. Treatment of systemic necrotizing vasculitides in patients ≥65 years old: results of the multicenter randomized CORTAGE trial (Abstract). Presse Med. 2013;42:679-80.

43. Généreau T, Lortholary O, Leclerq P, et al. Treatment of systemic vasculitis with cyclophosphamide and steroids: daily oral low-dose cyclophosphamide administration after failure of a pulse intravenous high-dose regimen in four patients. Br J Rheumatol. 1994;33:959-62.

44. Guillevin L, Cohen P, Mahr A, et al. Treatment of polyarteritis nodosa and microscopic polyangiitis with poor prognosis factors: a prospective trial comparing glucocorticoids and six or twelve cyclophosphamide pulses in sixty-five patients. Arthritis Rheum. 2003;49:93-100.

45. Samson M, Puéchal X, Devilliers H, et al. Long-term follow-up of a randomized trial on 118 patients with polyarteritis nodosa or microscopic polyangiitis without factors of poor prognosis. Autoimmun Rev. 2013: on line first: http://dx.doi.org/10.1016/j.autrev.2013.10.001.

CHAPTER 31

Granulomatosis with Polyangiitis (Wegener's Granulomatosis)

Aman Sharma, Pradeep Bambery

INTRODUCTION

Granulomatosis with polyangiitis (GPA), previously known as Wegener's granulomatosis, is a multisystem disease with a wide spectrum of clinical manifestations. Its classical histopathological triad consists of granulomatous inflammation, tissue necrosis and vasculitis. The first description was by Heinz Klinger in 1931, who described an old physician with constitutional symptoms, arthralgias, sinusitis, bloody nasal crusting, a "saddle nose deformity" and otitis media. At necropsy, he described crescentic glomerulonephritis and granulomatous inflammation of airways considering it to be a variant of polyarteritis nodosa.[1] It was Wegener, who after demonstration of histopathological changes on autopsy of three patients proposed that it was a distinct entity.[2] He had noted the upper airway involvement, granulomatous inflammation and vasculitis.[3]

CASE VIGNETTE

A 58-year-old male presented with history of sinusitis, nasal crusting, bloody nasal discharge and nasal septal perforation for four years and small joint polyarthritis for six months. Apart from mild swelling of two finger joints, physical examination was unremarkable. He had anemia (hemoglobin 9 mg/dL), leukocytosis (total leukocyte count of 13,560/µL), thrombocytosis (platelet count of 650,000/ µL), and elevated erythrocyte sedimentation rate (132 mm/h). Urinalysis showed 10–12 RBCs per high power field and 24 hours urine protein was 980 mg/total volume. Rheumatoid factor and ANCA were positive (c ANCA on indirect immunofluorescence, PR3 on ELISA). He had a normal serum creatinine. Chest X-ray was normal and kidney biopsy showed pauci-immune crescentic glomerulonephritis. A diagnosis of systemic GPA was made and he was started on pulse methylprednisolone (1000 mg/day for 3 days), followed by prednisolone (1 mg/kg/day) and pulse cyclophosphamide (15 mg/kg) according to the EUVAS regime. He had a good response with disappearance of joint symptoms, normalization of ESR and decrease in proteinuria. He achieved remission and was switched to azathioprine after 4 months. After 13 months, while on a holiday, he developed fever, painful redness of the right eye, decreased urine output, microscopic hematuria, and increased serum creatinine to 3.2 mg/dL, which increased further to 6.8 mg over the next four days. His ESR increased to 144 mm 1st hour. A major relapse with nodular scleritis and rapidly progressive renal failure was diagnosed, three pulses of methylprednisolone (1000 mg) administered and rituximab started at a dose of 375 mg/m^2 weekly for four weeks. Plasma exchange was also started for renal failure. Fever subsided in a few days but he remained anuric for three weeks. The serum creatinine gradually decreased to 2.4 over the next 5 weeks and then stabilized. He developed anemia of chronic disease and commenced on erythropoietin for it. Presently GPA is in remission but he carries the scars of septal perforation and chronic kidney disease.

CLASSIFICATION AND NOMENCLATURE

The American College of Rheumatology (ACR) set down the classification criteria for seven types of vasculitis including GPA (WG) in 1990.[4] Accordingly, for the purposes of a study, a diagnosis of GPA (WG) could be made if at least 2 of these 4 criteria were present.

1. *Nasal or oral inflammation:* Development of painful or painless oral ulcers or purulent or bloody nasal discharge.
2. *Abnormal chest radiograph:* Chest radiograph showing the presence of nodules, fixed infiltrates, or cavities.

3. *Urinary sediment:* Microhematuria (>5 red blood cells per high power field) or red cell casts in urine sediment.
4. *Granulomatous inflammation on biopsy:* Histologic changes showing granulomatous inflammation within the wall of an artery or in the perivascular or extravascular area (artery or arteriole).

These criteria had a sensitivity of 88.2% and a specificity of 92.0%. The Chapel Hill consensus conference nomenclature system provided the definition of GPA in 1994. According to this nomenclature system, GPA was characterized by granulomatous inflammation of the respiratory tract, along with necrotizing vasculitis of small and medium sized vessels (capillaries, venules, arterioles and arteries).[5]

The GPA has an association with ANCA and in the revised CHCC nomenclature system proposed in 2012, it has been put in a subgroup of ANCA associated vasculitis along with microscopic polyangiitis (MPA) and eosinophilic granulomatosis with polyangiitis (EGPA).[6]

EPIDEMIOLOGY

The estimates of prevalence of GPA have varied depending upon the study designs. A population based study, from England, reported an annual incidence of 8.5 per million.[7] The incidence of GPA seemed to increase after introduction of ANCA testing. However, studies done subsequently showed a stable incidence with no significant change during the 22 year observation period of the Norwich Vasculitis Cohort.[8] The incidence is higher in Northern Europe as compared to Southern Europe and Japan. The prevalence rates have also varied from 30 per million in a hospital based study in United States to 60 cases per million in a population based German study.[9,10] There is no gender predilection.

PATHOGENESIS

The GPA is an ANCA associated vasculitis. The details of pathogenesis are given in Chapter 7.

Briefly, the pathogenesis of AAV is multifactorial. The role of various environmental factors is suggested by the geographical distribution, relation with exposure to silica, hydrocarbons and various drugs.[11] Infections with *Ross river virus*, and *Staphylococcus aureus* have been incriminated in the development of AAV. *Staphylococcus aureus* infection has been implicated in relapses of GPA for a long-time. The link between infection and AAV is also suggested by the discovery of antilysosomal associated membrane protein 2 (LAMP2) antibodies in sera of patients with focal necrotizing glomerulonephritis (FNGN) and the induction of the same disease in animal models after immunization with LAMP2.[12]

Genetic associations with GPA have been studied in various populations. These include both HLA and non HLA associations. The association of HLA-DRB1*04, DPB1*0401, PRTN3 (A546G poly), AAT polymorphisms (SERPINA1) has been shown. There are unconfirmed, or conflicting, associations with IL2RA, IL10, LILRA2, CD226, and FCRIIIb.[13-19] The recent GVAS study has shown genetic association of HLA-DP, SERPINA1, PRTN3 with anti PR3AAV.[20]

Better understanding in this area now suggests that the future classification of AAV may be based upon antigen specificity and not phenotypic presentation. The same has been supported by the recent study of TLR 9 polymorphisms in PR3-ANCA vasculitis as opposed to MPO-ANCA vasculitis.[21]

Activated neutrophils and macrophages play an important role in the propagation of AAV. There is increase in the circulating levels of B-lymphocyte stimulator (BLys). Recent studies have shown T helper cell abnormalities like Th1 skewing in localized GPA; Th2 skewing and Th17 expansion in systemic GPA.[22,23]

Pathological features: The classical triad consists of granuloma, vasculitis and necrosis. One has to remember that the biopsy samples are generally small, and may not show all of these three features in one sample. The pathological changes in the lungs consist of granulomatous inflammation, granulomatous vasculitis and pulmonary capillaritis. The vasculitis may involve arteries, veins or capillaries. The details of pulmonary pathology are given in Chapter 9. The classical renal lesions are segmental necrotizing crescentic glomerulonephritis. This is *pauci-immune* as the immunofluorescence studies show very scant, if any, immune deposits in the renal biopsy tissues. The details of renal pathology are given in Chapter 10.

Antineutrophil cytoplasmic antibodies (ANCA): These are associated with GPA , MPA and EGPA. The details about ANCA, ANCA production, interaction of ANCA with target antigens, pathophysiology, pathogenic B-cell response and production of ANCA, aberrant T-cell response and granuloma formation, monocyte activation and AAV, ANCA-mediated interaction between neutrophils and endothelial cells, role of ANCA in the diagnosis of vasculitis and should ANCA titers may be used for the management of ANCA-vasculitis are given in Chapter 5.

CLINICAL FEATURES

Clinically, the disease shows very diverse manifestations ranging from a localized granulomatous respiratory inflammation to widespread systemic necrotizing granulomatous angiitis. The characteristic clinical phenotype is in the form of multisystem involvement with upper airway inflammation, lung nodules and glomerulonephritis. This must be considered amongst the differential diagnosis of renopulmonary syndrome. The various patterns of organ involvement in two large single center series are shown in Table 31.1.

Fever, arthralgia, weight loss and other constitutional symptoms are common in the generalized phase of the disease. Fever, during the course of disease may reflect either disease activity, or superadded infection. The transition from limited to generalized disease is usually associated with constitutional symptoms, elevated laboratory markers of inflammation and evidence of major organ involvement.

Articular involvement is usually in the form of arthralgia but true arthritis with active synovitis may also occur. The pattern of joint involvement may vary from oligoarticular, predominantly large joint involvement to symmetrical additive inflammatory small joint polyarthritis. It may be confused with rheumatoid arthritis (RA) as rheumatoid factor is positive in up to one-third of patients. Wegener, himself, had suspected that the disease may sometimes masquerade as RA.

UPPER AIRWAYS AND NOSE

Involvement of nose and paranasal sinuses is very common, seen in up to 60% patients.[24] The symptoms can be in the form of nasal congestion, nasal obstruction, rhinorrhea, pain over the dorsum of nose, anosmia, recurrent epistaxis and epiphora.[25] Chronic sinusitis is common and may present with headache, postnasal drip, chronic cough and sinus tenderness.[26] Chronic sinusitis, not responding to usual medical treatment, accompanied with nasal crusting should forcefully promote GPA among the differential diagnoses. Examination may reveal ulceration of nasal mucosa, nasal crusting and septal perforation (Fig. 31.1). Nasal endoscopy may show purulent discharge in the middle meatus, crusting over the septum and turbinates, friable nasal mucosa and rarely, nasal polyps.[27] Granulomatous inflammation may eventually result in "saddle nose deformity" (Fig. 31.2) and nasal airway stenosis.[28] Saddle nose deformity may be seen in 10-25% of patients with sino nasal involvement.[29] Involvement of larynx and trachea is also common.[30] Airway involvement is more common in the younger patients under 30 years of age and in females.[31] There may be ulceration, granuloma formation, pseudo membranes and cobble stone appearance of the mucosa of larynx and trachea. The symptoms are in the form of recurrent cough, change in voice, respiratory difficulty and hemoptysis. Subglottic stenosis is a rare complication and manifests as hoarseness of voice and stridor and can require emergency tracheostomy.[32] It is more commonly seen in association with generalized GPA. Biopsy from the subglottic area may occasionally confirm the diagnosis of GPA.[33]

Table 31.1 Patient's characteristics from two large single center cohorts for USA (Hoffman et al) and Germany (Reinhold keller et al)		
	Hoffman et al[50]	*Reinhold Keller et al*[80]
Total no. of patients	158 (24 years)	155
Male/Female (%)	50/50	49/51
Age at diagnosis (Mean) years	41	48
c ANCA	88%	84%
p ANCA	NA	NA
E (%)	79.3%	93.9%
K (%)	22.3%	77.1%
L (%)	52.9%	83.3%
EY (%)	28.8%	65.5%
Heart	NA/8	52% (13/25)
PNS	NA/15	52.5% (21/40)
CNS	NA/8	54.4% (6/11)
GI	NA	50% (3/6)
Skin	28% (13/46)	63.3% (21/33)
Cyc	89%	92%
Prednisolone	70%	70%
Death	20%	14%
Disease	12%	12%

Abbreviations: 'E'–upper airway involvement, K–kidney, L–lung, EY–eyes, PNS–peripheral nervous system, CNS–central nervous system, GI–gastrointestinal involvement, Cyc–cyclophosphamide, NA–not available

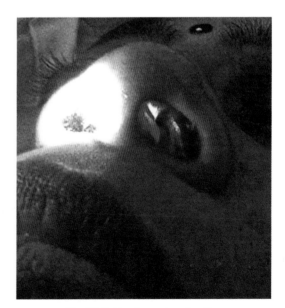

Fig. 31.1 Nasal septal perforation

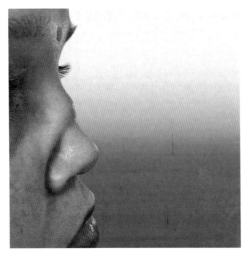

Fig. 31.2 Collapse of the nasal bridge

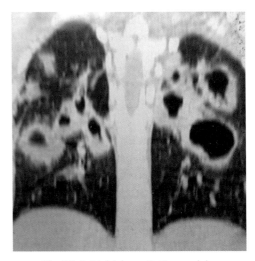

Fig. 31.4 Multiple cavitating nodules

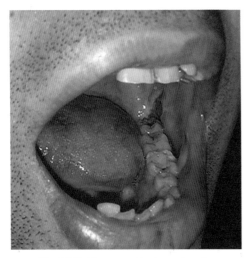

Fig. 31.3 Ulcer over the buccal cavity

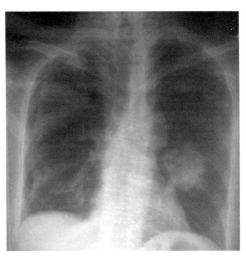

Fig. 31.5 Chest X-ray mimicking bronchogenic carcinoma in a patient with GPA

ORAL MANIFESTATIONS

Oral cavity involvement at presentation occurs in ≤ 6% of patients. "Strawberry" gingivitis, reddish to pinkish hyperplastic gingivitis with numerous petechiae, associated with pain and bleeding gums, is a classical manifestations. Mucosal ulcers over the tongue, buccal mucosa (Fig. 31.3), gums or palate, cobblestone like lesion over the palate, nonhealing extraction socket and oroantral fistula may be the other manifestations. Submandibular or parotid gland sialadenitis may be a presenting feature and simulate Sjögren syndrome.[34,35]

PULMONARY INVOLVEMENT

Pulmonary manifestations frequently dominate the clinical presentation. Lung involvement may vary from asymptomatic

lung nodules to catastrophic pulmonary hemorrhage. Nodules may be single or multiple (Fig. 31.4), solid or cavitory, fixed or migratory and can mimic lung abscess or even lung cancer (Fig. 31.5). Reticular or reticulonodular opacities, atelectasis and consolidation are less common. Pulmonary hemorrhage, due to capillaritis, may present with hemoptysis and pulmonary infiltrates (Fig. 31.6). Hemoptysis may be absent in some of these patients and the clue of pulmonary hemorrhage may come from fall in hemoglobin and lung infiltrates, which at time may be fleeting. Lymph node enlargement and pleural effusion are very rare.

RENAL MANIFESTATIONS

Kidney involvement is another major clinical manifestation. The most sinister presentation is in the form of rapidly progressive renal failure characterized by oliguria, microscopic hematuria, RBC casts and rapidly rising serum creatinine. The underlying renal pathology is usually pauci-immune crescentic glomerulonephritis. Renal involvement is harbinger of severe, active systemic disease necessitating aggressive management.

Eyes

The eyes may be involved in several ways. Necrotizing scleritis (Fig. 31.7), peripheral ulcerative keratitis and orbital pseudotumor (Fig. 31.8) are among the most prominent manifestations. Scleritis may begin with pain and redness and eventually cause "scleromalacia perforans" and loss of vision. PUK can also result in vision loss due to "corneal melt" resulting in perforation. The orbital pseudotumor like presentation can cause proptosis, pain, and vision loss. This is usually refractory to therapy. The description of GPA from India, is in the form of small case series and case reports.[36-39]

Other Manifestations

Skin manifestations include nodules, palpable purpura, ulcers, hemorrhagic bullae, or digital infarcts. Neurological manifestations include peripheral nervous system (PNS) or central nervous system (CNS) involvement. The PNS involvement is more common and usually manifests as mononeuritis multiplex or distal sensorimotor neuropathy. The CNS involvement is rare, usually in the form of cranial neuropathies, pachymeningitis (Fig. 31.9) or mass lesions. Rarer manifestations include diabetes insipidus due to pituitary involvement, bowel manifestations resembling

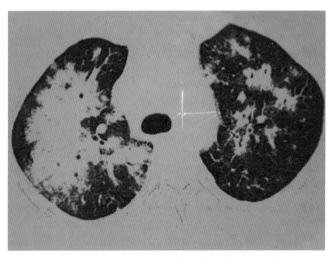

Fig. 31.6 CT scan showing diffuse alveolar hemorrhage

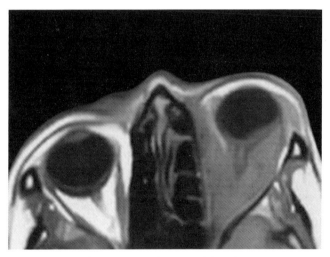

Fig. 31.8 Pseudotumor of the orbit

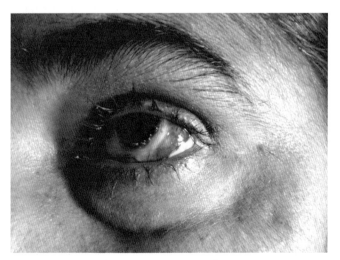

Fig. 31.7 Necrotizing scleritis

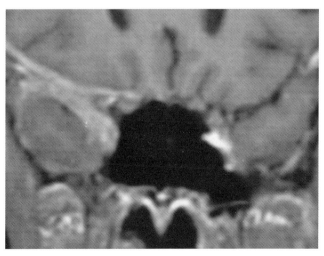

Fig. 31.9 Pachymeningitis

ischemic bowel and inflammatory bowel disease, prostatic vasculitis and "mass" lesions in the muscles and breasts.[40]

Diagnosis

In the absence of validated diagnostic criteria, the diagnosis of GPA is clinical. The key to the diagnosis is high index of suspicion in the appropriate clinical settings, especially when there is multisystem involvement. This is supported by ANCA along with histopathological evidence of GPA. It must be considered among the differential diagnosis of patients with a wide variety of clinical symptoms listed above, in the setting of an inflammatory process. Disseminated infection like infective endocarditis is a close clinical mimic and must be reasonably excluded.

Laboratory tests: No single test or laboratory finding can help in making the diagnosis. In the appropriate clinical setting, several relevant investigations need to be carried out. Acute phase reactants like ESR and CRP are generally elevated. There may be leukocytosis and thrombocytosis. Severe thrombocytopenia, at the time of presentation, is rare and may necessitate the need to look for other differential diagnosis more closely. The elevation of acute phase reactants and leukocytosis, by themselves, cannot differentiate between disease activity and infection. Rheumatoid factor may be positive in up to 50% patients. Urinalysis and renal function tests show abnormalities in renal involvement. Mild increase in transaminases may also be observed. The international consensus statement on reporting of ANCA recommends both IIF and ELISA assay as 5% of IIF negative results are ELISA positive.[41] The main target antigens of ANCA are located in the neutrophils and monocytes cytoplasm.[42] Two main target antigens are proteinase 3 (PR3) and myeloperoxidase (MPO).[43,44]

Imaging

Imaging plays an important role in the diagnosis. It does not only show the nature of involvement, but also suggests a site to biopsy. Computed tomography of nose and paranasal sinuses may show bone destruction with generalized mucosal thickening. Bone destruction typically commences in the midline affecting the nasal septum and turbinate's initially, spreading laterally, symmetrically to involve the maxillary antrum and other sinuses with sclerotic changes of the walls.[45] The end result is single large cavity with loss of nasal septum, turbinates and walls of the maxillary antrum.[46]

Magnetic resonance imaging shows high signal intensity of T1 weighted sequence and evidence of fat signal from the sclerotic walls of the sinus.[47] Though conventional X-rays would show nodules and infiltrates in widespread disease, CT scan of the chest has a better sensitivity than plain chest X-ray in demonstrating changes in patients with milder involvement. HRCT chest can show changes like small nodules, linear opacities and ground glass opacities. Angiographic studies have no role in demonstrating small vessel disease in GPA, but can demonstrate medium vessel involvement, e.g. in patients with mesenteric ischemia. Positron emission tomography is an upcoming modality. Its usefulness in systemic vasculitides is better studied in large vessel vasculitis. Recent studies have evaluated its role in GPA.[48] It was shown that the upper respiratory tract and lung lesions were more clearly detected by FDG PET/CT fusion imaging than by nonenhanced CT alone. These lesions also showed that there was decreased FDG uptake after treatment. The FDG uptakes in addition can also indicate the biopsy site. This modality would require further validation of its usefulness in day to day practice in the future.

FIBEROPTIC ENDOSCOPY AND BRONCHOSCOPY

Nasal endoscopy in patients with sinus involvement may show purulent discharge in the middle meatus, crusting over the septum and turbinates, friable nasal mucosa and rarely nasal polyps.[27] Nasal mucosal biopsy can be taken by fiberoptic endoscopy. The FESS may be required in refractory cases of chronic sinusitis. Septal perforation repair and correction of saddle nose deformity may be required, when the disease is in remission.

Bronchoscopy can demonstrate abnormalities like ulcerative bronchitis, inflammatory pseudotumors and bronchial stenosis. Bronchoalveolar lavage (BAL) can help in excluding infection in patients with pulmonary involvement.

MEASUREMENT OF DISEASE ACTIVITY

The details of assessment of disease activity are given in Chapter 25. The best theoretical way to assess disease activity would be to do the biopsy, but that is not feasible and even the yield of biopsy may be different from different sites. The objective assessment of disease activity and damage is important for better patient outcomes. This helps in planning therapy, and preventing undue immunosuppression as some symptoms may be due to accrual, rather than disease activity. Birmingham vasculitis activity score (BVAS) is a validated measure of disease activity. The BVAS version 3 is presently being used. There is a shorter GPA specific BVAS score. The validated measure of disease damage is vasculitis damage index (VDI). Though PR 3 ANCA levels rise in patients with reactivation of GPA, up to one-third of patients may have a rise in these titers without any clinical consequence. A recent study on relevance of monitoring PR3-ANCA titers in predicting relapse in GPA patients showed that no strict clinical-immunological correspondence was observed for 25% of the patients. It was concluded that GPA management cannot be based on ANCA levels alone.

Treatment

The prognosis in GPA was universally poor, till the addition of cyclophosphamide to corticosteroids. Median survival of untreated GPA was five months. Corticosteroids alone, improved this median survival to almost one year. Fauci and Wolff combined daily low dose oral cyclophosphamide (CYC) with corticosteroids. This combination dramatically improved the survival rates to 80%.[49] The problem with this regimen, however, was drug toxicity observed in 42% patients, including transition cell carcinoma of bladder in 6% patients.[50] The toxicity of CYC was related to the total cumulative dose. The next advancement was the introduction of intravenous pulses of CYC in doses of 0.75–1.0 mg/m^2 when it was observed that intermittent pulses of CYC were also effective.[51] A recent "Cyclops trial" showed that compared with oral daily CYC, the remission rates with intravenous CYC were similar, with somewhat greater risk of nonlife threatening relapses.[52,53] With the currently available treatment, this once invariably fatal condition has changed into a relapsing remitting, chronic disease. The present therapeutic concerns include the prevention of relapse, and minimizing damage due to disease activity and drugs.

Current treatment recommendations are based upon the disease severity. The European Vasculitis Study Group (EUVAS) recommends five grades of disease severity of AAV. These are (a) localized—upper or lower airway disease without other systemic involvement or constitutional symptoms, (b) early systemic disease—or systemic disease without organ or life threatening disease, (c) generalized—renal or other organ threatening disease, serum creatinine level ≤ 5.6 mg/dL, (d) severe-renal or other organ failure, serum creatinine ≥ 5.6 mg/dL, (e) refractory-progressive disease unresponsive to glucocorticoids and cyclophosphamide.[54]

Remission induction: In generalized or severe disease the drug of choice for remission induction remains CYC. Pulse CYC, (15 mg/kg) is administered every two weeks initially and then every three weeks for 3–6 months till remission is achieved. The dose is modified in the presence of renal failure and in old age. Mesna should be used to decrease bladder

toxicity of CYC, especially if oral CYC is used. In patients who have contraindication for CYC, like infection, cytopenia, intolerance, malignancy or fertility protection, rituximab (RTX) may be used an alternative agent for remission induction.

Rituximab is a chimeric anti CD20 monoclonal antibody shown to be effective to induce remission in GPA. The two back to back randomized controlled trails "The rituximab for ANCA associated vasculitis' (RAVE) and 'rituximab versus cyclophosphamide in ANCA associated renal vasculitis" (RITUXVAS) were published in 2010.[55,56] Both these trails showed that in nonlife threatening disease, RTX was not inferior to CYC for induction of remission. Long-term follow-up of RAVE study showed that those patients who achieved remission with a single course of RTX remained in remission for long.[57] Two dosing schedules are used for remission induction in AAV; 375 mg/m^2 weekly for four weeks or two 1000 mg pulses two weeks apart. Efficacy of the two weekly regime seems to be similar to the regime with four weekly pulses. There are reports of PMLE due to JC virus infection in patients receiving RTX.[58] A small recent study from Dublin showed that even a single infusion of RTX (375 mg/m^2) was a reasonable and cost effective method for remission induction.[59] Further studies would be required before this regime can be recommended for remission induction.

In patients with mild localized disease, a combination of methotrexate (MTX) 15-25 mg/week and prednisolone may be tried. The initial results of NORAM trial showed that in a nonlife threatening disease, treatment outcomes in the methotrexate arm were similar to the CYC arm.[60] This effect, however, was not sustained. Long-term follow-up data from the same study showed increased need of corticosteroids and CYC for relapse, as well as increased chances of infection in the MTX arm.[61]

Remission maintenance: Once remission is achieved, its maintenance can be achieved with drugs like azathioprine, mycophenolate mofetil (MMF) of methotrexate. CYCAZERAM trial showed that withdrawal of CYC and replacement with azathioprine did not result in increased relapse and it could be used for maintenance of remission. IMPROVE trial showed that mycophenolate mofetil (MMF) was inferior to azathioprine in remission maintenance in AAV, and should be considered in the maintenance if azathioprine has failed.[62] MMF has also been compared with CYC for remission induction. It showed similar results for remission induction but had increased rates of relapse.[63]

Rituximab has also been used in remission maintenance at 4-6 monthly intervals.[64,65] MAINRITSAN study has shown that after the initial induction with CYC, RTX (Initial one gram followed by 500 mg every 6 months) is better than azathioprine in remission maintenance.[66] RITAZAREM study is presently underway to compare fixed interval repeat dose RTX with azathioprine for patients receiving rituximab as treatment of relapsing GPA or MPA. The RTX can be planned provided IgG levels are ≥ 7 g/L, otherwise there may be increased risk of infections. A pretreat with intravenous immunoglobulins may be planned to raise the levels of IgG levels before giving RTX but there is little evidence for this treatment as of now.

Plasma Exchange

MEPEX trial showed that plasma exchange improved the chances of renal recovery in patients with serum creatinine ≥ 5.8 mg/dL. There was, however, no survival benefit. Its role in patients with lower serum creatinine and diffuse alveolar hemorrhage is uncertain.[67]

A recent meta analysis did not show any survival benefit or decrease in progression to end stage renal disease.[68] Prexivas study, currently underway, will assess the role of plasma exchange in decreasing death and end stage renal disease in AAV patients with renal involvement and alveolar hemorrhage.[69] The problems with plasma exchange are electrolyte abnormalities like hypocalcemia and increased risk of infections.

Treatment of Relapses/Refractory Disease

Relapses are common in GPA and this risk is higher than in MPA. Rituximab for ANCA-associated vasculitis study showed that in the subgroup of relapsing disease, RTX was better than CYC. The RTX should be considered in patients relapsing on CYC or having persistence of disease activity after three pulses of CYC. Oral CYC can also be considered as a rescue therapy for patients refractory to intravenous CYC. In the Granulomatosis-Entretien (WEGENT) trial, 75% of the patients with induction refractory disease on intravenous CYC achieved remission or low disease activity with oral CYC.[70] There was independent association of alveolar hemorrhage and a creatinine level >200 µmol/L with induction-refractory disease. Intravenous immunoglobulins can also be considered for use in patients with refractory disease though the evidence is only in form of small studies.[71,72]

Due to good safety and tolerability profile, it may be considered along with other therapeutic options for treatment with refractory disease. This, however, should not be considered with patients with glomerular filtration rate lower than 30 mL/min.

Wegener's granulomatosis etanercept (WGET) trial failed to show the efficacy of etanercept in AAV and there was also an increased risk of malignancies.[73,74] There are some reports of efficacy of infliximab in refractory AAV.[75,76] 15 deoxyspergualin (now called gusperimus) is another non-standard drug used in refractory or relapsing disease. In an open label study involving 45 patients, partial and complete remission was achieved in 95% and 45% patients respectively. This remission however, was not sustained.[77] The details of newer and future therapies of vasculitis are discussed by David Jayne in Chapter 26.

MORBIDITY

Despite significant advances in management, significant morbidity and mortality associated with AAV in patients, compared to matched background population, persists.[78] Increased morbidity is due to both the disease per se, and the treatment received. Various studies have identified advanced renal failure and increasing age as markers of poor prognostic.[79,80] Ear nose and throat disease has a high risk of local damage. Nasal inflammation can cause collapse of nasal bridge, recurrent local infections. These patients can benefit from regular nasal douching and application of local antibiotic ointment.[81] Twenty percent of patients with renal involvement will develop end stage renal disease over five years.[82] Eustachian tube obstruction, recurrent otitis media may result in hearing loss. Repeated episode of airway inflammation may cause subglottic, tracheal and bronchial stenosis. These might require repeated dilatation procedures. Lung hemorrhage generally recovers without a squeal, with only a minority developing lung fibrosis that occasionally might progress to respiratory failure.[83]

There are increased chances of deep venous thrombosis.[84] Despite control of disease activity, these patients have poor quality of life, with fatigue being a major contributor.[85] There is significant morbidity due to the treatment per se. There are increased chances of infection like *Pneumocystis jirovecii*, *Herpes zoster varicella (HZV)*. The RTX has been associated with increased risk of progressive multifocal leukoencephalopathy. The predictors for development of infection are age, severity of renal dysfunction, leukopenia and intensity and duration of immunosuppression.[86,87] The side effects of CYC include infections, cytopenias, hemorrhagic cystitis, and infertility. The frequency of hemorrhagic cystitis is 0.5/100 patient-years and is associated with oral cyclophosphamide use and total cumulative dose.[88] There is increased risk of malignancies due to exposure to cytotoxic therapies. This risk is two-fold as compared to general population.[89] These patients also have poor bone health and increase in atherosclerosis.[90,91]

KEY POINTS

- GPA is an ANCA associated vasculitis, classically characterized by upper airway involvement, lung nodules and renal failure clinically, and granuloma formation, necrosis and vasculitis on histopathology.
- The clinical manifestations vary from limited/localized disease to severe life-threatening multisystem involvement.
- The prognosis of this once universally fatal disease has improved significantly with the availability of various therapeutic options.
- Objective assessment of disease activity and damage with validated tools like BVAS and VDI helps in better patient outcomes.
- Combination of corticosteroids and CYC has been the standard of care for systemic disease though recent studies have shown that RTX may also be as effective in remission induction.
- Present major concerns of therapy are to find out ways to decrease morbidity due to frequent relapses, prevent damage due to disease or therapy and to improve quality of life.

REFERENCES

1. Klinger H. Grenzformen der polyarteritis nodosa. Frankfurter Zeitschrift für Pathologie. 1931;42:455-80.
2. Wegener F. Über generalisierte, septische gefäßerkrankungen. Verh Dtsch Ges Pathol. 1936;29:202-10.
3. Wegener F. Über eine eigenartige rhinogene granulomatose mit besonderer beteiligung des arteriensysytems und der nieren. Beitr Path Anat. 1939;102:36-8.
4. Leavitt RY, Fauci AS, Bloch DA, et al. The American college of rheumatology 1990 criteria for the classification of Wegener's granulomatosis. Arthritis Rheum. 1990;33:1101-7.
5. Jennette JC, Falk RJ, Andrassy K, et al. Nomenclature of systemic vasculitides. Proposal of an international consensus conference. Arthritis Rheum. 1994;37:187-92.
6. Jennette JC, Falk RJ, Bacon PA, et al. 2012 revised international chapel hill consensus conference nomenclature of vasculitides. Arthritis Rheum. 2013;65:1-11.
7. Watts RA, Carruthers DM, Scott DG. Epidemiology of systemic vasculitis: Changing incidence or definition? Semin Arthritis Rheum. 1995;25:28-34.
8. Watts RA, Mooney J, Skinner J, et al. The contrasting epidemiology of granulomatosis with polyangiitis (Wegener's) and microscopic polyangiitis. Rheumatology (Oxford). 2012;51:926-31.
9. Cotch MF, Hoffman GS, Yerg DE, et al. The epidemiology of Wegener's granulomatosis. Estimates of the five-year period prevalence, annual mortality, and geographic disease distribution from population-based data sources. Arthritis Rheum. 1996;39:87-92.
10. Reinhold-Keller E, Herlyn K, Wagner-Bastmeyer R, et al. Stable incidence of primary systemic vasculitides over five years: Results from the German vasculitis register. Arthritis Rheum. 2005;53:93-9.
11. Mahr AD, Neogi T, Merkel PA. Epidemiology of Wegener's granulomatosis: Lessons from descriptive studies and analyses of genetic and environmental risk determinants. Clin Exp Rheumatol. 2006;24:S82-91.
12. Kain R, Exner M, Brandes R, et al. Molecular mimicry in pauci-immune focal necrotizing glomerulonephritis. Nat Med. 2008;14:1088-96.
13. Cao Y, Schmitz JL, Yang J, et al. Drb1*15 allele is a risk factor for pr3-anca disease in african americans. J Am Soc Nephrol. 2011;22:1161-7.
14. Carr EJ, Niederer HA, Williams J, et al. Confirmation of the genetic association of ctla4 and ptpn22 with anca-associated vasculitis. BMC Med Genet. 2009;10:121.
15. Gencik M, Borgmann S, Zahn R, et al. Immunogenetic risk factors for anti-neutrophil cytoplasmic antibody (anca)-associated systemic vasculitis. Clin Exp Immunol. 1999;117:412-7.
16. Gencik M, Meller S, Borgmann S, et al. Proteinase 3 gene polymorphisms and Wegener's granulomatosis. Kidney Int. 2000;58:2473-7.
17. Mahr AD, Edberg JC, Stone JH, et al. Alpha(1)-antitrypsin deficiency-related alleles z and s and the risk of Wegener's granulomatosis. Arthritis Rheum. 2010;62:3760-7.
18. Morris H, Morgan MD, Wood AM, et al. Anca-associated vasculitis is linked to carriage of the z allele of alpha(1) antitrypsin and its polymers. Ann Rheum Dis. 2011;70:1851-6.
19. Tsuchiya N, Kobayashi S, Kawasaki A, et al. Genetic background of Japanese patients with antineutrophil cytoplasmic antibody-associated vasculitis: association of hla-drb1*0901 with microscopic polyangiitis. J Rheumatol. 2003;30:1534-40.
20. Lyons PA, Rayner TF, Trivedi S, et al. Genetically distinct subsets within anca-associated vasculitis. N Engl J Med. 2012;367:214-23.
21. Husmann CA, Holle JU, Moosig F, et al. Genetics of toll like receptor 9 in anca associated vasculitides. Ann Rheum Dis. 2014;73:890-6.
22. Free ME, Bunch DO, McGregor JA, et al. Patients with antineutrophil cytoplasmic antibody-associated vasculitis have defective treg cell function exacerbated by the presence of a suppression-resistant effector cell population. Arthritis Rheum. 2013;65:1922-33.
23. Wilde B, Thewissen M, Damoiseaux J, et al. T cells in anca-associated vasculitis: what can we learn from lesional versus circulating t cells? Arthritis Res Ther. 2010;12:204.
24. Rasmussen N. Management of the ear, nose, and throat manifestations of wegener granulomatosis: An otorhinolaryngologist's perspective. Curr Opin Rheumatol. 2001;13:3-11.
25. McDonald TJ, DeRemee RA. Wegener's granulomatosis. Laryngoscope. 1983;93:220-31.
26. McCaffrey TV. Nasal manifestations of systemic diseases. Otolaryngol Pol. 2009;63:228-35.

27. McDonald TJ, DeRemee RA, Kern EB, et al. Nasal manifestations of Wegener's granulomatosis. Laryngoscope. 1974;84:2101-12.

28. Rijuneeta, Panda N, Bambery P, et al. Nasal polyposis in Wegener's granulomatosis: a rare presentation. The Internet Journal of Otorhinolaryngology. 2005;4:28.

29. Martinez Del Pero M, Walsh M, Luqmani R, et al. Long-term damage to the ENT system in Wegener's granulomatosis. Eur Arch Otorhinolaryngol. 2011;268:733-9.

30. Lebovics RS, Hoffman GS, Leavitt RY, et al. The management of subglottic stenosis in patients with Wegener's granulomatosis. Laryngoscope. 1992;102:1341-5.

31. Alaani A, Hogg RP, Drake Lee AB. Wegener's granulomatosis and subglottic stenosis: Management of the airway. J Laryngol Otol. 2004;118:786-90.

32. Langford CA, Sneller MC, Hallahan CW, et al. Clinical features and therapeutic management of subglottic stenosis in patients with Wegener's granulomatosis. Arthritis Rheum. 1996;39:1754-60.

33. Devaney KO, Travis WD, Hoffman G, et al. Interpretation of head and neck biopsies in Wegener's granulomatosis: a pathologic study of 126 biopsies in 70 patients. Am J Surg Pathol. 1990;14:555-64.

34. Ah-See KW, McLaren K, Maran AG. Wegener's granulomatosis presenting as major salivary gland enlargement. J Laryngol Otol. 1996;110:691-3.

35. Specks U, Colby TV, Olsen KD, et al. Salivary gland involvement in Wegener's granulomatosis. Arch Otolaryngol Head Neck Surg. 1991;117:218-23.

36. Bambery P, Sakhuja V, Gupta A, et al. Wegener's granulomatosis in north India: an analysis of eleven patients. Rheumatol Int. 1987;7:243-7.

37. Bambery P, Sakhuja V, Bhusnurmath SR, et al. Wegener's Granulomatosis: clinical experience with eighteen patients. J Assosc Phys. 1992;40:597-600.

38. Malaviya AN, Kumar A, Singh YN, et al. Wegener's granulomatosis in India: not so rare. Br J Rheumatol. 1990;29:499-500.

39. Kumar A, Pandhi A, Menon A, et al. Wegener's granulomatosis in India: clinical features, treatment and outcome of twenty-five patients. Ind J Chest Dis Allied Sci. 2001;43:197-204.

40. Sharma A, Gopalakrishan D, Nada R, et al. Uncommon presentations of primary systemic necrotizing vasculitides: The great masquerades. Int J Rheum Dis. 2013;doi: 10.1111/1756-185X.12223.

41. Savige J, Gillis D, Benson E, et al. International consensus statement on testing and reporting of antineutrophil cytoplasmic antibodies (ANCA). Am J Clin Pathol. 1999;111:507-13.

42. Bartunkova J, Tesar V, Sediva A. Diagnostic and pathogenetic role of antineutrophil cytoplasmic autoantibodies. Clin Immunol. 2003;106:73-82.

43. Falk RJ, Jennette JC. Anti-neutrophil cytoplasmic autoantibodies with specificity for myeloperoxidase in patients with systemic vasculitis and idiopathic necrotizing and crescentic glomerulonephritis. N Engl J Med. 1988;318:1651-7.

44. Jenne DE, Tschopp J, Ludemann J, et al. Wegener's autoantigen decoded. Nature. 1990;346:520.

45. Lloyd G, Lund VJ, Beale T, et al. Rhinologic changes in Wegener's granulomatosis. J Laryngol Otol. 2002;116:565-9.

46. Simmons JT, Leavitt R, Kornblut AD, et al. CT of the paranasal sinuses and orbits in patients with Wegener's granulomatosis. Ear Nose Throat J. 1987;66:134-40.

47. Provenzale JM, Allen NB. Wegener granulomatosis: CT and MR findings. AJNR Am J Neuroradiol. 1996;17:785-92.

48. Ito K, Minamimoto R, Yamashita H, et al. Evaluation of Wegener's granulomatosis using 18f-fluorodeoxyglucose positron emission tomography/computed tomography. Ann Nucl Med. 2013;27:209-16.

49. Fauci AS, Haynes BF, Katz P, et al. Wegener's granulomatosis: Prospective clinical and therapeutic experience with 85 patients for 21 years. Ann Intern Med. 1983;98:76-85.

50. Hoffman GS, Kerr GS, Leavitt RY, et al. Wegener granulomatosis: an analysis of 158 patients. Ann Intern Med. 1992;116:488-98.

51. Bacon PA. Vasculitis—clinical aspects and therapy. Acta Med Scand Suppl. 1987;715:157-63.

52. de Groot K, Harper L, Jayne DR, et al. Pulse versus daily oral cyclophosphamide for induction of remission in antineutrophil cytoplasmic antibody-associated vasculitis: a randomized trial. Ann Intern Med. 2009;150:670-80.

53. Harper L, Morgan MD, Walsh M, et al. Pulse versus daily oral cyclophosphamide for induction of remission in ANCA-associated vasculitis: Long-term follow-up. Ann Rheum Dis. 2012;71:955-60.

54. Mukhtyar C, Guillevin L, Cid MC, et al. Eular recommendations for the management of primary small and medium vessel vasculitis. Ann Rheum Dis. 2009;68:310-7.

55. Jones RB, Tervaert JW, Hauser T, et al. Rituximab versus cyclophosphamide in ANCA-associated renal vasculitis. N Engl J Med. 2010;363:211-20.

56. Stone JH, Merkel PA, Spiera R, et al. Rituximab versus cyclophosphamide for ANCA-associated vasculitis. N Engl J Med. 2010;363:221-32.

57. Specks U, Merkel PA, Seo P, et al. Efficacy of remission-induction regimens for ANCA-associated vasculitis. N Engl J Med. 2013;369:417-27.

58. Jones RB, Ferraro AJ, Chaudhry AN, et al. A multicenter survey of rituximab therapy for refractory antineutrophil cytoplasmic antibody-associated vasculitis. Arthritis Rheum. 2009;60:2156-68.

59. Turner-Stokes T, Sandhu E, Pepper RJ, et al. Induction treatment of ANCA-associated vasculitis with a single dose of rituximab. Rheumatology (Oxford). 2014;53:1395-403.

60. De Groot K, Rasmussen N, Bacon PA, et al. Randomized trial of cyclophosphamide versus methotrexate for induction of remission in early systemic antineutrophil cytoplasmic antibody-associated vasculitis. Arthritis Rheum. 2005;52:2461-9.

61. Faurschou M, Westman K, Rasmussen N, et al. Brief report: Long-term outcome of a randomized clinical trial comparing methotrexate to cyclophosphamide for remission induction in early systemic antineutrophil cytoplasmic antibody-associated vasculitis. Arthritis Rheum. 2012;64:3472-7.

62. Hiemstra TF, Walsh M, Mahr A, et al. Mycophenolate mofetil vs azathioprine for remission maintenance in antineutrophil

cytoplasmic antibody-associated vasculitis: A randomized controlled trial. JAMA. 2010;304:2381-8.

63. Hu W, Liu C, Xie H, et al. Mycophenolate mofetil versus cyclophosphamide for inducing remission of ANCA vasculitis with moderate renal involvement. Nephrol Dial Transplant. 2008;23:1307-12.

64. Smith RM, Jones RB, Guerry MJ, et al. Rituximab for remission maintenance in relapsing antineutrophil cytoplasmic antibody-associated vasculitis. Arthritis Rheum. 2012;64:3760-9.

65. Rhee EP, Laliberte KA, Niles JL. Rituximab as maintenance therapy for antineutrophil cytoplasmic antibody-associated vasculitis. Clin J Am Soc Nephrol. 2010;5:1394-1400.

66. Terrier B, Pagnoux C, Karras A, et al. Rituximab versus azathioprine for maintenance in antineutrophil cytoplasmic antibodies (ANCA)-associated vasculitis (MAINRITSAN): Follow-up at 34 months. La Presse Médicale. 2013;42:778-9.

67. Jayne DR, Gaskin G, Rasmussen N, et al. Randomized trial of plasma exchange or high-dosage methylprednisolone as adjunctive therapy for severe renal vasculitis. J Am Soc Nephrol. 2007;18:2180-8.

68. Walsh M, Catapano F, Szpirt W, et al. Plasma exchange for renal vasculitis and idiopathic rapidly progressive glomerulonephritis: a meta-analysis. Am J Kidney Dis. 2011;57:566-74.

69. Walsh M, Merkel PA, Peh CA, et al. Plasma exchange and glucocorticoid dosing in the treatment of anti-neutrophil cytoplasm antibody associated vasculitis (PEXIVAS): protocol for a randomized controlled trial. Trials. 2013;14:73.

70. Seror R, Pagnoux C, Ruivard M, et al. Treatment strategies and outcome of induction-refractory Wegener's granulomatosis or microscopic polyangiitis: Analysis of 32 patients with first-line induction-refractory disease in the WEGENT trial. Ann Rheum Dis. 2010;69:2125-30.

71. Mouthon L, Kaveri SV, Spalter SH, et al. Mechanisms of action of intravenous immune globulin in immune-mediated diseases. Clin Exp Immunol. 1996;104:3-9.

72. Richter C, Schnabel A, Csernok E, et al. Treatment of anti-neutrophil cytoplasmic antibody (ANCA)-associated systemic vasculitis with high-dose intravenous immunoglobulin. Clin Exp Immunol. 1995;101:2-7.

73. The Wegener's granulomatosis etanercept trial (WGET) research group. Etanercept plus standard therapy for Wegener's granulomatosis. N Engl J Med. 2005;352:351-61.

74. Stone JH, Holbrook JT, Marriott MA, et al. Solid malignancies among patients in the Wegener's granulomatosis etanercept trial. Arthritis Rheum. 2006;54:1608-18.

75. Bartolucci P, Ramanoelina J, Cohen P, et al. Efficacy of the anti-TNF-alpha antibody infliximab against refractory systemic vasculitides: An open pilot study on 10 patients. Rheumatology (Oxford). 2002;41:1126-32.

76. Josselin L, Mahr A, Cohen P, et al. Infliximab efficacy and safety against refractory systemic necrotising vasculitides: Long-term follow-up of 15 patients. Ann Rheum Dis. 2008;67:1343-6.

77. Flossmann O, Baslund B, Bruchfeld A, et al. Deoxyspergualin in relapsing and refractory Wegener's granulomatosis. Ann Rheum Dis. 2009;68:1125-30.

78. Flossmann O, Berden A, de Groot K, et al. Long-term patient survival in ANCA-associated vasculitis. Ann Rheum Dis. 2011;70:488-94.

79. Hogan SL, Nachman PH, Wilkman AS, et al. Prognostic markers in patients with antineutrophil cytoplasmic autoantibody-associated microscopic polyangiitis and glomerulonephritis. J Am Soc Nephrol. 1996;7:23-32.

80. Reinhold-Keller E, Beuge N, Latza U, et al. An interdisciplinary approach to the care of patients with Wegener's granulomatosis: Long-term outcome in 155 patients. Arthritis Rheum. 2000;43:1021-32.

81. Laudien M, Lamprecht P, Hedderich J, et al. Olfactory dysfunction in Wegener's granulomatosis. Rhinology. 2009; 47:254-9.

82. Booth AD, Almond MK, Burns A, et al. Outcome of ANCA-associated renal vasculitis: A 5-year retrospective study. Am J Kidney Dis. 2003;41:776-84.

83. Arulkumaran N, Periselneris N, Gaskin G, et al. Interstitial lung disease and ANCA-associated vasculitis: A retrospective observational cohort study. Rheumatology (Oxford). 2011;50:2035-43.

84. Merkel PA, Lo GH, Holbrook JT, et al. Brief communication: High incidence of venous thrombotic events among patients with Wegener granulomatosis: the Wegener's clinical occurrence of thrombosis (WECLOT) study. Ann Intern Med. 2005;142:620-6.

85. Basu N, Jones GT, Fluck N, et al. Fatigue: a principal contributor to impaired quality of life in ANCA-associated vasculitis. Rheumatology (Oxford). 2010;49:1383-90.

86. Harper L, Savage CO. ANCA-associated renal vasculitis at the end of the twentieth century—a disease of older patients. Rheumatology (Oxford). 2005;44:495-501.

87. Charlier C, Henegar C, Launay O, et al. Risk factors for major infections in Wegener granulomatosis: analysis of 113 patients. Ann Rheum Dis. 2009;68:658-63.

88. Le Guenno G, Mahr A, Pagnoux C, et al. Incidence and predictors of urotoxic adverse events in cyclophosphamide-treated patients with systemic necrotizing vasculitides. Arthritis Rheum. 2011;63:1435-45.

89. Westman KW, Bygren PG, Olsson H, et al. Relapse rate, renal survival, and cancer morbidity in patients with Wegener's granulomatosis or microscopic polyangiitis with renal involvement. J Am Soc Nephrol. 1998;9:842-52.

90. Boomsma MM, Stegeman CA, Kramer AB, et al. Prevalence of reduced bone mineral density in patients with anti-neutrophil cytoplasmic antibody associated vasculitis and the role of immunosuppressive therapy: A cross-sectional study. Osteoporos Int. 2002;13:74-82.

91. de Leeuw K, Sanders JS, Stegeman C, et al. Accelerated atherosclerosis in patients with Wegener's granulomatosis. Ann Rheum Dis. 2005;64:753-9.

CHAPTER 32

Microscopic Polyangiitis

Chetan Mukhtyar, P Sharma

INTRODUCTION

Microscopic polyangiitis (MPA) was traditionally considered to be a part of polyarteritis nodosa (PAN). The terms PAN, MPA, and microscopic polyarteritis were often used interchangeably.[1] At the 1994 Chapel Hill Consensus Conference, MPA was formally recognized as a distinct entity and the nomenclature was accepted universally.[2] Microscopic polyangiitis is characterized by the presence of antibodies directed against antigenic targets in the neutrophil cytoplasm—the antineutrophil cytoplasm antibodies (ANCA). Together with granulomatosis with polyangiitis and eosinophilic granulomatosis with polyangiitis, it is classified under the umbrella term of ANCA-associated vasculitis (AAV). Microscopic polyangiitis is defined as a necrotizing vasculitis, with few or no immune deposits, predominantly affecting small vessels. Necrotizing arteritis involving small and medium arteries may be present. Necrotizing glomerulonephritis is very common. Pulmonary capillaritis often occurs. Granulomatous inflammation is absent.[3]

CASE VIGNETTE

A 74-year-old lady presented acutely to the acute medical unit with arthralgia and acute onset floppiness of the right leg. The arthralgia had been slowly progressive over the previous several months. On further questioning, she admitted to paresthesia in a stocking distribution over the previous year. She admitted to a single episode of hemoptysis a week prior to presentation. She was currently being investigated for a hypochromic microcytic anemia, and had a history of a resected meningioma 2 years prior. She had a 20-cigarette pack-year history that she had quit 30 years ago. She had been treated for hypothyroidism.

Clinical examination demonstrated a right foot drop, and urinalysis demonstrated 3+ proteinuria and 3+ hematuria. Systemic vasculitis was considered as a probable diagnosis.

Laboratory Investigations

She was anemic with hemoglobin of 11.4 g/dL microcytic hypochromic pattern. Serum creatinine was normal at 67 μmol/L, but had raised from 56 μmol/L over the previous 4 weeks. Serum calcium and other electrolytes were within the normal range. There was a marked inflammatory response with an erythrocyte sedimentation rate of 101 mm in the first hour, a serum C-reactive protein of 40 mg/L, and a platelet count of 428×10^9/L. Antineutrophil cytoplasm antibodies were positive in a perinuclear pattern on indirect immunofluorescence (IIF) with ELISA positivity for myeloperoxidase (MPO) in a titer of 105 U/mL. Chest X-ray was normal, with no evidence of vasculitis on a high-resolution CT scan of the chest or a CT scan of the sinuses. Nerve conduction testing demonstrated patchy axonal sensorimotor neuropathy in both the lower limbs. The renal biopsy confirmed focal segmental glomerulonephritis with crescents, and fibrinoid necrotizing vasculitis in an extraglomerular blood vessel. There were no immune deposits in the basement membrane.

A diagnosis of MPA was made and she was commenced on pulsed intravenous cyclophosphamide and oral prednisolone to induce remission. After six pulses over 13 weeks, she was ANCA-negative and in remission. At the last follow-up, 4 years after the diagnosis, she remains in remission with the help of methotrexate 15 mg per week as remission maintenance therapy. She gradually stopped prednisolone 3 years after the diagnosis. Since the diagnosis of MPA, she has developed peripheral vascular disease needing angioplasty of the posterior tibial artery and hypertension. The peripheral vascular disease is not believed to be related to the vasculitis.

EPIDEMIOLOGY

Microscopic polyangiitis has an annual incidence of 2.5–10/million.[4] It may have a latitudinal variation in incidence in the Northern Hemisphere, with increasing incidence in the more southern latitudes.[5] With increasing recognition and improved survival, the prevalence of MPA is increasing. The point prevalence is variable and has been observed to be 94/million in south Sweden,[6] 37/million in New Zealand,[5] and 24/million in Paris.[7] Microscopic polyangiitis is common in the Caucasian population,[8] and the age-corrected incidence in the elderly is significantly higher.[9] In Japan, MPA is the exclusive AAV with an annual incidence of 15/million, rising to 45/million in the population over 65.[10]

DIAGNOSIS

There are no diagnostic criteria for establishing the diagnosis of MPA. The diagnosis is based on grounds of clinical evidence of small-vessel vasculitis (purpura, mononeuritis multiplex, alveolar hemorrhage, nephritic proteinuria, and hematuria, etc). Once small-vessel vasculitis is suspected, it is recommended that the classification of the vasculitis is performed as set out by Watts et al.[11] In the presence of clinical features of medium- and/or small-vessel vasculitis typical of AAV or PAN, a biopsy of the affected organ should be undertaken unless there is a contraindication. The presence of fibrinoid necrosis or crescentic glomerulonephritis is highly suggestive of MPA or other AAV. The surrogate markers for GPA in the algorithm are X-ray evidence of fixed pulmonary infiltrates, nodules, or cavitations present for >1 month; bronchial stenosis; bloody nasal discharge and crusting for >1 month, or nasal ulceration; chronic sinusitis, otitis media, or mastoiditis for >3 months; retro-orbital mass or inflammation (pseudotumor); subglottic stenosis; saddle nose deformity/destructive sinonasal disease. The surrogate markers for renal vasculitis in the algorithm are hematuria associated with red cell casts or >10% dysmorphic erythrocytes; or 2+ hematuria and 2+ proteinuria on urinalysis.

CLINICAL FEATURES

Constitutional symptoms are common at diagnosis. Fever >38°C, weight loss >2 kg, arthralgia, and myalgia are reported in the majority of patients.

About 80% of patients with MPA present with renal involvement. Rapidly progressive glomerulonephritis can be a presenting feature. Most patients will have early hematuria and proteinuria with few other clinical manifestations, which may flare explosively. The presence of glomerulosclerosis on kidney biopsy at diagnosis is suggestive of the presence of smoldering disease prior to clinical presentation. Patients may present with oliguria/anuria and need dialysis at diagnosis. Proteinuria in the nephrotic range is not usual but is seen in about 15% of patients.[12]

Pulmonary involvement can be catastrophic, in the form of alveolar hemorrhage.[13] It is seen in about 10% of patients,[14] and has a poor prognosis. Most patients with pulmonary hemorrhage have coexistent glomerulonephritis. Pulmonary fibrosis is seen in about a third of patients with MPA,[14] and may be a function of the MPO-ANCA serotype.[15] CT scan imaging shows ground-glass changes, consolidation, and thickening of bronchovascular bundles.[15]

Neurological involvement is usually in the form of mononeuritis multiplex, which is observed in the majority of patients at diagnosis. Axonal sensorimotor neuropathy and cranial nerve involvement have also been documented as in the case illustrated above.[12] Other commonly witnessed clinical features include cutaneous changes such as purpura, ulcers, and digital gangrene; mucosal involvement such as mouth or genital ulcers; ocular involvement in the form of retinal vasculitis, scleritis, episcleritis, blepharitis, conjunctivitis, keratitis, and uveitis; rarely heart involvement in the form of pericarditis, myocardial infarction, and congestive cardiac failure; gastrointestinal involvement in the form of mesenteric ischemia, gastrointestinal bleeding, and perforation.

INVESTIGATIONS

Anemia and thrombocytosis are common. Renal abnormality of some form is nearly universal. The mean serum creatinine in the largest cohort of patients with MPA was 2.54 (SD 2.96) mg/dL at diagnosis.[12] The creatine kinase may be elevated in a small number of patients with muscle involvement.

Urine analysis abnormalities include hematuria, varying degrees of proteinuria, and red cell casts.

Antineutrophil cytoplasm antibodies are present in most patients at diagnosis. It can be detected either by IIF or by specific ELISA to test for antibodies directed against either proteinase 3 (PR3) or MPO. IIF uptake in a perinuclear (P) pattern or a diffuse cytoplasmic (C) pattern may be seen. ELISA is usually positive for MPO or PR3. P/MPO ANCA or a C/PR3 ANCA is over 98% specific for a diagnosis of AAV.[16] An international body of experts have suggested that ANCA testing should be carried out by both IIF and ELISA.[17] Patients with MPA are more likely to have the P/MPO ANCA than the C/PR3 ANCA. Serial ANCA measurement cannot be used to guide treatment.

Antibodies directed against lysosomal-associated membrane protein-2 have been shown to be pathogenic and may be of value in serial monitoring, but is currently of academic interest and requires further work.[18]

Chest imaging in the form of plain radiographs and CT scan is of value in documenting silent chest disease.

Histopathology remains the gold standard of diagnosis. Renal biopsy is highly sensitive for the diagnosis and when possible should be preferentially sampled. Sural nerve, muscle, and skin can be biopsied as well. The characteristic changes of MPA include focal segmental glomerulonephritis in the kidney with the presence of crescents in nearly all patients. There is little or no immune complex deposition. The other tissues may demonstrate fibrinoid necrosis of small and medium vessels. Granulomas are not a feature of MPA.

DIAGNOSTIC APPROACH

Microscopic polyangiitis should be suspected in patients with involvement of more than one organ system that includes the kidneys. Patients are typically unwell, and may have been investigated for chronic symptoms such as the case above who was being investigated for anemia.

In the absence of a diagnostic test, every effort should be made to obtain tissue biopsy prior to initiating treatment. In patients with an inconclusive/negative biopsy and negativity for P/MPO or C/PR3 ANCA, alternative differentials include systemic lupus erythematosus, infective endocarditis, cancer, antiglomerular basement membrane disease, and the other AAV.

MANAGEMENT

Remission Induction

Mild Localized Disease

Patients with no evidence of end-organ involvement can be treated with a combination of methotrexate 15–25 mg/week and prednisolone.[19] The dose of prednisolone is not set in stone, but most physicians with a vasculitis interest use up to 1 mg/kg/day to a maximum of 60 mg/day. The aim should be to taper the steroids down to 15 mg/day by the end of 3 months. There are very few patients with MPA who will fall into this staging of disease.[19] Most patients with MPA will have developed renal impairment by diagnosis and will need more aggressive treatment.

Systemic Non-life-threatening Disease

The majority of patients with MPA will have evidence of end-organ involvement in the form of nephritis, mononeuritis, lung involvement, etc. Cyclophosphamide has reduced the risk of mortality by over five-fold in these group of patients compared to those who are treated with glucocorticoids alone.[20] In addition to prednisolone as for mild disease, cyclophosphamide can be used orally in a dose of 2 mg/kg/day, but increasingly most experts prefer pulsed intravenous cyclophosphamide 15/mg/kg/pulse at week 0, 2, 4, 7, 10, and 13.[21] The risk of adverse events is significantly reduced with pulsed administration, but there may be an increased risk of relapse.[22] Patients with a contraindication to cyclophosphamide can be treated with rituximab 375 mg/m^2/week for 4 weeks combined with standard glucocorticoid therapy as for mild disease.[23] There is no difference in the adverse events or median time to remission between cyclophosphamide and rituximab.[24] Therefore, there is currently no merit in substituting rituximab for cyclophosphamide due to lack of long-term data.

Severe Disease

When the presentation of MPA is explosive in the form of rapidly progressive renal failure (serum creatinine >5.6 mg/dL, or oliguria, or need for dialysis) or lung hemorrhage with shifting pulmonary infiltrates, plasmapheresis may have an adjunctive role to cyclophosphamide or rituximab with oral prednisolone in preventing organ failure,[25] but not necessarily a survival advantage.[26] Plasma filtration or centrifugation techniques may be used. One preferred regimen is exchanging 60 mL/kg body weight with 3–5% albumin replacement per session for seven daily or alternate day sessions. Currently, a multinational randomized controlled clinical trial is underway to determine the efficacy of plasma exchange in reducing all cause mortality and progression to end-stage renal disease.[27] Where plasmapheresis is not available or at the clinicians' discretion, intravenous methylprednisolone 1 g daily for 3 days has been used to quickly stabilize the patient.

Remission Maintenance

The choice of remission maintenance agent depends on the choice of remission induction agent. When methotrexate has been used to induce remission, it can be continued as the remission maintenance agent. However, there is emerging evidence that the relapse rate may tend to be higher in this group of patients as compared to patients receiving oral cyclophosphamide.[28] There is no survival advantage with cyclophosphamide, and therefore, the authors still prefer methotrexate as the remission maintenance agent in this group of patients.

Where cyclophosphamide has been used as the remission induction agent, azathioprine is the remission maintenance agent of choice in a dose of 2 mg/kg/day.[29] In patients intolerant to azathioprine, alternative remission maintenance agents include leflunomide or methotrexate.[30] Mycophenolate mofetil can be used but has a higher relapse rate compared to azathioprine (55 versus 38% in one randomized controlled trial).[31]

When remission has been induced with rituximab, the current evidence suggests that rituximab should be used periodically at 4–6 months as a remission maintenance agent.[32,33] This can be continued for long-term as long as the IgG levels remain over 7 g/L. In the presence of low IgG levels, a risk-benefit analysis would have to be carried out to assess the threat of infections versus the risk of relapse. In those patients with a high risk of relapse, it would be reasonable to pretreat with intravenous immunoglobulins to raise the levels of IgG. There is little evidence for this course of treatment.

Treating Relapse

A minor relapse (no organ or life-threatening involvement) can be treated with an increase in oral prednisolone. A major relapse will need either retreatment with cyclophosphamide or rituximab. In one randomized controlled trial in patients with ANCA-associated vasculitis, relapsing disease was more effectively treated by rituximab than by cyclophosphamide. Sixty-seven percent in the rituximab arm, as compared to 42% in the cyclophosphamide arm achieved remission ($P = 0.01$).[23]

Treating Refractory Disease

In situations where the disease fails to improve or gets worse by the third pulse of cyclophosphamide, an alternative strategy has to be employed. The alternatives in this situation are either rituximab or 15-deoxyspergualin. In a multicenter survey of the treatment of 65 refractory patients with AAV, 49 patients achieved complete remission following rituximab, and a further 15 achieved partial remission.[34]

15-deoxyspergualin has only been subjected to one open-label trial in GPA.[35] There is no evidence for its use in MPA.

PROGNOSIS

Relapse

Relapse is common in MPA, albeit less frequent than in GPA.[36] It increases with time—8% at 18 months[29] rising to 34% at 70 months.[12]

Comorbidities

There is an increase in the risk of coronary artery disease and hypertension in patients with treated MPA. This may be due to impaired renal function, but the treatment with high-dose prednisolone may also have a role to play. In a follow-up study of 254 patients with MPA, there was a 16% incidence of cardiovascular events (myocardial infarctions, cerebrovascular accidents, or coronary revascularization procedures) at 5 years.[37] The risk is higher in those patients with MPO-ANCA positivity as compared to PR3-ANCA positivity (odds ratio 0.4 for PR3-ANCA versus MPO-ANCA).[37]

Survival

Survival of 1 and 5 years is 82–92% and 45–76%, respectively.[36] Microscopic polyangiitis survival may be worse compared to GPA, but this may be an artifact of worse renal involvement in MPA.[38,39] The presence of significant renal impairment is known to confer a hazard ratio of 3.69 (95% confidence intervals 1.006 to 13.4) for mortality.[40]

KEY POINTS

- P-ANCA directed against MPO is characteristic.
- Biopsy should always be obtained prior to treatment, if possible.
- Focal segmental necrotizing glomerulonephritis with crescents and without immune deposition is typical of MPA. Granulomas are never seen in MPA.
- Cyclophosphamide and prednisolone are the mainstay of therapy, but plasmapheresis may assist renal survival.
- Rituximab has an increasing role in difficult to treat disease.

REFERENCES

1. Niles JL. Value of tests for antineutrophil cytoplasmic autoantibodies in the diagnosis and treatment of vasculitis. Curr Opin Rheumatol. 1993;5:18-24.
2. Jennette JC, Falk RJ, Andrassy K, et al. Nomenclature of systemic vasculitides. Proposal of an International Consensus Conference. Arthritis Rheum. 1994;37:187-92.
3. Jennette JC, Falk RJ, Bacon PA, et al. Revised International Chapel Hill Consensus Conference Nomenclature of Vasculitides. Arthritis Rheum. 2012;65:1-11.
4. Mohammad AJ, Jacobsson LT, Westman KW, et al. Incidence and survival rates in Wegener's granulomatosis, microscopic polyangiitis, Churg–Strauss syndrome and polyarteritis nodosa. Rheumatology (Oxford). 2009;48:1560-5.
5. Gibson A, Stamp LK, Chapman PT, et al. The epidemiology of Wegener's granulomatosis and microscopic polyangiitis

in a Southern Hemisphere region. Rheumatology (Oxford). 2006;45:624-8.

6. Mohammad AJ, Jacobsson LT, Mahr AD, et al. Prevalence of Wegener's granulomatosis, microscopic polyangiitis, polyarteritis nodosa and Churg–Strauss syndrome within a defined population in southern Sweden. Rheumatology (Oxford). 2007;46:1329-37.

7. Mahr A, Guillevin L, Poissonnet M, et al. Prevalences of polyarteritis nodosa, microscopic polyangiitis, Wegener's granulomatosis, and Churg-Strauss syndrome in a French urban multiethnic population in 2000: a capture-recapture estimate. Arthritis Rheum. 2004;51:92-9.

8. Lane SE, Watts R, Scott DG. Epidemiology of systemic vasculitis. Curr Rheumatol Rep. 2005;7:270-5.

9. Watts RA, Lane SE, Bentham G, et al. Epidemiology of systemic vasculitis: a ten-year study in the United Kingdom. Arthritis Rheum. 2000;43:414-9.

10. Fujimoto S, Uezono S, Hisanaga S, et al. Incidence of ANCA-associated primary renal vasculitis in the Miyazaki Prefecture: the first population-based, retrospective, epidemiologic survey in Japan. Clin J Am Soc Nephrol. 2006;1:1016-22.

11. Watts R, Lane S, Hanslik T, et al. Development and validation of a consensus methodology for the classification of the ANCA-associated vasculitides and polyarteritis nodosa for epidemiological studies. Ann Rheum Dis. 2007;66:222-7.

12. Guillevin L, Durand-Gasselin B, Cevallos R, et al. Microscopic polyangiitis: clinical and laboratory findings in eighty-five patients. Arthritis Rheum. 1999;42:421-30.

13. Lauque D, Cadranel J, Lazor R, et al. Microscopic polyangiitis with alveolar hemorrhage. A study of 29 cases and review of the literature. Groupe d'Etudes et de Recherche sur les Maladies "Orphelines" Pulmonaires (GERM"O"P). Medicine (Baltimore). 2000;79:222-33.

14. Tzelepis GE, Kokosi M, Tzioufas A, et al. Prevalence and outcome of pulmonary fibrosis in microscopic polyangiitis. Eur Respir J. 2010;36:116-21.

15. Ando Y, Okada F, Matsumoto S, et al. Thoracic manifestation of myeloperoxidase-antineutrophil cytoplasmic antibody (MPO-ANCA)-related disease. CT findings in 51 patients. J Comput Assist Tomogr. 2004;28:710-6.

16. Choi HK, Liu S, Merkel PA, et al. Diagnostic performance of antineutrophil cytoplasmic antibody tests for idiopathic vasculitides: meta-analysis with a focus on antimyeloperoxidase antibodies. J Rheumatol. 2001;28:1584-90.

17. Savige J, Gillis D, Benson E, et al. International consensus statement on testing and reporting of antineutrophil cytoplasmic antibodies (ANCA). Am J Clin Pathol. 1999;111:507-13.

18. Kain R, Exner M, Brandes R, et al. Molecular mimicry in pauci-immune focal necrotizing glomerulonephritis. Nat Med. 2008;14:1088-96.

19. De Groot K, Rasmussen N, Bacon PA, et al. Randomized trial of cyclophosphamide versus methotrexate for induction of remission in early systemic antineutrophil cytoplasmic antibody-associated vasculitis. Arthritis Rheum. 2005;52:2461-9.

20. Hogan SL, Nachman PH, Wilkman AS, et al. Prognostic markers in patients with antineutrophil cytoplasmic autoantibody-associated microscopic polyangiitis and glomerulonephritis. J Am Soc Nephrol. 1996;7:23-32.

21. de Groot K, Harper L, Jayne DR, et al. Pulse versus daily oral cyclophosphamide for induction of remission in antineutrophil cytoplasmic antibody-associated vasculitis: a randomized trial. Ann Intern Med. 2009;150:670-80.

22. Harper L, Morgan MD, Walsh M, et al. Pulse versus daily oral cyclophosphamide for induction of remission in ANCA-associated vasculitis: long-term follow-up. Ann Rheum Dis. 2012;71:955-60.

23. Stone JH, Merkel PA, Spiera R, et al. Rituximab versus cyclophosphamide for ANCA-associated vasculitis. N Engl J Med. 2010;363:221-32.

24. Jones RB, Tervaert JW, Hauser T, et al. Rituximab versus cyclophosphamide in ANCA-associated renal vasculitis. N Engl J Med. 2010;363:211-20.

25. Jayne DR, Gaskin G, Rasmussen N, et al. Randomized trial of plasma exchange or high-dosage methylprednisolone as adjunctive therapy for severe renal vasculitis. J Am Soc Nephrol. 2007;18:2180-8.

26. Guillevin L, Cevallos R, Durand-Gasselin B, et al. Treatment of glomerulonephritis in microscopic polyangiitis and Churg–Strauss syndrome. Indications of plasma exchanges, Meta-analysis of 2 randomized studies on 140 patients, 32 with glomerulonephritis. Ann Med Interne (Paris). 1997;148:198-204.

27. Walsh M, Merkel PA, Peh CA, et al. Plasma exchange and glucocorticoid dosing in the treatment of anti-neutrophil cytoplasm antibody associated vasculitis (PEXIVAS): protocol for a randomized controlled trial. Trials. 2013;14:73.

28. Faurschou M, Westman K, Rasmussen N, et al. Brief Report: long-term outcome of a randomized clinical trial comparing methotrexate to cyclophosphamide for remission induction in early systemic antineutrophil cytoplasmic antibody-associated vasculitis. Arthritis Rheum. 2012;64:3472-7.

29. Jayne D, Rasmussen N, Andrassy K, et al. A randomized trial of maintenance therapy for vasculitis associated with antineutrophil cytoplasmic autoantibodies. N Engl J Med. 2003;349:36-44.

30. Mukhtyar C, Guillevin L, Cid MC, et al. EULAR recommendations for the management of primary small and medium vessel vasculitis. Ann Rheum Dis. 2009;68:310-7.

31. Hiemstra TF, Walsh M, Mahr A, et al. Mycophenolate mofetil vs azathioprine for remission maintenance in antineutrophil cytoplasmic antibody-associated vasculitis: a randomized controlled trial. JAMA. 2010;304:2381-8.

32. Smith RM, Jones RB, Guerry MJ, et al. Rituximab for remission maintenance in relapsing antineutrophil cytoplasmic antibody-associated vasculitis. Arthritis Rheum. 2012;64:3760-9.

33. Rhee EP, Laliberte KA, Niles JL. Rituximab as maintenance therapy for anti-neutrophil cytoplasmic antibody-associated vasculitis. Clin J Am Soc Nephrol. 2010;5:1394-400.

34. Jones RB, Ferraro AJ, Chaudhry AN, et al. A multicenter survey of rituximab therapy for refractory antineutrophil

cytoplasmic antibody-associated vasculitis. Arthritis Rheum. 2009;60:2156-68.

35. Flossmann O, Baslund B, Bruchfeld A, et al. Deoxyspergualin in relapsing and refractory Wegener's granulomatosis. Ann Rheum Dis. 2009;68:1125-30.

36. Mukhtyar C, Luqmani R. Disease-specific quality indicators, guidelines, and outcome measures in vasculitis. Clin Exp Rheumatol. 2007;25:120-9.

37. Suppiah R, Judge A, Batra R, et al. A model to predict cardio-vascular events in patients with newly diagnosed Wegener's granulomatosis and microscopic polyangiitis. Arthritis Care Res (Hoboken). 2011;63:588-96.

38. Mukhtyar C, Flossmann O, Hellmich B, et al. Outcomes from studies of antineutrophil cytoplasm antibody associated vasculitis: a systematic review by the European League against rheumatism systemic vasculitis task force. Ann Rheum Dis. 2008;67:1004-10.

39. Flossmann O, Berden A, de Groot K, et al. Long-term patient survival in ANCA-associated vasculitis. Ann Rheum Dis. 2011;70:488-94.

40. Bourgarit A, Le Toumelin P, Pagnoux C, et al. Deaths occurring during the first year after treatment onset for polyarteritis nodosa, microscopic polyangiitis, and Churg–Strauss syndrome: a retrospective analysis of causes and factors predictive of mortality based on 595 patients. Medicine (Baltimore). 2005;84:323-30.

CHAPTER **33**

Eosinophilic Granulomatosis with Polyangiitis (Churg-Strauss Syndrome)

Christian Pagnoux, Corisande Baldwin

INTRODUCTION

Eosinophilic granulomatosis with polyangiitis (EGPA), formerly or also named Churg-Strauss syndrome, is a small-sized vessel systemic necrotizing vasculitis.[1-4] It is the rarest of the three main antineutrophil cytoplasm antibody (ANCA)-associated vasculitides, and whether it should remain part of this vasculitis subgroup is increasingly being discussed.[5-7] Epidemiologically, most characteristic manifestations of EGPA, such as asthma and eosinophilia, and the main pathogenic mechanisms of EGPA differ from those of microscopic polyangiitis (MPA) and granulomatosis with polyangiitis (GPA). In addition, ANCAs, mainly antimyeloperoxidase (anti-MPO) ANCAs, are detected in the sera of only 30–40% of EGPA patients, whose clinical features differ from those of ANCA-negative patients.[8-10]

However, the clinical characteristics of EGPA are well known. Since the first reported cases of probable EGPA, in the mid-1910s[11] and the extensive description of the disease by Jacob Churg and Lotte Straussin 1951,[4] several large series have been published, with now substantial follow-up durations and information on therapeutic responses and outcomes. The diagnosis of EGPA is easy to establish in an anti-MPO-positive adult who presents with late-onset asthma and sinus polyposis followed by eosinophilic lung infiltrates as well as vasculitis manifestations such as purpuric skin lesions and mononeuritis multiplex. Conversely, the distinction between EGPA and primary hypereosinophilic syndrome or neoplasms as well as between "simple" asthma and/or allergic sinusitis exacerbations and an early vasculitis flare in a patient known to have EGPA can be challenging in the numerous patients who present less typical vasculitis and EGPA features.[12,13] The precise and detailed pathogenic mechanisms of EGPA are for the most part unknown, and

therefore, good diagnostic or prognostic biomarkers to help physicians ascertain EGPA diagnosis or flare are not available.

The treatment decisions and short-term outcomes for EGPA patients depend on the presence or not of major organ involvement. Cardiac, gastrointestinal, renal, and/or central nervous system involvement represent more severe disease that should be treated aggressively. Glucocorticoids (GCs) are the cornerstone of treatment for all EGPA patients and for the most severely affected patients, combined with a potent immunosuppressant (i.e. cyclophosphamide [CYC]). We lack a validated alternative to these agents in newly diagnosed patients. Patients with less severe EGPA can be treated first with GCs alone.[14,15] Immunosuppressants such as azathioprine or methotrexate can be added for patients who are GC-dependent because of vasculitis manifestations or, more often, persistent asthma or allergic rhinitis. The addition of these latter drugs to first-line GCs for some patients with nonsevere EGPA, such as those with peripheral nervous system involvement, can be considered and is indeed under investigation.[12,14] Several other and/or new agents or biological agents have been used or are also currently under evaluation for patients with refractory or GC-dependent EGPA, with some promising results that still need to be confirmed.

CASE VIGNETTE

A 54-year-old construction worker with a history of arterial hypertension and glucose intolerance began to complain of shortness of breath and wheezing 5 years ago and was diagnosed with asthma. He quit smoking when he was 30-year-old. Nasal obstruction due to sinus polyposis developed, with recurrent sinusitis and otitis media, which led to some conductive hearing loss, mainly on the right side. Three years ago, he underwent nasal polypectomy, with some transient relief of the nasal congestion. Histology of polyps showed mucosal and submucosal eosinophilic and neutrophilic infiltrates, without vasculitis, granuloma, or malignant cells. He had been using regular antiasthma inhalers since then.

Two years ago, the patient had lingering pneumonia that did not respond well to antibiotics, then arthralgia of the knees, ankles, and elbows developed and, more recently, a papular erythematous rash on the legs. Laboratory tests revealed hypereosinophilia at 10,000/mm³, hemoglobin level 112

g/L, C-reactive protein level 86 mg/L, and normal creatinine and urine analysis findings. CT of the sinuses showed pansinusitis and chest CT showed some patchy alveolar and ground-glass opacities (Figs 33.1 and 33.2). Echocardiography and electrocardiography (ECG) findings were normal.

The patient was positive for anti-MPO ANCAs (> 8 IU/L) on ELISA (with an atypical labeling pattern 1/80 on indirect immunofluorescence), thus diagnosed with EGPA. Because he showed no peripheral nerve, renal, gastrointestinal, or cardiac involvement, he was started on prednisone, 80 mg per day (1 mg/kg per day), with calcium and vitamin

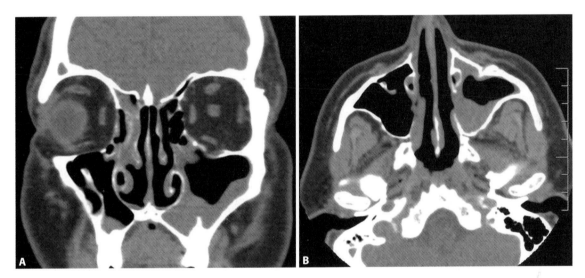

Figs 33.1A and B Sinus CT of a patient with eosinophilic granulomatosis with polyangiitis (EGPA) (coronal and horizontal views). Bilateral, nonerosive sinusitis (clearly predominating on the left maxillary sinus, with some fluid consolidation in right ethmoidosphenoidal sinus)

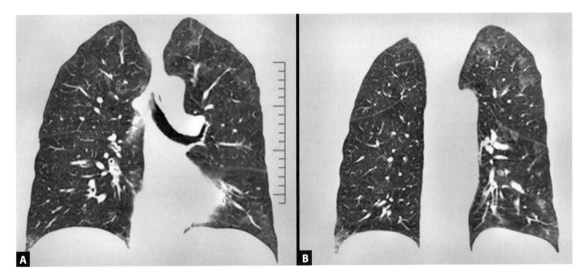

Figs 33.2A and B Chest CT of a patient with EGPA (frontal views). Multiple patchy ground-glass opacities, mainly in the left apex and bases

D supplementation. His condition improved rapidly. The skin rash disappeared within 24 hours, the pneumonia resolved, and the eosinophil count returned to normal within a week. The prednisone dose was tapered, but asthma and sinusitis symptoms recurred every time the dose was reduced to < 10 mg per day, with moderate and concurrent increase in C-reactive protein level to 10–25 mg/L and blood eosinophil count to 750–1,250/mm^3. The patient was started on methotrexate, which allowed for tapering the prednisone to 7.5 mg per day but not lower. He gained 11 kg while on prednisone and type 2 diabetes mellitus developed, which required therapy with oral antidiabetic agents.

EPIDEMIOLOGY

Eosinophilic granulomatosis with polyangiitis is one of the rarest primary systemic necrotizing vasculitides. Its prevalence ranges from 7 to 22 per million inhabitants. A few studies have reported a slightly higher prevalence in northern versus southern Europe and urban versus rural regions, but in general, the geographical distribution shows no pattern.[7,16,17] A few epidemiological studies of ANCA-associated vasculitis suggested that EGPA is rare in Asia, but some large series have recently been reported from Japan and Korea.[7,16-19]

The annual incidence of EGPA varies from 0 to 6.8 per million inhabitants (i.e. one-fifth to one-tenth the incidence of GPA or MPA). In asthma patients, the average annual incidence is not surprisingly higher, because asthma can be considered a predisposing condition for EGPA or a first phase of the disease; the EGPA incidence has been estimated at about 34 per million patients with asthma and up to 60–64.4 per million in those requiring a leukotriene-receptor antagonist or other nonleukotriene-modifying asthma drugs.[20-23] These numbers remain low and widely vary depending on the definitions used for EGPA and/or asthma and the populations analyzed. Importantly, no validated test is available for the early detection of patients with asthma who are at risk of EGPA. A recent study suggested an association of the human leukocyte antigen DRB4 (*HLA-DRB4*) and severe asthma, sinusitis, nasal polyposis, and eosinophils, which may help in the early identification of some patients at risk of EGPA.[24] The presence of blood eosinophilia in a patient with difficult-to-control and late-onset asthma or allergic sinusitis should certainly alert physicians but is not sufficient to establish a diagnosis of EGPA. Late-onset asthma is almost always present in EGPA patients and preceded the first vasculitis manifestations by a mean of 6.7–8.9 years in the French studies and a median of 4 years in the study by Keogh et al.[8,25,26]

Mean age at diagnosis of EGPA patients is about 50 years. Diagnosis of EGPA in children is rare, but a few case series have been reported, as well as in older adults.[19,27] There is no sex preponderance.

The exact cause(s) of EGPA remains unknown. Inhaled allergens, desensitization, or drugs (e.g., macrolides, carbamazepine, and quinine) have been implicated as potential triggers and/or precipitating cofactors for EGPA onset or flares as have several medications to treat asthma such as leukotriene-receptor antagonists or omalizumab.[23,28-30] A direct triggering role of these antiasthma drugs cannot be excluded, but more likely in reported cases, they provided the opportunity for substantial tapering or withdrawal of GCs in patients with asthma, thereby unmasking an underlying "forme fruste" of EGPA, which had been controlled by GCs. For a long time, vaccinations have been considered potential triggers of EGPA or EGPA flare. Recent studies of vaccinations in vasculitis patients have been more reassuring.[31,32]

Asthma often clusters in families, whereas familial cases of EGPA are exceptional. However, genetic studies, all of limited size, suggested some predisposing hereditary factors, mainly common *HLA-DRB1*04* and *HLA-DRB1*07* alleles and the *HLA-DRB4* gene in EGPA patients as compared with healthy controls, as well as an association with the interleukin *IL10.2* haplotype, associated with enhanced interleukin 10 (IL-10) expression, and, possibly, the *CD226 Gly 307S* polymorphism and the increased frequency of the potentially less active leptin receptor *LEPR 656As* allele.[13,33-38]

PATHOGENESIS

As detailed in the chapter on the pathogeny of ANCA-associated vasculitides, the understanding of the pathogenesis of EGPA is much less advanced than that of GPA or MPA, for multiple reasons. Eosinophilic granulomatosis with polyangiitis is a rare disease, no animal model of EGPA is available, and multiple pathways are likely involved—ANCAs and autoimmunity, eosinophils, and T-helper type-2 (Th2) lymphocytes—but with various roles in each patient.[39-41]

T-helper type-2 lymphocytes seem to be the main actors in asthma and allergic manifestations, via the release of cytokines such as IL-4, IL-5, and IL-13. IL-5, in association with IL-3, and granulocyte/macrophage colony-stimulating factor, is important in regulating eosinophil proliferation. IL-25, produced by eosinophils, further enhances the production of Th2 cytokines by activating peripheral blood mononuclear cells.[42]

Eosinophils infiltrate tissues, especially the lung, myocardium and/or gastrointestinal tract, and can exert their toxicity. The pathogenic effects of eosinophils are mainly linked to the release of their cytotoxic enzymes, including major basic protein, eosinophilic cationic protein, eosinophil-derived neurotoxin, and eosinophil peroxidase.[43]

Antineutrophil cytoplasm antibodies may play a role in the development of necrotizing vasculitis and some manifestations that are more typical of other ANCA-associated vasculitis, such as pauci-immune crescentic glomerulonephritis. However, eosinophilia has not been reported in anti-MPO ANCA animal models and not all patients have ANCAs.[44] The reasons and mechanisms of production of ANCAs in EGPA patients remain unknown. Whether B cells have a pathogenic role in EGPA is unclear, although disease in a few patients, including some ANCA-negative patients, has been effectively treated with rituximab, a monoclonal anti-CD20 anti–B-cell antibody.[45-47] Other mechanisms are likely involved in the break of immune tolerance in EGPA that may lead to the production of ANCAs, such as skewed regulatory and active T-cell balance or endothelial or regulatory T-cell function abnormalities.

The respective roles of each of these latter mechanisms likely to vary during the disease and among individuals. Several other subtle and, as yet, unidentified immunological signals are suggested to orchestrate these different pathways. Recently, several groups reported elevated serum levels of immunoglobulin G4 (IgG4) in patients with active EGPA, associated with the number of organ manifestations and disease activity, and infiltration of IgG4-positive plasmacytes has been observed in tissues such as kidneys in some EGPA patients.[48,49]

DIAGNOSIS

As described above and illustrated in the case vignette, the diagnosis of EGPA can be relatively simple. However, in many patients, especially ANCA-negative patients and/or those without histological evidence of (granulomatous and eosinophilic) vasculitis, several alternative diagnoses must be considered and ruled out. The most difficult diagnoses to exclude are primary hypereosinophilic syndrome, mainly with its lymphocytic subsets, and lymphomas, mostly T-cell types. Other differential diagnoses include those listed in Table 33.1 and are easier to screen for and rule out, but none must be forgotten.[12]

CLINICAL FEATURES

The diagnostic criteria for Churg-Strauss syndrome devised by Lanham in the mid-1980s are not used in practice for diagnosis of EGPA because they are too broad and not specific.[50,51] However, they remain of interest and are worth mentioning because they underscored, probably for the first time clearly, the three prototypical successive phases of the disease. The prodromal phase begins with asthma and allergic manifestations; the second stage is characterized by blood eosinophilia > 10% (1500/mm³) and tissue eosinophilia affecting visceral organs such as the lung; and the last stage involves the development of vasculitis features (involving two or more extrapulmonary organs) such as those affecting the skin (purpura) and peripheral nerves. The three phases do not systematically occur successively, because they can overlap in time. In the absence of overt clinical vasculitis manifestations (third phase), the diagnosis of EGPA remains uncertain and should likely not be concluded. We lack other diagnostic criteria at this time, although international efforts to develop criteria are under way.[52] The 1990 American College of Rheumatology classification criteria of Churg-Strauss vasculitis (Table 33.2) are for classification purposes.[3] The 2012 revised Chapel Hill Nomenclature of EGPA (Table 33.3) provided an updated definition of the disease.[2] Importantly, none of these criteria should be used to support a diagnostic impression because they are not diagnostic criteria and are specific to only patients with already established and proven vasculitis.

The frequencies of the most common manifestations in EGPA, according to some of the largest published studies, are in Table 33.4.[8,9,18,19,25,51,53-56] Constitutional symptoms such as arthralgias, myalgias, weight loss and/or fever are frequent at diagnosis. Ear, nose, and throat (ENT) manifestations, such as rhinitis or sinus polyposis, and/or asthma are present in almost all EGPA patients. Lung infiltrates, which would be predominantly eosinophilic if a bronchoalveolar lavage fluid examination is performed, are present in 35–75% of patients, depending on the series, and eosinophilic pleural effusion is present in 7–30%. Hilar and/or mediastinal lymphadenopathy are possible, although their presence should raise concerns about a possible underlying lymphoproliferative disorder. Alveolar hemorrhage and nodules are rare in EGPA. Interstitial lung fibrosis is a rare complication of anti-MPO ANCA-associated vasculitis, including MPA and EGPA.[57]

Skin and peripheral nerve involvement are the next most common manifestations, the former occurring in 30–75% of patients, mainly palpable purpura or maculopapules, often with an urticarial appearance and, sometimes, migratory pattern (Figs 33.3 and 33.4). Cutaneous nodules, livedo reticularis, ulcerations, erythema multiforme, scalp erythematous macular lesions (Fig. 33.5), nail-fold infarctions, vesicles or bullae, toe or finger ischemia, deep pannicular vasculitis, and facial edema have been reported. Mononeuritis multiplex, with asymmetric motor and/or

Table 33.1 Main differential diagnoses of eosinophilic granulomatosis with polyangiitis (adapted from reference 12)

Other systemic vasculitides (sometimes with low degree hypereosinophilia)

    Microscopic polyangiitis

    Granulomatosis with polyangiitis

    Polyarteritis nodosa

    Giant cell arteritis

    Henoch–Schönlein purpura

    Others: cutaneous leukocytoclastic vasculitis, cryoglobulinemic vasculitis, etc.

Hypersensitivity reactions

    Hypersensitivity vasculitis (mainly drug-related)

    DRESS (drug rash with eosinophilia and systemic symptoms)

    Eosinophilic/hypersensitivity pneumonitis (drugs, pneumallergens, etc.)

Allergic and/or hypereosinophilic asthma (can be associated with nonspecific systemic manifestations but without vasculitis features; can be difficult to distinguish from a "forme fruste" or an early stage of EGPA)

Idiopathic chronic eosinophilic pneumonia (Carrington's disease)

Allergic bronchopulmonary aspergillosis

Infections

    Helminthiases/nematodes (toxocarosis/larva migrans, anguillulosis, ankylostomiasis, trichinosis, ascaridiasis, oxyuriasis, trichocephalosis, etc.)

    Other parasitic infections with blood and/or tissue eosinophilia (liver distomatosis, bilharziasis, filarioses, onchocercosis, taeniases, hydatidosis, alveolar echinococcosis, myases, anisakiasis, gnathostomiasis, rarely toxoplasmosis)

    Human immunodeficiency virus infection (and/or hepatitis C virus infection)

(Primary) Hypereosinophilic syndrome (blood eosinophilia > 1500/mm^3 for > 6 months)

    Lymphoid hypereosinophilic syndrome (a circulating T-cell clone can sometimes be detected, but this is not totally specific)

    Myeloid hypereosinophilic syndrome (FIP1L1–PDGFRA gene fusion can be detected in some patients)

Other malignant hemopathies and solid cancers

    Lymphomas (mainly T and Hodgkin lymphomas)

    Myeloproliferative neoplasms

    Myelodysplastic syndromes

    Acute or chronic leukemias

    Solid cancers––mainly gastrointestinal tract, breast, or lung cancers (blood eosinophilia and, more rarely, authentic paraneoplastic vasculitis)

Miscellaneous

    Eosinophilic esophagitis and/or gastritis (can sometimes be the first manifestation of EGPA)

    IgG4-related syndrome (common pathogenic mechanisms and/or association with EGPA are possible)

    Eosinophilic fasciitis (Shulman syndrome)

    L-Tryptophan-related eosinophilia–myalgia syndrome and toxic oil syndrome

    Other systemic disease, with or without associated vasculitis (rheumatoid arthritis, dermatomyositis, etc.)

    Crohn's disease, ulcerative colitis

    Sarcoidosis (Löfgren's syndrome)

    Systemic mastocytosis

    Cholesterol emboli syndrome

    Gleich syndrome

    Kimura disease

sensory signs, is the most frequent and characteristic feature of peripheral nerve involvement. The peroneal and tibial branches of the sciatic, ulnar, and median nerves are the most commonly affected nerves. Polyneuropathy, symmetrical or not, is rarer.

Cardiac manifestations occur in 10–50% of patients, depending on the series, with definitions and/or cardiac investigations described.[50,58,59] The mechanisms of EGPA cardiac manifestations may combine eosinophilic and/or granulomatous infiltration of the myocardium, eosinophil-derived protein toxicity in heart tissues, possibly leading to fibrosis, and/or coronary artery and small myocardial vessel vasculitis, causing ischemic lesions. Cardiomyopathy has been associated with increased mortality in earlier series of EGPA and justifies an aggressive therapeutic management. Eosinophilic pericardial effusion is frequent, in up to 20% of patients, as are conduction disorders and supraventricular arrhythmias. Intraventricular thrombi, dysautonomic manifestations, or cardiac valve involvement are rare.[60]

Table 33.2 1990 American College of Rheumatology criteria for the classification of Churg-Strauss syndrome (adapted from reference 3)

Criteria	Definition
1. Asthma	History of wheezing or diffuse high-pitched rales on expiration
2. Eosinophilia	Eosinophilia > 10% of white blood cell differential count
3. Mononeuropathy or polyneuropathy	Development of mononeuropathy, multiple mononeuropathies, or polyneuropathy (i.e., glove/stocking distribution) attributable to vasculitis
4. Pulmonary infiltrates, nonfixed	Migratory or transitory pulmonary infiltrates on radiographs (not including fixed infiltrates), attributable to systemic vasculitis
5. Paranasal sinus abnormality	History of acute or chronic paranasal sinus pain or tenderness or radiographic opacification of the paranasal sinuses
6. Extravascular eosinophils	Biopsy including artery, arteriole or venule, showing accumulations of eosinophils in extravascular areas

For classification purposes, a patient with vasculitis shall be said to have CSS if at least four of these six criteria are present. The presence of any four or more criteria yields a sensitivity of 85% and a specificity of 99.7%.

Table 33.3 Place and definition of eosinophilic granulomatosis with polyangiitis according to the 2012 revised Chapel Hill Nomenclature (adapted from reference 2)

Small vessel vasculitis (SVV)
Antineutrophil cytoplasmic antibody (ANCA)–associated vasculitis
Microscopic polyangiitis (MPA)
Granulomatosis with polyangiitis (Wegener's) (GPA)
Eosinophilic granulomatosis with polyangiitis (Churg-Strauss) (EGPA)
Eosinophil-rich and necrotizing granulomatous inflammation often involving the respiratory tract, and necrotizing vasculitis predominantly affecting small to medium vessels, and associated with asthma and eosinophilia. ANCA is more frequent when glomerulonephritis is present.

Other possible manifestations include cranial nerve palsy, central nervous system involvement (intracranial and/or subarachnoid hemorrhage, cerebral infarction, pachymeningitis), which usually occur later during the course of the disease, and gastrointestinal manifestations (abdominal pain, vomiting or diarrhea, eosinophilic granulomatous colitis or esogastritis, and of more concern, bleeding, mesenteric artery branch vasculitis, with the risk of bowel infarction and perforation). Kidney involvement (mainly focal segmental and pauci-immune glomerulonephritis) and urological manifestations (urethral or ureteral stenosis, prostatitis) are not as frequent as in GPA. Ophthalmologic manifestations (uveitis, episcleritis, or retinal vasculitis) and venous thromboembolic events, including pulmonary embolism, mainly during the active phase of the vasculitis, are other possible manifestations.[61,62]

Several retrospective studies have reported that ANCA-positive patients differ clinically from ANCA-negative patients. Antineutrophil cytoplasm antibody-positive patients tend to have a higher frequency of renal involvement, constitutional symptoms, purpura, alveolar hemorrhage and/or mononeuritis multiplex, whereas ANCA-negative patients more frequently have cardiomyopathy, pericarditis, livedo and/or pulmonary infiltrates.[8-10,25,26] Furthermore, vasculitis in histological specimens from ANCA-negative patients seems to be less frequent, whereas eosinophil tissue infiltration is more often prominent. Outcomes for patients seem similar regardless of ANCA status at diagnosis but with a limited follow up of 3–5 years; some studies with a longer follow-up suggested a possible higher relapse rate of the vasculitis manifestations (differentiated from "simple" asthma exacerbations) but lower mortality in ANCA-positive than negative patients.[9,25,63]

Investigations

Biology

C-reactive protein level or erythrocyte sedimentation rate are usually increased during active phases of the disease. Blood eosinophilia is almost constant during active disease, usually > 1,000/mm^3, and can exceed 50,000/mm^3. Serum IgE level is elevated in most patients, as a simple surrogate marker of eosinophilia (its measurement does not seem to add much to the diagnosis or monitoring disease). Antineutrophil cytoplasm antibodies can be detected in up to 40% of EGPA patients, usually generating a perinuclear immunofluorescent-labeling pattern, most frequently anti-MPO, on ELISA.[6,12,25,26]

Serum levels of eosinophil cationic protein, IL-5, IL-25, vascular endothelial growth factor, eotaxin-3 (CCL26), and several other chemokines or cytokines are high but are not tested on a routine basis.[41,64-66] We lack good markers or combinations of markers to help distinguish between EGPA and primary hypereosinophilic syndrome. The role of other biomarkers of common asthma such as periostin or sputum eosinophil count is not yet well defined for the diagnosis or

Table 33.4 Frequencies (%) of clinical features in eosinophilic granulomatosis with polyangiitis according to the main series in the literature including more than 30 adult patients

Reference	UK + literature – Lanham[51]	Spain – Solans et al.[53]	USA – Keogh et al.[25]	Italy –Sinico et al.[9]	Italy –Baldini et al.[10]	Japan – Uchiyama et al. + Japan literature[19]	USA (FDA) – Healy et al.[55]	Germany – Moosig et al.[56]	France – Comarmond et al.[8]	Korea –Kim et al.[18]
	1984	2001	2003	2005	2009	2011	2012	2012	2013	2014
Clinical features										
Number of patients	138	32	91	93	38	123	93	150	383	52
Sex Male	72	9	51	39	17	46	—	76	199	29
Female	66	23	40	54	21	77	—	74	184	23
Age (year) Mean	38	42	49 ± 16	51.7	48.7 ± 15	54.7 ± 16.5	—	49.1 ± 1.2	50.3 ± 15.7	49
Range	—	(17–85)	—	(18–86)	(21–76)	(15–85)	—	—	—	(14–79)
General symptoms	—	69	—	67.7	—	—	62.4	17, initial	—	34.6
Arthritis, arthralgias	46	—	30	—	48	—	35.5	16, initial 51.3, overall	29.8	—
Myalgias	—	—	—	—	48	—	33.3	—	38.1	—
Allergic rhinitis and/or ear, nose and throat involvement	69	—	74	77.4	79	—	63.4	57, initial 93.3, overall	48	61.5
Asthma	100	100	99	95.7	100	96	100	92.7	91.1	78.8
Pulmonary infiltrates	74	53	58	50.5	53	44	64.5	58	38.6	61.5
Pleural effusion	29	19	—	—	—	—	12.9	7.3	8.9	—
Skin involvement	—	69	57	52.7	—	—	67.7	19, initial 49.3, overall	39.7	41.9
Purpura	46	—	—	—	21	43	43	34.7	22.5	13.5
Peripheral nervous system involvement (mainly mononeuritis multiplex)	64	44	76	64.5	53	76 (more common in > 60 years old)	51.6	35, initial 56, overall	51.4	61.5
Central nervous system involvement	—	6	11	14	—	4	12.9	3	5.2	7.7
Digestive involvement	62	38	31	21.5	42	28 (more common in > 60 years old)	17.2	8, initial 28.7, overall	23.2	30.8
Cardiac involvement	52	28	13 cardio-myopathy (7 pericarditis)	16.1	13–16	12	28	17, initial 46.7, overall	27.4	11.5
Renal involvement	42	13	25	26.9	7	11	17.2	5, initial 18.7, overall	21.7	13.5

*Previous series from the FVSG (French vasculitis study group) are not listed in this table, as this series included those patients previously reported.

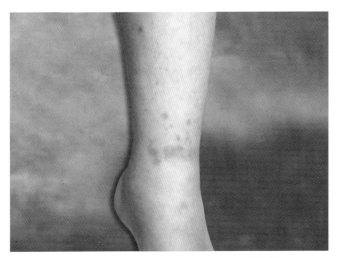

Fig. 33.3 Purpuric macular skin lesions on the leg, above the ankle, in a patient with EGPA

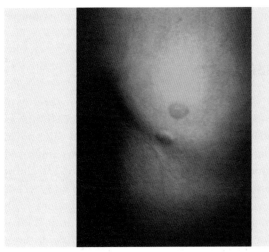

Fig. 33.4 Maculopapular pseudo-urticarial lesion in the scapular area in a patient with EGPA

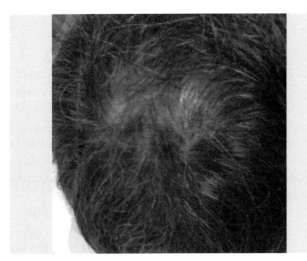

Fig. 33.5 Erythematomacular skin lesions of the scalp, superficially eroded, in a patient with EGPA

monitoring of EGPA.[67-69] Conversely, several other routine tests and investigations should be performed, depending on patient characteristics and presentation, to rule out some of the differential diagnoses (listed in Table 33.1).

Radiology

Patients suspected of having EGPA should undergo a chest X-ray and CT scan and a sinus CT scan. Imaging of the sinus may reveal nondestructive sinusitis and/or sinus polyposis (Fig. 33.1). Chest radiographs can show pulmonary infiltrates, most often transient, labile, and patchy, with an alveolar pattern (Figs 33.2 and 33.6). A diffuse interstitial infiltrative pattern or massive bilateral nodular infiltrates may be seen, as well as pleural effusion.

Cardiac imaging should probably be systematic at diagnosis with ultrasound and/or MRI. However, the clinical and prognostic significance of subtle abnormalities disclosed only on MRI in patients with no cardiac symptoms and no ECG abnormalities remain undetermined (Fig. 33.7).[8-10,25,26] Decisions for other radiological investigations are based on the clinical presentation.

Histopathology

When possible, the diagnosis of EGPA should be substantiated by biopsy of an involved tissue. The three main histological lesions of EGPA include: (1) Vessel wall infiltrates (mainly with eosinophils) with fibrinoid necrosis (vasculitis), (2) Extravascular eosinophilic infiltrates, and (3) Extravascular necrotizing granulomas (mainly with eosinophils). However, these three types of histological lesions are found together in only a few cases.[39,70]

Skin biopsies are easy to obtain when patients have cutaneous lesions. Lung and/or muscle and peripheral nerve biopsies are more invasive. The yield of ENT biopsies is low; the histology of polyps is often nonspecific (eosinophilic infiltrates, as in more common allergic polyposis). Endomyocardial biopsy is not often done during diagnostic work-up, but its sensitivity seems high in patients with cardiomyopathy. Gastrointestinal tract endoscopic biopsies must be deep extensive to be informative, thereby carrying a non-negligible risk of perforation.[8]

Diagnostic Approach

Diagnosis relies on the combination of suggestive clinical manifestations, as described above, and biological parameters, including eosinophilia and, in up to 40% of patients, positive-ANCA test results. Ideally, diagnosis is

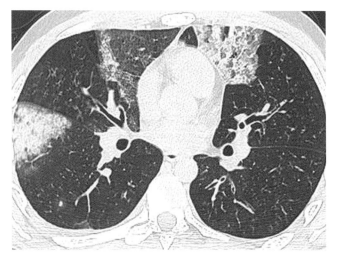

Fig. 33.6 Chest CT of a patient with EGPA (horizontal view). Multiple patchy opacities and consolidation

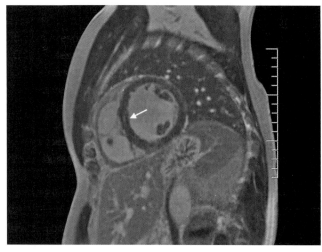

Fig. 33.7 Cardiac MRI for a patient with EGPA and cardiac involvement (parasagittal view, late postgadolinium phase-sensitive inversion recovery sequence). The left-ventricular volume is in the upper limit of normal. A small, linear, late gadolinium enhancement (arrow) in the basal and mid septum involves the mesocardium. Dynamic sequences reveal mild reduction in left ventricle systolic function with mild hypokinesis of the septum consistent with mild dilated cardiomyopathy

supported by biopsy findings when feasible. The main alternative diagnoses are in Table 33.1. Sometimes, diagnosis of EGPA can be confirmed and that of chronic eosinophilic pneumonia or primary eosinophilic syndrome ruled out only after several months or years of follow-up. Circulating lymphocyte immunophenotyping, T-cell clonal and cytogenetic studies, and molecular analyses to detect Fip1-like 1 (FIP1L1) platelet-derived growth factor receptor-α (PDGFRA) gene fusion should be performed for patients with

suspected EGPA, but who are ANCA-negative and/or without histologically proven vasculitis to detect lymphoid or myeloid neoplasms associated with eosinophilia. However, these screening tests are not entirely sensitive and the presence of a circulating but simply reactive T-cell clone is possible during active phases of obvious EGPA.[6,10,12,39,71] More specific tests and screening for other *PDGFRA*, *PDGFRB*, or *FGFR1* fusion gene should be discussed with hematologists.

Once the diagnosis of EGPA is established, disease severity should be thoroughly evaluated. Chest X-ray and/ or CT should be systematic as should perhaps sinus CT at diagnosis. Importantly, investigations to search for cardiac (echocardiography and ECG systematically and, perhaps, MRI and Holter-ECG) and renal (serum creatinine and urine analysis and microscopy) are mandatory. Investigations for nervous system or gastrointestinal involvement should be based on clinical findings. Treatment for patients with life-threatening and/or major organ involvement must not be delayed.

MANAGEMENT

Treatment should be adapted to the type and severity of disease and should combine immunosuppressants as needed and local antiasthma therapies (inhaled GCs and/or bronchodilators). Globally, EGPA outcomes have improved greatly within the past four decades. Remission rates now peak at more than 80% and the 10-year survival rate exceeds 75%. However, death can occur, especially in patients with cardiomyopathy; vasculitis relapse occurs in up to 35% of patients and asthma persists in more than 70% of those who may require continuing low doses of GCs, inhaled GCs and/or GC-sparing agents.[8,14,56] Finally, damage is frequent and may result from vasculitic peripheral neuropathy, congestive heart failure, or side effects of long-term treatments.[14,60,72,73]

Notably, the definitions of remission and EGPA flare lack consensus, mainly because most patients must continue to receive GCs for asthma control. As well, whether asthma exacerbations should be considered a manifestation of EGPA when all other vasculitis manifestations (e.g., cutaneous purpura or alveolar hemorrhage) have disappeared remains debated. Several patients in apparent clinical remission may show persistently mild, isolated, and fluctuating eosinophilia.

Patients without severe manifestations can initially receive GCs alone.[14,15] More than 90% will achieve remission, but 35% will experience vasculitis relapse, mainly during the first year of treatment, and 80% of those in remission will continue to require low-dose GCs to control their asthma or allergic sinusitis.[15] Whether adding a GC-sparing agent such as azathioprine, methotrexate, mycophenolate mofetil, or leflunomide for patients such as in our case vignette, with GC-dependent asthma, is effective is not known. Although a common practice, their efficacy and the relative superiority of individual agents is not clear.[74,75] However, whether the addition of an immunosuppressant other than CYC at diagnosis would be helpful in such patients, is under investigation.[12]

Patients with severe manifestations must receive a combination of GCs (starting with a prednisone-equivalent dose of 1 mg/kg per day, preceded by methylprednisolone intravenous [IV] pulses – 0.5 to 1 g per day for 1–3 consecutive days—in most severe cases, then gradually tapered to 20 mg per day at about month 3, then 5 mg per day at month 5, if possible) and a potent immunosuppressant, primarily CYC, for induction (CYC, 15 mg/kg IV every two weeks for 1 month, then every three weeks or 2 mg/kg per day when given orally, adjusted for age and renal function).[14,76] Similar to treatment for MPA and GPA, CYC should be switched after a maximum of 3–6 months to a less toxic immunosuppressant, such as azathioprine (orally, 2 mg/kg per day) or methotrexate (orally or subcutaneously, 0.3 mg/kg per week with a maximum dose of 25 mg per week), once remission has been achieved. The optimal duration of this entire staged strategy is unknown but should be at least 18–24 months. Again, although more than 85% of patients will achieve remission with this strategy, vasculitis relapses will occur in more than one third of the survivors and 60–80% will remain GC-dependent because of asthma, allergic sinusitis, or rhinitis (mean dose about 8 mg per day, after a mean follow-up of 8 years).

Intravenous immunoglobulins (2 g/kg per month) may be an alternative to immunosuppressants in pregnant women and have been beneficial in few patients with refractory EGPA.[77] Plasma exchange should be considered in patients with severe glomerulonephritis and/or alveolar hemorrhage.[78-81]

We need other drugs that limit GC exposure, treat refractory disease and/or lingering and GC-dependent respiratory symptoms, and optimize the functional recovery of patients with cardiac and/or peripheral nerve involvement. Interferon-alpha (3 MU thrice weekly, up to 21 MU per week) can reverse Th2-mediated immune responses and has been used in a few patients with refractory EGPA. However, the treatment has potential cardiac toxicity and responses were generally only transient.[82,83] Omalizumab, a murine monoclonal antibody directed against human IgE, can be used to treat allergic asthma and showed some benefits for

asthma control in few EGPA patients. However, development of full-blown EGPA in patients with "common" asthma after receiving omalizumab has been reported, likely due to the GC-sparing effect of the biological agent that allowed EGPA with a "forme fruste" of EGPA to become overt, similar to what was previously reported with antileukotriene-receptor antagonists.[84-88] Rituximab was used in a few CSS patients, mainly, but not only, ANCA-positive positive, with some interesting results, at least in the short term and for eosinophil counts.[45-47,89] Conversely, the drug was found ineffective and caused severe bronchospasms in two ANCA-negative patients.[90] Use of mycophenolate mofetil, hydroxyurea, cyclosporin A, tyrosine-kinase inhibitors such as imatinib, or TNF-α blockers such as infliximab or etanercept to treat EGPA has been anecdotal.[91-98] One randomized controlled study of mepolizumab, a humanized monoclonal anti-IL-5 antibody, is including patients with refractory, relapsing or GC-dependent EGPA manifestations after promising results were observed in small open studies of such patients.[99-101] Studies with other and newer drugs or monoclonal antibodies will likely be conducted in the future.

Besides receiving immunosuppressive therapy, EGPA patients must receive appropriate antiasthma treatment and general prophylactic treatments to limit damage of long-term GC use and prevent infections such as pneumocystosis (in patients receiving CYC or rituximab) or flu (influenza vaccination is safe in EGPA, according to recent studies).[31,102] Follow-up and management of conventional cardiovascular risk factors is mandatory; long-term cardiovascular mortality appears increased in vasculitis patients because of treatments received as well as, likely, the disease.

CONCLUSION

Eosinophilic granulomatosis with polyangiitis is one of the rarest systemic vasculitis. Its clinical manifestations are well known, but we need to better understand its pathogenic mechanisms followed by treatment optimization. In the mid-2010s, GCs and conventional immunosuppressants such as CYC, azathioprine, or methotrexate remain the cornerstones of management. With the appropriate use of these agents, the mortality rate is < 15% at 10 years. However, persistent and/or recurrent disease manifestations and/or asthma exacerbations require that most patients remain under treatment for years, thereby increasing the frequency of numerous side effects. Sustained, collaborative and international efforts are needed to complete the picture and are indeed under way.

KEY POINTS

- Eosinophilic granulomatosis with polyangiitis is rare, with prevalence of 7–22 per million inhabitants and an annual incidence of 0–6.8 per million inhabitants.
- Most characteristic manifestations of EGPA are well known but overlap with those of primary hypereosinophilic syndrome and T-cell lymphoma, which remain difficult to exclude in the absence of specific biomarkers.
- Antineutrophil cytoplasm antibodies, mainly antimyeloperoxidase ANCAs, are detected in the sera of only 30–40% of patients, whose clinical features differ from those of ANCA-negative patients.
- Patients with cardiac, gastrointestinal, renal, and/or central nervous system involvement should receive a combination of GCs and a potent immunosuppressant.
- Rituximab and mepolizumab treatments have been promising but need to be confirmed, in patients with refractory or glucocorticoid-dependent EGPA.

REFERENCES

1. Jennette JC, Falk RJ, Andrassy K, et al. Nomenclature of systemic vasculitides. Proposal of an international consensus conference. Arthritis Rheum. 1994;37:187-92.
2. Jennette JC, Falk RJ, Bacon PA, et al. 2012 Revised International Chapel Hill Consensus Conference Nomenclature of Vasculitides. Arthritis Rheum. 2013;65:1-11.
3. Masi AT, Hunder GG, Lie JT, et al. The American College of Rheumatology 1990 criteria for the classification of Churg-Strauss syndrome (allergic granulomatosis and angiitis). Arthritis Rheum. 1990;33:1094-100.
4. Churg J, Strauss L. Allergic granulomatosis, allergic angiitis, and periarteritis nodosa. Am J Pathol. 1951;27:277-301.
5. Kallenberg CG. Churg-Strauss syndrome: just one disease entity? Arthritis Rheum. 2005;52:2589-93.
6. Pagnoux C, Guillevin L. Churg-Strauss syndrome: evidence for disease subtypes? Curr Opin Rheumatol. 2010;22:21-8.
7. Mahr A, Moosig F, Neumann T, et al. Eosinophilic granulomatosis with polyangiitis (Churg-Strauss): evolutions in classification, etiopathogenesis, assessment and management. Curr Opin Rheumatol. 2014;26:16-23.
8. Comarmond C, Pagnoux C, Khellaf M, et al. Eosinophilic granulomatosis with polyangiitis (Churg-Strauss): clinical characteristics and long-term follow-up of the 383 patients enrolled in the French Vasculitis Study Group cohort. Arthritis Rheum. 2013;65:270-81.
9. Sinico RA, Di Toma L, Maggiore U, et al. Prevalence and clinical significance of antineutrophil cytoplasmic antibodies in Churg-Strauss syndrome. Arthritis Rheum. 2005;52:2926-35.
10. Baldini C, Della Rossa A, Grossi S, et al. [Churg-Strauss syndrome: outcome and long-term follow-up of 38 patients from a single Italian centre]. Reumatismo. 2009;61:118-24.
11. Lamb AR. Periarteritis nodosa—a clinical and pathological review of the disease: with a report of two cases. Arch Intern Med (Chic). 1914;XIV:481-516.
12. Pagnoux C. Churg-Strauss syndrome: evolving concepts. Discov Med. 2010;9:243-52.
13. Vaglio A, Buzio C, Zwerina J. Eosinophilic granulomatosis with polyangiitis (Churg-Strauss): state of the art. Allergy. 2013;68:261-73.
14. Samson M, Puechal X, Devilliers H, et al. Long-term outcomes of 118 patients with eosinophilic granulomatosis with polyangiitis (Churg-Strauss syndrome) enrolled in two prospective trials. J Autoimmun. 2013;43:60-9.
15. Ribi C, Cohen P, Pagnoux C, et al. Treatment of Churg-Strauss syndrome without poor-prognosis factors: a multicenter, prospective, randomized, open-label study of seventy-two patients. Arthritis Rheum. 2008;58:586-94.
16. Mohammad AJ, Jacobsson LT, Mahr AD, et al. Prevalence of Wegener's granulomatosis, microscopic polyangiitis, polyarteritis nodosa and Churg-Strauss syndrome within a defined population in southern Sweden. Rheumatology (Oxford). 2007;46:1329-37.
17. Mohammad AJ, Jacobsson LT, Westman KW, et al. Incidence and survival rates in Wegener's granulomatosis, microscopic polyangiitis, Churg-Strauss syndrome and polyarteritis nodosa. Rheumatology (Oxford). 2009;48:1560-5.
18. Kim MY, Sohn KH, Song WJ, et al. Clinical features and prognostic factors of Churg-Strauss syndrome. Korean J Intern Med. 2014;29:85-95.
19. Uchiyama M, Mitsuhashi Y, Yamazaki M, et al. Elderly cases of Churg-Strauss syndrome: case report and review of Japanese cases. J Dermatol. 2011;39:76-9.
20. Harrold LR, Andrade SE, Eisner M, et al. Identification of patients with Churg-Strauss syndrome (CSS) using automated data. Pharmacoepidemiol Drug Saf. 2004;13:661-7.
21. Harrold LR, Andrade SE, Go AS, et al. Incidence of Churg-Strauss syndrome in asthma drug users: a population-based perspective. J Rheumatol. 2005;32:1076-80.
22. Harrold LR, Patterson MK, Andrade SE, et al. Asthma drug use and the development of Churg-Strauss syndrome (CSS). Pharmacoepidemiol Drug Saf. 2007;16:620-6.
23. Wechsler ME, Pauwels R, Drazen JM. Leukotriene modifiers and Churg-Strauss syndrome: adverse effect or response to corticosteroid withdrawal? Drug Saf. 1999;21:241-51.
24. Bottero P, Motta F, Bonini M, et al. Can HLA-DRB4 help to identify asthmatic patients at risk of Churg-Strauss syndrome? ISRN Rheumatol. 2014;2014:843804.
25. Keogh KA, Specks U. Churg-Strauss syndrome: clinical presentation, antineutrophil cytoplasmic antibodies, and leukotriene receptor antagonists. Am J Med. 2003;115:284-90.
26. Keogh KA, Specks U. Churg-Strauss syndrome: update on clinical, laboratory and therapeutic aspects. Sarcoidosis Vasc Diffuse Lung Dis. 2006;23:3-12.
27. Zwerina J, Eger G, Englbrecht M, et al. Churg-Strauss syndrome in childhood: A systematic literature review and clinical comparison with adult patients. Semin Arthritis Rheum. 2009;39:108-15.

28. Bottero P, Bonini M, Vecchio F, et al. The common allergens in the Churg-Strauss syndrome. Allergy. 2007;62:1288-94.

29. Wechsler ME, Finn D, Gunawardena D, et al. Churg-Strauss syndrome in patients receiving montelukast as treatment for asthma. Chest. 2000;117:708-13.

30. Wechsler ME, Wong DA, Miller MK, et al. Churg-Strauss syndrome in patients treated with omalizumab. Chest. 2009;136:507-18.

31. Kostianovsky A, Charles P, Alves JF, et al. Immunogenicity and safety of seasonal and 2009 pandemic A/H1N1 influenza vaccines for patients with autoimmune diseases: a prospective, monocentre trial on 199 patients. Clin Exp Rheumatol. 2012;30:S83-9.

32. Duggal T, Segal P, Shah M, et al. Antineutrophil cytoplasmic antibody vasculitis associated with influenza vaccination. Am J Nephrol. 2013;38:174-8.

33. Vaglio A, Martorana D, Maggiore U, et al. HLA-DRB4 as a genetic risk factor for Churg-Strauss syndrome. Arthritis Rheum. 2007;56:3159-66.

34. Wieczorek S, Hellmich B, Arning L, et al. Functionally relevant variations of the interleukin-10 gene associated with antineutrophil cytoplasmic antibody-negative Churg-Strauss syndrome, but not with Wegener's granulomatosis. Arthritis Rheum. 2008;58:1839-48.

35. Wieczorek S, Hellmich B, Gross WL, et al. Associations of Churg-Strauss syndrome with the HLA-DRB4 locus, and relationship to the genetics of antineutrophil cytoplasmic antibody-associated vasculitides: comment on the article by Vaglio et al. Arthritis Rheum. 2008;58:329-30.

36. Wieczorek S, Hoffjan S, Chan A, et al. Novel association of the CD226 (DNAM-1) Gly307 Ser polymorphism in Wegener's granulomatosis and confirmation for multiple sclerosis in German patients. Genes Immun. 2009;10:591-5.

37. Wieczorek S, Holle JU, Bremer JP, et al. Contrasting association of a nonsynonymous leptin receptor gene polymorphism with Wegener's granulomatosis and Churg-Strauss syndrome. Rheumatology (Oxford). 2010;49:907-14.

38. Wieczorek S, Holle JU, Epplen JT. Recent progress in the genetics of Wegener's granulomatosis and Churg-Strauss syndrome. Curr Opin Rheumatol. 2010;22:8-14.

39. Vaglio A, Moosig F, Zwerina J. Churg-Strauss syndrome: update on pathophysiology and treatment. Curr Opin Rheumatol. 2012;24:24-30.

40. Zwerina J, Axmann R, Jatzwauk M, et al. Pathogenesis of Churg-Strauss syndrome: Recent insights. Autoimmunity. 2009;42:376-9.

41. Zwerina J, Bach C, Martorana D, et al. Eotaxin-3 in Churg-Strauss syndrome: a clinical and immunogenetic study. Rheumatology (Oxford). 2011;50:1823-7.

42. Terrier B, Bieche I, Maisonobe T, et al. Interleukin-25: a cytokine linking eosinophils and adaptive immunity in Churg-Strauss syndrome. Blood. 2010;116:4523-31.

43. Guilpain P, Auclair JF, Tamby MC, et al. Serum eosinophil cationic protein: a marker of disease activity in Churg-Strauss syndrome. Ann N Y Acad Sci. 2007;1107:392-9.

44. Xiao H, Heeringa P, Hu P, et al. Antineutrophil cytoplasmic autoantibodies specific for myeloperoxidase cause glomerulonephritis and vasculitis in mice. J Clin Invest. 2002;110:955-63.

45. Koukoulaki M, Smith KG, Jayne DR. Rituximab in Churg-Strauss syndrome. Ann Rheum Dis. 2006;65:557-9.

46. Thiel J, Hassler F, Salzer U, et al. Rituximab in the treatment of refractory or relapsing eosinophilic granulomatosis with polyangiitis (Churg-Strauss syndrome). Arthritis Res Ther. 2013;15:R133.

47. Pepper RJ, Fabre MA, Pavesio C, et al. Rituximab is effective in the treatment of refractory Churg-Strauss syndrome and is associated with diminished T-cell interleukin-5 production. Rheumatology (Oxford). 2008;47:1104-5.

48. Yamamoto M, Takahashi H, Suzuki C, et al. Analysis of serum IgG subclasses in Churg-Strauss syndrome—the meaning of elevated serum levels of IgG4. Intern Med. 2010;49:1365-70.

49. Vaglio A, Strehl JD, Manger B, et al. IgG4 immune response in Churg-Strauss syndrome. Ann Rheum Dis. 2012;71:390-3.

50. Lanham JG, Cooke S, Davies J, et al. Endomyocardial complications of the Churg-Strauss syndrome. Postgrad Med J. 1985;61:341-4.

51. Lanham JG, Elkon KB, Pusey CD, et al. Systemic vasculitis with asthma and eosinophilia: a clinical approach to the Churg-Strauss syndrome. Medicine. 1984;63:65-81.

52. Luqmani RA, Suppiah R, Grayson PC, et al. Nomenclature and classification of vasculitis--update on the ACR/EULAR Diagnosis and Classification of Vasculitis Study (DCVAS). Clin Exp Immunol. 2011;164(Suppl 1):11-3.

53. Solans R, Bosch JA, Perez-Bocanegra C, et al. Churg-Strauss syndrome: outcome and long-term follow-up of 32 patients. Rheumatology (Oxford). 2001;40:763-71.

54. Sehgal M, Swanson JW, DeRemee RA, et al. Neurologic manifestations of Churg-Strauss syndrome. Mayo Clin Proc. 1995;70:337-41.

55. Healy B, Bibby S, Steele R, et al. Antineutrophil cytoplasmic autoantibodies and myeloperoxidase autoantibodies in clinical expression of Churg-Strauss syndrome. J Allergy Clin Immunol. 2013;131:571-6.

56. Moosig F, Bremer JP, Hellmich B, et al. A vasculitis centre based management strategy leads to improved outcome in eosinophilic granulomatosis and polyangiitis (Churg-Strauss, EGPA): monocentric experiences in 150 patients. Ann Rheum Dis. 2013;72:1011-7.

57. Hervier B, Pagnoux C, Agard C, et al. Pulmonary fibrosis associated with ANCA-positive vasculitides. Retrospective study of 12 cases and review of the literature. Ann Rheum Dis. 2009;68:404-7.

58. Mavrogeni S, Tsirogianni AK, Gialafos EJ, et al. Detection of myocardial inflammation by contrast-enhanced MRI in a patient with Churg-Strauss syndrome. Int J Cardiol. 2009;131:e54-5.

59. Marmursztejn J, Guillevin L, Trebossen R, et al. Churg-Strauss syndrome cardiac involvement evaluated by cardiac magnetic resonance imaging and positron-emission tomography: a

prospective study on 20 patients. Rheumatology (Oxford). 2013;52:642-50.

60. Pagnoux C, Guillevin L. Cardiac involvement in small and medium-sized vessel vasculitides. Lupus. 2005;14:718-22.

61. Allenbach Y, Seror R, Pagnoux C, et al. High frequency of venous thromboembolic events in Churg-Strauss syndrome, Wegener's granulomatosis and microscopic polyangiitis but not polyarteritis nodosa: a systematic retrospective study on 1130 patients. Ann Rheum Dis. 2009;68:564-7.

62. Ames PR, Roes L, Lupoli S, et al. Thrombosis in Churg-Strauss syndrome. Beyond vasculitis? Br J Rheumatol. 1996;35:1181-3.

63. Sable-Fourtassou R, Cohen P, Mahr A, et al. Antineutrophil cytoplasmic antibodies and the Churg-Strauss syndrome. Ann Intern Med. 2005;143:632-8.

64. Hellmich B, Csernok E, Gross WL. Proinflammatory cytokines and autoimmunity in Churg-Strauss syndrome. Ann N Y Acad Sci. 2005;1051:121-31.

65. Khoury P, Zagallo P, Talar-Williams C, et al. Serum biomarkers are similar in Churg-Strauss syndrome and hypereosinophilic syndrome. Allergy. 2012;67:1149-56.

66. Polzer K, Karonitsch T, Neumann T, et al. Eotaxin-3 is involved in Churg-Strauss syndrome—a serum marker closely correlating with disease activity. Rheumatology (Oxford). 2008;47:804-8.

67. Rose DM, Hrncir DE. Primary eosinophilic lung diseases. Allergy Asthma Proc. 2013;34:19-25.

68. Meziane H, Maakel ML, Vachier I, et al. Sputum eosinophilia in Churg-Strauss syndrome. Respir Med. 2001;95:799-801.

69. Parulekar AD, Atik MA, Hanania NA. Periostin, a novel biomarker of TH2 -driven asthma. Curr Opin Pulm Med. 2014;20:60-5.

70. Noth I, Strek ME, Leff AR. Churg-Strauss syndrome. Lancet. 2003;361:587-94.

71. Gotlib J. World health organization—defined eosinophilic disorders: 2014 update on diagnosis, risk stratification, and management. Am J Hematol. 2014;89:325-37.

72. Little MA, Nightingale P, Verburgh CA, et al. Early mortality in systemic vasculitis: relative contribution of adverse events and active vasculitis. Ann Rheum Dis. 2010;69:1036-43.

73. Groh M, Masciocco G, Kirchner E, et al. Heart transplantation in patients with eosinophilic granulomatosis with polyangiitis (Churg-Strauss syndrome). J Heart Lung Transplant. 2014 (Aug.);33:842-50.

74. Metzler C, Hellmich B, Gause A, et al. Churg-Strauss syndrome-- successful induction of remission with methotrexate and unexpected high cardiac and pulmonary relapse ratio during maintenance treatment. Clin Exp Rheumatol. 2004;22:S52-61.

75. Iatrou C, Zerbala S, Revela I, et al. Mycophenolate mofetil as maintenance therapy in patients with vasculitis and renal involvement. Clin Nephrol. 2009;72:31-7.

76. Cohen P, Pagnoux C, Mahr A, et al. Churg-Strauss syndrome with poor-prognosis factors: a prospective multicenter trial comparing glucocorticoids and six or twelve cyclophosphamide pulses in forty-eight patients. Arthritis Rheum. 2007;57:686-93.

77. Danieli MG, Cappelli M, Malcangi G, et al. Long term effectiveness of intravenous immunoglobulin in Churg-Strauss syndrome. Ann Rheum Dis. 2004;63:1649-54.

78. Cordier JF, Cottin V. Alveolar hemorrhage in vasculitis: primary and secondary. Semin Respir Crit Care Med. 2011;32:310-21.

79. Guillevin L, Pagnoux C. Indications of plasma exchanges for systemic vasculitides. Ther Apher Dial. 2003;7:155-60.

80. Guillevin L, Lhote F, Cohen P, et al. Corticosteroids plus pulse cyclophosphamide and plasma exchanges versus corticosteroids plus pulse cyclophosphamide alone in the treatment of polyarteritis nodosa and Churg-Strauss syndrome patients with factors predicting poor prognosis. A prospective, randomized trial in sixty-two patients. Arthritis Rheum. 1995;38:1638-45.

81. Guillevin L, Lhote F. Treatment of polyarteritis nodosa and Churg-Strauss syndrome: indications of plasma exchanges. Transfus Sci. 1994;15:371-88.

82. Metzler C, Lamprecht P, Hellmich B, et al. Leucoencephalopathy after treatment of Churg-Strauss syndrome with interferon {alpha}. Ann Rheum Dis. 2005;64:1242-3.

83. Metzler C, Schnabel A, Gross WL, et al. A phase II study of interferon-alpha for the treatment of refractory Churg-Strauss syndrome. Clin Exp Rheumatol. 2008;26:S35-40.

84. Giavina-Bianchi P, Agondi R, Kalil J. One year administration of anti-IgE to a patient with Churg-Strauss syndrome. Int Arch Allergy Immunol. 2008;146:176.

85. Giavina-Bianchi P, Giavina-Bianchi M, Agondi R, et al. Omalizumab and Churg-Strauss syndrome. J Allergy Clin Immunol. 2008;122:217.

86. Giavina-Bianchi P, Giavina-Bianchi M, Agondi RC, et al. Anti-IgE in Churg-Strauss syndrome. Thorax. 2009;64:272.

87. Pabst S, Tiyerili V, Grohe C. Apparent response to anti-IgE therapy in two patients with refractory "Forme fruste" Of Churg-Strauss syndrome. Thorax. 2008;63:747-8.

88. Hanania NA, Wenzel S, Rosen K, et al. Exploring the effects of omalizumab in allergic asthma: an analysis of biomarkers in the extra study. Am J Respir Crit Care Med. 2013;187:804-11.

89. Jones RB, Ferraro AJ, Chaudhry AN, et al. A multicenter survey of rituximab therapy for refractory antineutrophil cytoplasmic antibody-associated vasculitis. Arthritis Rheum. 2009;60:2156-68.

90. Bouldouyre MA, Cohen P, Guillevin L. Severe bronchospasm associated with rituximab for refractory Churg-Strauss syndrome. Ann Rheum Dis. 2009;68:606.

91. Assaf C, Mewis G, Orfanos CE, et al. Churg-Strauss syndrome: successful treatment with mycophenolate mofetil. Br J Dermatol. 2004;150:598-600.

92. Lee RU, Stevenson DD. Hydroxyurea in the treatment of Churg-Strauss syndrome. J Allergy Clin Immunol. 2009;124:1110-1.

93. Josselin-Mahr L, Werbrouck-Chiraux A, Garderet L, et al. Efficacy of imatinib mesylate in a case of Churg-Strauss syndrome: evidence for the pathogenic role of a tyrosine kinase? Rheumatology (Oxford). 2014;53:378-9.

94. Tiliakos At, Shaia S, Hostoffer R, et al. The use of infliximab in a patient with steroid-dependent Churg-Strauss syndrome. J Clin Rheumatol. 2004;10:96-7.

95. Arbach O, Gross WL, Gause A. Treatment of refractory Churg-Strauss syndrome (CSS) by TNF-alpha blockade. Immunobiology. 2002;206:496-501.

96. El-Gamal Y. Churg-Strauss syndrome in the pediatric age group. World Allergy Organ J. 2008;1:34-40.

97. Lou J, Xu WB. Churg-Strauss syndrome: clinical features and long-term follow-up of 16 patients. Zhonghua Yi Xue Za Zhi. 2009;89:524-8.

98. McDermott EM, Powell RJ. Cyclosporin in the treatment of Churg-Strauss syndrome. Ann Rheum Dis. 1998;57:258-9.

99. Kim S, Marigowda G, Oren E, et al. Mepolizumab as a steroid-sparing treatment option in patients with Churg-Strauss syndrome. J Allergy Clin Immunol. 2010;125:1336-43.

100. Herrmann K, Gross WL, Moosig F. Extended follow-up after stopping mepolizumab in relapsing/refractory Churg-Strauss syndrome. Clin Exp Rheumatol. 2012;30:S62-5.

101. Moosig F, Gross WL, Herrmann K, et al. Targeting interleukin-5 in refractory and relapsing Churg-Strauss syndrome. Ann Intern Med. 2011;155:341-3.

102. Pagnoux C, Guillevin L. How can patient care be improved beyond medical treatment? Best Pract Res Clin Rheumatol. 2005;19:337-44.

CHAPTER 34

Immunoglobulin A Vasculitis

Deepti Suri, Vikas Suri

INTRODUCTION

Immunoglobulin A vasculitis (IgAV), more commonly known as Henoch-Schönlein purpura (HSP), is an IgA-mediated small vessel leukocytoclastic vasculitis predominantly affecting the skin, joints, gastrointestinal system and the kidneys. It is often a self-limited disease in young children but can result in serious morbidity in older children and adults. Clinically, it is characterized by triad of nonthrombocytopenic palpable purpura, mostly located on the dependent parts like lower extremities and buttocks along with arthralgia or arthritis, abdominal pain secondary to bowel angina. Renal involvement may occur manifesting as hematuria or proteinuria.

CASE VIGNETTE

A 4-year-old boy presented with abdominal pain and pain in joints for a day. The next day, he was noted to have progressive rash over the lower limbs and buttocks. There was history of short febrile illness a week back. On examination, he was afebrile with normal vital signs. Palpable purpuric eruptions were noted on both the legs and buttocks. Mild periarticular swelling around right knee was noted and movements were restricted. A clinical diagnosis of HSP/IgAV was made. Blood counts showed mild polymorphonuclear leukocytosis, thrombocytosis and raised erythrocyte sedimentation rate (ESR). Serial urine examinations were normal. Skin biopsy showed leukocytoclastic vasculitis with IgA deposits confirming the diagnosis of IgA vasculitis. The child was managed conservatively with nonsteroidal anti-inflammatory drugs for arthritis. Rash subsided in a few days and serial urine examinations on follow-up did not reveal any renal involvement. Child remained well and no recurrences were noted.

The above case highlights the usual course and management of a child with IgA vasculitis. However, there are exceptions and not all children with IgA vasculitis have a benign self-limiting course.

Epidemiology

Henoch-Schönlein purpura (HSP) was first described in 1837 as a triad of purpura rash, arthritis, and abnormalities of the urinary sediment by a German physician Johann Lukas Schönlein.[1] In 1874, his student Edward Heinrich Henoch described the association of purpuric rash and gastrointestinal involvement.[2]

In 1990, American College of Rheumatology (ACR) established criteria to classify seven types of vasculitides including HSP.[3] The criteria for HSP/IgAV included at least two of four items: age < 20 years, palpable purpura, and abdominal pain or vessel wall granulocytes on biopsy. But these ACR criteria proved to be inappropriate for pediatric as well as adult populations and the classification underwent various modifications. In 2005, pediatric consensus criteria were developed by the European League against Rheumatism (EULAR) and the Paediatric Rheumatology European Society (PRES) and were subsequently validated in conjunction with the Paediatric Rheumatology International Trials Organization (PRINTO). In 2010, the EULAR/PRINTO/PRES classification criteria for HSP[4] were formally published and are summarized in Table 34.1.

The HSP/IgAV is the most common form of systemic vasculitis in children. It has a pronounced predilection for children between 3 and 12 years of age. There is a male predominance with reported male-to-female ratios of 1.2:1 to 1.8:1. About half of the cases of IgAV are preceded by an upper respiratory infection, especially those caused by *Streptococcus*. Other infectious agents, vaccinations, and

Table 34.1 EULAR/PRES classification criteria for Henoch-Schönlein purpura

Palpable purpura as an essential criterion, along with at least one of the following criteria:

1. Diffuse abdominal pain
2. Leukocytoclastic vasculitis with predominant IgA deposits on skin biopsy
3. Acute arthritis or arthralgias in any joint
4. Renal involvement as evidenced by proteinuria and/or hematuria.

Abbreviations: EULAR–Eurpoean League Against Rheumatism; PRES–Paediatric Rheumatology Eurpoean Society

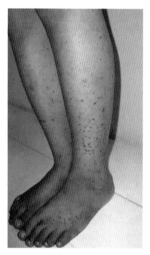

Fig. 34.1 Palpable purpuric rash on lower limbs: HSP/IgAV

insect bites also have been implicated as possible triggers for HSP/IgAV. In adults, the mean age at diagnosis varies from 45 to 50 years with a similar male predominance as the childhood disease. In adults, IgAV has been linked to cancer, most common with solid malignancies, but this linkage needs further validation.[5-7]

Clinical Features in Children

The HSP/IgAV includes the tetrad of palpable purpura (Fig. 34.1) without thrombocytopenia and coagulopathy, arthritis/arthralgia, abdominal pain and renal disease.

Palpable purpura: The rash often begins with erythematous, macular or urticarial wheals. These wheals then evolve into the typical lesions that include ecchymoses, petechiae, and palpable purpura. This rash commonly appears in crops, is symmetrically distributed, and is located primarily in gravity/pressure-dependent areas of the body, such as the lower

extremities. Common sites involved are buttocks in toddlers, and the face, trunk, and upper extremities in nonambulatory children. Localized subcutaneous edema in these areas may also be observed, especially in younger children (<3 years of age).

Arthritis/arthralgia: It is the presenting symptom in about 15% children. It generally precedes the appearance of purpura, though usually by no more than one or two days. Arthritis may be transient or migratory, is commonly oligoarticular and non-deforming. The joints most commonly affected are the lower extremity large joints (hips, knees, and ankles), or less commonly the upper extremities (elbows, wrists, and hands).[8] There is often a prominent periarticular swelling and tenderness, but it is usually without joint effusion, erythema, or warmth. There may be considerable pain and limitation of motion and younger children with lower extremity involvement may even refuse to ambulate, thus giving a false impression of paresis.

Gastrointestinal symptoms occur in about 50% of children with HSP/IgAV. These may range from mild nausea, vomiting, abdominal pain, and transient paralytic ileus but may occasionally result in life-threatening gastrointestinal hemorrhage, bowel ischemia with/without necrosis, intussusception and gastrointestinal perforation.

Gastrointestinal symptoms typically develop within 8 days of the appearance of the rash but may precedes the rash in about 15–35% of cases, thus making the diagnosis of HSP/IgAV difficult in these patients.[9] Gastrointestinal symptoms without the appearance of cutaneous purpura at any time also have been described in case reports.

Intussusception is the most common gastrointestinal complication of HSP/IgAV. It is generally limited to the small bowel in about 60% of cases, in contrast to idiopathic intussusception, which is typically ileocolic. It should be suspected in any child with severe gastrointestinal pain and/or requiring hospitalization.[10] Rarer gastrointestinal manifestations include acute pancreatitis, gallbladder involvement, bowel perforation, and, in children, a protein-losing enteropathy.

Renal involvement has been reported in 20–54% of children with HSP/IgAV. The most common presentation is hematuria with or without red cell casts and no or mild proteinuria. Nephrotic range proteinuria, an elevated serum creatinine, and/or hypertension, which are present in a minority of patients, are associated with an increased risk of progressive disease.[11]

Renal involvement is typically noted within a few days to one month after the onset of systemic symptoms, but is not predictably related to the severity of extrarenal involvement.

The risk factors for renal involvement are male sex and age more than 5 years. Renal biopsy is indicated if there is significant proteinuria, azotemia, or gross hematuria. The findings on renal biopsy are identical to those in IgA nephropathy that include mesangial IgA deposition on immunofluorescence. In addition, immunofluorescence may reveal IgG, IgM, fibrinogen, and C3 in the glomeruli. Strong immunofluorescence staining for C1q should suggest the possibility of lupus nephritis. By electron microscopy, electron-dense deposits may typically found in the mesangial areas, occasionally extending out into the peripheral capillary loops.

Other organ systems also may be involved with increasing reports of scrotal involvement,[12] central and peripheral nervous system (headaches, seizures, focal neurologic deficits, intracerebral hemorrhage and central and peripheral neuropathy),[13-15] respiratory tract (impaired lung diffusion capacity with mild interstitial changes, pulmonary hemorrhage) and involvement of eye (keratitis/uveitis).[16]

Clinical Features in Adults

Adult patients with HSP/IgAV present with clinical manifestations similar to those that occur in children. There are two main differences between adults and children, intussusception is rare in adults and they are at increased risk for developing significant renal involvement including end-stage renal disease.[17]

Recurrent Disease

Recurrence of HSP/IgAV is reported in about one-third of affected children and generally occurs within four months of the initial episode. Recurrences tend to be milder and briefer than the initial episode, and they occur more commonly in patients with nephritis, in those with evidence of acute inflammation. These findings suggest that patients who have a more severe course of HSP/IgAV are at increased risk of recurrence.

Diagnosis

The diagnosis of HSP/IgAV is usually based upon clinical manifestations of the disease. In patients with incomplete or unusual presentations, a biopsy of an affected organ (skin or kidney) that demonstrates leukocytoclastic vasculitis with a predominance of IgA deposition confirms the diagnosis.

Platelet counts are normal or elevated, despite the purpura. There is a moderately raised white blood count and acute phase reactants. About half will have raised serum IgA.

Urinalysis may show red or white cells, cellular casts, and proteinuria. In general, these findings reflect the degree of renal involvement. Serum creatinine should be obtained in all adult patients. As renal involvement may occur much later (6 months) after the initial manifestations of HSP, so the urinary screening should be continued beyond the acute presentation.

Treatment

Management of HSP/IgAV is divided into supportive care, symptomatic therapy, and targeted treatment to decrease the risk of complications. Supportive care includes adequate hydration, rest, and symptomatic relief of pain. Patients with renal disease may be hypertensive and require antihypertensive therapy.

Hospitalization is indicated if there is inability to maintain adequate hydration with oral intake, severe abdominal pain, significant gastrointestinal bleeding, altered sensorium, severe joint involvement limiting ambulation and/or self-care, renal insufficiency (elevated creatinine), hypertension, and/or nephrotic syndrome.

Symptomatic treatment for abdominal and joint pain in patients with HSP/IgAV includes the use of acetaminophen or nonsteroidal anti-inflammatory drugs (NSAIDs). The risk of gastrointestinal hemorrhage resulting from bowel vasculitis has not been shown to increase when inhibitors of cyclooxygenase are used, so these agents are not contraindicated in HSP (IgAV).

In patients with active gastrointestinal bleeding or glomerulonephritis, however, NSAIDs may be contraindicated because of their effects on platelets and renal perfusion. Naproxen, 10–20 mg/kg divided into two doses per day, may be used because of its ease of dosing. In adolescents and adults, a maximum total daily dose of 1500 mg may be used for a few days.

The use of glucocorticoids in patients with HSP/IgAV is controversial. Various studies have proven beyond doubt that glucocorticoids shorten the duration of abdominal pain, decrease the risk of intussusception, gastrointestinal procedures, recurrence and renal involvement.[18,19]

It is recommended that prednisone (1–2 mg/kg per day, maximum dose of 60 to 80 mg per day) be used only in patients with symptoms severe enough to affect their oral intake, interfere with their ability to ambulate and perform activities of daily living, and/or who require hospitalization. In patients who cannot tolerate oral medications, equivalent doses of parenteral methylprednisolone may be administered (0.8–1.6 mg/kg per day, maximum dose of 64 mg per day).

Intravenous methylprednisolone may be more beneficial early in the disease course when patients have active gastrointestinal disease due to submucosal edema and hemorrhage altering absorption of oral medications. It is not recommended to use of glucocorticoids to prevent renal disease, since the available data do not support such a role for this intervention. But it is important to keep in mind that after glucocorticoid use inflammation may be ameliorated, but the pathophysiology of the disease does not appear to be affected. Therefore the glucocorticoid dose must be lowered very slowly, typically over four to eight weeks, otherwise a disease flare be precipitated by overly aggressive medication tapering.

Specific treatment of HSP/IgAV nephritis should be considered only in patients with marked proteinuria and/or impaired renal function during the acute episode. It is recommended to obtain a renal biopsy as the severity of the histologic lesions (particularly the degree of crescent formation) is the best indicator of prognosis. Conventional doses of glucocorticoids have no beneficial effect in patients with HSP/IgAV with a renal involvement. On the contrary, high dose methylprednisolone (250–1000 mg per day for three days) followed by oral prednisone (1 mg/kg per day for three months) may be beneficial in patients with advanced disease, which is usually defined as crescentic nephritis. Cyclophosphamide alone or with glucocorticoids does not appear to reduce protein excretion or improve or preserve renal function neither. Other drugs used alone or along with glucocorticoids include cyclosporine, azathioprine, and dipyridamole.

Promising results have been observed with plasmapheresis especially in patients with severe, usually crescentic, disease with rapidly progressive renal failure but data are still not conclusive. Intravenous immune globulin has been tried in a small number of patients with IgA nephropathy or HSP (IgAV) nephritis with heavy proteinuria and a progressive decline in glomerular filtration rate but more data are required to confirm benefit.

Renal transplantation can be performed in those patients who progress to end-stage renal disease, although recurrent disease can occur.

Prognosis

The short- and long-term outcomes of children with HSP/IgAV, are very encouraging and the initial episode resolves within one month provided there is no renal involvement. In only one-third of patients, recurrence is seen at least once, typically within four months of the initial presentation but each of these subsequent episodes has similar clinical findings but is generally milder and/or shorter in duration than the preceding one.[20,21]

Morbidity in the initial phase of HSP/IgAV is primarily a result of gastrointestinal complications, including intussusception and, less commonly, bowel ischemia, bowel perforation, or pancreatitis.

The long-term morbidity in patients with HSP/IgAV is a result of renal disease. The risk of progressive renal disease is increased in adults. The severity of the renal involvement correlates with the severity of the initial renal presentation and histologic changes seen on renal biopsy. Risk factors for a worse renal prognosis include nephrotic range proteinuria, elevated serum creatinine, hypertension, crescentic glomerulonephritis (>50%) and tubulointerstitial fibrosis.

Follow-up

Ninety percent of children who develop renal involvement do so within 2 months of onset, and 97% within six months.[22] Therefore, all patients with HSP/IgAV should be followed with urinalysis and blood pressure monitoring weekly or biweekly for the first one to two months after presentation. Once the disease appears to be subsiding, additional follow-up for urine and blood pressure monitoring should be scheduled monthly at first, then every other month until one year after the initial presentation. To identify patients, who may develop late renal disease, continued screening (urinalysis and blood pressure measurements) should be performed by the primary care clinician during subsequent well-child visits.

Patients with persistent proteinuria, hypertension, or renal insufficiency should be referred to a nephrologist for further evaluation and treatment. In addition, pregnant women with a history of HSP/IgAV should be monitored closely, as they have a higher risk of hypertension

KEY POINTS

- IgA vasculitis is the most common childhood vasculitis.
- It commonly affects the skin, GI system and kidneys.
- There is deposition of IgA and C3 in small vessel walls.
- Treatment is mostly supportive but some manifestations require aggressive immunosuppressive treatment.

REFERENCES

1. Therapie, vol. 2. Herisau,Germany: Literatur-Comptoir; 1837.
2. Henoch EH. Uber ein eigenthumliche Form von Purpura. Berl Klin Wochenschr. 1874;11:641-3.

3. Mills JA, Michel BA, Bloch DA, et al. The American College of Rheumatology 1990 criteria for the classification of vasculitis. Arthritis Rheum. 1990;33:1114-21.

4. Ozen S, Pistorio A, Iusan SM, et al. EULAR/PRINTO/PRES criteria for Henoch–Schönlein purpura, childhood polyarteritis nodosa, childhood Wegener granulomatosis and childhood Takayasu arteritis: Ankara 2008. Part II: final classification criteria. Ann Rheum Dis. 2010;69:798-806.

5. Piram M, Mahr A. Epidemiology of immunoglobulin A vasculitis (Henoch-Schönlein): current state of knowledge. Curr Opin Rheumatol. 2013;25:171.

6. Gardner-Medwin JM, Dolezalova P, Cummins C, et al. Incidence of Henoch-Schönlein purpura, Kawasaki disease, and rare vasculitides in children of different ethnic origins. Lancet. 2002;360:1197.

7. Saulsbury FT. Epidemiology of Henoch-Schönlein purpura. Cleve Clin J Med. 2002;69:SII87.

8. Trapani S, Micheli A, Grisolia F, et al. Henoch Schönlein purpura in childhood: epidemiological and clinical analysis of 150 cases over a 5-year period and review of literature. Semin Arthritis Rheum. 2005;35:143.

9. Feldt RH, Stickler GB. The gastrointestinal manifestations of anaphylactoid purpura in children. Proc Staff Meet Mayo Clin. 1962;37:465.

10. Chang WL, Yang YH, Lin YT, et al. Gastrointestinal manifestations in Henoch-Schönlein purpura: a review of 261 patients. Acta Paediatr. 2004;93:1427.

11. Coppo R, Andrulli S, Amore A, et al. Predictors of outcome in Henoch-Schönlein nephritis in children and adults. Am J Kidney Dis. 2006;47:993.

12. Chamberlain RS, Greenberg LW. Scrotal involvement in Henoch-Schönlein purpura: a case report and review of the literature. Pediatr Emerg Care. 1992;8:213.

13. Belman AL, Leicher CR, Moshé SL, et al. Neurologic manifestations of Henoch-Schönlein purpura: report of three cases and review of the literature. Pediatrics. 1985;75:687.

14. Misra AK, Biswas A, Das SK, et al. Henoch-Schönlein purpura with intracerebral haemorrhage. J Assoc Physicians India. 2004;52:833.

15. Bulun A, Topaloglu R, Duzova A, et al. Ataxia and peripheral neuropathy: rare manifestations in Henoch-Schönlein purpura. Pediatr Nephrol. 2001;16:1139.

16. Muqit MM, Gallagher MJ, Gavin M, et al. Henoch-Schönlein purpura with keratitis and granulomatous anterior uveitis. Br J Ophthalmol. 2005;89:1221.

17. Pillebout E, Thervet E, Hill G, et al. Henoch-Schönlein purpura in adults: outcome and prognostic factors. J Am Soc Nephrol. 2002;13:1271.

18. Weiss PF, Feinstein JA, Luan X, et al. Effects of corticosteroid on Henoch-Schönlein purpura: a systematic review. Pediatrics. 2007;120:1079.

19. Rosenblum ND, Winter HS. Steroid effects on the course of abdominal pain in children with Henoch-Schönlein purpura. Pediatrics. 1987;79:1018.

20. Saulsbury FT. Henoch-Schönlein purpura in children. Report of 100 patients and review of the literature. Medicine (Baltimore). 1999;78:395.

21. Meadow SR. The prognosis of Henoch-Schönlein nephritis. Clin Nephrol. 1978;9:87.

22. Narchi H. Risk of long term renal impairment and duration of follow up recommended for Henoch-Schönlein purpura with normal or minimal urinary findings: a systematic review. Arch Dis Child. 2005;90:916.

CHAPTER 35

Primary Angiitis of Central Nervous System

Atul Khasnis, Leonard Calabrese

INTRODUCTION

Primary angiitis of the central nervous system (PACNS) is a rare illness (2.4 cases/1,000,000 person-years) characterized by exclusive CNS vascular inflammation (brain and spinal cord). Diagnosing PACNS is often challenging and relies on a combination of clinical features, such as cerebrospinal fluid (CSF) analysis, CNS imaging and angiography, or CNS histopathology. Mimics of PACNS are more common than PACNS itself. Treatment involves potentially toxic immunosuppression, and therefore diagnosis is the key. The Calabrese and Mallek diagnostic criteria (1988) continue to be used to date.[1] Advances have been made in understanding of clinical disease and imaging, but disease mechanisms and epidemiologic investigation still remain obscure due to rarity of disease and limited access to tissue.[2]

CASE VIGNETTE[3]

The median age at diagnosis is 32–47 years, with a slight male predominance. Common presenting symptoms include chronic headache, cognitive difficulties, focal neurological deficits (hemiparesis, aphasia, sensory abnormalities, numbness, and ataxia), seizures, and visual symptoms. Uncommon manifestations include extrapyramidal involvement, urinary retention, and cauda equina involvement. Systemic symptoms are unusual. The onset is typically insidious; other presentations include acute, waxing and waning, unilateral chronic relapsing and prolonged disease quiescence with eventual relapse. Laboratory tests such as complete blood count, metabolic panel, erythrocyte sedimentation rate, and C-reactive protein levels are commonly normal compared with other forms of systemic vasculitis. Serologic testing for autoantibodies may help exclude other systemic autoimmune conditions in appropriate

clinical presentations. The most indispensable test with true diagnostic utility is CSF analysis, being abnormal in 81–88% of cases demonstrating a picture of chronic aseptic meningitis with a slight lymphocytic pleocytosis and elevated protein, either alone or in combination. The median CSF WBC count reported in series ranges from 5 to 60 cells/mm^3 and median protein level ranges from 72 to 118 mg/dL. A CSF WBC > 250 cells/mm^3 with neutrophilic predominance or a very low CSF glucose level should lead to aggressive work-up for infection or other etiologies. Although CSF findings are nonspecific, its main utility is in excluding other diagnoses. A combination of normal MRI brain and normal CSF carries a very high negative predictive for the diagnosis of PACNS. Clinical variants of PACNS include mass/pseudotumor lesions, spinal cord involvement including cauda equina, and rapidly progressive PACNS with increased morbidity and mortality.[4]

IMAGING

Neuroimaging involves imaging the brain parenchyma (CT/MRI) and cerebral vasculature (CT/MR angiography or conventional dye angiography). CT is 50% sensitive but findings are often nonspecific, leading to the increased use of MRI. Indirect signs on MRI include infarcts of varying duration in multiple vascular territories on T2 and diffusion-weighted imaging (DWI). Indirect visualization of the CNS vasculature by magnetic resonance angiography (MRA) may reveal multifocal stenosis. Medium-sized vessels may be unaffected and MRA can therefore be normal. High-resolution 3 T MR appears to be a feasible tool with potential to demonstrate "vascular inflammation" (concentric wall enhancement and thickening) but needs further study.[5] Dye angiographic findings are also neither sensitive nor specific for the diagnosis. In a retrospective analysis by

Duna et al.[6] cerebral angiography had < 30% specificity and MRI was sensitive but lacked specificity. PACNS may involve small-sized blood vessels only, beyond the resolution of conventional angiography. Salvarani et al.[7] have reported this "angiography negative" subset of patients with PACNS with a possibly favorable outcome compared to the "angiography positive" group. Newer imaging modalities such as functional DWI may have a role, but reflect microvascular ischemia, which in itself is not pathognomonic of PACNS.

BIOPSY AND PATHOLOGY

Biopsy of the CNS tissue and leptomeninges remains the diagnostic gold standard, when appropriate staining and studies are performed to exclude mimics. Tissue biopsies demonstrate patchy inflammation of medium and small arteries and arterioles in the brain and meninges making sampling error possible. The presence of inflammatory cells within the vessel wall with or without architectural distortion is convincing histologic evidence of vasculitis (Fig. 35.1). Infiltrating cells include lymphocytes, plasma cells, macrophages, neutrophils, and eosinophils with or without formation of granulomas and giant cells, but this classic granulomatous pathology is observed in less than 50% of biopsies. Biopsies are more likely to be positive when performed on an abnormal region. The combination biopsy of leptomeninges and brain tissue increases the diagnostic yield. If a focal abnormal area cannot be targeted, the biopsy of the nondominant temporal lobe tip and overlying meninges is recommended. Rare findings on biopsies include transmural vascular eosinophilic infiltrates, perivascular granulomatous infiltrates resulting in "cuffing," venulitis,

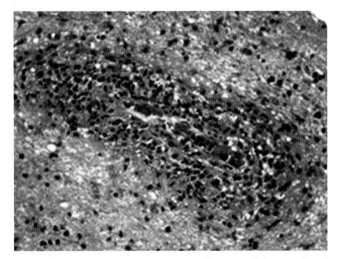

Fig. 35.1 Brain biopsy demonstrating infiltration of the vessel wall by inflammatory cells resulting in destruction of the wall architecture consistent with a true definition of vasculitis

and accompanying cerebral amyloid angiopathy. Biopsy is also central to excluding mimics. In a study by Alrawi et al.[8] retrospective analysis of data from 61 consecutive patients with suspected PACNS, PACNS was detected in 22 (36%), alternative diagnoses in 24 (39%), and no diagnosis in 15 (25%).

MIMICS

As mentioned previously, mimics of PACNS are much more common than the disease itself.[9] Some mimics such as infection are absolutely necessary to exclude, since immunosuppression can be associated with unfortunate outcomes. It is not possible to discuss mimics of PACNS. Infections that can mimic PACNS include but are not limited to *Varicella zoster virus*, HIV, *Hepatitis C virus*, *Treponema pallidum*, *Rickettsia* species, *Mycobacterium tuberculosis,* and *Bartonella* species. Progressive multifocal leukoencephalopathy due to *JC virus* can present with progressive cognitive decline, altered mental status, neurologic deficits, and subcortical white matter changes on MRI. Testing for organisms and serologies in the CSF may be helpful. Reversible cerebral vasoconstriction syndromes (RCVS) are idiopathic vasospastic disorders affecting the cerebral vasculature characterized by acute onset, severe, recurrent thunderclap headaches, with or without additional neurological signs and symptoms such as transient or permanent visual or neurological deficits. They may be idiopathic or associated with pregnancy, medications, illicit drug use, metabolic disorders, trauma, neurosurgery or following catheter-based vascular intervention. Severe cerebral vasoconstriction may result in either ischemic or hemorrhagic stroke and rarely death. The CSF tends to be normal or near normal and vascular imaging shows multifocal segmental arterial narrowing (beading) that is reversible within 12 weeks. There is no vasculitis on biopsies. Subsequent reversal of vascular abnormalities at serial imaging is essential to secure the diagnosis of RCVS (Fig. 35.2).[10] Premature atherosclerosis, a common cause of cerebral angiographic abnormalities, is associated with vascular risk factors (diabetes, hypertension, hyperlipidemia, and smoking). Unlike PACNS, the CSF is normal and headache is not a prominent symptom. While atherosclerosis can cause multiple infarcts, the infarcts are usually restricted to a single vascular territory. However, large-artery atherosclerosis or small-vessel occlusion may cause acute multiple infarcts in the different cerebral vascular territories. Fibromuscular dysplasia and Moyamoya disease are other causes of angiographic abnormalities, but are distinguished based upon their characteristic angiographic appearances.

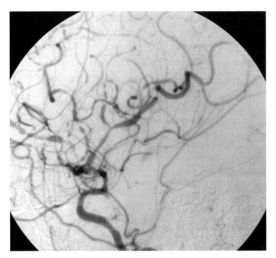

Fig. 35.2 Multifocal stenosis and dilatation noted on cerebral angiogram in a patient with RCVS (reversal of angiographic abnormalities demonstrated at 12 weeks). A single abnormal angiogram does not in itself make the diagnosis of PACNS or RCVS

The small, scattered ischemic lesions on neuroimaging can be difficult to discriminate from the demyelinating lesions of multiple sclerosis. Primary intravascular CNS lymphoma and gliomatosis cerebri can mimic MRI as well as cerebral angiographic appearance of PACNS. A positive family history can suggest genetic etiologies such as cerebral autosomal dominant arteriopathy with subcortical infarcts and leukoencephalopathy or retinal vasculopathy with cerebral leukodystrophy.[11] Susac's syndrome should be considered in patients with concomitant visual deficits and hearing loss. Amyloid-beta-related angiitis (ABRA) is a treatable cause of progressive dementia to be considered especially in adults over the age of 60 years.[12]

DIAGNOSING PACNS

Diagnosing PACNS can be very challenging given the nonspecific clinical presentation, lack of specific laboratory testing, imaging findings, and even biopsy findings. The diagnosis may be invoked in patients with progressive neurologic decline, multiple strokes without any identifiable cause, chronic meningitis, or an abnormal cerebral angiogram or MRI brain. Adding to the diagnostic complexity is the relatively high false-negative rate of brain biopsy, and the absence of serological tests or biomarkers. PACNS should be distinguished from "secondary" CNS angiitis related to rheumatologic disorders or other conditions such as ABRA. Family history can be useful in suggesting genetic etiologies. Ultimately a high degree of clinical suspicion, and a well-planned, thorough work-up, serves well to exclude mimics and firmly establish the diagnosis.

TREATMENT

The treatment is empiric given the lack of controlled trials.[9] The therapeutic approach is adapted from treatment paradigm for other primary systemic vasculitides. The standard induction phase consists of high-dose glucocorticoids with or without cyclophosphamide (CYC). Granulomatous PACNS usually requires a combination of CYC and glucocorticoids. Cyclophosphamide is typically used for 3–6 months. Prednisone is usually maintained at 1 mg/kg for the first month and then tapered. Once remission is achieved, CYC is switched to another immunosuppressant such as azathioprine or mycophenolate mofetil. Methotrexate is sometimes used, but its CNS penetration is suboptimal. All patients on high-dose glucocorticoids should get individualized bone health protection and be considered for *Pneumocystis jirovecii* prophylaxis. Assessing disease activity is very challenging and often involves the same approach as taken for initial diagnosis. Any new manifestation in an immunosuppressed patient should be rigorously evaluated for infection. The need for close clinical and laboratory monitoring and regular follow-up in patients whose disease continues to stay in remission is emphasized.

KEY POINTS

- Mimics of PACNS are more common than PACNS itself.
- CSF analysis is an absolute requirement when evaluating a patient with PACNS.
- Neuroimaging is neither sensitive nor specific for diagnosing PACNS.
- Brain biopsy may be valuable in excluding alternative diagnoses.
- An atypical response to therapy warrants further work-up for other diagnostic possibilities rather than escalation of immunosuppression.

REFERENCES

1. Calabrese LH, Mallek JA. Primary angiitis of the central nervous system. Report of 8 new cases, review of the literature, and proposal for diagnostic criteria. Medicine (Baltimore). 1988;67:20-39.
2. Calabrese LH. Primary angiitis of the central nervous system: reflections on 20 years of investigation. Clin Exp Rheumatol. 2009;27:S3-4.
3. Salvarani C, Brown RD Jr, Calamia KT, et al. Primary central nervous system vasculitis: analysis of 101 patients. Ann Neurol. 2007;62:442-51.
4. Salvarani C, Brown RD Jr, Calamia KT, et al. Rapidly progressive primary central nervous system vasculitis. Rheumatology (Oxford). 2011;50:349-58.

5. Obusez EC, Hui F, Hajj-Ali RA, et al. High-resolution MRI vessel wall imaging: spatial and temporal patterns of reversible cerebral vasoconstriction syndrome and central nervous system vasculitis. AJNR Am J Neuroradiol. 2014. [Epub ahead of print]

6. Duna GF, Calabrese LH. Limitations of invasive modalities in the diagnosis of primary angiitis of the central nervous system. J Rheumatol. 1995;22:662-7.

7. Salvarani C, Brown RD Jr, Calamia KT, et al. Angiography-negative primary central nervous system vasculitis: a syndrome involving small cerebral vessels. Medicine (Baltimore). 2008;87:264-71.

8. Alrawi A, Trobe JD, Blaivas M, et al. Brain biopsy in primary angiitis of the central nervous system. Neurology. 1999;53:858-60.

9. Hajj-Ali R. Primary angiitis of the central nervous system: differential diagnosis and treatment. Best Pract Res Clin Rheumatol. 2010;24:413-26.

10. Calabrese LH, Dodick DW, Schwedt TJ, et al. Narrative review: reversible cerebral vasoconstriction syndromes. Ann Intern Med. 2007;146:34-44.

11. Shahane A, Khasnis A, Hajj Ali R. Three unusual mimics of primary angiitis of the central nervous system. Rheumatol Int. 2012;32:737-42.

12. Danve A, Grafe M, Deodhar A. Amyloid beta-related angiitis-A case report and comprehensive review of literature of 94 cases. Semin Arthritis Rheum. 2014. [Epub ahead of print]

CHAPTER 36

Behçet's Disease

Fatma Alibaz-Oner, Haner Direskeneli

INTRODUCTION

Behçet's disease (BD) is a chronic, multisystemic, inflammatory disease characterized by recurrent attacks of mucocutaneous, ocular, musculoskeletal, vascular, central nervous system (CNS), and gastrointestinal (GI) manifestations. The disease was first described by Behçet, a Turkish dermatologist, as a triple complex with oral, genital ulcers (GUs), and hypopyon uveitis in 1937.[1] Behçet's disease has a disease course with remission and relapses; complete remission is observed in at least 60% of the patients at 20 years.[2]

The major genetic risk factor for BD is HLA-B*51. Recent studies have expanded the list of genetic loci, which now also includes interleukin (IL)10, IL23R, HLA-A*26, CCR1, STAT4, ERAP1, UBAC2, Cw6, GIMAP and, most recently, TLR4 and MEFV.[3-7] Oral microorganisms, associated with dental/periodontal diseases, are implicated as environmental causes of BD. Inflammation in BD can be triggered by autoimmune responses resulting from inappropriate adaptive immune activation and broken self-tolerance against local autoantigens such as mucosal or retinal proteins. Although HLA-B*51 is a class I HLA molecule activating cytotoxic T-cell responses, recent genetic studies mentioned before have also clearly linked hyperactive innate immune mechanisms to BD risk, also supporting an autoinflammatory contribution to its pathogenesis.[8]

Mixed neutrophilic and mononuclear cell infiltrations are usually observed in tissue specimens in BD. Nonspecific hyper-reactivity such as "pathergy" test (skin reaction to simple trauma) is possibly associated with proinflammatory cytokine responses such as IL-1 and IL-6. Increased γδT cells secreting tumor necrosis factor (TNF)-α and interferon (IFN) γ in tissue infiltrates are also a consistent finding, suggesting the role of innate immunity.[9,10] Immune cross-reactivity due to molecular mimicry between bacterial and human molecules, such as heat-shock proteins, is suggested to drive T- and B-cell responses with a proinflammatory and Th1-type cytokine profile (TNF-α and IL-12). Recently, increased IL-17, IL-22, and IL-23 expressions are also observed, expanding the immune spectrum with Th17-type responses.[11]

CASE VIGNETTE

A 25-year-old male was referred to our clinic due to pain and swelling on his right leg for 3 days. He had been on colchicine therapy (1.5 mg daily) for 2 years with a history of recurrent oral aphthous ulcers and erythema nodosum (EN) together with a positive pathergy test. On physical examination, there was obvious swelling and pain on his right calf. He had an elevated erythrocyte sedimentation rate (ESR): 45 mm/h and c-reactive protein (CRP): 14.1 mg/dL. An acute venous thrombosis was detected in his right popliteal vein with venous Doppler ultrasonography. Methylprednisolone (MP) 0.5 mg/kg daily and azathioprine (AZA) 150 mg daily were prescribed. The symptoms completely resolved in a few weeks. After a 1-year follow-up, the patient stopped his treatment during clinical remission. After 9 months, the patient came back to emergency ward with hemoptysis and was diagnosed to have a pulmonary aneurysm with CT angiogram. He was put on 1000 mg per day MP infusions for 3 days, then on 1 mg/kg daily MP, and cyclophosphamide 1000 mg monthly infusions for 6 months. In his last visit after 5 years of follow-up, he was on AZA 150 mg per day with an ESR: 11 mm/h and CRP: 0.4 mg/dL.

EPIDEMIOLOGY

Behçet's disease has a distinct geographical distribution. It is more prevalent in countries around the Mediterranean basin and East Asia (Japan, Korea and China). The prevalences were reported to be 20–421/10[5] in Turkey,[12-14] 80/10[5] in Iran, 15/10[5] in Israel, 13.5/10[5] in Japan, 0.64/10[5] in England, and 3.8/10[5] in Italy.[15-19]

The course of BD is more severe in males and in patients having a young disease onset (<25 years old).[20,21] The disease most frequently starts in second and third decades. The disease onset can be in pediatric ages, but onset after 50 years is very rare.[22-24] Some of the manifestations of BD also show regional differences. Gastrointestinal findings are common in Japanese and Korean patients, but rather infrequent in Turkey and the Middle East. In contrast, vascular disease is rare in East Asia. Pathergy test, the nonspecific hypersensitivity of the skin to a needle prick, is less commonly positive in North European and North American Caucasian patients.[25]

DIAGNOSIS

There is no specific diagnostic test for BD and the diagnosis depends on clinical features. International Study Group (ISG) for BD developed a set of classification criteria in 1990. ISG criteria were validated and are widely used for BD, with a sensitivity and specificity >90%. The diagnosis requires recurrent oral ulcers and at least two GUs, erythema nodosum-like lesions, folliculitis, uveitis (anterior or panuveitis), and pathergy test (Table 36.1).[26]

Table 36.1 International criteria for classification of Behçet's disease
Recurrent oral ulceration:
• Minor aphthous, major aphthous, or herpetiform ulceration observed by a physician or reported reliably by patient
• Recurrent at least three times in one 12-month period
Plus 2 of:
Recurrent genital ulceration
• Recurrent genital aphthous ulceration or scarring, especially in males, observed by a physician or reported reliably by patient
Eye lesions
• Anterior uveitis
• Posterior uveitis
• Cells in vitreous on slit lamp examination or retinal vasculitis observed by qualified physician
Skin lesions
• Erythema nodosum-like lesions observed by a physician or reported reliably by patient
• Pseudofolliculitis
• Papulopustular lesions or acneiform nodules consistent with BD
Positive pathergy test
• An erythematous papule,>2 mm, at the prick site after the application of a sterile needle, 20–22 gauge, which obliquely penetrated avascular skin to a depth of 5 m, read by a physician at 48 h.

Note: Findings are applicable if no other clinical explanation is present.

CLINICAL FEATURES

Mucocutaneous Involvement

Recurrent Aphthous Ulcers

Recurrent aphthous (oral) ulcers are seen in 95–97% of patients and are usually the first disease manifestation of BD, preceding the diagnosis by an average of 6–7 years. They often present as painful, erythematous, circular, and slightly raised areas evolving into oval or round ulcers within 48 hours (Fig. 36.1). Oral ulcers are frequently observed on the mucous membranes of the lips, gingivae, cheeks, and tongue, perhaps more posteriorly than ordinary aphthae. They usually heal in about 10–15 days without scarring.[27-30] In a long-term routine follow-up, oral aphthous ulcers were observed to be the main cause of ongoing clinical activity.[31]

Genital Ulcers

Genital ulcers are another major manifestations of BD. They are also the most specific (95%) mucocutaneous sign of BD.[26] The frequency of GUs ranges between 50 and 85%. They are usually located on the scrotum in males and on the major and minor labia in females (Fig. 36.2). They usually begin as papules or pustules that ulcerate after a short time[26-29] and usually heal in 10–30 days if they are not secondarily infected, leaving scars in about 60% of the patients.[32]

Cutaneous Lesions

Other types of cutaneous lesions in BD can be grouped into three categories.[33]

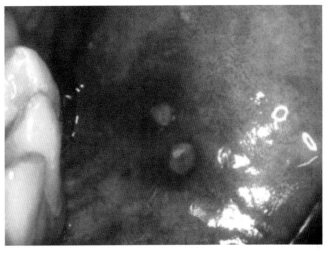

Fig. 36.1 Oral ulcers in Behçet's disease
[*Source:* Professor (Dr) Tulin Ergun]

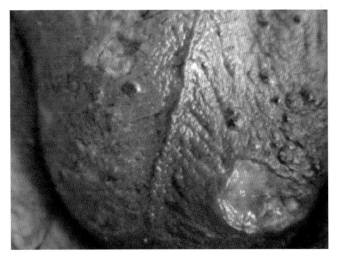

Fig. 36.2 Genital ulcer in Behçet's disease
[*Source:* Professor (Dr) Tulin Ergun]

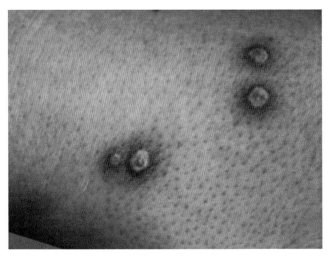

Fig. 36.3 Papulopustular lesions in Behçet's disease
[*Source:* Professor (Dr) Tulin Ergun]

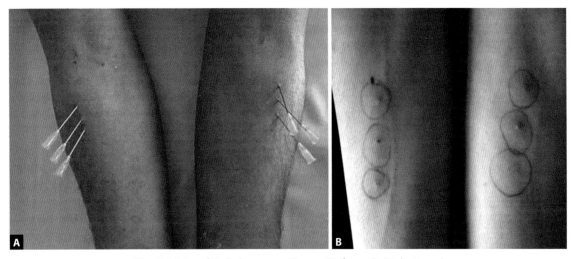

Figs 36.4A and B Pathergy test [*Source:* Professor (Dr) Tulin Ergun]

1. EN-like lesions and superficial thrombophlebitis (ST)
2. Papulopustular and acneiform lesions
3. Other lesions such as skin ulcers and Sweet syndrome

Erythema nodosum-like lesions are red, tender, erythematous nonulcerating nodules that are frequently located on the legs and generally resolve with pigmentation.[26-28] Erythema nodosum-like lesions are observed in approximately 50% of BD patients and are more frequently present in females.[21] Superficial thrombophlebitis is the most common type of venous involvement[34] and it can be difficult to differentiate ST and EN in some cases. It presents as palpable, painful subcutaneous nodules that are string-like hardenings with erythema of the overlying skin.[35]

Papulopustular lesions are frequently indistinguishable from ordinary acne. They are seen at usual acne sites such as face, upper chest and back, and additionally on the legs and arms (Fig. 36.3).[36] Other cutaneous lesions, such as skin ulcers and Sweet syndrome, can also be observed in BD.

Pathergy Reaction

Pathergy test is a nonspecific hyper-reactivity in response to minor trauma in the skin and is quite specific for BD. It is usually used as a diagnostic test and is performed by inserting a 20–22 gauge needle into the dermis of the forearm of the patient (Fig. 36.4A). The presence of a papule or pustule at 48 h is considered positive (Fig. 36.4B).[37]

Eye Involvement

Eye involvement is one of the main causes of morbidity in BD. It is observed in up to 50% of patients. Generally, a chronic, relapsing bilateral uveitis is present. Ocular inflammation is commonly a panuveitis and retinitis. However, some patients can present with an isolated anterior uveitis. Retinal lesions consist of exudates, hemorrhages, papilledema, and macular disease. Postinflammatory changes, such as synechiae and retinal scars, are important determinants of prognosis in eye involvement.[37] In the 20-year Cerrahpaşa Outcome Survey, eye involvement was bilateral in 80% of the males and 64% of females at the first visit. At the end of 20 years of follow-up, 87% of males and 71% of females had bilateral eye disease.[2]

Musculoskeletal Disease

Arthritis or arthralgia is seen in about 50% of patients with BD. It is usually manifested as a nondeforming, nonerosive peripheral oligoarthritis involving the knees, ankles, hands, and wrists in decreasing order. It usually resolves in a couple of days to weeks.[38] Sacroiliitis is not a prominent part of the clinical picture, but the coexistence of acne, arthritis, and enthesopathies suggests that at least a subgroup of patients have reactive arthritis-like features.[39]

Vascular Involvement

Vasculitis is a main pathological finding in BD. Vessels of all sizes can be involved, both in the arterial and venous systems.[40,41] Major vessel involvement consists of arterial occlusion, arterial aneurysms, and major vein occlusions (Fig. 36.5). Vascular involvement is seen in up to 40% of the patients with BD, especially in young males and is one of the major causes of mortality and morbidity. Venous involvement (80%) is reported to be more common than arterial disease.[10] Lower extremity vein thrombosis is the most frequent form of vascular involvement (Fig. 36.6).[2] Although venous thrombosis is seen primarily in the lower extremities, it may affect many different sites including inferior and superior vena cava, pulmonary artery, suprahepatic vessels, and cardiac cavities. Up to 17% of the mortality in BD is reported to be associated with venous involvement such as pulmonary embolism or Budd-Chiari syndrome.[42] There have been sporadic reports of valvular lesions, myocarditis, coronary

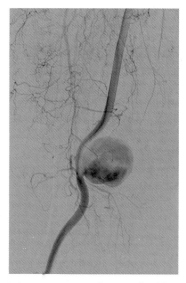

Fig. 36.5 A pseudoaneurysm in right superficial femoral artery in BD

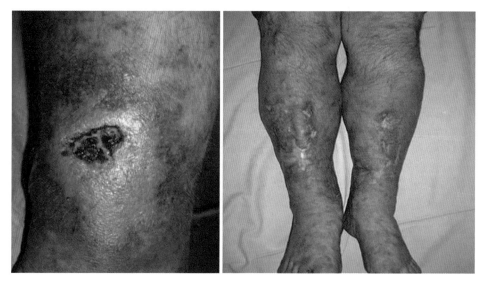

Fig. 36.6 Lower extremity venous insufficiency and ulcers [*Source:* Professor (Dr) Tulin Ergun]

vasculitis, ventricular aneurysms, and intracavitary thrombus formation, but overall cardiac involvement is uncommon in BD.[37]

Neurologic Involvement

Central nervous system involvement is seen in 5% of patients with BD. There are two main forms of CNS disease: vascular and parenchymal. Parenchymal disease leads to inflammatory lesions in the brainstem, diencephalon, basal ganglia and, less frequently, the spinal cord and cerebellum. The cerebral cortices seem to be spared. They usually manifest with bilateral pyramidal signs, unilateral hemiparesis, behavioral changes, sphincter disturbances, and headache. Brainstem signs and sensory disturbances are less common. Abnormal cerebrospinal fluid findings such as pleocytosis and increased cellularity are found in 60% of patients with parenchymal involvement. The second form of neurological involvement is dural sinus thrombosis, mainly characterized by headache and papilledema. It usually associates with deep vein thrombi in other areas and has a better prognosis than parenchymal involvement.[43,44]

Gastrointestinal Involvement

Gastrointestinal involvement is seen in one-third of BD patients in Japan and Korea, but is rare in Mediterranean countries (<5%). It is characterized by mucosal ulcerations primarily in the terminal ileum and the cecum, with vomiting, abdominal pain, and diarrhea being the main symptoms. A mass is often palpable in the abdomen during exacerbations, and ileocecal perforations may rarely occur. It is sometimes difficult to distinguish the findings of GI BD from those of Crohn's disease.[37,45] Younger age at diagnosis is associated with a more severe disease course and a poorer prognosis.[46]

Other Clinical Findings

Renal involvement such as glomerulonephritis is rarely reported as sporadic cases in BD. AA-type amyloidosis can occasionally be seen.[47] As a cause of testicular pain, epididymitis can be observed in male patients.[48] A recent study from Turkey also reported increased incidence of varicocele in BD.[49]

INVESTIGATIONS

There is no characteristic or pathognomonic investigation in BD. ESR and CRP are usually mildly elevated, mainly in cases with arthritis, EN-like lesions, or vascular disease. Autoantibodies such as rheumatoid factor, antinuclear, anticardiolipin, and antineutrophil cytoplasmic antibodies are generally absent. However, BD patients having GI involvement have higher levels of anti-*Saccharomyces cerevisiae* antibodies.[50]

DIAGNOSTIC APPROACH

As a clinical entity with mainly mucocutaneous features, BD requires a differential diagnosis from other disorders with frequent oral ulcers, such as spondyloarthropathies, especially inflammatory bowel disease. Posterior uveitis should be differentiated from tuberculosis and sarcoidosis and vascular disease from vasculitides.

MANAGEMENT

Treatment of BD changes according to organ involvement, gender, and age of the patient. Major organ involvement such as uveitis, vascular, neurologic, and GI disease needs a more aggressive approach with long-term immunosuppressive treatments. Young males are in the group with the highest risk regarding major organ disease.[2]

Mucocutaneous and Musculoskeletal Involvement

Colchicine is the most widely used agent for the treatment of mucocutaneous involvement. However, in a 2-year, double-blind study, it was found to be superior compared to placebo only for GU and EN in women.[51] Colchicine is also widely used without an evidence-based approach in OU. In a study of our group, majority of BD patients are not in complete remission in the long-term, routine follow-up, mainly due to oral ulcer presence in spite of colchicine usage in most patients.[27] Topical corticosteroids can be used in mild OU and GU. Another topical agent, sucralfate, was also found to be effective for OU and GU.[52] Thalidomide was found effective for all mucocutaneous symptoms in a controlled study, but side effects such as neuropathy and teratogenicity limit its use.[53] Azathioprine and IFN-α can be used in refractory mucocutaneous lesions.[54,55] The efficacy of TNF-α inhibitors was also shown in some reports.[56,57] In a recent phase II study, apremilast, which is an oral phosphodiesterase 4 inhibitor, decreased the number and pain of oral ulcers in BD.[58]

Arthritis in BD is usually nonerosive and self-limiting. Colchicine was found effective for joint problems in BD.[49] Corticosteroids and nonsteroidal anti-inflammatory drugs may be used during acute arthritis.[59] In addition to sulfasalazine and methotrexate, IFN-α and TNF-α inhibitors can be used in refractory patients.

Major Organ Disease

Azathioprine and systemic corticosteroids were suggested as the first choice for treatment in ocular involvement, especially with posterior segment disease according to the European League Against Rheumatism (EULAR) management recommendations. In refractory patients, cyclosporine-A (CsA), TNF-α inhibitors or IFN-α can be considered as alternative options.[59-61] There are case series showing the efficacy of Gevokizumab (XOMA 052) and canakinumab, both IL-1-inhibitors, in ocular involvement.[62,63]

Currently, there are no controlled studies for the management of major vascular involvement (VBD) in BD. According to EULAR recommendations for the management of BD, only immunosuppressive (IS) agents such as corticosteroids, AZA, cyclophosphamide, or Cs-A are recommended for VBD. Azathioprine with a moderate dose of corticosteroids (prednisolone 0.5 mg/kg per day) is usually preferred as the initial IS treatment for venous thrombosis. In more serious cases such as superior vena caval thrombosis or Budd-Chiari syndrome, monthly pulse cyclophosphamide should be considered. Despite a high frequency of venous thrombosis, as pulmonary embolism is rare and a coexisting pulmonary aneurysm might result in fatal bleeding, anticoagulants (ACs), antiplatelet, or antifibrinolytic agents are not recommended.[59] Cyclosporine-A, IFN-α, methotrexate, TNF-α inhibitors can also be used in refractory patients with vascular involvement.[64]

There are also no controlled studies in the management of CNS involvement in BD. According to EULAR recommendations, corticosteroids are recommended for neurologic involvement (both parenchymal involvement and dural sinus thrombosis) of BD.[59] The current approach includes AZA together with oral corticosteroids as a first-line therapy. Acute stage of neurologic involvement is treated with high-dose, pulse IV corticosteroids for 5–10 days.[65] Anticoagulant treatment for dural sinus thrombosis is controversial. In a recent consensus report, while half of the neurologists suggest AC treatment, the other half did not.[66] Cyclosporine-A should not be preferred in patients with CNS involvement because of its potential neurotoxicity.[59] There are satisfactory data about the efficacy of infliximab in refractory patients with neurologic involvement.[67,68] There are also case reports showing efficacy of adalimumab,[69] etanercept,[70] and tociluzumab in neurologic involvement of BD.[71,72]

5-aminosalicylic acid (ASA) derivatives may be used in mild cases with GI disease—with or without corticosteroids.[73] Azathioprine may be an alternative in resistant patients to 5-ASA derivatives or as first-line therapy in more severe patients with GI involvement.[74] Thalidomide and TNF-α inhibitors may be used in refractory cases.[75]

KEY POINTS

- Behçet's disease has a distinct geographical distribution. It is more prevalent in countries around the Mediterranean basin and East Asia (Japan and Korea).
- Recurrent aphthous ulcers are observed in >95% of the patients and are usually the first disease manifestation. However, genital ulcers are the most specific disease manifestation.
- Young (<25 years old), male patients consist the group with the highest risk for morbidity and mortality. Major organ disease requires high-dose corticosteroid and immunosuppressives such as AZA, cyclophosphamide, and cyclosporine-A. IFN-α and TNF-α inhibitors are preferred in refractory cases. Anti-IL-1 therapies and phosphodiesterase 4 inhibitors are also under investigation.

REFERENCES

1. Behçet H. Uber rezidiverende, aphthose, durch ein virus verursachte Gescgwure am Mund, um Auge und an den Genitalen. Derm Woch. 1937;105:1152-7.
2. Kural-Seyahi E, Fresko I, Seyahi N, et al. The long-term mortality and morbidity of Behçet syndrome: a 2-decade outcome survey of 387 patients followed at a dedicated center. Medicine (Baltimore). 2003;82:60-76.
3. Remmers EF, Cosan F, Kirino Y, et al. Genome-wide association study identifies variants in the MHC class I, IL10, and IL23R-IL12RB2 regions associated with Behçet's disease. Nature Genet. 2010;42(8):698-702.
4. Mizuki N, Meguro A, Ota M, et al. Genome-wide association studies identify IL23R-IL12RB2 and IL10 as Behçet's disease susceptibility loci. Nature Genet. 2010;42:703-6.
5. Kirino Y, Bertsias G, Ishigatsubo Y, et al. Genome-wide association analysis identifies new susceptibility loci for Behçet's disease and epistasis between HLA-B*51 and ERAP1. Nature Genet. 2013;45:202-7.
6. Kirino Y, Zhou Q, Ishigatsubo Y, et al. Targeted resequencing implicates the familial Mediterranean fever gene MEFV and the toll-like receptor 4 gene TLR4 in Behçet disease. Proc Natl Acad Sci USA. 2013;110:8134-9.
7. Hughes T, Coit P, Adler A, et al. Identification of multiple independent susceptibility loci in the HLA region

in Behçet's disease. Nature Genet. 2013;45:319-24. doi: 10.1038/ng.2551.

8. Ombrello MJ, Kirino Y, de Bakker PI, et al. Behçet disease-associated MHC class I residues implicate antigen binding and regulation of cell-mediated cytotoxicity. Proc Natl Acad Sci USA. 2014 (May). Epub ahead of print.

9. Direskeneli H. Behçet's disease: infectious etiology, new auto-antigens and HLA-B51. Ann Rheum Dis. 2001;60:996-1002.

10. Sakane T, Takeno M, Suzuki N, et al. Behçet's disease. N Engl J Med. 1999;341:1284-91.

11. Krause I, Weinberger A. Behçet's disease. Curr Opin Rheumatol. 2008;20:82-7.

12. Yurdakul S, Günaydin I, Tüzün Y, et al. The prevalence of Behçet's syndrome in a rural area in northern Turkey. J Rheumatol. 1988;15:820-2.

13. Azizlerli G, Köse AA, Sarica R, et al. Prevalence of Behçet's disease in Istanbul, Turkey. Int J Dermatol. 2003;42:803-6.

14. Cakir N, Dervis E, Benian O, et al. Prevalence of Behçet's disease in rural western Turkey: a preliminary report. Clin Exp Rheumatol. 2004;22:S53-55.

15. Davatchi F, Jamshidi AR, Banihashemi AT, et al. WHO-ILAR COPCORD Study (Stage 1, Urban Study) in Iran. J Rheumatol. 2008;35:1384.

16. Krause I, Yankevich A, Fraser A, et al. Prevalence and clinical aspects of Behçet's disease in the north of Israel. Clin Rheumatol. 2007;26:555-60.

17. Nakae K, Masaki F, Hashimoto T, et al. Recent epidemiological features of Behçet's Disease in Japan. In: Wechsler B, Godeau P (Eds). Behçet Disease. Amsterdam: Excerpta Medica. pp. 145-52.

18. Chamberlain MA. Behçet's syndrome in 32 patients in Yorkshire. Ann Rheum Dis. 1977;36:491-9.

19. Salvarani C, Pipitone N, Catanoso MG, et al. Epidemiology and clinical course of Behçet's disease in the Reggio Emilia area of northern Italy: a seventeen-year population-based study. Arthritis Rheum. 2007;57:171-8.

20. O'Neill TW, Rigby AS, Silman AJ, et al. Validation of the International Study Group criteria for Behçet's disease. Br J Rheumatol. 1994;33:115-7.

21. Yazici H, Tüzün Y, Pazarli H, et al. Influence of age of onset and patient's sex on the prevalence and severity of manifestations of Behçet's syndrome. Ann Rheum Dis. 1984;43:783-9.

22. Colin GB. History and diagnosis. In: Yazıcı Y, Yazıcı H (Eds). Behçet's Disease. New York: Springer; 2010. pp. 7-34.

23. Shafaie N, Shahram F, Davatchi F, et al. Behçet's disease in children. In: Wechsler B, Godeau P (Eds). Behçet's Disease (International Congress series 1037). Amsterdam: Excerpta Medica; pp. 381-3.

24. Zouboulis CC, Kötter I, Djawari D, et al. Epidemiological features of Adamantiades–Behçet's disease in Germany and in Europe. Yonsei Med J. 1997;38:411-22.

25. Fresko F, Stübiger N, Tascilar K. Behçet's syndrome, relapsing polychondritis and eye involvement in rheumatic disease (Modül 25). Eular on-line course on rheumatic diseases. (2007-2012).

26. International Study Group for Behçet's Disease. Criteria for diagnosis of Behçet's disease. Lancet. 1990;335:1078-80.

27. Idil A, Gürler A, Boyvat A, et al. The prevalence of Behçet's disease above the age of 10 years. The results of a pilot study conducted at the Park Primary Health Care Center in Ankara, Turkey. Ophthalmic Epidemiol. 2002;9:325-31.

28. Alpsoy E, Donmez L, Onder M, et al. Clinical features and natural course of Behçet's disease in 661 cases: a multicentre study. Br J Dermatol. 2007;157:901-6.

29. Saylan T, Mat C, Fresko I, et al. Behçet's disease in the Middle East. Clin Dermatol. 1999;17:209-23; discussion 105-6.

30. Bang D, Hur W, Lee ES, et al. Prognosis and clinical relevance of recurrent oral ulceration in Behçet's disease. J Dermatol. 1995;22:926-9.

31. Alibaz-Oner F, Mumcu G, Kubilay Z, et al. Unmet need in Behçet's disease: most patients in routine follow-up continue to have oral ulcers. Clin Rheumatol. 2014 (April). Epub ahead of print.

32. Mat MC, Goksugur N, Engin B, et al. The frequency of scarring after genital ulcers in Behçet's syndrome: a prospective study. Int J Dermatol. 2006;45:554-6.

33. Mat C, Bang D, Melikoğlu M. The mucocutaneous manifestations and pathergy reaction in Behçet's disease. In: Yazıcı Y, Yazıcı H (Eds). Behçet's Syndrome, 1st edition. New York, USA: Springer; 2010.

34. Kuzu MA, Ozaslan C, Köksoy C, et al. Vascular involvement in Behçet's disease: 8-year audit. World J Surg. 1994;18:948-53; discussion 953-4.

35. Alpsoy E, Zouboulis CC, Ehrlich GE. Mucocutaneous lesions of Behçet's disease. Yonsei Med J. 2007;48:573-85.

36. Jorizzo JL, Abernethy JL, White WL, et al. Mucocutaneous criteria for the diagnosis of Behçet's disease: an analysis of clinicopathologic data from multiple international centers. J Am Acad Dermatol. 1995;32:968-76.

37. Yurdakul S, Hamuryudan V, Fresko I, et al. Behçet's syndrome. In: Hochberg MC, Silman AJ, Smolen JS, Weinblatt WE, Weisman MH (Eds). Rheumatology, 4th edition. Philadelphia, USA; 2008.

38. Yurdakul S, Yazici H, Tüzün Y, et al. The arthritis of Behçet's disease: a prospective study. Ann Rheum Dis. 1983;42:505-15.

39. Hatemi G, Fresko I, Tascilar K, et al. Increased enthesopathy among Behçet's syndrome patients with acne and arthritis: an ultrasonography study. Arthritis Rheum. 2008;58:1539-45. doi: 10.1002/art.23450.

40. Calamia KT, Schirmer M, Melikoglu M. Major vessel involvement in Behçet's disease: an update. Curr Opin Rheumatol. 2011;23:24-31.

41. Yazici H, Yurdakul S, Hamuryudan V. Behçet disease. Curr Opin Rheumatol. 2001;13:18-22.

42. Saadoun D, Wechsler B, Desseaux K, et al. Mortality in Behçet's disease. Arthritis Rheum. 2010;62:2806-12.

43. Akman-Demir G, Serdaroglu P, Tasçi B. (The Neuro-Behçet Study Group). Clinical patterns of neurological involvement in Behçet's disease: evaluation of 200 patients. Brain. 1999;122:2171-82.

44. Siva A, Kantarci OH, Saip S, et al. Behçet's disease: diagnostic and prognostic aspects of neurological involvement. J Neurol. 2001;248:95-103.

45. Korman U, Cantasdemir M, Kurugoglu S, et al. Enteroclysis findings of intestinal Behçet's disease: a comparative study with Crohn disease. Abdom Imaging. 2003;28:308-12.

46. Park JJ, Kim WH, Cheon JH. Outcome predictors for intestinal Behçet's disease. Yonsei Med J. 2013;54:1084-90. doi: 10.3349/ymj.2013.54.5.1084.

47. Melikoğlu M, Altiparmak MR, Fresko I, et al. A reappraisal of amyloidosis in Behçet's syndrome. Rheumatology (Oxford). 2001;40:212-5.

48. Cetinel B, Akpinar H, Tüfek I, et al. Bladder involvement in Behçet's syndrome. J Urol. 1999;161:52-56.

49. Yilmaz O, Yilmaz S, Kisacik B, et al. Varicocele and epididymitis in Behçet's disease. J Ultrasound Med. 2011;30:909-13.

50. Fresko I, Ugurlu S, Ozbakir F, et al. Anti-Saccharomyces cerevisiae antibodies (ASCA) in Behçet's syndrome. Clin Exp Rheumatol. 2005;23:S67-70.

51. Yurdakul S, Mat C, Tüzün Y, et al. A double-blind trial of colchicine in Behçet's syndrome. Arthritis Rheum. 2001; 44:2686-92.

52. Alpsoy E, Er H, Durusoy C, et al. The use of sucralfate suspension in the treatment of oral and genital ulceration of Behçet disease: a randomized, placebo-controlled, double-blind study. Arch Dermatol. 1999;135:529-32.

53. Hamuryudan V, Mat C, Saip S, et al. Thalidomide in the treatment of the mucocutaneous lesions of the Behçet syndrome. A randomized, double-blind, placebo-controlled trial. Ann Intern Med. 1998;128(6):443-50.

54. Yazici H, Pazarli H, Barnes CG, et al. A controlled trial of azathioprine in Behçet's syndrome. N Engl J Med. 1990; 322:281-5.

55. Alpsoy E, Durusoy C, Yilmaz E, et al. Interferon alfa-2α in the treatment of Behçet disease: a randomized placebo-controlled and double-blind study. Arch Dermatol. 2002;138:467-71.

56. Melikoglu M, Fresko I, Mat C, et al. Short-term trial of etanercept in Behçet's disease: a double blind, placebo controlled study. J Rheumatol. 2005;32:98-105.

57. Arida A, Fragiadaki K, Giavri E, et al. Anti-TNF agents for Behçet's disease: analysis of published data on 369 patients. Semin Arthritis Rheum. 2011;41:61-70.

58. Hatemi G, Melikoglu M, Tunc R, et al. Apremilast for the treatment of Behçet's syndrome: a phase II randomized, placebo-controlled, double-blind study. Arthritis Rheum. 2013;65:S322.

59. Hatemi G, Silman A, Bang D, et al. EULAR Expert Committee. EULAR recommendations for the management of Behçet disease. Ann Rheum Dis. 2008;67:1656-62. doi: 10.1136/ard.2007.080432.

60. Okada AA, Goto H, Ohno S, et al. Ocular Behçet's Disease Research Group of Japan. Multicenter study of infliximab for refractory uveoretinitis in Behçet disease. Arch Ophthalmol. 2012;130:592-8.

61. Sfikakis PP, Kaklamanis PH, Elezoglou A, et al. Infliximab for recurrent, sight-threatening ocular inflammation in Adamantiades–Behçet disease. Ann Intern Med. 2004;140:404-6.

62. Gul A, Tugal-Tutkun I, Dinarello CA, et al. Interleukin-1b-regulating antibody XOMA 052 (gevokizumab) in the treatment of acute exacerbations of resistant uveitis of Behçet's disease: an open-label pilot study. Ann Rheum Dis. 2012;71:563-6.

63. Ugurlu S, Ucar D, Seyahi E, et al. Canakinumab in a patient with juvenile. Behçet's syndrome with refractory eye disease. Ann Rheum Dis. 2012;71:1591-2.

64. Ozguler Y, Hatemi G, Yazici H. Management of Behçet's syndrome. Curr Opin Rheumatol. 2014;26:285-91. doi: 10.1097/BOR.0000000000000050.

65. Akman-Demir G, Saip S, Siva A. Behçet's disease. Curr Treat Options Neurol. 2011;13:290-310.

66. Kalra S, Silman A, Akman-Demir G, et al. Diagnosis and management of Neuro-Behçet's disease: international consensus recommendations. J Neurol. 2013. Epub ahead of print.

67. Giardina A, Ferrante A, Ciccia F, et al. One year study of efficacy and safety of infliximab in the treatment of patients with ocular and neurological Behçet's disease refractory to standard immunosuppressive drugs. Rheumatol Int. 2011;31:33-37. doi: 10.1007/s00296-009-1213-z.

68. Fasano A, D'Agostino M, Caldarola G, et al. Infliximab monotherapy in neuro-Behçet's disease: four year follow-up in a long-standing case resistant to conventional therapies. J Neuroimmunol. 2011;239:105-7.

69. Olivieri I, Leccese P, D'Angelo S, et al. Efficacy of adalimumab in patients with Behçet's disease unsuccessfully treated with infliximab. Clin Exp Rheumatol. 2011;29:S54-57.

70. Alty JE, Monaghan TM, Bamford JM. A patient with neuro-Behçet's disease is successfully treated with etanercept: further evidence for the value of TNF alpha blockade. Clin Neurol Neurosurg. 2007;109:279-81.

71. Shapiro LS, Farrell J, Haghighi AB. Tocilizumab treatment for neuro-Behçet's disease: the first report. Clin Neurol Neurosurg. 2012;114:297-8.

72. Urbaniak P, Hasler P, Kretzschmar S. Refractory neuro-Behçet treated by tocilizumab: a case report. Clin Exp Rheumatol. 2012;30:S73-75.

73. Jung YS, Hong SP, Kim TI, et al. Long-term clinical outcomes and factors predictive of relapse after 5-aminosalicylate or sulfasalazine therapy in patients with intestinal Behçet disease. J Clin Gastroenterol. 2012;46:e38-45.

74. Jung YS, Cheon JH, Hong SP, et al. Clinical outcomes and prognostic factors for thiopurine maintenance therapy in patients with intestinal Behçet's disease. Inflamm Bowel Dis. 2012;18:7507.

75. Hatemi I, Hatemi G, Erzin Y, et al. Characteristics, treatment and outcome of gastrointestinal involvement of Behçet's syndrome: experience in dedicated center. Ann Rheum Dis. 2012;71:391.

CHAPTER 37

Cryoglobulinemic Vasculitis

Cloé Comarmond, Patrice Cacoub

INTRODUCTION

Cryoglobulinemia are immune complexes that may induce systemic cryoglobulinemic vasculitis (Cryovas), a small-vessel vasculitis involving the skin, the joints, the peripheral nerve system, and the kidneys.[1,2] During the last 20 years, progresses have been made with the discovery that the hepatitis C virus (HCV) is the main etiologic agent of mixed cryoglobulinemia (MC).[3-5] Besides HCV infection, B-cell lymphoproliferative disorders, autoimmune diseases, and other infections represent the main causes. Cryoglobulins are immunochemically characterized into three types by the method of Brouet et al.[6] Type I cryoglobulins are single monoclonal immunoglobulins always linked to a B-cell lymphoproliferative disorder. Type II cryoglobulins consist of polyclonal immunoglobulin G (IgG) with monoclonal immunoglobulin M (IgM) with rheumatoid factor (RF) activity. Type III cryoglobulins are comprised of polyclonal IgG and polyclonal IgM with RF activity. Type II and III are often referred to as MC, and may be linked to B-cell lymphoproliferative disorders, autoimmune disorders, and/or infections. In the absence of identified etiologic factor, Cryovas is defined as essential or idiopathic.

CASE VIGNETTE

A 54-year-old woman was admitted to the hospital because of headache and transient visual problems. The patient had been well until approximately 4 weeks before admission, when fever, arthralgias, and muscle weakness developed, attributed to a "flu-like syndrome." Blood tests were normal.

About 3 days before admission, she began to have episodes of monocular blindness that involved either eye. The patient had two daughters and had a blood transfusion at the second delivery.

On examination, the blood pressure was 180/100 mm Hg, the pulse 101 beats/min, and the temperature 37.4°C; other vital signs were normal. There was evidence of a purpuric rash on her legs. An electrocardiogram was normal. A magnetic resonance imaging study of the brain showed normal findings. The urine was positive (++) for protein.

Renal vascular ultrasonography revealed no dilatation and no evidence of renal artery stenosis. Cytologic examination of the urine showed red-cell casts and no malignant cells. Culture of the urine was sterile. The creatininemia level was 350 μmol/L, associated with moderate anemia (hemoglobin level 10.4 g/dL). Kidney biopsy revealed a typical membranoproliferative glomerulonephritis.

Test for hepatitis C antibodies was positive and viral load positivity was confirmed by polymerase chain reaction. Tests for hepatitis B and HIV antibodies were negative. Tests for antinuclear antibodies and RF were positive. Anti-double-stranded DNA, anticentromere, anti-Ro, anti-La, anti-Sm, anti-U1-RNP, anti-neutrophil cytoplasmic antibody, and antimitochondrial antibodies were negative. C3 and C4 serum levels were low. Cryoglobulinemia was positive. Immunofixation of the cryoprecipitate showed two monoclonal IgM kappa bands, together with polyclonal IgG, findings that categorized the process as a type II MC.

In summary, this patient presented with Cryovas related to a chronic HCV infection revealed by rapidly progressive glomerulonephritis and purpura.

EPIDEMIOLOGY

Mixed cryoglobulinemia is considered to be a rare disorder, but no adequate epidemiological studies of its overall prevalence have been carried out. Numerous cohort studies of a series of patients from different countries suggest that the prevalence of MC is geographically heterogeneous. The disease is more common in southern Europe than in northern Europe or northern America. It is more common in women than men (female-to-male ratio of 3:1), while the disease onset is particularly common in the fourth to fifth decades and older people, but rarely seen in young people.

The epidemiology of MC associated with HCV infection has been examined by cohort studies focusing on HCV-infected subjects, which reported circulating mixed cryoglobulins in more than 70% of cases, while overt cryoglobulinemic syndrome developed in about 5–10%. Hepatitis C virus infection is particularly diffuse worldwide; therefore, a growing incidence of MC and of other HCV-related extrahepatic manifestations can be expected, especially in underdeveloped countries where HCV in the general population is prevalent.

In contrast, the prevalence of "essential" MC is generally seen in a significantly lower proportion of patients with MC, being quite rare in some geographical areas, such as southern Europe, where the whole MC is prevalent.

DIAGNOSIS

In 1989, the Italian Group proposed preliminary criteria for MC classification for the study of cryoglobulinemias, successively revised by including clinicopathological and virological findings.[7] This classification is mainly based on the serological and clinical hallmarks of the disease—namely, circulating mixed cryoglobulins, low C4, and orthostatic skin purpura. Leukocytoclastic vasculitis, involving medium and, more often, small-sized blood vessels (arterioles, capillaries, and venules) is the typical pathological finding of affected tissues. It is easily detectable by a skin biopsy of recent vasculitic lesions (within the first 24–48 hours).

More recently, preliminary classification criteria for Cryovas have been developed by a cooperative study using a standardized methodology.[8] If formally validated in MC patients referred to experts from a larger number of countries, these criteria may be usefully employed in epidemiological and clinicopathogenetic studies, as well as in therapeutical trials.

In all cases, the cryoglobulin detection in the serum is necessary for a definite classification of MC syndrome and their characterization as type II (IgG+IgM monoclonal) or type III (IgG+IgM polyclonal) mixed cryoglobulins. Unfortunately, there are no universally accepted methodologies for cryoglobulin measurements, but simple standardized indications are often sufficient for testing for cryoglobulinemia. Cryoglobulins are characterized by high thermal instability. For a correct evaluation of serum cryoglobulins, it is necessary to avoid false-negative results due to immunoglobulin cold precipitation that also occurs at room temperature. Blood sampling for cryoglobulin detection should be done at once or blood should be rapidly transported to the laboratory using a thermostable device (37°C). In general, to avoid the possible loss of cryoglobulins, the first steps (blood sampling, clotting, and serum separation by centrifugation) should always be carried out at 37°C. On the contrary, isolated serum for cryoglobulin determination and characterization should be managed at 4°C. The serum with cryoglobulins should be tested for reversibility of the cryoprecipitate by rewarming an aliquot at 37°C for 24 hours. Cryocrit measurement is usually done in serum sample stored at 4°C for 7 days. The cryocrit corresponds to the percentage of packed cryoglobulins with reference to the total serum after centrifugation at 4°C; it should be determined on blood samples without anticoagulation to avoid false-positive results due to cryofibrinogen or heparin-precipitable proteins. Without the above relatively simple precautions, not only will the quantities of cryoglobulins measured be incorrect but also the test may completely fail to detect cryoglobulins.

After isolating and washing the cryoprecipitate, the identity of cryoglobulin components can be determined by immunoelectrophoresis or immunofixation. These analyses must be performed at 37°C to avoid precipitation and hence loss of the cryoglobulin during the procedures. More sophisticated methodologies, such as immunoblotting or two-dimensional polyacrylamide gel electrophoresis, may be used for laboratory investigations. Although the detection of serum cryoglobulins is fundamental for the diagnosis of MC, the levels of serum cryoglobulins do not necessarily correlate with the severity and prognosis of the disease. Very low levels of cryocrit, often difficult to quantify, can be associated with severe and/or active cryoglobulinemic syndrome; in contrast, high cryocrit values may characterize a mild or asymptomatic disease course. In rare cases, very high cryocrit levels, possibly associated with a cryogel phenomenon, may be associated with classical hyperviscosity syndrome. A sudden decrease or disappearance of serum mixed cryoglobulins, with or without abnormally high levels of C4, should be regarded as alarming signal of complicating B-cell malignancy.

Box 37.1 summarizes the clinicoserological investigations at a patient's first evaluation in order to classify the MC syndrome correctly and to identify possible overlapping disorders or comorbidities, or both. The prevalence of the latter, in particular atherosclerosis, may be correlated with

Box 37.1 Clinicodiagnostic assessment of mixed cryoglobulinemia syndrome

Clinical and serological investigations at a patient's first evaluation

- Past clinical history, physical examination
- Chest X-ray examination, ECG, abdominal ultrasonography (US), blood chemistry, and urine analysis
- Cryoglobulin detection and characterization (see Table 37.1)
- Rheumatoid factor activity, C3–C4, antinuclear antibodies (abs), antiextractable nuclear antigen abs, antineutrophil cytoplasmic abs, antismooth muscle abs, antimitochondrial abs, antiliver/kidney microsome type I abs, other autoabs
- *Virological markers:* HCV (viremia, genotyping), hepatitis B virus, others
- Evaluate possible comorbidities (cardiovascular, endocrine/metabolic, etc.)
- MC classification (definite, essential, and secondary)

Diagnosis and monitoring of major MC complications

- *Chronic hepatitis, cirrhosis, hepatocellular carcinoma:*
  - Monitoring (every 6–12 months) of alanine aminotransferase, alkaline phosphatase
  - Liver US (biopsy, CT scan)
- *Glomerulonephritis:*
  - Monitoring of urine analysis and serum creatinine (kidney US, biopsy)
- *Peripheral neuropathy:*
  - Clinical monitoring
  - Electromyography
- *Skin ulcers:*
  - Exclusion of vascular comorbidities (arteriovenous Doppler evaluation)
- *Sicca syndrome:*
  - Differential diagnosis with primary Sjögren syndrome
- *Arthritis:*
  - Differential diagnosis with rheumatoid arthritis
- *Thyroid involvement:*
  - Hormones
  - Autoantibodies
  - Neck US
  - Fine-needle aspiration
- *B-cell lymphoma:*
  - Clinical monitoring
  - Bone marrow/lymph node biopsies
  - Total body CT scan

Table 37.1 Main clinical and biological features of 250 mixed cryoglobulinemic patients

Features	Value
Clinical features:	
• Age at disease onset (years), mean (SD) [range]	54 (13) [29–72]
• Female/male ratio	3
• Disease duration (years), mean (SD) [range]	12 (10) [1–40]
• Purpura	98%
• Weakness	98%
• Arthralgias	91%
• Arthritis (non-erosive)	8%
• Raynaud's phenomenon	32%
• Sicca syndrome	51%
• Peripheral neuropathy	81%
• Renal involvement	31%
• Liver involvement	73%
• B-cell non-Hodgkin's lymphoma	11%
• Hepatocellular carcinoma	3%
Serological and virological features:	
• Cryocrit (%), mean (SD)	4.4 (12)
• Type II/type III mixed cryoglobulins	2/1
• C3 (mg/dL), mean (SD) (normal 60–130)	93 (30)
• C4 (mg/dL), mean (SD) (normal 20–55)	10 (12)
• Antinuclear antibodies	30%
• Antimitochondrial antibodies	9%
• Anti-smooth muscle antibodies	18%
• Anti-extractable nuclear antigen antibodies	8%
• Anti-HCV antibodies ± HCV RNA	92%
• Anti-HBV antibodies	32%
• HBsAg	1%

CLINICAL FEATURES

The most frequently target organs are skin, joints, nerves, and kidneys.[5] The disease expression is variable, ranging from mild clinical symptoms (purpura, arthralgia) to fulminant life-threatening complications (glomerulonephritis, widespread vasculitis).[9] The main clinical and biological signs are summarized in Table 37.1.

Purpura

Skin is the most frequently involved target organ. It is the direct consequence of the small-size vessel vasculitis. The main sign is a palpable purpura that is reported in 70–90% of patients, but cutaneous ulcers may occur. It always begins at the lower limbs and may extend to the abdominal area, less frequently to the trunk and upper limbs. It persists 3–10 days

the disease duration, and with cumulative side effects of prolonged treatments. Diagnosis and monitoring of the major MC manifestations is essential for their timely treatment, especially for life-threatening liver, renal, and/or neoplastic complications.

with a residual brownish pigmentation. Raynaud's syndrome and acrocyanosis, which may evolve to digital ulcerations, can also occur.

Arthralgia

Arthralgia is reported in about 40% of patients. Joint pains are bilateral and symmetric, nondeforming and involved mainly great articulations, knees, and hands, more seldom elbows, and ankles. Frank arthritis is rarely reported, being present in less than 10% of patients.

Neuropathy

Neurologic manifestations range from pure sensory axonopathy to mononeuritis multiplex. The most frequently described form is a distal sensory or sensory-motor polyneuropathy. Polyneuropathy usually presents with painful, asymmetric paresthesia that later become symmetric. Motor deficit is inconsistent and mainly affects the lower limbs, appearing a few months to a few years after sensory symptoms.

Renal Involvement

Renal manifestations are reported in 20–35% of patients. The most frequent clinical and pathological picture is that of acute or chronic type I membranoproliferative glomerulonephritis with subendothelial deposits. It represents more than 80% of cryoglobulinemic renal diseases. It is strongly associated with the presence of type II cryoglobulinemia with IgMk RF. The most frequent presentation (about 55%) is proteinuria with microscopic hematuria and a variable degree of renal insufficiency.

Other Manifestations

Sicca syndrome has been reported in 20–40% of patients. However, those meeting most definitions of definite Sjögren's syndrome are rarely encountered. Other organs may more rarely be involved. Abdominal pains and gastrointestinal bleeding secondary to mesenteric vasculitis has been described. Lungs can be involved more frequently without clinical symptoms, but some patients may present moderate exercise dyspnea, dry cough, interstitial lung fibrosis, pleural effusions, or hemoptysis, which can be the consequence of pulmonary intra-alveolar hemorrhages. Cardiac involvement including mitral valvular damage, coronary vasculitis complicated by myocardial infarction, pericarditis, or congestive cardiac failure all have been described.

DIAGNOSTIC APPROACH

Cryoglobulinemic vasculitis is classified among small-vessel systemic vasculitides. The disease is a combination of serological findings (mixed cryoglobulins with RF activity and frequent low C4) and clinicopathological features (purpura, leukocytoclastic vasculitis with multiple organ involvement).

The disease can be correctly identified on the basis of typical orthostatic purpura with the histological pattern of leukocytoclastic vasculitis on skin samples taken within the first 24–48 hours, detection of serum mixed (IgG-IgM) cryoglobulins, low-complement C4, and RF+.

The production of cryoglobulins is most often the consequence of an underlying disorder that needs an etiological check-up. It depends, at least in part, on the immunochemical determination. Main causes are summarized in Table 37.2.

The diagnostic management is mainly determined by the immunochemical characterization. Type I cryoglobulins are always linked to a B-cell lymphoproliferative disorder, i.e. multiple myeloma, Waldenström macroglobulinemia, chronic lymphocytic leukemia, B-NHL, and hairy cell leukemia. Type I Cryovas presentation is often severe, in part because of high cryoglobulin levels, with frequent cutaneous and renal involvement. Type II and III mixed cryoglobulins may be linked to B-cell lymphoproliferative disorder, autoimmune disorders, and/or infections. As indicated previously, HCV infection is the most frequent cause of MC, representing 80% of Cryovas cases. In the absence of identified etiologic factor (20%), Cryovas is defined as essential or idiopathic.

MANAGEMENT

The therapeutic management of Cryovas must be individualized according to the underlying disorder and the severity of disease.

Type I Cryovas is life-threatening because of the severity of cutaneous and visceral involvement and the underlying hematological disorder. Specific treatment may also be indicated, including plasma exchange, corticosteroids, rituximab, or ilomedine. Outcome and prognosis of mixed cryoglobulinemic (type II or III) vasculitis is variable according to the extent of systemic vasculitis, in particular the renal involvement, and the occurrence of complications such as lymphoma.

With the discovery that the HCV is the main etiologic agent of MC, new opportunities and problems in developing therapy for HCV-Cryovas have emerged. The cornerstone of HCV therapy has been interferon-alpha, which has

Table 37.2 Main diseases responsible for/or associated with cryoglobulin

B-cell lymphoproliferation (type I or type II cryoglobulin):
- Multiple myeloma
- Waldenström macroglobulinemia
- Plasmocytoma
- B-cell non-Hodgkin lymphoma
- Chronic lymphocytic leukemia
- Hairy cell leukemia

Autoimmune disorders (type II or type III cryoglobulin):
- Sjögren's syndrome
- Systemic lupus erythematosus
- Dermatopolymyositis

Systemic sclerosis:
- Autoimmune thyroiditis
- Primary biliary cirrhosis
- Autoimmune hepatitis
- Celiac disease
- Polyarteritis nodosa
- Granulomatosis with polyangiitis (formerly Wegener's)
- Henoch-Schönlein purpura
- Rheumatoid arthritis
- Behçet's disease
- Sarcoidosis
- Pemphigus vulgaris

Mediterranean fever

Infection (type II or type III cryoglobulin)

Virus:
- Hepatitis C virus
- Hepatitis B virus
- Human immunodeficiency virus
- Epstein-Barr virus
- Cytomegalovirus
- Adenovirus
- B19 Parvovirus

Bacteria:
- Endocarditis
- Super-infection of atrioventricular shunt
- Syphilis
- Lyme disease
- Brucellosis
- Acute post-streptococcal glomerulonephritis
- Leprosy

Parasitosis and fungi diseases:
- Malaria
- Toxoplasmosis
- Leishmaniosis
- Schistosomiasis
- Echinococcosis
- Coccidioidomycosis

Others (type II or type III cryoglobulin):
- Extracapillary glomerulonephritis
- Cancers

the potential to exacerbate autoimmune disease states.[10] Recent advances using a triple combination with pegylated interferon, ribavirin, and a protease inhibitor in patients infected by the genotype 1 virus have shown promising results. More recently, interferon-free strategies have been developed with promising results.[11] In more severe cases, combination therapy with rituximab and optimal HCV treatment appears logical, as it may target both mixed cryoglobulin producing B-cells and the viral trigger.

THERAPEUTIC GUIDELINES FOR HCV-MC

Aggressive optimal antiviral therapy should be considered as induction therapy for HCV-Cryovas patients with mild-to-moderate disease severity and activity (i.e. without rapidly progressive nephritis, motor neuropathy, or other life-threatening complications) (Flow chart 37.1). The type of antivirals and the duration of therapy have not yet been rigorously determined with new direct anti-HCV therapies (interferon-free). Current treatment duration in HCV-Cryovas patients is 24 weeks for all HCV genotypes.

In patients presenting with more severe HCV-Cryovas disease (i.e. worsening of renal function, mononeuritis multiplex, extensive skin disease including ulcers and distal necrosis), an immunosuppression induction phase is often necessary while awaiting the response to antiviral treatments. The following therapeutic schedule is recommended: (1) Weekly administration of four intravenous infusions of rituximab at 375 mg/m² (on days 1, 8, 15, and 22) over a one-month period; and (2) Antiviral combination starting after the last rituximab infusion for 12 months.

Flow chart 37.1 Therapeutic options in patients with HCV-induced mixed Cryovas

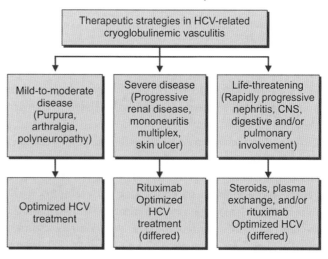

For patients presenting with the fulminant forms (catastrophic HCV-Cryovas disease) including peripheral necrosis of the extremities, rapidly progressive nephritis, digestive, cardiac, pulmonary, and/or central nervous system involvement, and/or signs and symptoms of hyperviscosity, apheresis can have immediate beneficial effects but must be combined with immunosuppression. The combination of rituximab, fludarabine, and cyclophosphamide appeared to be an effective salvage treatment for refractory Cryovas associated with lymphoma.

In patients who failed to respond or have contraindication to an optimal antiviral therapy, rituximab may be used alone. The following therapeutic schedule is therefore recommended: (1) Weekly administration of four intravenous infusions of rituximab at 375 mg/m² (on days 1, 8, 15, and 22) over a one-month period; and (2) Administration of one infusion of rituximab, every 6–9 months period, at a dose of 200–500 mg.

Biologic treatment with B-cell-directed therapy is promising in the treatment of HCV-Cryovas, but many questions remain regarding the appropriate role of this strategy in treatment. The duration of effect appears finite, with response duration typically lasting 6–12 months, and it is necessary to combine it with antiviral drugs. The safety of repeated therapy in HCV-Cryovas requires further investigation.

Follow-up

Clinical Observations

During immunosuppressive and/or antiviral treatment (for HCV-related cryoglobulinemia), signs and symptoms gradually improve, varying from weeks (i.e. purpura, glomerulonephritis, and arthralgia) to months (peripheral neuropathy).

Expectations

With treatment, most patients can achieve a partial or complete remission. In HCV-related Cryovas, the clinical and immunological response is closely related to the viral response.

Long-term outcome is also dependent on the occurrence of complications. Patients with non-HCV-related MC vasculitis have an increased risk of death, primarily due to sepsis, and a fourfold increased risk of developing B-cell non-Hodgkin lymphoma. In HCV-related MC vasculitis, the overall risk of B-cell non-Hodgkin lymphoma is about 35 times higher than in the general population. In the absence of antivirals, these patients are also exposed to HCV chronic infection-induced liver disease, i.e. liver fibrosis, cirrhosis, and hepatocellular carcinoma.

Blood Tests

During treatment, biological improvement can be assessed by the quantification of cryoglobulinemia and other surrogate markers (C4 and CH50 serum levels, rheumatoid factor activity).

In the case of HCV-related MC, the time course of HCV viral load also represents a major predictive factor of long-term outcome.

CONCLUSION

Cryoglobulinemic vasculitis is a heterogeneous disease regarding its etiology and its clinical presentation, ranging from mild to severe and life-threatening manifestations. Hepatitis C virus is now well recognized as the main etiologic agent of mixed Cryovas. Antiviral therapy with should be considered as induction therapy for HCV-Cryovas with mild to moderate disease severity and activity. An early virologic response to antiviral therapy is correlated with a complete clinical response of HCV-Cryovas. In patients presenting with more severe disease (i.e. worsening of renal function, mononeuritis multiplex, extensive skin disease including ulcers and distal necrosis), an immunosuppression induction phase is often necessary while awaiting the generally slow response to antiviral treatments. Combination therapy with rituximab plus an optimal antiviral combination is recommended, as it may target both the downstream B-cell arm of autoimmunity and the viral trigger. In contrast to HCV-related MC, demographical, clinical, and therapeutic data on essential or idiopathic Cryovas are scarce. Idiopathic Cryovas has a poor outcome and an increased risk of developing B-NHL. The use of corticosteroids and immunosuppressant agents is frequently required. Rituximab could represent an interesting alternative therapeutic option, with a particular caution regarding the risk of severe infections.

KEY POINTS

- Cryoglobulinemia vasculitis is a heterogeneous disease regarding its etiology and its clinical presentation, ranging from mild to severe and life-threatening manifestations.
- Mixed cryoglobulinemia (MC) vasculitis may be associated with well-defined immunological, infectious, or neoplastic disorders; when isolated, it

represents a distinct disease, the so-called essential MC. After the discovery of a striking association between MC and hepatitis C virus (HCV) infection, the term "essential" is now used to refer to a minority of patients (<20%).

- The main clinical features of cryoglobulinemic vasculitis are the typical triad—purpura, arthralgias, and weakness. Liver and renal involvement, peripheral neuropathy, skin ulcers, and the possible development of malignancies, mainly B-cell lymphomas, generally as late complication, may also be seen.

- Liver and/or renal involvement, as well as neoplastic complications, may severely affect the overall prognosis of MC. These patients, more often women, aged 50–60 at the time of diagnosis, have a worse prognosis than the general population.

- Hepatitis C virus (HCV) is both a hepatotropic and a lymphotropic virus; it may exert a chronic stimulus on the immune system with both T- and B-lymphocyte alterations. "Benign" B-cell lymphoproliferation is responsible for different autoantibody production, mainly RF and cryoglobulins. Besides cryoglobulinemic vasculitis, HCV may trigger different immune-mediated extrahepatic disorders (thyroiditis, diabetes type II, polyarthritis, glomerulonephritis, porphyria cutanea tarda, sicca syndrome, etc.), as well as some malignancies, mainly B-cell lymphomas.

REFERENCES

1. Damoiseaux J, Cohen Tervaert JW. Diagnostics and treatment of cryoglobulinaemia: it takes two to tango. Clin Rev Allergy Immunol. 2013.
2. Ramos-Casals M, Stone JH, Cid MC, et al. The cryoglobulinaemias. Lancet. 2012;379:348-60.
3. Cacoub P, Poynard T, Ghillani P, et al. Extrahepatic manifestations of chronic hepatitis C. Multivirc group. Multidepartment virus C. Arthritis Rheum. 1999;42:2204-12.
4. Sansonno D, Dammacco F. Hepatitis C virus, cryoglobulinaemia, and vasculitis: immune complex relations. Lancet Infect Dis. 2005;5:227-36.
5. Trejo O, Ramos-Casals M, Garcia-Carrasco M, et al. Cryoglobulinemia: study of etiologic factors and clinical and immunologic features in 443 patients from a single center. Medicine (Baltimore). 2001;80:252-62.
6. Brouet JC, Clauvel JP, Danon F, et al. Biologic and clinical significance of cryoglobulins: a report of 86 cases. Am J Med. 1974;57:775-88.
7. Ferri C, Zignego AL, Pileri SA. Cryoglobulins. J Clin Pathol. 2002;55:4-13.
8. De Vita S, Soldano F, Isola M, et al. Preliminary classification criteria for the cryoglobulinaemic vasculitis. Ann Rheum Dis. 2011;70:1183-90.
9. Ramos-Casals M, Robles A, Brito-Zeron P, et al. Life-threatening cryoglobulinemia: clinical and immunological characterization of 29 cases. Semin Arthritis Rheum. 2006;36:189-96.
10. Misiani R, Bellavita P, Fenili D, et al. Interferon alfa-2a therapy in cryoglobulinemia associated with hepatitis c virus. N Engl J Med. 1994;330:751-6.
11. Liang TJ, Ghany MG. Current and future therapies for hepatitis C virus infection. N Engl J Med. 2013;368:1907-17.

CHAPTER 38

Relapsing Polychondritis

Aman Sharma, Arjun D Law, Kusum Sharma, Rohini Handa

INTRODUCTION

Recurrent inflammation and subsequent destruction of cartilaginous and proteoglycan-containing tissues are the hallmarks of relapsing polychondritis (RP). It was first described in literature in 1923 by the Austrian physician von Jaksch-Wartenhorst who used the term "polychondropathia" to describe this entity.[1] The currently accepted terminology of "relapsing polychondritis" was first employed in a series of 12 patients by Pearson et al. in 1960.[2] Many reports describing the various systemic and organ-specific manifestations of RP have since appeared and there is an ever increasing body of literature.

EPIDEMIOLOGY

Patients typically develop symptoms in the fifth decade of life, with most patients being between 44 and 51 years at the time of diagnosis.[3] Cases have been described at extremes of age as well. The childhood presentation of RP shares many features with the adult form as concluded in a review of 37 pediatric RP patients.[4] Although many studies report an equal gender distribution,[5,6] one study by Trentham and Le[3] showed a 3:1 female preponderance. The racial distribution of RP is controversial. Most data exist for Caucasian populations; however, there is an increasing body of literature from Asia. The clinical features and organ involvement were shown to be different in Caucasian patients as compared to patients of Asian ethnicities in a series of reports. In a case series of southeast Asian patients, the disease course was similar to that in Caucasian patients; however, there were more airway-related complications and a lower incidence of renal, nervous, or cutaneous involvement.[7] The spectrum of clinical manifestations in a series from north India was similar to that seen in Caucasians; however, the incidence of laryngeotracheal involvement was less frequent.[8] A series from southern India reported a lower incidence of auricular and cutaneous involvement.[9] No familial or geographical clustering of cases has been reported to date. One case report exists of the child of an RP patient being born with a saddle nose and self-limiting recurrent arthritis.[10] A study of 25 pregnancies in 11 patients with RP did not reveal any features of RP in the offspring, and the course of the disease was not modified by the pregnancy in any case.[11]

ETIOPATHOGENESIS

No clear etiology has been described for RP. Changes in both cellular and antibody-mediated immune mechanisms may contribute to pathogenesis.

Macrophage migration inhibition and lymphocyte transformation techniques have been used to demonstrate cellular immune reactivity toward cartilage extracts.[12] The presence of T cell clones that have specificity for peptides corresponding to residues 261–273 on the type II collagen molecule has also been described in RP patients.[13] An imbalance of T-lymphocyte subsets and exaggerated cellular responses to cartilage proteoglycans has been described as well.[14]

Tissue deposition of immune complexes as well as the presence of circulating antibodies has been noted in RP patients. This may be directed against major cartilage constituents including collagen type II (native and denatured) as well as collagen types IX and XI.[15] The titers of circulating antibodies to type II collagen have also been shown to correspond to disease activity.[16] These may be seen in 33% of patients with active disease.[17] Autoantibodies to type II collagen have also been detected in patients with other autoimmune diseases such as systemic lupus erythematosus (SLE) and rheumatoid arthritis (RA); however, the epitope specificity may differ in these cases.[18,19] Antibodies directed against the cartilage-specific protein matrilin-1 have also been identified in patients with RP and are likely to be associated with tracheobronchial disease.[20,21]

An association with HLA class II molecules may also be present in RP patients. When compared to controls, increased HLA-R4 antigen frequency was seen in RP patients albeit without a subtype predominance.[22] The extent of organ involvement in RP patients was found to be negatively correlated with HLA-DR6 in a series of 62 cases.[23]

Animal models of RP have been described in experimental studies on mice. These induced forms of RP closely mimic human disease.[24,25]

CLINICAL FEATURES

A characteristic clinical picture and abrupt onset of symptoms are the hallmarks of RP; however, unusual presentations have been described. The onset of the disease is usually abrupt, and there is characteristic clinical picture.

AURICULAR AND VESTIBULAR INVOLVEMENT

Auricular chondritis is seen in most patients and has a characteristic pattern of involvement with inflammatory changes in the cartilaginous portion of the pinna and sparing of the lobule (Figs 38.1A to C). Local signs of inflammation are clearly evident in the affected area, and a tender, swollen,

and red ear is a frequent presenting feature.[26] External ear deformities may occur as a result of cartilage destruction and the pinna may assume a nodular or verrucous appearance or lose shape and become soft and flabby. Subsequently, conductive hearing loss may occur as a result of auricular collapse, external auditory meatus obstruction, eustachian tube dysfunction and edema, and serous otitis media. Stapedial footplate fixation may be present and is surgically correctable.[27] Sensorineural hearing loss and vestibular symptoms such as nausea, vomiting, and ataxia may be seen as a consequence of vestibular inflammation or vasculitic changes of the internal auditory artery.[28-30]

JOINT INVOLVEMENT

Joint pain is the initial presenting symptom in 33% patients with RP and is seen in 50–75% cases over the course of the disease, making it the second most common manifestation.[31] The metacarpophalangeal, proximal interphalangeal, knee, and wrist joints are most commonly affected although any joint may be inflamed. The classic presentation is an episodic, asymmetric, usually migratory, nonerosive and nondeforming polyarthritis or oligoarthritis with or without synovitis that is self-remitting over a period of weeks to months.

NASAL INVOLVEMENT

Sudden onset of pain and tenderness, sometimes with mild epistaxis or serosanguinous exudation, is the usual presenting

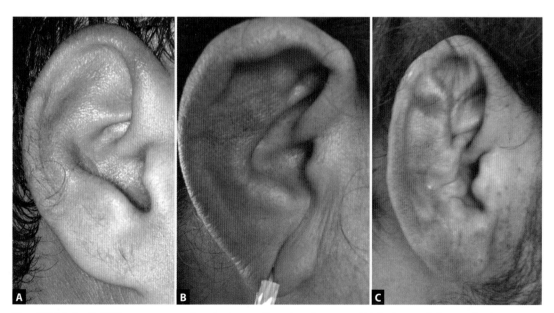

Figs 38.1A to C Different stages of auricular cartilage involvement: (A) Redness of the cartilaginous area characteristically sparing the ear lobule; (B) Thickening and redness of the ear with sparing of lobule in a patient with disease for 3 years; (C) Mutilating involvement of the ear in the later stages after 10 years of illness

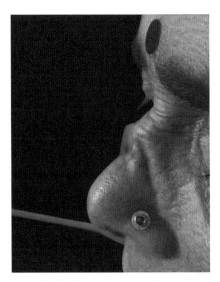

Fig. 38.2 Saddle nose deformity

feature of nasal chondritis.[32] Nasal involvement may be seen at presentation in 24% of cases and is seen in 53% over the course of the disease.[33] Destruction of the cartilaginous portion of the nasal septum may result in flattening of the nasal tip or cause a characteristic nasal bridge "saddle nose" deformity (Fig. 38.2). Such deformities are more frequently observed in females and in patients younger than 50 years of age.[3,6]

RESPIRATORY TRACT INVOLVEMENT

Involvement of the respiratory tract is a major cause of morbidity and mortality in RP, and laryngeotracheal involvement is seen in about 50% of patients.[5] Initial complaints may include local pain and tenderness over the thyroid cartilage and trachea. Hoarseness, nonproductive cough, dyspnea, stridor, and wheezing may occur following inflammation of cartilaginous structures in the larynx and tracheobronchial tree.[5,34] Acute collapse of the upper airway may lead to respiratory distress necessitating emergency tracheostomy. Subglottic stenosis may result following chronic inflammation.[35] Involvement of rib cartilage may result in costochondritis, dislocation, or flail chest.[36] Pulmonary function may be impaired due to airway and chest wall involvement and result in ineffective clearing of airway secretion leading to lung collapse and infection.[37] Respiratory involvement is a leading cause of mortality, and incidence varies from 10% to 50%. Notably, a lower incidence has been reported in north Indian populations.[3,6,8]

CARDIOVASCULAR INVOLVEMENT

Cardiovascular involvement is the second most frequent cause of mortality after respiratory tract involvement in RP patients and is seen in 24–52% patients during the course of the disease.[3,6,38] Any vessel may be affected by vasculitis and the range of clinical manifestations ranges from cutaneous leucocytoclastic vasculitis to involvement of major vessels. Aneurysmal dilatation of the thoracic and abdominal aorta may be seen (Figs 38.3A and B).[39] A case of RP with auricular chondritis and Takayasu arteritis has also been described.[40] Thrombotic complications affecting arterial

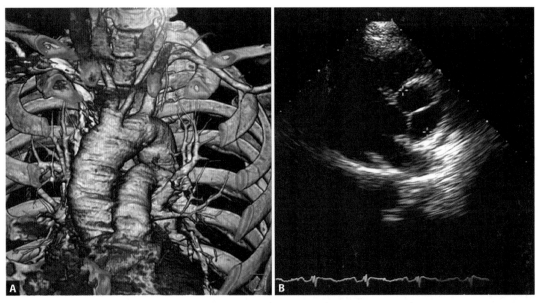

Figs 38.3A and B CT reconstructed and echocardiographic image showing dilatation of aortic root and ascending aorta

and venous circulations have been described in association with the antiphospholipid syndrome as well as secondary to vasculitis.[41,42] Valvular involvement is noted in 5–10% of cases, with aortic regurgitation seen in 4–6% and mitral regurgitation or mitral valve prolapse in 2–4%.[5,6] Electrical rhythm abnormalities may include incidentally detected changes, paroxysmal atrial tachycardia, first-degree heart block, and complete heart block.[6,33,43] Ischemic heart disease secondary to coronary artery vasculitis has been described.[44] Myocarditis, pericarditis, and silent myocardial infarction have also been described.[45-47]

OCULAR INVOLVEMENT

Ocular involvement is frequent and may be seen in over half of all patients with RP during the course of the disease.[3,6] Common manifestations of ocular involvement include scleritis (Fig. 38.4), episcleritis, and conjunctivitis.[5,32,48-51] Ocular adnexal involvement in the form of periorbital edema causing proptosis or extraocular muscle palsy secondary to vasculitis affecting the muscle or its nerve supply may also be seen.[5,48,51] Diffuse anterior scleritis is the most common variant reported although severe necrotizing forms causing globe perforation have also been seen. Uveitis in the form of sclerouveitis or iridocyclitis is seen in upto 25% of patients.[52] Corneal involvement in the form of thinning and ulceration is seen in 10% of patients.[49,50] Severe inflammation causing macropannus formation and corneomalacia have also been described. Retinal involvement,[33] ischemic optic neuropathy,[28] cystoid macular edema, and cataract have also been described, either due to disease activity or as a complication of treatment.

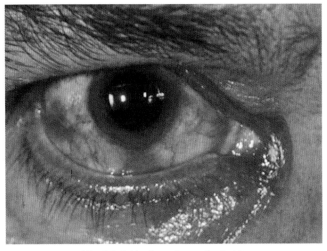

Fig. 38.4 Healing phase of scleritis

NEUROLOGIC INVOLVEMENT

Vasculitis affecting the central or peripheral nervous system is responsible for the neurological manifestations of RP. These include headache, cranial neuropathies, seizures, organic brain syndrome, aseptic meningitis, meningoencephalitis, and cerebral aneurysms.[53] Stroke may be an unusual presenting symptom.[54] Optic neuropathy is the most common type of cranial nerve involvement in RP.[55] Lymphocytic infiltration of the perivascular pia and cerebral white matter was shown in the autopsy of one such case.[56]

RENAL INVOLVEMENT

Renal involvement in RP may be due to the disease process per se or secondary to an associated condition such as systemic vasculitis or SLE.[57-60] Elevated serum creatinine may be seen in 10% of RP cases, and abnormal urinalysis is described in 26%. A mild mesangial expansion and cellular proliferation may be seen on histopathology.[3] Crescentic glomerulonephritis, glomerulosclerosis, tubular loss, IgA nephropathy, and tubulointerstitial nephritis have been described as well.[57] Immunofluorescence studies show mesangial deposits of C3, IgG, or IgM. Any type of lupus nephritis may be seen if concomitant SLE is present. The presence of renal involvement, despite its relative rarity, portends a grave prognosis in RP patients with a reported 10-year survival rate of 10%.[60]

DERMATOLOGICAL INVOLVEMENT

Approximately 35% of patients with RP may have cutaneous lesions that predate the development of chondritis.[61] These nonspecific lesions include purpura, papules, macules, vesicles, bullae, aphthosis, panniculitis, nodules over the extremities, livedo reticularis, and superficial thrombophlebitis.[33] Cutaneous involvement is more frequent in males and may progress independent of other systemic manifestations of RP.[3] Rarely, erythema multiforme and Sweet's syndrome may be presenting features of RP.[62,63] The association of Sweet's syndrome in patients with RP and an associated myelodysplastic syndrome has also been described.[64] The distinct entity, mouth and genital ulcers with inflamed cartilage syndrome represents a unique subset of patients with RP who also have features of Behçet's disease.[65,66]

OTHER SYMPTOMS

Fever, fatigue, weight loss, lethargy, and other constitutional symptoms may be present at diagnosis as well as during flares of the disease. Rarely, fever may be the only presenting feature.[67]

PROGNOSIS

Most patients with RP have a fluctuating course with frequent exacerbations of inflammation. Sites and severity of inflammation rarely remain constant. Many patients experience the persistence of some symptoms in between acute exacerbations. Most deaths in patients with RP occur secondary to infections, airway or cardiovascular involvement, and advanced systemic vasculitis.[6] The overall survival of patients with RP has improved from a dismal 55% at 10 years in 1986 to 94% at 8 years in 1998.[3,5] With better physician and patient awareness in addition to improved management of complications, survival is likely to increase even further.

ASSOCIATED CONDITIONS

Other systemic conditions and, more frequently, autoimmune disorders are present in 25–35% of RP patients.[5] Vasculitis is the most frequently associated condition and is noted in 12–18% cases. The severity may range from mild cutaneous lesions to life-threatening or organ-threatening systemic vasculitis.[3,5] Vasculitis may occur in the context of RP itself or associated with primary vasculitides like polyarteritis nodosa, eosinophilic granulomatosis and polyangiitis (GPA), GPA, or Behçet's disease. Vessels of all sizes may be affected. Large-vessel involvement causing aortic ring dilatation or aneurysmal dilatation of the ascending aorta is common although involvement of the thoracic and abdominal aorta is also seen.[68] Other autoimmune conditions such as SLE,[69] sarcoidosis,[70] and rheumatoid arthritis[71] are known to coexist.

DIAGNOSTIC CRITERIA

Initial diagnostic criteria for RP were developed by McAdam et al. in 1976.[5] In 1979, an expansion of these criteria was suggested by Damiani and Levine.[72] The case series by Michet et al. used a modification of these criteria for inclusion of cases.[6] These criteria are shown in Table 38.1.

The diagnosis may be missed in initial stages due to nonspecific presentations. The mean delay in diagnosis may be as high as 2.9 years.[3]

DIFFERENTIAL DIAGNOSIS

Auricular chondritis can occur with trauma and infection, but sparing of the ear lobule, bilateral involvement, and

Table 38.1 Diagnostic criteria for relapsing polychondritis

Author	Criteria	Requirement
McAdam et al.[5]	Recurrent chondritis of both auricles Nonerosive inflammatory polyarthritis Chondritis of nasal cartilages Inflammation of auricular structures (conjunctivitis/keratitis/scleritis/uveitis) Chondritis of respiratory tract (laryngeal/tracheal cartilages) Cochlear and/or vestibular damage (neurosensory hearing loss/tinnitus/vertigo)	Three of six
Damiani and Levine.[72]	Three of six McAdam et al. criteria One of six McAdam et al. criteria and a positive hostologic confirmation Two of six McAdam et al. criteria and a response to corticosteroid or dapsone	Any of these
Michet et al.[6]	Proven inflammation in two of three auricular, nasal or laryngotracheal cartilages Proven inflammation in one of the above and two other signs among ocular inflammation, hearing loss, vestibular dysfunction or seronegative inflammatory arthritis	Any of these

spontaneous remission tilt the balance in favor of RP, especially in the presence of other associated features. Nasal chondritis and saddle nose need to be differentiated from various infections, congenital syphilis, leprosy, and GPA. When another condition is associated, the clinical picture of RP generally follows the onset of the other disease.

INVESTIGATIONS

The diagnosis of RP is largely based on the clinical features, and the role of laboratory investigations is purely supportive. However, the utility of investigations to rule out other associated conditions must be considered.

Hematological investigations show normocytic–normochromic anemia, leukocytosis, and thrombocytosis. Elevated erythrocyte sedimentation rate, C-reactive protein levels, and polyclonal hypergammaglobulinemia are consistent with an inflammatory state. Urinalysis is usually normal, but patients with renal involvement manifest proteinuria or active sediments that may be accompanied by raised serum creatinine. Cerebrospinal fluid (CSF) analysis may show abnormalities in patients with CNS involvement, especially those with aseptic meningitis. Neutrophilic pleocytosis and reduced glucose levels may mimic the picture of pyogenic meningitis.[73] Antiglutamate receptor epsilon2 (NR2B) autoantibodies have been reported in the CSF and serum of a patient with RP and limbic encephalitis.[74]

Radiographs may reveal calcification of the pinna in cases presenting late. This nonspecific finding is also seen in frost bite, Addison's disease, acromegaly, and ochronosis. In chronic RP, the nasal and tracheal cartilage might also show calcification. Joint radiographs may reveal narrowing of the joint space due to involvement of the articular cartilage, but cysts and erosions are seen rarely.[61] Computed tomography (CT) can identify early laryngotracheal disease or bronchial cartilage involvement. In a recent series, the major abnormal CT findings noted were airway wall thickening, airway stenosis, airway wall calcification, and air trapping. Mediastinal lymph nodes were found in 12 patients.[75] Magnetic resonance imaging (MRI) or spiral CT provides better resolution and also helps to differentiate upper airway disease from vascular involvement. Magnetic resonance imaging of the joints can also help to differentiate the arthropathy of RP from other causes by identifying its characteristic pattern of inflammation affecting the perichondrium and chondroepiphysis preferentially.[76] Positron emission tomography (PET) is a potentially valuable tool in the diagnosis of RP and may also serve to quantify the sites and extent of disease.[77,78] Virtual bronchoscopy can help in the assessment of airway lesions in patients with lung involvement.[79] Pulmonary function testing is abnormal in advanced lower respiratory tract disease. Laryngoscopy and bronchoscopy may be useful but are associated with a risk of exacerbating the inflammation. Endobronchial ultrasonography can reveal soft tissue changes in the tracheobronchial cartilage in the initial stages of the disease.[80] Echocardiography is used to assess the valves and aortic root in patients with suspected cardiovascular involvement.

Histopathological examination of involved cartilage may be useful in occasional patients where the diagnosis is uncertain. However, it is important to remember that no biopsy finding is diagnostic of RP and may contribute to further cartilage damage. Bone scintigraphy usually reveals the increased for uptake of 99m technetium-methylene diphosphonate in the inflamed cartilages and can help locate the site for biopsy.[81] Meticulous sampling of the inflamed perichondral tissue is required for demonstration of the characteristic histologic picture, failing which only nonspecific granulation tissue will be visualized.[3] The initial change is the loss of basophilia in the cartilage matrix, corresponding to loss of matrix proteoglycans. Cellular infiltrates by lymphocytes, neutrophils, and plasma cells are most evident in the cartilage—soft tissue interface, and reduced number of chondrocytes are seen in areas of cartilage destruction.[3]

ASSESSMENT OF DISEASE ACTIVITY

Circulating anticollagen type II antibodies may be present in the acute phase of the disease, and the titers have been found to correlate with disease activity.[82,83] The level of urinary glycosaminoglycans may also be elevated.[84] The levels of urinary collagen type II neoepitope, a specific marker of catabolism of hyaline cartilage rich in type II collagen, have been found to be elevated in active inflammation and can also be used to assess response to treatment.[85] Serum levels of cartilage oligomeric matrix protein were found to be elevated during disease flares in a retrospective study and may be used as a marker of disease activity.[86] Serum levels of soluble triggering receptor expressed on myeloid cells-1 have been found to be potential biomarkers of disease activity in RP patients.[87]

The Relapsing Polychondritis Disease Activity Index (RPDAI) has been developed recently by a worldwide panel of RP experts.[88] The experts rated the physician's global assessment of disease activity (the physician's evaluation of disease activity for a given test case) of the test cases involved in the study who were diagnosed with RP based on Michet's criteria (Table 38.1). This index, which comprises of 27 variables, is a promising step in objective clinical assessment of activity and response to treatment and is yet to be used widely in clinical trials and routine clinical practice.

MANAGEMENT

Management issues in RP are largely related to providing symptomatic care and preventing complications. Due to its rarity, no standard treatment protocols exist for RP. Nonlife-threatening symptoms such as mild auricular or nasal chondritis and arthralgia are generally treated with nonsteroidal anti-inflammatory drugs. Dapsone and colchicine may also be used in these patients. Dapsone in doses of 50–200 mg/day has been advocated as an effective initial therapy in patients without cardiorespiratory involvement,[89-91] but Trentham and Le[3] observed that it was not effective in most patients and resulted in a number of adverse reactions. Organ-threatening diseases, including severe polychondritis, ocular or laryngotracheal involvement, and systemic vasculitis, require rapid treatment with corticosteroids. Oral prednisolone or its equivalent is generally employed in doses of 0.5–1 mg/kg of body weight per day. High-dose steroid therapy or intravenous pulse therapy may be required in severe cases. Doses may be tapered after the acute flare. Many patients require low-dose steroids in between attacks for control of residual symptoms although there are insufficient data to recommend this. Long-term steroid therapy may reduce the frequency and severity of the acute episodes but is not known to affect disease progression or prevent vital organ involvement.[92] Inhalational corticosteroids provide rapid and marked symptomatic relief in patients with obstructive airway disease due to RP. They may also reduce the amount of systemic steroid required for disease control.[93] Oral colchicine and indomethacin have also been proven to be useful in the remission phase in some reports.[94]

Immunosuppressive therapy is often necessary for patients that are unresponsive or intolerant to steroid therapy. Methotrexate, azathioprine, cyclosporine, and chlorambucil may be used in these patients. Trentham and Le observed that methotrexate was the most effective nonsteroid drug in causing symptomatic benefit and reducing the steroid requirement at an average dose of 17.5 mg/week.[3] Minocycline, an antibiotic with immunomodulatory activity, has been used effectively in a patient who was intolerant to methotrexate.[95] Intravenous cyclophosphamide and plasmapheresis are used in patients with life-threatening or organ-threatening disease including acute airway obstruction or glomerulonephritis.[96] Letko et al. report that scleritis is a marker of disease activity and advocate cyclophosphamide as the initial therapy of choice in patients with RP and necrotizing scleritis.[92] They also observed that in patients with diffuse scleritis, methotrexate alone or in combination with steroids was sufficient. Leflunomide has been tried in some patients but data regarding its safety and efficacy in RP are inadequate.[7]

Biological agents are increasingly being used in the management of RP, especially in refractory cases. An anti-CD4 monoclonal antibody was the first biological agent used with some efficacy in RP.[97,98] There are isolated case reports of a favorable response to rituximab in patients not responding to immunosuppressive therapy.[99,100] However, a retrospective study of nine patients treated with rituximab showed that at the end of 12 months of therapy, no patient was in partial or complete remission, even though depletion of B cells was demonstrated.[101] Anti-TNF agents such as infliximab, adalimumab, and etanercept have been used in patients not responding to conventional immunosuppression. There are several reports of infliximab (3–10 mg/kg every 4–8 weeks) being used with good or partial response in improvement of chondritis and respiratory complications.[100,102-106]

Etanercept[107-109] and adalimumab[110,111] have been used in some cases with encouraging responses. Anakinra, the IL-1 receptor antagonist,[112,113] and abatacept, the CTLA4-IgG1 fusion protein,[114] are the other agents that have been utilized. Kawai et al. have reported satisfactory responses to the anti-interleukin-6 receptor antibody, tocilizumab, in two patients with refractory RP.[115] Tocilizumab was also used with gratifying results in a refractory RP patient with cardiovascular involvement.[116] The data for the use of biological agents in RP are mostly in the form of case reports and small series. Larger trials are necessary before any clear consensus can be reached regarding the optimal use of these novel agents.

MANAGEMENT OF COMPLICATIONS AND SEQUELAE

Patients with tracheal stricture or collapse may require stenting or tracheal dilatation by interventional bronchoscopy.[117,118] Silicon T-tubes are an effective treatment measure for preserving airway patency in patients with tracheal stenosis due to the disease.[119] Extensive respiratory involvement may require surgical reconstruction of the laryngotracheal region.[120] Bronchial rupture, tension pneumothorax, and tension pneumoperitoneum may occur due to procedural complications.[121,122] Glottic bamboo nodules may be associated with RP and may be treated with potassium-titanyl-phosphate laser.[123] Cochlear implant surgeries can restore hearing in patients with sensorineural hearing loss.[124] Reconstructive rhinoplasty can correct nasal bridge or septal abnormalities such as the saddle nose deformity.[125] Bone grafting from the iliac crest may be useful for reconstructive surgery, as autologous cartilage harvesting may lead to disease flares at the site of cartilage exposure.[126] In patients with regurgitant valvular lesions requiring valve replacement, recurrent perivalvular regurgitation and valve dehiscence are common due to the dilated aortic root and adjacent inflamed tissue. Sharma et al. reported a case of RP in which aggressive early therapy prevented the progression of aortic regurgitation.[127] In vivo immunoablation in combination with autologous hematopoietic stem cell transplantation has been shown to cause complete remission in a patient with refractory RP.[128] In RP associated with myelodysplastic syndrome, there are isolated case reports of both autologous and allogeneic hematopoietic stem cell transplant resulting in the improvement of symptoms.[129] In a case report of RP associated with hepatitis C virus (HCV) infection, treatment with pegylated interferon and ribavirin resulted in suppression of HCV and remission of difficult-to-treat RP with azathioprine.[130]

KEY POINTS

- Relapsing polychondritis is a rare inflammatory disorder of cartilaginous and proteoglycan rich structures.
- The manifestations vary from mild to life- and organ-threatening complications.
- Rapid diagnosis and initiation of potent immuno-suppressive therapy is important.
- Newer diagnostic modalities such as PET scanning and the use of disease activity scores such as the RPDAI are likely to improve diagnosis and stratification of disease severity.

REFERENCES

1. Jaksch-Wartenhorst R. Polychondropathy. Wien Arch Inn Med. 1923;6:93-100.
2. Pearson CM, Kline HM, Newcomer VD. Relapsing polychondritis. N Engl J Med. 1960;263:51-58.
3. Trentham DE, Le CH. Relapsing polychondritis. Ann Intern Med. 1998;129:114-22.
4. Belot A, Duquesne A, Job-Deslandre C, et al. Pediatric-onset relapsing polychondritis: case series and systematic review. J Pediatr. 2010;156:484-9.
5. McAdam LP, O'Hanlan MA, Bluestone R, et al. Relapsing polychondritis: prospective study of 23 patients and a review of the literature. Medicine (Baltimore). 1976;55:193-215.
6. Michet CJ, Jr., McKenna CH, Luthra HS, et al. Relapsing polychondritis. Survival and predictive role of early disease manifestations. Ann Intern Med. 1986;104:74-78.
7. Kong KO, Vasoo S, Tay NS, et al. Relapsing polychondritis—an oriental case series. Singapore Med J. 2003;44:197-200.
8. Sharma A, Bambery P, Wanchu A, et al. Relapsing polychondritis in north India: a report of 10 patients. Scand J Rheumatol. 2007;36:462-5.
9. Ananthakrishna R, Goel R, Padhan P, et al. Relapsing polychondritis—case series from south India. Clin Rheumatol. 2009;28:S7-10.
10. Arundell FW, Haserick JR. Familial chronic atrophic polychondritis. Arch Dermatol. 1960;82:439-41.
11. Papo T, Wechsler B, Bletry O, et al. Pregnancy in relapsing polychondritis: twenty-five pregnancies in eleven patients. Arthritis Rheum. 1997;40:1245-9.
12. Saxne T, Heinegard D. Serum concentrations of two cartilage matrix proteins reflecting different aspects of cartilage turnover in relapsing polychondritis. Arthritis Rheum. 1995;38:294-6.
13. Buckner JH, Van Landeghen M, Kwok WW, et al. Identification of type II collagen peptide 261-273-specific T cell clones in a patient with relapsing polychondritis. Arthritis Rheum. 2002;46:238-44.
14. Rajapakse DA, Bywaters EG. Cell-mediated immunity to cartilage proteoglycan in relapsing polychondritis. Clin Exp Immunol. 1974;16:497-502.
15. Yang CL, Brinckmann J, Rui HF, et al. Autoantibodies to cartilage collagens in relapsing polychondritis. Arch Dermatol Res. 1993;285:245-9.
16. Giroux L, Paquin F, Guerard-Desjardins MJ, et al. Relapsing polychondritis: an autoimmune disease. Semin Arthritis Rheum. 1983;13:182-7.
17. Foidart JM, Abe S, Martin GR, et al. Antibodies to type II collagen in relapsing polychondritis. N Engl J Med. 1978;299:1203-7.
18. Terato K, Shimozuru Y, Katayama K, et al. Specificity of antibodies to type II collagen in rheumatoid arthritis. Arthritis Rheum. 1990;33:1493-500.
19. Burkhardt H, Koller T, Engstrom A, et al. Epitope-specific recognition of type II collagen by rheumatoid arthritis antibodies is shared with recognition by antibodies that are arthritogenic in collagen-induced arthritis in the mouse. Arthritis Rheum. 2002;46:2339-48.
20. Hansson AS, Heinegard D, Piette JC, et al. The occurrence of autoantibodies to matrilin 1 reflects a tissue-specific response to cartilage of the respiratory tract in patients with relapsing polychondritis. Arthritis Rheum. 2001;44:2402-12.
21. Hansson AS, Johannesson M, Svensson L, et al. Relapsing polychondritis, induced in mice with matrilin 1, is an antibody- and complement-dependent disease. Am J Pathol. 2004;164:959-66.
22. Lang B, Rothenfusser A, Lanchbury JS, et al. Susceptibility to relapsing polychondritis is associated with HLA-DR4. Arthritis Rheum. 1993;36:660-4.
23. Zeuner M, Straub RH, Rauh G, et al. Relapsing polychondritis: clinical and immunogenetic analysis of 62 patients. J Rheumatol. 1997;24:96-101.
24. Taneja V, Griffiths M, Behrens M, et al. Auricular chondritis in NOD.DQ8.Abetao (Ag7-/-) transgenic mice resembles human relapsing polychondritis. J Clin Invest. 2003;112:1843-50.
25. Hansson AS, Heinegard D, Holmdahl R. A new animal model for relapsing polychondritis, induced by cartilage matrix protein (matrilin-1). J Clin Invest. 1999;104:589-98.
26. Sharma A, Bambery P, Wanchu A, et al. A woman with abnormal ears and an unusual voice. Med J Aust. 2007;186:424.
27. Takwoingi YM. Relapsing polychondritis associated with bilateral stapes footplate fixation: a case report. J Med Case Rep. 2009;3:8496.
28. Cody DT, Sones DA. Relapsing polychondritis: audiovestibular manifestations. Laryngoscope. 1971;81:1208-22.
29. Tsuda T, Nakajima A, Baba S, et al. A case of relapsing polychondritis with bilateral sensorineural hearing loss and perforation of the nasal septum at the onset. Mod Rheumatol. 2007;17:148-52.
30. Rampelberg O, Gerard JM, Namias B, et al. ENT manifestations of relapsing polychondritis. Acta Otorhinolaryngol Belg. 1997;51:73-77.
31. Arkin CR, Masi AT. Relapsing polychondritis: review of current status and case report. Semin Arthritis Rheum. 1975;5:41-62.
32. McCaffrey TV, McDonald TJ, McCaffrey LA. Head and neck manifestations of relapsing polychondritis: review of 29 cases. Otolaryngology. 1978;86:ORL473-8.

33. Isaak BL, Liesegang TJ, Michet CJ Jr. Ocular and systemic findings in relapsing polychondritis. Ophthalmology. 1986;93:681-9.

34. Gibson GJ, Davis P. Respiratory complications of relapsing polychondritis. Thorax. 1974;29:726-31.

35. Cansiz H, Yilmaz S, Duman C. Relapsing polychondritis: a case with subglottic stenosis and laryngotracheal reconstruction. J Otolaryngol. 2007;36:E82-84.

36. Lim MC, Chan HL. Relapsing polychondritis—a report on two Chinese patients with severe costal chondritis. Ann Acad Med Singapore. 1990;19:396-403.

37. Mohsenifar Z, Tashkin DP, Carson SA, et al. Pulmonary function in patients with relapsing polychondritis. Chest. 1982;81:711-7.

38. Del Rosso A, Petix NR, Pratesi M, et al. Cardiovascular involvement in relapsing polychondritis. Semin Arthritis Rheum. 1997;26:840-4.

39. Giordano M, Valentini G, Sodano A. Relapsing polychondritis with aortic arch aneurysm and aortic arch syndrome. Rheumatol Int. 1984;4:191-3.

40. Kobak S. Relapsing polychondritis-associated Takayasu's arteritis. Folia Med (Plovdiv). 2009;51:49-52.

41. Empson M, Adelstein S, Garsia R, et al. Relapsing polychondritis presenting with recurrent venous thrombosis in association with anticardiolipin antibody. Lupus. 1998;7:132-4.

42. Quere I, Biron C, Dubois A. Lupus anticoagulant and thrombosis in relapsing polychondritis. J Rheumatol. 1996;23:946-7.

43. Bowness P, Hawley IC, Morris T, et al. Complete heart block and severe aortic incompetence in relapsing polychondritis: clinicopathologic findings. Arthritis Rheum. 1991;34:97-100.

44. Stein JD, Lee P, Kuriya B, et al. Critical coronary artery stenosis and aortitis in a patient with relapsing polychondritis. J Rheumatol. 2008;35:1898-900.

45. Higgins JV, Thanarajasingam U, Osborn TG. A unique case of relapsing polychondritis presenting with acute pericarditis. Case Rep Rheumatol. 2013;2013:287592.

46. Watanabe M, Suzuki H, Ara T, et al. Relapsing polychondritis complicated by giant cell myocarditis and myositis. Intern Med. 2013;52:1397-402.

47. Dolan DL, Lemmon GB, Jr, Teitelbaum SL. Relapsing polychondritis. Analytical literature review and studies on pathogenesis. Am J Med. 1966;41:285-99.

48. Rucker CW, Ferguson RH. Ocular manifesations of relapsing polychondritis. Arch Ophthalmol. 1965;73:46-48.

49. Barth WF, Berson EL. Relapsing polychondritis, rheumatoid arthritis and blindness. Am J Ophthalmol. 1968;66:890-6.

50. Bergaust B, Abrahamsen AM. Relapsing polychondritis. Report of a case presenting multiple ocular complications. Acta Ophthalmol (Copenh). 1969;47:174-81.

51. McKay DA, Watson PG, Lyne AJ. Relapsing polychondritis and eye disease. Br J Ophthalmol. 1974;58:600-5.

52. Matas BR. Iridocyclitis associated with relapsing polychondritis. Arch Ophthalmol. 1970;84:474-6.

53. Willis J, Atack EA, Kraag G. Relapsing polychondritis with multifocal neurological abnormalities. Can J Neurol Sci. 1984;11:402-4.

54. Bouton R, Capon A. Stroke as initial manifestation of relapsing polychondritis. Ital J Neurol Sci. 1994;15:61-63.

55. Killian PJ, Susac J, Lawless OJ. Optic neuropathy in relapsing polychondritis. JAMA. 1978;239:49-50.

56. Imamura E, Yamashita H, Fukuhara T, et al. Autopsy case of perivasculitic meningoencephalitis associated with relapsing polychondritis presenting with central nervous system manifestation. Rinsho Shinkeigaku. 2009;49:172-8.

57. Neild GH, Cameron JS, Lessof MH, et al. Relapsing polychondritis with crescentic glomerulonephritis. Br Med J. 1978;1:743-5.

58. Espinoza LR, Richman A, Bocanegra T, et al. Immune complex-mediated renal involvement in relapsing polychondritis. Am J Med. 1981;71:181-3.

59. Dalal BI, Wallace AC, Slinger RP. IgA nephropathy in relapsing polychondritis. Pathology. 1988;20:85-89.

60. Chang-Miller A, Okamura M, Torres VE, et al. Renal involvement in relapsing polychondritis. Medicine (Baltimore). 1987;66:202-17.

61. Frances C, el Rassi R, Laporte JL, et al. Dermatologic manifestations of relapsing polychondritis. A study of 200 cases at a single center. Medicine (Baltimore). 2001;80:173-9.

62. Jain VK, Arshdeep, Ghosh S. Erythema multiforme: a rare skin manifestation of relapsing polychondritis. Int J Dermatol. 2014; 53(10):1272-4.

63. Astudillo L, Launay F, Lamant L, et al. Sweet's syndrome revealing relapsing polychondritis. Int J Dermatol. 2004;43:720-2.

64. Diamantino Fda E, Raimundo PM, Fidalgo AI. Sweet's Syndrome and relapsing polychondritis signal myelodysplastic syndrome. An Bras Dermatol. 2011;86:S173-7.

65. Firestein GS, Gruber HE, Weisman MH, et al. Mouth and genital ulcers with inflamed cartilage: MAGIC syndrome. Five patients with features of relapsing polychondritis and Behçet's disease. Am J Med. 1985;79:65-72.

66. Orme RL, Nordlund JJ, Barich L, et al. The MAGIC syndrome (mouth and genital ulcers with inflamed cartilage). Arch Dermatol. 1990;126:940-4.

67. Samanta A, McLeod BK, Nichol FE. Relapsing polychondritis: an unusual cause of PUO in an Asian lady. Br J Rheumatol. 1988;27:483-5.

68. Michet CJ. Vasculitis and relapsing polychondritis. Rheum Dis Clin North Am. 1990;16:441-4.

69. Job-Deslandre C, Delrieu F, Delbarre F, et al. Relapsing polychondritis and systemic lupus erythematosus. J Rheumatol. 1983;10:666-8.

70. Pasquet F, Cottin V, Sivova N, et al. Coexisting relapsing polychondritis and sarcoidosis: an unusual association. Rheumatol Int. 2010;30:1507-9.

71. Hussain T, Memon AR, Tauheed S, et al. Relapsing polychondritis associated with rheumatoid arthritis. J Pak Med Assoc. 1995;45:249-50.

72. Damiani JM, Levine HL. Relapsing polychondritis—report of ten cases. Laryngoscope. 1979;89:929-46.

73. Yaguchi H, Tsuzaka K, Niino M, et al. Aseptic meningitis with relapsing polychondritis mimicking bacterial meningitis. Intern Med. 2009;48:1841-4.

74. Kashihara K, Kawada S, Takahashi Y. Autoantibodies to glutamate receptor GluRepsilon2 in a patient with limbic

encephalitis associated with relapsing polychondritis. J Neurol Sci. 2009;287:275-7.

75. Lin ZQ, Xu JR, Chen JJ, et al. Pulmonary CT findings in relapsing polychondritis. Acta Radiol. 2010;51:522-6.

76. Rohena-Quinquilla IR, Mullens F, Chung EM. MR findings in the arthropathy of relapsing polychondritis. Pediatr Radiol. 2013;43:1221-6.

77. Yamashita H, Takahashi H, Kubota K, et al. Utility of fluorodeoxyglucose positron emission tomography/computed tomography for early diagnosis and evaluation of disease activity of relapsing polychondritis: a case series and literature review. Rheumatology (Oxford). 2014;53:1482-90.

78. Honne K, Nagashima T, Onishi S, et al. Fluorodeoxyglucose positron emission tomography/computed tomography for diagnostic imaging in relapsing polychondritis with atypical manifestations. J Clin Rheumatol. 2013;19:104-5.

79. Yasutake T, Nakamoto K, Ohta A, et al. Assessment of airway lesions using "virtual bronchoscopy" in a patient with relapsing polychondritis. Nihon Kokyuki Gakkai Zasshi. 2010;48:86-91.

80. Miyazu Y, Miyazawa T, Kurimoto N, et al. Endobronchial ultrasonography in the diagnosis and treatment of relapsing polychondritis with tracheobronchial malacia. Chest. 2003;124:2393-5.

81. Imanishi Y, Mitogawa Y, Takizawa M, et al. Relapsing polychondritis diagnosed by Tc-99m MDP bone scintigraphy. Clin Nucl Med. 1999;24:511-3.

82. Alsalameh S, Mollenhauer J, Scheuplein F, et al. Preferential cellular and humoral immune reactivities to native and denatured collagen types IX and XI in a patient with fatal relapsing polychondritis. J Rheumatol. 1993;20:1419-24.

83. Buckner JH, Wu JJ, Reife RA, et al. Autoreactivity against matrilin-1 in a patient with relapsing polychondritis. Arthritis Rheum. 2000;43:939-43.

84. Passos CO, Onofre GR, Martins RC, et al. Composition of urinary glycosaminoglycans in a patient with relapsing polychondritis. Clin Biochem. 2002;35:377-81.

85. Kraus VB, Stabler T, Le ET, et al. Urinary type II collagen neoepitope as an outcome measure for relapsing polychondritis. Arthritis Rheum. 2003;48:2942-8.

86. Kempta Lekpa F, Piette JC, Bastuji-Garin S, et al. Serum cartilage oligomeric matrix protein (COMP) level is a marker of disease activity in relapsing polychondritis. Clin Exp Rheumatol. 2010;28:553-5.

87. Sato T, Yamano Y, Tomaru U, et al. Serum level of soluble triggering receptor expressed on myeloid cells-1 as a biomarker of disease activity in relapsing polychondritis. Mod Rheumatol. 2014;24:129-36.

88. Arnaud L, Devilliers H, Peng SL, et al. The relapsing polychondritis disease activity index: development of a disease activity score for relapsing polychondritis. Autoimmun Rev. 2012;12:204-9.

89. Barranco VP, Minor DB, Soloman H. Treatment of relapsing polychondritis with dapsone. Arch Dermatol. 1976;112:1286-8.

90. Martin J, Roenigk HH, Lynch W, et al. Relapsing polychondritis treated with dapsone. Arch Dermatol. 1976;112:1272-4.

91. Ridgway HB, Hansotia PL, Schorr WF. Relapsing polychondritis: unusual neurological findings and therapeutic efficacy of dapsone. Arch Dermatol. 1979;115:43-45.

92. Letko E, Zafirakis P, Baltatzis S, et al. Relapsing polychondritis: a clinical review. Semin Arthritis Rheum. 2002;31:384-95.

93. Tsuburai T, Suzuki M, Tsurikisawa N, et al. Use of inhaled fluticasone propionate to control respiratory manifestations of relapsing polychondritis. Respirology. 2009;14:299-301.

94. Mark KA, Franks AG Jr. Colchicine and indomethacin for the treatment of relapsing polychondritis. J Am Acad Dermatol. 2002;46:S22-24.

95. Trentham DE, Dynesius-Trentham RA. Antibiotic therapy for rheumatoid arthritis. Scientific and anecdotal appraisals. Rheum Dis Clin North Am. 1995;21:817-34.

96. Botey A, Navasa M, del Olmo A, et al. Relapsing polychondritis with segmental necrotizing glomerulonephritis. Am J Nephrol. 1984;4:375-8.

97. Choy EH, Chikanza IC, Kingsley GH, et al. Chimaeric anti-CD4 monoclonal antibody for relapsing polychondritis. Lancet. 1991;338:450.

98. van der Lubbe PA, Miltenburg AM, Breedveld FC. Anti-CD4 monoclonal antibody for relapsing polychondritis. Lancet. 1991;337:1349.

99. McCarthy EM, Cunnane G. Treatment of relapsing polychondritis in the era of biological agents. Rheumatol Int. 2010;30:827-8.

100. Ratzinger G, Kuen-Spiegl M, Sepp N. Successful treatment of recalcitrant relapsing polychondritis with monoclonal antibodies. J Eur Acad Dermatol Venereol. 2009;23:474-5.

101. Leroux G, Costedoat-Chalumeau N, Brihaye B, et al. Treatment of relapsing polychondritis with rituximab: a retrospective study of nine patients. Arthritis Rheum. 2009;61:577-82.

102. Mpofu S, Estrach C, Curtis J, et al. Treatment of respiratory complications in recalcitrant relapsing polychondritis with infliximab. Rheumatology (Oxford). 2003;42:1117-8.

103. Saadoun D, Deslandre CJ, Allanore Y, et al. Sustained response to infliximab in 2 patients with refractory relapsing polychondritis. J Rheumatol. 2003;30:1394-5.

104. Jabbarvand M, Fard MA. Infliximab in a patient with refractory necrotizing scleritis associated with relapsing polychondritis. Ocul Immunol Inflamm. 2010;18:216-7.

105. Marie I, Lahaxe L, Josse S, et al. Sustained response to infliximab in a patient with relapsing polychondritis with aortic involvement. Rheumatology (Oxford). 2009;48:1328-9.

106. Richez C, Dumoulin C, Coutouly X, et al. Successful treatment of relapsing polychondritis with infliximab. Clin Exp Rheumatol. 2004;22:629-31.

107. Schrader C, Lohmann J. Successful therapy with etanercept in relapsing polychondritis. Z Rheumatol. 2010;69:356-8.

108. Subrahmanyam P, Balakrishnan C, Dasgupta B. Sustained response to etanercept after failing infliximab, in a patient with relapsing polychondritis with tracheomalacia. Scand J Rheumatol. 2008;37:239-40.

109. Carter JD. Treatment of relapsing polychondritis with a TNF antagonist. J Rheumatol. 2005;32:1413.

110. Seymour MW, Home DM, Williams RO, et al. Prolonged response to anti-tumour necrosis factor treatment with adalimumab (Humira) in relapsing polychondritis complicated by aortitis. Rheumatology (Oxford). 2007;46:1738-9.

111. Lahmer T, Knopf A, Treiber M, et al. Treatment of relapsing polychondritis with the TNF-alpha antagonist adalimumab. Clin Rheumatol. 2010;29:1331-4.

112. Vounotrypidis P, Sakellariou GT, Zisopoulos D, et al. Refractory relapsing polychondritis: rapid and sustained response in the treatment with an IL-1 receptor antagonist (anakinra). Rheumatology (Oxford). 2006;45:491-2.

113. Buonuomo PS, Bracaglia C, Campana A, et al. Relapsing polychondritis: new therapeutic strategies with biological agents. Rheumatol Int. 2010;30:691-3.

114. Moulis G, Sailler L, Astudillo L, et al. Abatacept for relapsing polychondritis. Rheumatology (Oxford). 2010;49:1019.

115. Kawai M, Hagihara K, Hirano T, et al. Sustained response to tocilizumab, anti-interleukin-6 receptor antibody, in two patients with refractory relapsing polychondritis. Rheumatology (Oxford). 2009;48:318-9.

116. Stael R, Smith V, Wittoek R, et al. Sustained response to tocilizumab in a patient with relapsing polychondritis with aortic involvement: a case based review. Clin Rheumatol. 2014 (May).

117. Mendez-Flores S, Vera-Lastra O, Osnaya-Juarez J. Tracheal stenosis as a initial manifestation of relapsing polychondritis. Case report. Rev Med Inst Mex Seguro Soc. 2009;47:673-6.

118. Faul JL, Kee ST, Rizk NW. Endobronchial stenting for severe airway obstruction in relapsing polychondritis. Chest. 1999;116:825-7.

119. Nakayama T, Horinouchi H, Asakura K, et al. Tracheal stenosis due to relapsing polychondritis managed for 16 years with a silicon T-tube covering the entire trachea. Ann Thorac Surg. 2011;92:1126-8.

120. Karaman E, Duman C, Cansz H, et al. Laryngotracheal reconstruction at relapsing polychondritis. J Craniofac Surg. 2010;21:211-2.

121. Lin YT, Zuo Z, Lo PH, et al. Bilateral tension pneumothorax and tension pneumoperitoneum secondary to tracheal tear in a patient with relapsing polychondritis. J Chin Med Assoc. 2009;72:488-91.

122. Chapron J, Wermert D, Le Pimpec-Barthes F, et al. Bronchial rupture related to endobronchial stenting in relapsing polychondritis. Eur Respir Rev. 2012;21:367-9.

123. Childs LF, Rickert S, Wengerman OC, et al. Laryngeal manifestations of relapsing polychondritis and a novel treatment option. J Voice. 2012;26:587-9.

124. Seo YJ, Choi JY, Kim SH, et al. Cochlear implantation in a bilateral sensorineural hearing loss patient with relapsing polychondritis. Rheumatol Int. 2012;32:479-82.

125. Tobisawa Y, Shibata M. A case of saddle nose deformity caused by relapsing polychondritis: a long-term follow-up report after iliac bone grafting. J Plast Reconstr Aesthet Surg. 2013;66:1621-2.

126. Haug MD, Witt P, Kalbermatten FD, et al. Severe respiratory dysfunction in a patient with relapsing polychondritis: should we treat the saddle nose deformity? J Plast Reconstr Aesthet Surg. 2009;62:e7-10.

127. Sharma A, Mittal T, Kumar S, et al. Successful treatment of aortic root dilatation in a patient with relapsing polychondritis. Clin Rheumatol. 2013;32:S59-61.

128. Rosen O, Thiel A, Massenkeil G, et al. Autologous stem-cell transplantation in refractory autoimmune diseases after in vivo immunoablation and ex vivo depletion of mononuclear cells. Arthritis Res. 2000;2:327-36.

129. Tomomatsu J, Hamano Y, Ando J, et al. Non-myeloablative allogenic BMT for myelodysplastic syndrome successfully controlled accompanying relapsing polychondritis. Bone Marrow Transplant. 2012;47:742-3.

130. Hemmati I, Yoshida E, Shojania K. Relapsing polychondritis associated with hepatitis C virus infection. Clin Rheumatol. 2012;31:391-4.

CHAPTER 39

IgG4 Disease

M Vishnu Vardhan Reddy

INTRODUCTION

Immunoglobulin (Ig) G4-related disease is a novel systemic fibroinflammatory and clinical entity characterized by a tendency to form tumefactive mass lesions, frequent elevations in serum IgG4, unique histopathology, and striking response to glucocorticoids.[1]

The disease was recognized as a systemic condition in 2003, when extrapancreatic manifestations were identified in patients with autoimmune pancreatitis. Although initially recognized in Japan, it is now being increasingly reported from other parts of the world.

How Concept of IgG4-RSD Had Evolved?

The IgG4 concept is analogous to sarcoidosis, in that it affects virtually all organ systems, unified by a distinctive histologic appearance regardless of the organ involved.[2]

This concept is framed based on four major observations:

1. Identification of autoimmune pancreatitis in early to mid-1990s.
2. Elevations in the serum IgG4 concentration in autoimmune pancreatitis.
3. Similarity of histopathologic findings across a spectrum of organ systems infiltrated by IgG4-bearing plasma cells.
4. The frequent co-occurrence of similar disease processes within at least two organs of the same patient.

Immunoglobulin G4-related systemic disease (IgG4-RSD) spectrum unified a large number of eponymic diagnoses known for decades previously thought to be confined to single-organ systems (Table 39.1).

The nomenclature for IgG4-RD continues to evolve.[3] However, the ubiquity of IgG4 positive plasma cells within involved organs led to the present acceptance of the term "IgG4-related disease" as the name of the disease (Table 39.2).

Table 39.1 Eponymic conditions that comprise (or may comprise) parts of the IgG4-RD spectrum

- Mikulicz's disease
- Kuttner tumor
- Riedel thyroiditis
- Eosinophilic angiocentric fibrosis
- Multifocal fibrosclerosis
- Lymphoplasmacytic sclerosing pancreatitis/autoimmune pancreatitis
- Inflammatory pseudotumor
- Fibrosing mediastinitis
- Sclerosing mesenteritis
- Retroperitoneal fibrosis (Ormond disease)
- Periaortitis/periarteritis
- Inflammatory aortic aneurysm
- Cutaneous pseudolymphoma
- Idiopathic hypertrophic pachymeningitis
- Idiopathic tubulointerstitial nephritis
- Idiopathic hypocomplementemic tubulointerstitial nephritis
- With extensive tubulointerstitial deposits
- Idiopathic cervical fibrosis

Abbreviations: IgG4-RD, immunoglobulin G4-related disease.

Table 39.2 Different names employed to refer to IgG4-related disease

- IgG4-related autoimmune disease
- IgG4-associated multifocal systemic fibrosis
- IgG4-related sclerosing disease
- IgG4-related systemic disease
- IgG4 syndrome
- Hyper-IgG4 disease
- IgG4-related multiorgan lymphoproliferative syndrome
- Systemic IgG4-plasmacytic syndrome
- IgG4-related disease

The spectrum of IgG4-RD includes diseases that are as follows:

- Immune-mediated
- Fibroinflammatory
- Often tumefactive (responsible for pseudotumor lesions and/or focal inflammation)
- Likely to cause organ dysfunction and failure if inadequately treated.

As IgG4-RD affects various organs, its clinical symptoms vary, and each patient with IgG4-RD may visit specialists addressing organ-specific lesions. This review aims to provide the rheumatologist with a set of practical guidelines for the diagnosis and management of IgG4-RD, and also addresses the many controversies associated with this disease (Table 39.3).

EPIDEMIOLOGY

Unlike other autoimmune diseases, most IgG4-RSD patients are male (60–80%) and older than 50 years of age. However, for IgG4-related dacryoadenitis and sialadenitis the gender ratio is almost equal.

Virtually all studies pertaining to the epidemiology of the disease come from Japan and Asia and focus on autoimmune pancreatitis. The estimated prevalence of autoimmune pancreatitis is 0.8 cases per 100,000 persons in Japan, where this disorder is believed to account for up to 6% of all cases of chronic pancreatitis.

PATHOGENESIS

IgG4 Antibody

Immunoglobulin G4 is the least abundant subclass, representing about 5% of total IgG in serum of healthy adults (0.5 g/L, normal range: 0.05–1.4 g/L). However, IgG4 antibody can represent up to 80% of total IgG antibody after chronic exposure to antigen. In addition, 3–7% of healthy population have elevated serum IgG4 levels, but rarely they have more than two times above the upper limit of normal.

Why IgG4 Antibodies are Counterinflammatory?

Immunoglobulin G4 antibodies undergo half-antibody exchange *in vivo* resulting in bispecific and functionally monovalent antibodies with two different Fab arms. Since these antibodies can only bind to antigen with one Fab arm, they cannot cross-link antigens and are unable to form

Table 39.3 Spectrum of IgG4-RSD and its mimics

Organ	IgG4-RSD	Mimics
Pancreas	AIP—autoimmune pancreatitis	Carcinoma pancreas, chronic pancreatitis
Submandibular glands	Kuttner tumor	Sjögren's syndrome, lymphoma, sarcoidosis
Orbits	Eosinophilic angiocentric fibrosis	Lymphoma
Eyes	Chronic sclerosing dacryoadenitis	Sjögren's syndrome, lymphoma, sarcoidosis
Mediastinum	Mediastinal fibrosis	Tuberculosis, histoplasmosis, drug-induced fibrosis
Aorta	Inflammatory aortic aneurysm	Takayasu's arteritis, Behçet's disease, atherosclerotic
Retroperitoneum	Retroperitoneal fibrosis	Idiopathic fibrosis, malignancy-related fibrosis
Breast	Sclerosing mastitis	Carcinoma beast
CNS	Infundibular hypophysitis, hypertrophic pachymeningitis, intracerebral pseudotumor	Rheumatoid arthritis vasculitis, sarcoidosis
Heart	Pericarditis (sometimes constrictive)	—
Lung	Inflammatory pseudotumor Interstitial pneumonia	Interstitial lung disease, metastases, sarcoidosis, infectious pneumonia
Bile ducts	Sclerosing cholangitis	Primary sclerosing cholangitis
Thyroid	Reidel's thyroiditis and Hashimoto thyroiditis	Anaplastic thyroid carcinoma
Kidney	Tubulointerstitial nephritis, inflammatory pseudotumor	Renal cell carcinoma, pyelonephritis
Prostate	Prostatitis	BPH
Lymph node	Lymphadenopathy	Castleman's disease, lymphoma

Abbreviations: IgG4-RSD, immunoglobulin G4-related systemic disease.

large-immune complexes. Also IgG4 have low affinity for C1q and Fc receptors.

Pathophysiological Mechanisms

Why High Fibrosis?

Autoimmunity and infectious agents are potential immunologic triggers in IgG4-RD. Immunoglobulin G4 production is controlled primarily by T helper 2 (Th 2) cells. T helper 2 cytokines interleukin-4 (IL-4) and IL-13 enhance the production of IgG4 and IgE. However, regulatory T (T reg) cells derived cytokines IL-10, IL-12, and IL-21 shift the balance between IgG4 and IgE, favoring IgG4. Thus, selective IgG4 induction is referred to as the combined effect of Th 2 and T reg cells (Fig. 39.1).

It remains to be clarified whether the IgG4 hypergammaglobulinemia and IgG4+ plasma cell infiltration into involved organs are pathogenic or just "innocent bystanders". So far, convincing support for the hypothesis that (auto-) antibody activity of IgG4 is driving the pathology is lacking.

Although several candidate autoantibodies were described that were directed against pancreatic trypsin inhibitor, lactoferrin, and carbonic anhydrase, mainly in patients with pancreatic involvement, they were mostly not of the IgG4 subclass.

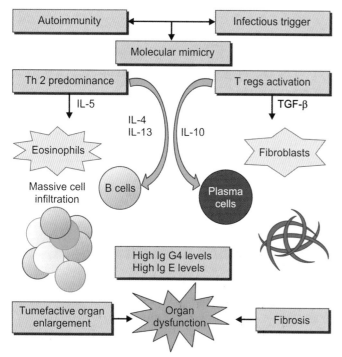

Fig. 39.1 Pathogenetic mechanisms in immunoglobulin G4-related disease

DIAGNOSIS

In order to diagnose IgG4-RD by excluding its mimics, it is critical to have a collaboration between the pathologist and the treating physician.

- *Serology findings:* Polyclonal hypergammaglobulinemia, elevated serum IgE, and hypocomplementemia. Sometimes low titer positivity for antinuclear antibody, rheumatoid factor, normal C-reactive protein, erythrocyte sedimentation rate, and normal LDH.

- *Serum IgG4:* A serum IgG4 >135 mg/dL has been widely accepted as a cutoff value for diagnosis of IgG4-RD. In patients with multiple organ involvement, the polyclonal serum IgG4 can be elevated up to 5–50 times the upper limit of normal.

Some of the queries related to IgG4 are as follows:

- Can IgG4 level be normal in a biopsy proved case of IgG4-RSD?

  Yes. And the reasons are as follows:

  - *Truly negative:* Approximately 20–40% of patients with biopsy-proven IgG4-RD have normal serum IgG4 concentrations at the time of diagnosis, even before the institution of therapy.

  - *False negative:* Prozone phenomenon *(hook effect)*—in the presence of very high levels of IgG4, serum assays using nephelometry, and radial immunodiffusion underestimate serum IgG4 level. The prozone phenomenon should be considered when the serum IgG4 appears discordant with the clinician's assessment of disease activity.

- Can we use serial measurement of serum IgG4 levels for disease activity follow-up?

  Serum concentrations of IgG4 are unreliable as diagnostic markers of IgG4-RD, as indicators of disease activity, and as measures of response to treatment. Although they become lower with treatment, they still remain above baseline in many patients. Serum IgG4 can be elevated despite disease remission.

- Can serum IgG4 levels predict relapse?

  Monitoring will help to identify some patients who relapse. Only one-third patients with persistent elevated IgG4 levels will relapse. However, in 10% of patients the disease will relapse despite normal serum IgG4 levels.

- Which conditions other than IgG4-RSD have elevated serum IgG4 levels?

  - Chronic antigenic exposure like bee keepers
  - Human filariasis
  - Atopic dermatitis
  - Pemphigus vulgaris, and pemphigus foliaceus
  - Carcinoma pancreas.

Multiple non-IgG4-RD conditions are associated with elevated serum IgG4, leading to poor specificity and low positive predictive value for this test.

Neither doubling the cut-off for serum IgG4 nor examining the serum IgG4/IgG ratio improves the overall test characteristics for the diagnosis of IgG4-RD.

HISTOPATHOLOGICAL FEATURES OF IgG4-RELATED DISEASE

The sine qua non of the diagnosis is increased numbers of infiltrating IgG4-bearing plasma cells within involved organs.

The three major histopathological features associated with IgG4-RD are as follows:
1. Dense lymphoplasmacytic infiltrate.
2. Fibrosis, arranged at least focally in a storiform pattern.
3. Obliterative phlebitis.

Other histopathological features associated with IgG4-RD are:
- Phlebitis without obliteration of the lumen
- Increased numbers of eosinophils.

Histopathological features inconsistent with IgG4-RSD are as follows:
- Epithelioid cell granulomas
- Prominent neutrophilic infiltrate.

The severity of fibrosis is dependent on the individual organs involved. For example, storiform fibrosis a characteristic of IgG4-related autoimmune pancreatitis is seldom found in patients with IgG4-related Mikulicz's disease and IgG4-related lymphadenopathy.

QUANTITATIVE ASSESSMENT OF THE IgG4 STAIN

Immunoglobulin G4 immunostaining is an essential test for the pathological diagnosis of IgG4-RD especially in cases with normal levels of serum IgG4. The cutoff points, proposed vary from more than 10 to more than 200 IgG4-positive plasma cells per high-power field. However, the appropriate cutoff point differs from organ to organ because of the predominance of fibrosis at the time of diagnosis. For example, the cutoff for pancreas is > 10 and for lacrimal gland it is >200 IgG4 plasma cells per HPF.

The IgG4-to-IgG Ratio

By virtue of abundance of plasma cells, some inflammatory lesions even that are not IgG4-RD are associated with high numbers of IgG4 plasma cells.

To circumvent this caveat, the IgG4+/IgG-positive plasma cell ratio is proposed and considered more powerful tool than IgG4-positive plasma cell counts in establishing the diagnosis of IgG4-RD.

The Japanese Ministry of Health, Labour, and Welfare's 2011 guidelines adopted IgG4+/IgG+ plasma cell ratio >40% as a mandatory criterion for histological diagnosis of IgG4-RD.[4]

However, the same caveat that applies to IgG4 cell count also applies to IgG4/IgG-plasma cell ratio in that some immune mediated conditions associated with elevated serum interleukin-6 (IL-6) concentrations like multicentric Castleman's disease, rheumatoid arthritis, have abundant IgG4 + plasma cells within tissue (IgG4+/IgG+ plasma cell ratio>40%) and elevated serum IgG4 concentrations.

Isolated finding of elevated IgG4 positive cells or high IgG4/IgG ratio is not diagnostic of IgG4-RSD. Not every entity with increased IgG4 + plasma cells and a high IgG4/IgG ratio can be accepted as belonging to the spectrum of IgG4-RSD. A recent consensus statement on the pathology of IgG4-related disease emphasizes that certain light microscopy features, particularly storiform fibrosis, obliterative phlebitis, mild-to-moderate eosinophilia, and germinal center formation, and an appropriate clinical context are mandatory for diagnosis (Table 39.4).[5]

However, none of these conditions consistently shows IgG4-rich inflammation and all lack the characteristic histopathological features of IgG4-RD.

Malignancies and IgG4

Cancer tissue can be infiltrated by IgG4-positive plasma cells to various degrees.

Always low-grade B-cell lymphomas must be excluded in cases of possible IgG4-RD with florid lymphoplasmacytic infiltrates, especially if the plasma cells exhibit atypical features such as prominent nuclear or cytoplasmic inclusions.

However, plasma cell infiltration in malignant tissue is usually patchy, and not associated with other typical

Table 39.4 NonIgG4-related systemic disease conditions with elevated IgG4-positive cells

Multicentric Castleman's disease	ANCA-associated vasculitis
Rosai-Dorfman disease	Rheumatoid arthritis
Biliary xanthogranulomatous inflammation	Primary sclerosing cholangitis
	Inflammatory bowel disease
Cutaneous plasmacytosis	Pulmonary abscess
Autoimmune atrophic gastritis (pernicious anemia)	Oral inflammatory diseases

histological features of IgG4-RD (e.g. storiform fibrosis or obliterative phlebitis).

The lymphomas that can mimic IgG4-RD are extranodal marginal zone lymphomas, follicular lymphomas, and angioimmunoblastic lymphomas.

Occasionally peritumoral tissue rich in IgG4-positive plasma cells can mimic IgG4-RD. Thus, a needle biopsy sampling the periphery of a malignant neoplasm may be misdiagnosed as IgG4-RD. So to avoid this diagnostic pitfall, it is usually appropriate to obtain more tissue.

To make matters more confusing, IgG4-producing lymphoma also exists!

What we do not know at this time is whether cases reported as synchronous carcinoma and IgG4-RD represents a true association or nonspecific pericancerous IgG4 reaction.

Role of 18 F-FDG PET/CT

Fluorodeoxyglucose positron emission tomography computed tomography (18F-FDG PET/CT) provides metabolic information of the whole body in one scan. It helps to evaluate the systemic inflammatory disease and reflect the involvements in each organ and the activity in each lesion.

Advantages of PET/CT

*   Fluorodeoxyglucose positron emission tomography computed tomography identifies more lesions than conventional imaging by MRI/CT. Many patients thought to have single-organ disease on conventional imaging will be identified to harbor multiorgan involvement after a PET/CT.
*   It helps in selection of a minimal and adequate biopsy site in those with multiple lesions but without functional preference.
*   Helps to detect asymptomatic involvement that might lead to severe complications at the early stage like aortitis and retroperitoneal fibrosis.

IMAGE CHARACTERISTICS SUGGESTIVE OF IgG4-RELATED DISEASE ON 18 F-FDG PET/CT

*   Evenly, symmetrically distributed 18 F-FDG uptake in the salivary glands without signs of infection.
*   Diffusely enlarged pancreas with moderate to intense 18 F-FDG uptake without pancreaticobiliary duct obstruction.
*   Patchy thickness of aorta wall with moderate to intense 18 F-FDG uptake not limited to the vascular intima.

*   Patchy retroperitoneal lesion with moderate to intense 18 F-FDG uptakes.
*   The 18 F-FDG-avid lesions have more than 80% decrease of activity after 2–4 weeks of steroid-based treatment at a dosage of 40–50 mg prednisone per day.

Note:
*   FDG-PET is not a useful identifying renal involvement, because accumulation of radioisotope, which is excreted via the kidneys, is physiologically detected in normal kidneys.
*   Accumulation of FDG at sites atypical for IgG4-RD is strongly suggestive of underlying cancers.

Clinical Features

Clinical symptoms are relatively mild and vary depending on the affected organ. Swollen but painless organs are characteristic of IgG4-RD. However, some patients may experience serious complications, such as obstruction or compression symptoms due to organomegaly or hypertrophy, and organ dysfunction caused by cellular infiltration or fibrosis. Constitutional symptoms such as fever are unusual.

It is one of the few autoimmune conditions which predominantly affect male subjects in the fifth and sixth decades of life.

The organ involvement is two types in a given patient, either single or multiple (Flow chart 39.1). The lesions can be present simultaneously or arise metachronously.

Synchronous Lesions

Lesions at multiple sites at same time.

Metachronous Lesions

Lesions at a single site with a probable history of IgG4-RD at another site. For example, now patient has lacrimal gland swelling, however, sometime in the past had autoimmune pancreatitis.

Flow chart 39.1 Pattern of organ Involvement in immunoglobulin G4-related systemic disease

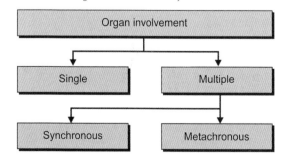

Diagnostic Approach

As clinical symptoms and pathological features depend on lesion location, it is probably impossible to establish criteria that include all patients with IgG4-RD.

The diagnosis of IgG4-RD is based on a combination of features that include clinical, imaging, serologic, histology, and immunohistochemistry. The gold standard for the diagnosis of IgG4-RD is histopathology. Guidelines for the pathologic diagnosis of this condition have been published by an international group of experts.

There are two types of criteria that have been defined for IgG4-RSD in Japanese populations:
1. Organ-specific criteria for autoimmune pancreas (AIP), MD, KD.
2. Comprehensive clinical-diagnostic criteria.

The organ-specific criteria are not suitable for diagnosing patients with other involved organs, and are not familiar to general clinicians and nonspecialists.

Comprehensive diagnostic criteria for IgG4-RD, including the involvement of various organs, are intended for the practical use of general physicians and nonspecialists.

It is appropriate to use, the comprehensive diagnostic criteria, concurrently with organ-specific diagnostic criteria to increase the sensitivity of these criteria.

The criteria that classify the disease in other populations are not available at present.

Comprehensive Clinical Diagnostic Criteria for IgG4-RD

- Clinical examination showing characteristic diffuse/localized swelling or masses in single or multiple organs (Flow chart 39.2).
- Hematological examination shows elevated serum IgG4 concentrations (> 135 mg/dL).
- Histopathologic examination shows
  – Marked lymphocyte and plasmacytic infiltration and fibrosis.
  – *Infiltration of IgG4+ plasma cells:* Ratio of IgG4+/IgG+ cells > 40% and >10 IgG4 + plasma cells/HPF.
  Definite: 1) + 2) + 3)
  Probable: 1) + 3)
  Possible: 1) + 2)

Conditions to be Excluded or Differentiated
- Malignancies (e.g. cancer, lymphoma) in involved organs.
- Similar diseases—Sjögren's syndrome, primary sclerosing cholangitis, multicentric Castleman's disease, idiopathic retroperitoneal fibrosis, Granulomatosis with polyangiitis

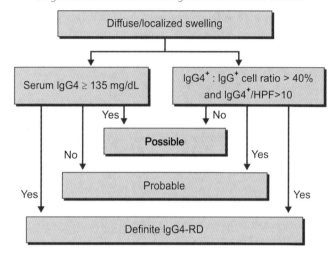

Flow chart 39.2 Diagnostic algorithm for comprehensive diagnostic criteria for immunoglobulin G4-related disease

(GPA) (Wegener's granulomatosis), sarcoidosis, and Eosinophilic GPA (Churg-Strauss syndrome).

Two great mimics of Ig4-RSD and even fulfill diagnostic criteria for IgG4-RSD:
1. Multicentric Castleman's disease.
2. GPA involving head and neck regions.

PANCREAS

Type 1 AIP (autoimmune pancreas) is regarded as a prototypical organ manifestation of IgG4-RD, which can occur alone or either simultaneously or metachronously with other organ complications. This disease is synonymous with IgG4-related sclerosing pancreatitis/lymphoplasmacytic sclerosing pancreatitis. Obstructive jaundice is the most common presenting symptom with pancreatic carcinoma being the most important differential diagnosis. It can also present as acute or chronic pancreatitis.

The hallmark finding on ERCP in patients with autoimmune pancreatitis is a focal, diffuse, or segmental attenuation of the main pancreatic duct and the disappearance of right-angled branches. The main pancreatic duct adjacent to or upstream of the strictures is minimally dilated. The typical imaging finding in AIP is a diffuse enlargement of the pancreas (also called "sausage-shaped" pancreas) with delayed enhancement.

Extrapancreatic Lesions

After the initial description of IgG4-RD in pancreas, it was identified in virtually every organ system: the biliary tree, salivary glands, orbital tissues (e.g. lacrimal gland, extraocular muscles, and retrobulbar space), kidneys, lungs, lymph nodes, meninges, aorta, breast, prostate, thyroid gland, pericardium, retroperitoneum, and skin.

Presence of extrapancreatic manifestations helps in strengthening the diagnosis.

IgG4-Related Sclerosing Cholangitis

The most common extrapancreatic system to be involved is the biliary tract (30–90%). This disease is characterized by sclerotic changes with diffuse or localized stenosis in the intrahepatic/extrahepatic bile duct and gallbladder. The distal common bile duct is the most common site of involvement. Patients present with obstructive jaundice. It is important to differentiate this condition from cholangiocarcinoma and primary sclerosing cholangitis because of dramatic response to steroid therapy.

IgG4-Related Lacrimal and Salivary-Gland Lesions

IgG4-related Mikulicz's disease is characterized by symmetrical (sometimes unilateral) swelling of any of the lacrimal, parotid, submandibular, sublingual glands, and some minor salivary glands. Mikulicz's disease can be diagnosed by the organ-specific diagnostic criteria for IgG4-related Mikulicz's disease established.

Similarities between IgG4-RD and primary Sjögren's syndrome:
- Systemic with multiple organs involvement, especially lacrimal and salivary glands
- Hypergammaglobulinemia
- Massive lymphocyte infiltration or sometimes generation of germinal centers
- Good respond well to corticosteroid therapy.

The dissimilarities between IgG4-RSD and Sjögren's syndrome are in Table 39.5.

Table 39.5 Dissimilarities between IgG4-RSD and Sjögren's syndrome

	IgG4-RSD	Sjögren's syndrome
Sex	More males	More females
Sicca severity	Milder	Mild severe
ESR and CRP	Not elevated	Often elevated
Eosinophilia	Yes	No
Anti-Ro, La	No	Yes
Salivary ducts	Intact	Lymphocytic infiltration
Steroid response	Dramatic	Mild to moderate

Abbreviations: IgG4-RSD, immunoglobulin G4-related systemic disease; ESR, erythrocyte sedimentation rate; CRP, C-reactive protein.

Diagnostic Criteria for IgG4 Mikulicz's Disease (Approved by the Japanese Society for Sjögren's Syndrome, 2008)

- Symmetrical swelling of at least two pairs of lachrymal, parotid, and submandibular glands continuing for more than 3 months
- Elevated serum IgG4 (135 mg/dL)
- Histopathological features including lymphocyte and IgG4+ plasma-cell infiltration (IgG4+ plasma cells/IgG+ plasma cells > 50%) with typical tissue fibrosis or sclerosis.

IgG4-Related Kuttner Tumor

Kuttner tumor, a unilateral sclerosing sialadenitis, is an IgG4-related disease involving only lacrimal gland or unilateral sub mandibular gland.

The classification of immune mediated sialadenitis is showing in Flow chart 39.3.

IgG4-Related Lymphadenopathy

IgG4-related lymphadenopathy is both an underdiagnosed and overdiagnosed entity.

Clinically, three types of lymphadenopathy are recognized.
1. Group A—involves enlarged regional nodes.
2. Group B—nonregional lymph node of organs affected by IgG4-RD.
3. Group C—cases of unexplained lymphadenopathy.

The histological patterns of IgG4-related lymphadenopathy are showing in the Table 39.6.

Clinical Features

- Middle to elderly age group with marked male predominance
- Absence of B symptoms/no fever

Flow chart 39.3 Classification of immune mediated sialadenitis

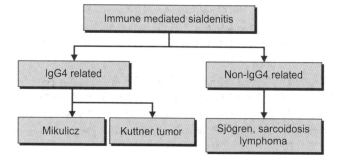

Table 39.6 Histologic patterns of IgG4-related lymphadenopathy

Pattern	Histological subtype	Distributive pattern of IgG4 + cells
Pattern 1	Castleman's disease like	Interfollicular
Pattern 2	Reactive follicular hyperplasia	Interfollicular
Pattern 3	Interfollicular plasmacytosis	Interfollicular
Pattern 4	Progressive transformation of germinal center like	Intragerminal center
Pattern 5	Inflammatory pseudotumor-like morphology	Interfollicular

- Systemic lymphadenopathy
- Lymph nodes are not very large (usually up to 2 cm)
- The exocrine or extranodal lesions may precede, follow, or present together with the lymph node swelling.

Laboratory Features

- Polyclonal hyperimmunoglobulinemia
- Raised serum IgG and IgE levels
- Elevation of serum soluble interleukin-2 (IL-2) receptor
- Presence of autoantibodies
- Normal CRP, IL-6, and LDH.

IgG4-RD often clinically and/or histologically mimics multicentric Castleman's disease or malignant lymphoma.

It is appropriate to diagnose IgG4-related lympha-denopathy only for patients with known IgG4-RD or in the presence of corroborating clinical and laboratory findings.

Outside these circumstances, a descriptive diagnosis of "reactive lymphoid hyperplasia with increased IgG4+ cells" accompanied by a recommendation for follow-up will be appropriate because IgG4-RD will likely ensue only in a minority of such patients.

IgG4-Related Thyroiditis

As of now two forms of thyroiditis are considered to be a part of IgG4-RSD spectrum.
1. Some cases of Riedel thyroiditis.
2. The fibrous variant of Hashimoto thyroiditis.

IgG4-related thyroiditis is often associated with massive enlargement of the thyroid due to lympho-cytic infiltration, necessitating surgical treatment in some patients.

IgG4-Related Lungs

Four categories of IgG4-related lung disease are defined till date:
1. GGO—ground glass opacities.
2. Thickening of bronchovascular bundles and interlobular septa.
3. Bronchiectasis.
4. A solitary large-nodular lesion that includes a mass.

They are frequently accompanied by mediastinal and hilar lymphadenopathy. Some patients have asthma-like symptoms. IgG4-RSD is an important differential diagnosis of malignant tumours, sarcoidosis, metastases, interstitial lung diseases, and pneumonias.

IgG4-Related Kidney Disease

IgG4-related kidney disease mainly manifests as tubulo-interstitial nephritis, whereas IgG4-related glomerulo-nephritis is rare. Almost all patients with IgG4-RD are asymptomatic as IgG4-related kidney disease is often focal. It is frequently detected synchronously when contrast enhanced CT is done for extrarenal lesions like sialadenitis, lymphadenopathy, or type 1 autoimmune pancreatitis. Renal involvement is present in about one-third of patients with autoimmune pancreatitis.

There are four disease patterns:
1. Round or wedge-shaped renal cortical nodules.
2. Peripheral cortical lesions.
3. Mass-like lesions.
4. Renal pelvic involvement.

Renal cortical nodules are composed of lympho-plasmacytic infiltrate. When round or wedge-shaped nodules are present, the differential diagnosis includes pyelonephritis or metastases. Rarely, renal disease manifests as a solitary lesion, which may mimic a neoplasm. Sometimes thickened lesions occur at the renal hilum, and about half of these patients develop hydronephrosis due to ureteral obstruction. A delay in treatment may result in irreversible renal failure.

Serology usually demonstrates high levels of serum total IgG and IgG4, and high levels of serum IgE and hypocomplementemia.

Since FDG-PET is not useful for examining renal involvement, a histological examination is mandatory in patients with renal abnormalities detected using CT imaging.

Note: Patients with idiopathic membranous nephropathy have IgG4 autoantibodies to the M-type phospholipase A2 receptor in the circulation and glomerular immune deposits, but is not considers a spectrum of IgG4-RSD.

AORTITIS

Noninfectious thoracic aortitis, inflammatory abdominal aortic aneurysms/abdominal periaortitis, and idiopathic retroperitoneal fibrosis are all chronic inflammatory conditions. A fraction of the cases is due to IgG4-RSD.

Because of the good response of IgG4-RSD to glucocorticoid treatment it should be ruled out in all patients with noninfectious aortitis.

The fibrosis in these locations may extend to involve the kidney, ureter and bowel mesentery with varying response to steroid therapy.

Pituitary Gland and Dura Mater Involvement

Infundibulohypophysitis (Inflammation of the Pituitary Gland)

The clinical picture includes patients presenting with hypopituitarism, diabetes insipidus, and/or symptomatic local mass effect. A pituitary mass and/or thickening of the pituitary stalk are identified on imaging studies.

IgG4-related Pachymeningitis (Inflammation of the Dura Mater)

Patients present with chronic headache and cranial neuropathy, such as visual loss and facial nerve palsy of the facial nerve. It needs to be differentiated from hypertrophic pachymeningitis, associated with rheumatoid vasculitis, tuberculosis, and mycosis.

PERIPHERAL NERVES

Infraorbital nerve enlargement, which is specific to IgG4-related ophthalmic disease, can be detected by MRI: coronal MRI analysis can reveal substantial enlargement of the infraorbital nerves. These neural lesions are radiologically characterized by nerve-centered distinct soft tissue masses and needs to be differentiated from a variety of diseases like malignant lymphoma, neurolymphomatosis, neurogenic tumors, and sarcoidosis.

Management

There is no standardized therapeutic protocol for this highly complex disease with varying severity. At the present time, we do not have a fully established evaluation system, making it difficult to outline the severity of the disease on presentation in an individual patient. One approach in AIP is to initiate treatment based on clinical symptoms rather than the severity and extent of the disease on imaging findings, although evidence is lacking.[6] Since there are no randomized control trials for IgG4-RD treatment to date, management is based currently on small-case series and observational studies. Prompt treatment is needed because the potential for reversibility of clinical glandular function is very good in the short-term.

Disease Activity and Damage

Before starting treatment, it is important to assess disease activity and damage, at baseline. Clinical symptoms and signs that are associated with activity and damage in each organ are to be separately recorded.

Disease activity refers to ongoing manifestations of IgG4-related inflammation within an organ.

"Damage" refers to organ system dysfunction that has occurred as a result of active IgG4-RD, whether or not the disease is still active in that organ system. Damage is a permanent organ/site "scar" that will not improve, even with appropriate treatment for IgG4-RD.

Patients may have both damage and activity in the same organ at the same time.

Measurement of disease activity is difficult in IgG4-RSD is difficult due to two reasons:
1. Because of the complex, multiorgan-system nature, it difficult to summarize the state of disease activity across all organs.
2. Stage of disease activity can vary across organs; a patient can have active inflammation likely in one organ (steroid responsive) and advanced fibrosis (less likely to respond to steroid) in another organ.

IgG4-Related Disease Responder Index

Immunoglobulin G4-related disease responder index is developed on the lines of the Birmingham vasculitis activity score for wegener's granulomatosis (BVAS/WG). It is designed to detect any changes in disease activity and identify improvement and worsening in the same and/or different organ systems. This allows objective quantification of the treatment response by providing standardized outcome measures. Assessing clinical response and not simply serologic response is increasingly important to establish endpoints in randomized control trials.

When to Start Treatment?

Sometimes even active widespread disease may not require immediate treatment like IgG4-related lymphadenopathy; in fact some may never need treatment.

However, even asymptomatic and localized disease like aortitis and liver/biliary tract involvement is severe enough to warrant urgent treatment to prevent organ dysfunction.

Treatment Options

Steroids: Typically corticosteroids are very effective at the outset. A common regimen: 40–60 mg daily for 2 weeks and then taper over 3 months. Sometimes, maintenance low-dose prednisone after tapering is needed.

The rate of relapse after tapering or discontinuing glucocorticosteroids is as high as 30–60%. For those intolerant of corticosteroids or unable to taper without flaring, numerous traditional steroid-sparing agents (azathioprine, mycophenolate mofetil, methotrexate) have been tried, but are generally ineffective.

Rituximab: B-cell depletion with rituximab should be considered in all patients with active and steroid refractory inflammation.[7] Patients treated with rituximab show a fast decline in serum IgG4 levels, accompanied by a rapid clinical and histological improvement.

Moreover, repeated courses of rituximab maintain their effectiveness and result in further decreases in IgG4 concentrations. The regimen consists of two 1 g infusions, 15 days apart. Rituximab may be used in place of steroids as induction therapy, especially for those with less severe disease not requiring urgent treatment. Organ-specific interventions such as ureteral or biliary stents may be necessary initially to manage disease. Often these can be removed when medications take effect.

CONCLUSION

Immunoglobulin G4-related disease is a new concept. Many questions remain regarding its pathogenesis, the establishment of diagnostic criteria, and the role of IgG4. Prospective studies of patients with IgG4-RD are required to clarify the natural history, long-term prognosis, and treatment approaches in this recently recognized condition.

KEY POINTS

- Any steroid responsive mass lesion should be examined for IgG4-RSD.
- A raised serum IgG4 level is not mandatory for the diagnosis.
- Serum IgG4 is not a perfect biomarker of IgG4-RSD.
- Not every entity with increased IgG4+ plasma cells and a high IgG4/IgG ratio should be diagnosed as IgG4-RSD.
- FDG PET/CT is a useful tool for assessing organ involvement, monitoring therapeutic response, and guiding interventional treatment of IgG4-RD.
- Corticosteroids are the cornerstone of initial treatment.
- A major determinant of treatment responsiveness is the degree of fibrosis within the affected organs.
- Rituximab is a promising agent in management of IgG4-RSD.
- Screen for underlying malignancies both during the diagnosis and follow-up of IgG4-related disease.

REFERENCES

1. Stone JH, Zen Y, Desphande V. IgG4-related disease. N Engl J Med. 2012;366:539-51.
2. Umehara H, Okazaki K, Masaki Y, et al. A novel clinical entity, IgG4-related disease (IgG4-RD): general concept and details. Mod Rheumatol. 2012;22:1-14.
3. Stone JH, Khosroshahi A, Deshpande V, et al. Recommendations for the nomenclature of IgG4-related disease and its individual organ system manifestations. Arthritis Rheum. 2012;64:3061-7.
4. Umehara H, Okazaki K, Masaki Y, et al. Comprehensive diagnostic criteria for IgG4-related disease (IgG4-RD), 2011. Mod Rheumatol. 2012;22:21-30.
5. Deshpande V, Zen Y, Chan JK, et al. Consensus statement on the pathology of IgG4-related disease. Mod Pathol. 2012;25:1181-92.
6. Yamamoto M, Takahashi H, Shinomura Y. Mechanisms and assessment of IgG4-related disease: lessons for the rheumatologist. Nat Rev Rheumatol. 2014;10:148-59.
7. Khosroshahi A, Carruthers MN, Deshpande V, et al. Rituximab for the treatment of IgG4-related disease: lessons from 10 consecutive patients. Medicine (Baltimore). 2012;91:57-66.

CHAPTER 40

Infection-associated Vasculitis

Neha Garg, Ajay Wanchu

INTRODUCTION

Several infections have been well known to be associated with some vasculitides, such as polyarteritis nodosa (PAN) induced by hepatitis B virus (HBV)[1-3] or cryoglobulinemic vasculitis[3,4] associated with hepatitis C virus (HCV). These vasculitides are discussed separately elsewhere in this book. Recently, revised nomenclature for vasculitis[5] identifies a specific group—vasculitis associated with probable etiology, and includes hepatitis B-associated PAN, hepatitis C-associated cryoglobulinemic vasculitis, and vasculitis-associated with syphilis. However, there are other infectious agents from all groups including bacteria, viruses, mycobacteria, fungi, and parasites, associated with various forms of vasculitis. Among viruses that have been associated with development of vasculitis such as human immunodeficiency virus (HIV),[6,7] Epstein-Barr virus (EBV), parvovirus B19,[8,9] cytomegalovirus (CMV),[10,11] and others. Most recently, Burkholderia-like strain has been isolated from temporal arteries of several patients with giant cell arteritis.[12] This chapter covers these rare vasculitides, which may have infectious agents as a causative factor. Septic phlebitis, vasculitis associated with rickettsia, and bacterial endocarditis are other infection-associated vasculitides we will discuss in this chapter.

VIRAL INFECTIONS AND VASCULITIS

Viruses are frequently considered as putative inciters of autoimmune vasculitis due to presence of circulating immune complexes found during many acute viral infections. Apart from HCV and HBV, most frequently reported associations exist for HIV, parvovirus B19, CMV, and EBV. The true prevalence, pathogenic mechanisms, clinical manifestations, and best treatment strategy are not well established.

HIV-ASSOCIATED VASCULITIS

Most common skin vasculitis in HIV patients is drug related hypersensitivity[13,14] such as didanosine and zidovudine.[15,16] Incidence of vasculitides associated with HIV is estimated at 1%.[7] HIV-associated vasculitis can be implicated in a wide spectrum of vasculitis involving any vessel size and occur in a nonspecific pattern.[17,18] Patients presenting with vasculitis should be tested routinely for HIV, hepatitis B, and hepatitis C infection. Incidence could be as high as 23% in symptomatic HIV patients[7] including hypersensitivity vasculitis, PAN, Henoch–Schönlein purpura, Kawasaki's disease (KD) both in children and adults, giant cell arteritis, granulomatosis with polyangiitis (GPA) (formerly known as Wegener's granulomatosis), cryoglobulinemic vasculitis and angiitis of the central nervous system, and infectious vasculitides.[19]

Polyarteritis Nodosa

Polyarteritis nodosa seems to be the most common form in HIV-infected individuals. Association with medium-vessel vasculitis like PAN is somewhat stronger as evidenced by a multitude of case reports of PAN in HIV positive but hepatitis B negative individuals.[20-26] In such cases, the most common manifestation is peripheral neuropathy and muscle disease, whereas the classic PAN features, such as fevers, cutaneous ulcers, renal, and gastrointestinal involvement are less common. Pathogenesis is largely unknown; however, CD8 T cells, macrophages, and IgM deposition have been seen[13] with immune complex deposition as a plausible mechanism of injury. Direct injury to vessel wall by the virus is less likely since virus is not universally isolated from such lesions. Kawasaki disease is a medium-vessel vasculitis typically seen in children less than 5 years of age. Kawasaki-like syndrome has been reported in HIV-positive individuals with a similar clinical picture to the idiopathic variety seen in children.[24-26] Mechanism of injury may involve IgA as IgA positive plasma cells are seen in vasculitis lesions.[24] Kawasaki-like syndrome has been reported at medium to severe immune dysfunction as well as after the introduction of highly active antiretroviral therapy (HAART).[27] Recently HIV-associated PAN has been described to differ significantly from classical (hepatitis B associated) PAN and that associated with hepatitis C virus infection[28] (Table 40.1).

Cryoglobulinemic Vasculitis

Prevalence of cryoglobulinemic vasculitis (mostly Type II and III mixed cryoglobulins) in HIV positive patients ranges from 1 to 27% but it is more frequent with HIV and hepatitis co-infection.[28-30] It is mostly asymptomatic and HIV infection does not seem to play a significant role in cryoglobulin production.[28] In patients with HIV and hepatitis C co-infection, cryoglobulinemic vasculitis presents with palpable purpura, mononeuritis multiplex, arthralgias, and nephritic syndrome. It responds well to hepatitis C treatment with ribavirin and interferon. Most recently, rituximab has been successfully used in the treatment of cryoglobulinemic vasculitis with or without hepatitis C.[31,32] It remains to be seen whether rituximab can be used in cryoglobulinemic vasculitis associated with HIV with or without HCV co-infection.

ANCA-Associated Small-vessel Vasculitis

Diagnostic evaluation of ANCA-associated small-vessel vasculitis in HIV-infected patients is complicated by the fact that ANCA are detected in HIV-positive individuals without clinical vasculitis.[33,34] Two distinct patterns of small-vessel vasculitis can be seen in HIV-infected patients depending on the severity of immune compromise.[7] In early, less severe stage, CD8+ T-cell infiltration or direct HIV virus mediated injury may be responsible for vascular injury. In later stage with CD4 T-cell counts below 200 cells/μL, coexisting infections might play an important role in the pathogenesis. Hence, therapeutic implications in early and late stage vasculitis might be different.

Central Nervous System Vasculitis

Among HIV patients with stroke, CNS vasculitis is a cause for cerebrovascular disease about 13% of the times. It can occur at any time during the course of HIV disease, immediately after HIV infection, or when CD4 count falls below 200 copies/μL. Cerebral aneurysms are well-recognized complications in HIV-infected young men presenting with recurrent strokes in the absence of established risk factors. Pathogenesis may be complex involving both HIV and varicella-zoster virus.[7] Histopathology shows vascular damage with destruction of the internal elastic lamina, fibrosis of the media as well as intimal hyperplasia, sparing the small arteries.[35] Intracranial aneurysms presenting with infarcts and hemorrhage have also been described in heavily immunosuppressed patients.[36]

Giant Cell Arteritis and Takayasu Arteritis

Association of large-vessel vasculitis such as giant cell arteritis (GCA) and Takayasu arteritis with HIV is based solely on rare case reports.[37-39] A focal necrotizing vasculitis of the aorta and large arteries has been reported in HIV patients from African descent. This can be rapidly progressive with aneurysm formation and rupture. Immune complex mediated leukocytoclastic vasculitis of vasa vasora or periadventitial vessels has been implicated in these young individuals.[40]

Table 40.1 Differences between different forms of polyarteritis nodosa			
	Classical PAN	*Nonclassical PAN*	*Nonclassical PAN*
Association	HBV	HIV	HCV
Symptoms	Waxing, waning	Acute	Acute
Organs involved	Renal, GI and CNS	Skin, joints	Skin and others like HBV
Response to therapy	Fair (steroids and cytotoxic)	Excellent (mostly steroids only; HAART)	Good (Rituximab); relapses common; Peg IFN+Ribavarin
Severity	Severe	Mild	Moderate
Relapses	Common	Uncommon	Very common
Prognosis	Poor (35% mortality)	Excellent	Fair (10% mortality)

Source: Scotto G, Cibelli DC, Saracino A, et al. Cryoglobulinemia in subjects with HCV infection alone, HIV infection and HCV/HIV coinfection. J Infect. 2006;52:294-9.

Vasculitis Related to Coinfections

Opportunistic infections occurring in HIV-infected individuals such as *Toxoplasma gondii, CMV, and Pneumocystis carinii* can also cause vasculitis.[7,11] Vasculitis resulting from CMV infection can result in prominent gastrointestinal and cutaneous manifestations and its inclusion bodies can be demonstrated by microscopy. In such cases, antiviral agents like ganciclovir or foscarnet should be started and any concomitant immunosuppressive therapy reduced. Any drugs that can cause hypersensitivity vasculitis must be withdrawn. Life-threatening complications affecting the lungs, kidneys, or the nervous system should be treated with steroids and immunosuppressive medications. Antiretroviral drugs may help and additional therapy in the form of prophylaxis for herpes zoster and *Pneumocystis pneumonia* must be instituted.

Treatment for vasculitis is along the lines of idiopathic systemic vasculitides with high-dose corticosteroids. *Pneumocystis jiroveci* prophylaxis should be given and CD4 counts should be carefully monitored. Addition of IVIG, cyclophosphamide or rituximab can be considered as appropriate for life-threatening vasculitis manifestations, in conjunction with HAART treatment and supplemented by treatment of concomitant infections.

PARVOVIRUS B19 ASSOCIATED VASCULITIS

The association of parvovirus B19 and vasculitis is limited to case reports.[8,9, 41-44] The most common clinical manifestation of B19 infection is erythema infectiosum (fifth disease). B19 infection is also associated with arthritis, chronic anemia to transient aplastic crisis and hydrops fetalis and fetal death.[43] Vasculitic manifestations have included multisystemic disease including glomerulonephritis, purpura and mononeuritis multiplex, PAN, and GPA.[44] CNS vasculitis,[45] Henoch-Schönlein purpura,[46-48] and Kawasaki disease[49,50] have also been reported.

Evidence of pathogenic role of parvovirus comes from seroconversion data from PCR amplification of parvovirus B19 from serum of individuals with vasculitis, and its presence detected in dermal and glomerular capillaries[46-48] and from temporal arteries in patients with GCA.[51] Clinical implication of ANCA antibodies should be ascertained with caution as transient rise in PR3-ANCAs can be seen during acute parvovirus B infection.[52] Chronicity of B19 infection can be assessed by enzyme immunoassay for IgG and IgM antibodies to B19 and polymerase chain reaction for B19 DNA in serum and tissue samples.[44] Controversy exists regarding the pathogenic role of parvovirus B19 since it is also isolated in tissue samples of patients without vasculitis for example from atherosclerotic carotid or aortic disease.[53]

The presence of parvovirus in such cases may alter expected response to treatment. Intravenous immunoglobulin (IVIG) has been used effectively in a few cases with complete to partial recovery.[43,44,52] It showed improvement in three cases that did not respond to corticosteroids or even to cyclophosphamide.[44] IVIG treatment resulted in clearance of viremia as well as resolution of signs and symptoms of vasculitis, allowing the eventual withdrawal of immunosuppressive therapy, without relapse. It has been postulated that since both B19 IgM antibodies and B19 DNA are rarely found in patients not infected with parvovirus, their presence suggests an association between B19 and the vasculitis.[43] Resolution of IgM antibodies and viral DNA correlated with success of treatment.

CYTOMEGALOVIRUS

Association with CMV and vasculitis outside of immunodeficiency is rare and limited to few case reports and has included PAN, pulmonary hemorrhage, and gut ulcers.[10,11] Clinical associations have been reported most commonly with gut and skin vasculitis,[11,54] as well as CNS lesions,[55] and Kawasaki-like disease with coronary aneurysms.[10] In these instances, it is important to confirm the diagnosis by demonstrating intranuclear inclusions characteristic of CMV infection. Cytomegalovirus induced allograft rejection in kidney transplant recipients may be mediated by endothelial damage raising the question of vasculitis. A more difficult diagnostic challenge occurs when CMV infection induced vasculitis occurs in patients receiving immunosuppression for other vasculitis such as GPA. Prompt cultures and mucosal biopsy specimens showing typical CMV lesions could help instituting correct treatment and should be obtained in these individuals with new skin, glomerular or gut lesions. Treatment has included glucocorticoids initially along with prompt institution of antiviral therapy.

EPSTEIN-BARR VIRUS

Epstein-Barr virus has a unique ability to modify our immune system due to its tropism for lymphoid cells. Evidence of association of EBV- and vasculitis-like responses comes from isolation of EBV DNA from the vessel walls of patients with large-,[56,57] medium-vessel KD-like[58-61] and immune-complex-mediated small-vessel vasculitides.[62] Transformation of lymphoid and NK cells induced by EBV has been linked to lesions of several vascular syndromes associated with angiocentric lymphoid proliferation such as lymphoid granulomatosis (LG) as evidenced by isolation of EBV DNA from B cells of these lesions.[63] Lymphoid granulomatosis is an uncommon mimic of vasculitis, especially GPA due to its propensity for lung involvement, but it usually occurs in immunocompromised patients.

VARICELLA-ZOSTER VIRUS

Varicella-Zoster virus-associated vasculitis has been reported mainly after an instance of zoster ophthalmicus weeks to months after the infection, in the form of large-vessel vasculitis within the CNS presenting as strokes in immunocompetent hosts[64] but has been reported without such an antecedent infection as well.[65] Multifocal small-vessel vasculitis affecting eyes, skin, gut, lungs, and kidneys also occur but more so in patients suffering from AIDS or other forms of immunodeficiency states. Cutaneous and ophthalmic involvement is less frequent in such cases and clinical course, if more often protracted.

BACTERIAL INFECTIONS AND VASCULITIS

Staphylococcus aureus and Granulomatosis with Polyangiitis

Chronic nasal carriage of *Staphylococcus (S.) aureus* is associated with relapses of GPA with highest risk of relapse for TSST-1 superantigen-positive *S. aureus*; suggesting a link between infection and PR3-ANCA associated GPA.[66-69] Treatment with trimethoprim-sulfamethoxazole has been shown to reduce the infections as well as the number of relapses in GPA.[70]

Transient elevation of PR3-ANCA can be seen in many infections, such as subacute bacterial endocarditis, parvovirus B19 infection, and chronic hepatitis C virus infection. Indeed, work with *S. aureus* has revealed convincing evidence of association between bacterial infections and generation of ANCA antibodies. Stimulation of peripheral blood mononuclear cells with unmethylated CpG oligonucleotides (constituent of bacterial DNA) results in production of ANCA in PR3-ANCA positive AAV-patients.[71,72] Potential mechanisms in the pathophysiology of ANCA-positive vasculitis include barrier dysfunction, danger-signals (CpG), superantigens (*S. aureus*) and neutrophil extracellular traps.[73]

Bacterial Endocarditis

S. aureus, S. lugdunensis, Streptococcus viridians, and other *S.* species can be detected in ANCA-positive (usually c-ANCA) patients with subacute bacterial endocarditis. Clinical manifestations include small-vessel systemic vasculitis such as glomerulonephritis; skin purpura, arthritis, pulmonary infiltrates, and can be seen in such cases.[74-76] Vasculitis similar to primary CNS vasculitis has also been reported[77,78] with hemorrhage and infarcts as consequences.

Infectious Aortitis

Infections reported to cause aortitis include streptococci (in the pre-antibiotic era), gram-negative bacteria and *S. aureus*. Infection usually arises from hematogenous spread of a preexisting aneurysm from infective endocarditis or from intravenous drug use. Pathology usually demonstrates acute inflammation superimposed on atherosclerosis.[78] Aortitis can occur with nontyphoidal *Salmonella* infections, most commonly abdominal aorta. Prognosis is poor with about 40% mortality.[79] It should be sought as a cause in younger individuals with recurrent aortitis. Common strains isolated include *S. typhimurium, S. enteritidis,* and *S. cholerasuis*.[79,80] Atherosclerosis is a strong predictor of endovascular infection with *Salmonella*. Other causes of aortitis include syphilis, tuberculosis, and leprosy.

Tuberculous mycotic aneurysm is very rare, as per a Korean report only 45 cases have been reported.[81] It usually occurs in descending thoracic aorta in the patient with disseminated tuberculosis. Contiguous spread from an adjacent pulmonary lesion is thought to be more common mechanism of spread to aorta than hematogenous spread from a distant source.[81] Caseating necrosis of the entire aortic wall can occur, and subsequently pseudoaneurysm formation, which can rupture at an unpredictable time in future. Initial presentation is chest pain, which in association with constitutional symptoms of fever, weight loss, and hemoptysis should lead to a high degree of suspicion in endemic areas. CT angiography of the chest can be very useful in these situations. Most of these pseudoaneurysms eventually rupture lead to hemorrhagic shock with a very high mortality. Tuberculous pseudoaneurysm might even develop despite antitubercular treatment; hence past history of TB should also lead to a high degree of suspicion in the right clinical setting. Management is challenging as it involves both medical and surgical approach. Early diagnosis with appropriate surgical repair of the lesion is essential for successful outcomes.

Syphilitic aortitis (caused by *Treponema palladium*) usually occurs in tertiary stage of syphilis when dermatological and constitutional symptoms are usually absent. Hence, the diagnosis is usually incidental. The incidence has declined dramatically as for other manifestations of tertiary syphilis with early detection and treatment of syphilis. Before the discovery of penicillin, syphilis was the most common cause of aortitis, occurring in 70–80% cases of untreated primary syphilis. Obliterative endarteritis of the vasa vasorum of the aorta is thought to be the underlying mechanism of necrotic inflammation. There has been concern for lower sensitivity of rapid plasma reagin (RPR) tests in late syphilis (about 70%), compared to treponema-specific tests such as TPHA, microhemagglutination test, fluorescent treponemal antibody absorption (FTA) test (94–96%).[82] Untreated cases can be life-threatening and 18-FDG-PET-CT or CT angiography may be very helpful in identifying an active subclinical lesion.[83] Surgical repair is mandatory since medical therapy alone is insufficient, and even with complete resection and eradication of organism, disease can recur, which make lifelong follow-up necessary.

In addition to aorta there may be periaortic fibrosis mimicking IgG4 related diseases. Current advances in arterial imaging techniques have greatly improved the detection of vessel wall enhancement. Magnetic resonance aortogram imaging with gadolinium enhancement, computed tomography angiography, or FDG-PET scanning are useful techniques to image large vessels, which may show vessel wall thickening and enhancement in a concentric pattern, distinct from aortic atherosclerosis. Surgical repair with prolonged antibiotics has led to less morbidity and mortality from these infections.[84]

Miscellaneous Associations

Septic thrombophlebitis from various bacteria (*Fusobacterium necrophorum, Bacteroides fragilis*) may be considered a form of infectious vasculitis and responds promptly to appropriate antibiotic treatment. Rocky Mountain spotted fever caused by *Rickettsia rickettsii* may be considered a form of infection-induced vasculitis caused by host immune system in response to rickettsial infection causing the characteristic viscerotropic rash, and frequently fatal systemic disease with meningoencephalitis, skin necrosis, respiratory distress syndrome, and rhabdomyolysis. Travel history and history of tick bite are crucial in identifying this disease and instituting prompt therapy with tetracyclines.

Nonhepatitis B- and C-related infectious vasculitides are less frequent when compared to other vasculitides described in this book. However, they constitute a definite category of disorders that need to be considered in a situation where the picture of vasculitis but does not conform to the classic vasculitides.

KEY POINTS

- Infectious vasculitis not associated with hepatitis B and C is relatively infrequent.
- These could be viral, bacterial, fungal, or parasitic in nature.
- These possibilities should be entertained when other more frequent causes are not found in the patient who presents with a multisystem disorder that is thought to be vasculitic in nature.

REFERENCES

1. Trepo C, Thivolet J. Hepatitis associated antigen and periarteritis nodosa (PAN). Vox Sang. 1970;19:410-1.
2. Gocke DJ, Hsu K, Morgan C, et al. Association between polyarteritis and Australia antigen. Lancet. 1970;2:1149-53.
3. Guillevin L, Mahr A, Callard P, et al. Hepatitis B virus-associated polyarteritis nodosa: clinical characteristics, outcome, and impact of treatment in 115 patients. Medicine (Baltimore). 2005;84:313-22.
4. Agnello V, Chung RT, Kaplan LM. A role for hepatitis C virus infection in type II cryoglobulinemia. N Engl J Med. 1992;327:1490-5.
5. Jennette JC, Falk RJ, Bacon PA, et al. 2012 Revised International Chapel Hill Consensus Conference Nomenclature of Vasculitides. Arthritis Rheum. 2013;65:1-11.
6. Gisselbrecht M, Cohen P, Lortholary O, et al. HIV-related vasculitis: clinical presentation and therapeutic approach on six patients. AIDS. 1997;11:121-3.
7. Guillevin L. Vasculitides in the context of HIV infection. AIDS. 2008;22:S27-33.
8. Bilge I, Sadikoglu B, Emre S, et al. Central nervous system vasculitis secondary to parvovirus B19 infection in a pediatric renal transplant patient. Pediatr Nephrol. 2005;20:529-33.
9. Leruez-Ville M, Lauge A, Morinet F, et al. Polyarteritis nodosa and parvovirus B19. Lancet. 1994;344:263-4.
10. Catalano-Pons C, Quartier P, Leruez-Ville M, et al. Primary cytomegalovirus infection, atypical Kawasaki disease, and coronary aneurysms in 2 infants. Clin Infect Dis. 2005;41:e53-6.
11. Golden MP, Hammer SM, Wanke CA, et al. Cytomegalovirus vasculitis. Case reports and review of the literature. Medicine (Baltimore). 1994;73:246-55.
12. Koening CL, Katz BJ, Hernandez-Rodriguez J, et al. Identification of a Burkholderia-like strain from temporal arteries of subjects with giant cell arteritis. Arthritis Rheum. 2012;64:S373.
13. Gherardi R, Belec L, Mhiri C, et al. The spectrum of vasculitis in human immunodeficiency virus-infected patients: a clinicopathologic evaluation. Arthritis Rheum. 1993;36:1164-74.
14. Patel N, Patel N, Khan T, et al. HIV infection and clinical spectrum of associated vasculitides. Curr Rheumatol Rep. 2011;6:506-12.

15. Torres RA, Lin RY, Lee M, et al. Zidovudine-induced leukocytoclastic vasculitis. Arch Intern Med. 1992;152:850-1.

16. Herranz P, Fernández-Díaz ML, et al. Cutaneous vasculitis associated with didanosine. Lancet. 1994;344:680.

17. Kaye B. Rheumatologic manifestations of HIV infection. Rev Allergy Immunol. 1996;14:385-416.

18. Guillevin L. Infections in vasculitis. Best Pract Res Clin Rheumatol. 2013;27:19-31.

19. Pagnoux C, Cohen P, Guillevin L. Vasculitides secondary to infections. Clin Exp Rheumatol. 2006;24:S71-81.

20. Conri C, Mestre C, Constans J, et al. Periarteritis nodosa-type vasculitis and infection with human immunodeficiency virus. Rev Med Interne. 1991;12:47-51.

21. Libman BS, Quismorio FP Jr, Stimmler MM. Polyarteritis nodosa-like vasculitis in human immunodeficiency virus infection. J Rheumatol. 1995;22:351-5.

22. Font C, Miro O, Pedrol E, et al. Polyarteritis nodosa in human immunodeficiency virus infection: report of four cases and review of the literature. Br J Rheumatol. 1996;35:796-9.

23. Chetty R. Vasculitides associated with HIV infection. J Clin Pathol. 2001;54:275-8.

24. Johnson RM, Barbarini G, Barbaro G. Kawasaki-like syndromes and other vasculitic syndromes in HIV-infected patients. AIDS. 2003;17:S77–82.

25. Johnson RM, Little JR, Storch GA. Kawasaki-like syndromes associated with human immunodeficiency virus infection. Clin Infect Dis. 2001;32:1628-34.

26. Velez AP, Menezez L, Crespo A. Kawasaki-like syndrome possibly associated with immune reconstitution inflammatory syndrome in an HIV-positive patient. AIDS Read. 2006;16:464-6.

27. Calabrese LH, Kirchner E, Shresta R. Rheumatic complications of human immunodeficiency virus infection in the era of highly active antiretroviral therapy: emergence of a new syndrome of immune reconstitution and changing patterns of disease. Semin Arthritis Rheum. 2005;35:166-74.

28. Scotto G, Cibelli DC, Saracino A, et al. Cryoglobulinemia in subjects with HCV infection alone, HIV infection and HCV/HIV coinfection. J Infect. 2006;52:294-9.

29. Kosmas N, Kontos A, Panayiotakopoulos G, et al. Decreased prevalence of mixed cryoglobulinemia in the HAART era among HIV-positive, HCV-negative patients. J Med Virol. 2006;78:1257-61.

30. Dimitrakopoulos AN, Kordossis T, Hatzakis A, et al. Mixed cryoglobulinemia in HIV-1 infection: the role of HIV-1. Ann Intern Med. 1999;130:226-30.

31. Michael CS, Zonghui H, Carol AL. A randomized controlled trial of rituximab following failure of antiviral therapy for hepatitis C virus-associated cryoglobulinemic vasculitis. Arthritis Rheum. 2012;64:835-42.

32. De Vita S, Quartuccio L, Isola M, et al. A randomized controlled trial of rituximab for the treatment of severe cryoglobulinemic vasculitis. Arthritis Rheum. 2012;64:843-85.

33. Cornely OA, Hauschild S, Weise C, et al. Seroprevalence and disease association of antineutrophil cytoplasmic autoantibodies and antigens in HIV infection. Infection. 1999;27:92-6.

34. Jansen TL, van Houte D, de Vries T, et al. ANCA seropositivity in HIV: a serological pitfall. Neth J Med. 2005;63:270-4.

35. Kossorotoff M, Touze E, Godon-Hardy S, et al. Cerebral vasculopathy with aneurysm formation in HIV-infected young adults. Neurology. 2006;66:1121-2.

36. Goldstein DA, Timpone J, Cupps TR. HIV associated intracranial aneurismal vasculopathy in adults. J Rheumatol. 2010;37:226-33.

37. Javed MA, Sheppard MN, Pepper J. Aortic root dilation secondary to giant cell aortitis in a human immunodeficiency virus-positive patient. Eur J Cardiothorac Surg. 2006;30:400-1.

38. Solinger AM, Hess EV. Rheumatic diseases and AIDS: is the association real? J Rheumatol. 1993;20:678-83.

39. Kalungi S, Kigonya E, Eyoku S, et al. Takayasu's arteritis (pulseless disease) in Uganda. Afr Health Sci. 2004;4:185-7.

40. Chetty R, Batitang S, Nair R. Large artery vasculopathy in HIV positive patients: another vasculitic enigma. Hum Pathol. 2000;31:374-9.

41. Sakalli H, Baskin E, Bayrakçi US, et al. Ozdemir BH Parvovirus B19-induced multisystemic vasculitis and acute endocapillary proliferative glomerulonephritis in a child. Ren Fail. 2010;32:506-9.

42. Shimohata H, Higuchi T, Ogawa Y, et al. Serum TNF-related and weak inducer of apoptosis levels in septic shock patients. Ther Apher Dial. 2011;15:342-8.

43. Torok TJ. Parvovirus B19 and human disease. Adv Intern Med. 1992;37:431-55.

44. Finkel TH, Torok TJ. Chronic parvovirus B19 infection and systemic necrotising vasculitis: Opportunistic infection or aetiological agent. Lancet. 1994;343:1255-8.

45. Bilge I, Sadikoglu B, Emre S, et al. Central nervous system vasculitis secondary to parvovirus B19 infection in a pediatric renal transplant patient. Pediatr Nephrol. 2005;20:529-33.

46. Ferguson PJ, Saulsbury F, Dowell SF, et al. Prevalence of human parvovirus B19 infection in children with Henoch–Schönlein purpura. Arthritis Rheum. 1996;39:880-1.

47. Veraldi S, Macuso R, Rizzitelli G, et al. Henoch–Schönlein syndrome associated with human parvovirus B19 primary infection. Eur J Dermatol. 1999;9:232-3.

48. Cioc A, Sedmak D, Nuovo G, et al. Parvovirus B19 associated with adult Henoch–Schönlein purpura. J Cutan Pathol. 2002;29:602-7.

49. Holm JM, Hansen LK, Oxhoj H. Kawasaki disease associated with parvovirus B19 infection. Eur J Pediatr. 1995;154:633-4.

50. Nigro G, Zerbini M, et al. Active or recent parvovirus B19 infection in children with Kawasaki disease. Lancet. 1994;343:1260-1.

51. Gabriel SE, Espy M, Erdman DD, et al. The role of parvovirus B19 in the pathogenesis of giant cell arteritis: a prelim evaluation. Arthritis Rheum. 1999;42:1255-8.

52. Hermann J, Demel U, Stünzner D, et al. Clinical interpretation of antineutrophil cytoplasmic antibodies: parvovirus B19 infection as a pitfall. Ann Rheum Dis. 2005;64:641-3.

53. Salvarani C, Farnetti E, et al. Detection of parvovirus B19 DNA by polymerase chain reaction in giant cell arteritis: a case-control study. Arthritis Rheum. 2004;46:3099-101.

54. Tatum ET, Sun PC, et al. Cytomegalovirus vasculitis and gut perforation in a patient with acquired immunodeficiency syndrome. Pathology. 1989;21:235-8.

55. Koeppen AH, Lansing LS, Peng SK, et al. Central nervous system vasculitis in cytomegalovirus infection. J Neurol Sci. 1981;51:395-410.

56. Ban S, Goto Y, et al. Systemic granulomatous arteritis associated with Epstein-Barr virus infection. Virchows Arch. 1999;434:249-54.

57. Murakami K, Ohsawa M, et al. Large vessel arteritis associated with chronic active Epstein-Barr virus infection. Arthritis Rheum. 1998;41:369-73.

58. Kikuta H, Matsumoto S, et al. Kawasaki disease and Epstein-Barr virus. Acta Paediatr Jpn. 1991;33:765-70.

59. Kikuta H, Nakanishi M, et al. Detection of Epstein-Barr virus sequences in patients with Kawasaki disease by means of polymerase chain reaction. Intervirology. 1992;33:1-5.

60. Kanegane H, Tsuji T, et al. Kawasaki disease and concomitant primary Epstein-Barr virus infection. Acta Paediatr Jpn. 1994;36:713-6.

61. Nakagawa A, Ito M, et al. Chronic active Epstein-Barr virus infection and giant coronary aneurysms. Am J Clin Pathol. 1996;105:733-6.

62. Lande M, Mowry JA, et al. Immune complex disease associated with Epstein-Barr virus infectious mononucleosis. Pediatr Nephrol. 1998;12:651-3.

63. Guinee D, Jaffe E, et al. Pulmonary lymphomatoid granulomatosis: evidence for a proliferation of Epstein–Barr virus infected B-lymphoctyes with a prominent T-cell component and vasculitis. Am J Surg Pathol. 1994;18:753-64.

64. Gilden D. Varicella zoster virus and central nervous system syndromes. Herpes. 2004;11:89A-94A.

65. Gilden DH, Kleinschmidt-DeMasters BK, et al. Varicella zoster virus: a cause of waxing and waning vasculitis: the New England Journal of Medicine case 5-1995 revisits. Neurology. 1996;47:1441-6.

66. Charlier C, Henegar C, Launay O, et al. Risk factors for major infections in Wegener granulomatosis: analysis of 113 patients. Ann Rheum Dis. 2009;68:658-63.

67. Popa ER, Stegeman CA, Kallenberg CG, et al. *Staphylococcus aureus* and Wegener's granulomatosis. Arthritis Res. 2002;4:77-9.

68. Stegman CA, Cohen-Tervaert JW, Sluiter WJ, et al. Association of chronic nasal carriage of *Staphylococcus aureus* and higher relapse rates in Wegener granulomatosis. Ann Intern Med. 1994;120:12-7.

69. Popa ER, Stegeman CA, Abdulahad WH, et al. Staphylococcal toxic-shock- syndrome-toxin-1 as a risk factor for disease relapse in Wegener's granulomatosis. Rheumatology (Oxford). 2007;46:1029-33.

70. Stegman CA, Cohen-Tervaert JW, de Jong PE, et al. For the Dutch co-trimoxazole Wegener study group. N Engl J Med. 1996;335:16-20.

71. Hurtado PR, Jeffs L, Nitschke J, et al. CpG oligodeoxynucleotide stimulates production of antineutrophil cytoplasmic antibodies in ANCA-associated vasculitis. BMC Immunol. 2008;9:34.

72. Tadema H, Abdulahad WH, Lepse N, et al. CpG triggers ANCA production by blood-derived B-cells from ANCA-associated vasculitis patients in clinical remission. APMIS 2009; 117:116.

73. Elena C, Peter L, Wolfgang LG. Clinical and immunological features of drug-induced and infection-induced proteinase 3-antineutrophil cytoplasmic antibodies and myeloperoxidase-antineutrophil cytoplasmic antibodies and vasculitis. Curr Opin Rheumatol. 2010;22:43-8.

74. Subra JF, Michelet C, Laporte J, et al. The presence of cytoplasmic antineutrophil cytoplasmic antibodies (C-ANCA) in the course of subacute bacterial endocarditis with glomerular involvement, coincidence or association. Clin Nephrol. 1998;49:15-8.

75. Choi HK, Lamprecht P, Niles JL, et al. Subacute bacterial endocarditis with positive cytoplasmic antineutrophil cytoplasmic antibodies and antiproteinase 3 antibodies. Arthritis Rheum. 2000;43:226-31.

76. Fukuda M, Motokawa M, Usami T, et al. PR3-ANCA-positive crescentic necrotizing glomerulonephritis accompanied by isolated pulmonic valve infective endocarditis, with reference to previous reports of renal pathology. Clin Nephrol. 2006;66:202-9.

77. Miller DV, Oderich GS, et al. Surgical pathology of infected aneusyms of descending thoracic and abdominal aorta: clinicopathological correlations in 29 cases. Hum Pathol. 2004;35:1112-20.

78. Lane GP, Cochrane AD, et al. *Salmonella* mycotic abdominal-aortic aneurysm. Med J Aust. 1988;149:95-7.

79. Soravia-Dunand VA, Loo VG, et al. Aortitis due to *Salmonella*: report of 10 cases and comprehensive review of the literature. Clin Infect Dis. 1999;29:862-8.

80. Oskoui R, Davis WA, et al. *Salmonella* aortitis, a report of successfully treated case with a comprehensive review of the literature. Arch Int Med. 1993;153:517-25.

81. Park SC, Moon IS, Koh YB. Tuberculous pseudoaneurysm of the descending thoracic aorta. Ann Vasc Surg. 2010;24:417. e11-417.

82. Larsen SA, Steiner BM, Rudolph AH. Laboratory diagnosis and interpretation of tests for syphilis. Clin Microbiol Rev. 1995;8:1-21.

83. Paulo N, Cascarejo J, Vouga L. Syphilitic aneurysm of the ascending aorta. Interact Cardiovasc Thorac Surg. 2012;14:223-5.

84. Fernandez Guerrero ML, Aguado JM, et al. The spectrum of cardiovascular infections due to *Salmonella enterica*: a review of clinical and factors determining outcome. Medicine (Baltimore). 2004;83:123-38.

Vasculitis Mimics

Subramanian Ramaswamy, Vinod Ravindran

INTRODUCTION

Vasculitis defines a spectrum of disorders wherein the primary pathology is inflammation of blood vessels as a sequel of which target organ damage ensues. The clinical features may, however, be heterogeneous and need not necessarily be confined to a territorial boundary of the supplying vessel. Vasculitic mimics, on the other hand, connote a spectrum of disorders, which may or may not cause inflammation of blood vessels but have myriad of presentations (clinically, on investigations and histologically) similar to primary systemic vasculitides (PSV). These are secondary to a systemic pathology either in the form of infection, malignancy, thrombotic disorders, and some rare causes (Table 41.1). Therapeutic implications of vasculitic mimics vis-à-vis PSV make it important to differentiate between these two conditions. Moreover, in cases of PSVs also, it is important to exclude vasculitic mimics, either clinically or by appropriate investigations.

CASE VIGNETTE

A 52-year-old male presented with fever of 1-month duration along with erythematous rashes in bilateral lower limbs, which were nonpruritic. The fever was high grade without any associated chills. There were no cardiac or respiratory complaints. His habits were clean. He had been treated for acute myeloid leukemia, M2 stage and was declared to be in clinical and molecular remission 6 months prior. On examination, he was febrile and with stable vitals. Maculopapular rashes were present on both lower limbs extending up to the knees. Hepatosplenomegaly was present but rest of the systemic examination was unremarkable.

Table 41.1 Vasculitis mimics	
Infections	*Bacterial:* Subacute bacterial endocarditis, mycobacterium, syphilis, Rickettsia *Viral:* Retrovirus, hepatitic viruses, CMV *Parasites:* Trichinellosis *Fungal:* Candidemia, sporotrichosis
Coagulopathies	Cholesterol embolism, atrial myxoma, antiphospholipid antibody syndrome, calciphylaxis, procoagulant states
Collagen disorders	Marfan's syndrome, pseudoxantoma elasticum, Loez-Dietz syndrome
Miscellaneous	Fibromuscular dysplasia, neurofibromatosis, segmental arterial mediolysis, scurvy Hematologic malignancies, paraneoplastic syndromes *Drugs:* Cocaine, hydralazine, minocycline, oxymetazoline, ergot, radiation

Investigations revealed hemoglobin 7.2 gm/dL, total leukocyte count of 15,200/cu mm, and platelet counts of 1.1×10^3/cu mm. Differential counts were neutrophils 82%, lymphocytes 12%, monocytes 6%, and basophils nil. No abnormal cells were noted on the peripheral smear. Creatinine was 1.7 mg/dL, and urine showed albuminuria ++ with active sediments (RBCs 25–30/hpf and WBC 10–12/hpf). Blood cultures were sterile (48 hours samples). Antinuclear antibody (ANA) was negative and pulmonary antineutrophil cytoplasmic antibody (ANCA) was positive. Skin biopsy showed evidence of leukocytoclastic vasculitis.

Based on this, patient was started on steroids at 1 mg/kg of prednisolone, and fever defervescence was seen in 72 hours but he then became dyspneic and orthopneic. At this time, jugular venous pulse (JVP) was elevated 12 cm above the sternal angle. S3 gallop was present. An emergency echocardiogram was performed, and vegetations were seen in the tricuspid valve leaflet. Blood culture on the fourth day had grown gram-positive cocci and culture yield was of *Staphylococcus aureus.*

Patient at this stage was now started on vancomycin with a diagnosis of acute bacterial endocarditis secondary to the central venous line infection after chemotherapy. Despite treatment, patient succumbed to congestive cardiac failure on the seventh day of admission.

WHEN TO SUSPECT VASCULITIC MIMICS?

In particular, two types of presentations should alert the clinician to the possibility of systemic vasculitis: (1) unexplained ischemia, such as claudication, limb ischemia, angina, transient ischemic attack, stroke, mesenteric ischemia, and cutaneous ischemia, particularly in a young patient or a patient without risk factors for atherosclerosis and (2) multiple organ dysfunction in a systemically ill patient, especially in the presence of other suggestive clinical features[1] with constitutional symptoms.

In this context, presence of one or more of the following should raise the question of vasculitis mimics.

- Extremes of age
- Immunocompromised patients
- Acute onset of symptoms with rapid deterioration of symptoms
- Patient on drugs known to cause vasculitis, e.g., hydralazine, propylthiouracil, and carbimazole
- Underlying established malignancy
- *Comorbid conditions:* Liver, kidney diseases.

INFECTIONS

A plethora of bacterial, fungal, and viral pathogens may occasionally have vasculitis as an initial presentation, and in most cases, it may not be the major clinical feature. The vascular insult may be a result of direct invasion of the pathogens or due to a bystander injury[2] as a result of immune-mediated hypersensitivity response, mainly type III. Direct endothelial injury may be caused by *Cytomegalovirus, Herpes simplex,* Rickettsiae, fungi, and bacteria.[3,4] *Candida* polysaccharides and fragments of gram-positive and gram-negative organisms can activate the alternate pathway and also lead to the inflammatory reaction characteristic of vasculitis.[3-5] *Streptococcus-* and staphylococcal-mediated vascular injury may be due to release of inflammatory cytokines such as tumor necrosis factor and various cytokines.

Infective Endocarditis

Infective endocarditis (IE) is an infection of the endocardial surface of the heart leading to valvular insufficiencies, intractable congestive cardiac failure, and myocardial abscess. Infective endocarditis also produces a wide variety of systemic signs and symptoms through several mechanisms, including both sterile and infected emboli and various immunological phenomena.[6,7] All cases of IE develop from a commonly shared process[8] as follows:

- Bacteremia (nosocomial or spontaneous) that delivers the organisms to the surface of the valve
- Adherence of the organisms
- Eventual invasion of the valvular leaflets.

Complications of subacute endocarditis result from embolization, slowly progressive valvular destruction, and various immunological mechanisms. Levels of agglutinating and complement-fixing bactericidal antibodies and cryoglobulins are markedly increased in patients with subacute endocarditis. Many of the extracardiac manifestations of this form of the disease are due to circulating immune complexes. These include glomerulonephritis, peripheral manifestations (e.g., Osler nodes, Roth spots, subungual hemorrhages), and, in some cases, various musculoskeletal abnormalities. Janeway lesions usually arise from infected microemboli. The microorganisms that most commonly cause endocarditis (*S. aureus, Streptococcus viridans*; group A, C, and G Streptococci; Enterococci) resist the bactericidal action of complement and possess fibronectin receptors for the surface of the fibrin–platelet thrombus. Among the many other characteristics of IE-producing bacteria demonstrated *in vitro* and *in vivo*, some features include the following:

- Increased adherence to aortic valve leaflet disks by enterococci, *S. viridans,* and *S. aureus*
- Mucoid-producing strains of *S. aureus*
- Dextran-producing strains of *S. viridans*
- *S. viridans* and enterococci that possess FimA surface adhesion
- Platelet aggregation by *S. aureus* and *S. viridans* and resistance of *S. aureus* to platelet microbicidal proteins.

Other Bacterial Infections

Various bacteria may cause vasculitis by the following:

- Direct bacterial invasion and formation of mycotic aneurysms are characteristics of *Staphylococcus, Streptococcus,* and *Salmonella* species.[9-11]

- Tropism for vascular endothelium is shown by Rickettsial group.[12] Infection results in widespread microvascular leak, local thrombosis, and ultimately multisystem failure, if untreated.[13,14]
- Mycobacterial or fungal pulmonary infections may mimic granulomatosis with polyangiitis (GPA) (Wegener's granulomatosis) or EGPA (Churg-Strauss vasculitis) in eliciting a granulomatous reaction in vessels. Spread of *Mycobacterium tuberculosis* to the aorta may be seen as a cause of tuberculous aortitis, coronary arteritis, and mycotic aneurysm.[15-17]
- *Coccidioides immitis* may also present as an immune-complex-mediated disease with erythema nodosum, periarthritis predominantly of the ankles, and bilateral hilar lymphadenopathy[18]
- *Neisseria* species may be associated with small-vessel vasculitis. In *Neisseria gonorrhea* infection, cutaneous papules vesiculate and then become necrotic. *Neisseria meningitides* can manifest in the skin and gastrointestinal tract with the endothelium showing necrosis and thrombosis.[19,20]

Viral Infections

- *Hepatitis C virus:* Patients may have a triad of arthritis, palpable purpura, and type II cryoglobulinemia. Extremities and skin are sufficiently cold so as to explain a predilection for small-vessel leukocytoclastic vasculitis of the skin; in addition, gravity enhances vascular injury in dependent distal vessels, giving rise to palpable purpura predominantly in the lower extremities. More severe cases may manifest visceral organ involvement including membranoproliferative glomerulonephritis and bowel involvement. Small- and medium-sized arteries may be involved as well, especially in the kidneys.[21]
- *Hepatitis B virus:* It provides the classic example of virally mediated immune-complex disease. A lymphocytic venulitis or neutrophilic vasculitis of small vessels with leukocytoclastic or fibrinoid changes presents typically as an "urticaria–arthritis syndrome."[22]
- *Human T lymphotropic virus:* Infection with this may cause retinal, cutaneous, or central nervous system vasculitis.[23-25]
- *Varicella zoster virus and Cytomegalovirus:* Both have been implicated in the etiopathogenesis of various vasculitides via numerous overlapping mechanisms including direct microbial invasion of endothelial cells, immune-complex-mediated vessel wall damage, and

stimulation of autoreactive B and/or T cells through molecular mimicry and superantigens.
- *Parvovirus B19:* This virus has been suggested as the causative agent of GPA and polyarteritis nodosa in a number of case reports and short case series.
- *Others:* Rare cases of vasculitis have similarly been reported following *Rubella* virus, *Adenovirus, Echovirus, Coxsackie virus, Parainfluenza* virus, *Herpes simplex* viruses, and hepatitis A virus infections.

DISORDERS OF THE CONNECTIVE TISSUE MATRIX

Marfan's syndrome caused by mutations in the gene for fibrillin-1, *Ehlers-Danlos syndrome* caused by type IV mutations in the type III procollagen gene (COL3A1), and *Loeys–Dietz syndrome* by the mutations in the TGF-β receptors (TGFBR 1 and 2) are a few inherited disorders that may present with stenotic or aneurysmal dilatation of the vessel wall mimicking large-vessel vasculitis such as Takayasu's aortoarteritis or giant cell arteritis. In addition, Loeys–Dietz syndrome can have abnormalities such as cleft lip, bifid uvula, and valvular regurgitant lesions. Cystic medial necrosis is a common finding in Marfan's and Ehlers-Danlos syndrome as also seen in granulomatous aortitis in large-vessel vasculitis.

Other inherited disorders such as neurofibromatosis type 1, Moyamoya disease, CADASIL fibromuscular dysplasia, and Grange syndrome may also mimic medium- and large-vessel vasculitis.

Scurvy is a less appreciated cause of rash that can resemble vasculitis. Findings included a purpuric skin rash, myalgias, and malaise. Some patients may present with fractures secondary to osteopenia. The patients have low vitamin C levels, and skin biopsy demonstrates noninflammatory perivascular extravasation of RBCs and hemosiderin deposits around the hair follicles.[26] The low levels of serum vitamin C may not necessarily indicate the levels of tissue vitamin C. Leukocyte vitamin C levels are more indicative of tissue stores, as these levels are not affected by circadian rhythm or dietary supplementation. These tests may not however be routinely available. The best method of diagnosis of scurvy is reassessment after supplementation.

DRUG-INDUCED VASCULITIS

Drugs such as hydralazine, minocycline, and cocaine can cause vasculitis mimicking ANCA-associated vasculitides.

Cocaine use may result in nasal mucosal irritation and necrosis, intense vasoconstriction leading to nasal septal perforation and collapse with a saddle-nose deformity. These patients can have a classical ANCA pattern on immunofluorescence and positive antiproteinase 3 testing by immunoassay. However, in cocaine-induced vasculitis, the epitope is human neutrophil elsastase.[27] Evidence of multisystem disease, however, favors ANCA-associated systemic vasculitis.

MALIGNANCY-ASSOCIATED VASCULITIS

Vasculitis as a result of an underlying malignancy may either occur with or precede the diagnosis of malignancy. It is more common with hematologic malignancies than in solid tumors.[28] It can also occur following chemotherapy, radiotherapy, or stem cell transplantation.[28] The etiopathogenesis of malignancy-associated vasculitic syndromes is, however, unknown. Interferon regulatory factor-1 has been postulated in some cases.

ATHEROTHROMBOTIC VASCULAR DISORDERS

Immune-mediated inflammatory processes are well known in the pathogenesis of plaque formation, rupture, and superadded thrombosis in atherosclerotic diseases, and the clinical consequence of these can have a vasculitic presentation. These syndromes, however, have a characteristic age group and have well-defined features of metabolic syndromes in the form diabetes, hypertension, dyslipidemia, and a strong family history. Prothrombotic states, be it inherited (protein C and S deficiency, antithrombin III deficiency, etc.) or acquired (antiphospholipid antibodies related), also have similar presentations in the form of a diffuse or systemic vasocclusive phenomena leading to organ ischemia and multisystem presentation.

MISCELLANEOUS

Calciphylaxis

Calciphylaxis is a poorly understood and highly morbid syndrome of vascular calcification and skin necrosis. Disorders that are most often implicated in the pathogenesis of calciphylaxis include chronic renal failure, obesity, diabetes mellitus, hypercalcemia, hyperphosphatemia, secondary hyperparathyroidism, and also a variety of hypercoagulable states. Calciphylaxis is an active form of osteogenesis with upregulation of bone morphogenic protein 2, Runx2, its target gene, and its indirect antagonist sclerostin2. Lesions of calciphylaxis typically develop suddenly and progress rapidly. Lesions may be singular or numerous, and they generally occur on the lower extremities. Early lesions of calciphylaxis manifest as nonspecific violaceous mottling as livedo reticularis or as erythematous papules, plaques, or nodules. More developed skin lesions have a stellate purpuric configuration with necrotic center. An intact peripheral pulse helps to distinguish acral calciphylaxis from atherosclerotic peripheral vascular disease.[29]

Cryofibrinogenemia

Cryofibrinogen is a cryoprotein in which the precipitate forms only in plasma and not in the serum, unlike in cryoglobulinemia. Cryofibrinogenemia may be primary (essential) or secondary to other underlying disorders, such as carcinoma, infection, vasculitis, collagen disease, or associated with cryoglobulinemia. It may manifest as cold intolerance, Raynaud's phenomenon, purpura, or livedo reticularis. Skin necrosis, acral ulcers, and gangrene can lead to surgery and amputation often as a result of occlusive thrombotic diathesis. Cryofibrinogenemia, however, is essentially a treatable and potentially reversible disease. In moderate forms, it can be treated by simply avoiding cold temperatures. Confirmation of diagnosis is however difficult due to lack of diagnostic criteria. Demonstration of cryofibrins in an appropriate clinical setting may give a clue. The use of corticosteroids in association with low-dose aspirin is the treatment of choice for moderate forms, although stanozolol is an alternative maintenance therapy. Immunosuppressive therapies, plasmapheresis, and/or intravenous fibrinolysis are useful at treating severe forms of cryofibrinogenemia.[30]

Ergot

Ergot and its derivatives can cause retroperitoneal fibrosis and pleuropericardial fibrosis or symptoms of occlusive vasculopathy. The major pharmacologic effects of the ergot alkaloids include smooth muscle stimulation, central sympatholytic activity, and peripheral alpha adrenergic blockade. The manifestations can be gangrenous or convulsive but the basic mechanism in both is severe vasospasm. Direct neurotoxication has not been confirmed. Discontinuation of treatment, heparinization, and sympathectomy may be considered depending on the severity of the manifestations.[31]

Cardiac Myxoma

Atrial myxomas are the most common primary heart tumors accounting for up to 45–50% of the cardiac tumors. Myxomas have been demonstrated to produce numerous growth factors and cytokines, including vascular endothelial growth factor, resulting in angiogenesis and tumor growth and an increased expression of the inflammatory cytokine, interleukin-6.[32-34]

The clinical manifestations may be that of heart failure or symptoms related to embolization. Embolic phenomena may have an occlusive vasculitis such as presentation including coronary, aortic, renal, visceral, or peripheral vessels, and may result in infarction or ischemia of the corresponding organ. On the right side of circulation, embolization results in pulmonary embolism and infarction leading to visceral ischemia. Constitutional symptoms such as fever and Raynauds may be secondary to release of cytokines such as IL-6. Paraneoplastic presentations such as bone lesions, visual loss, tinnitus, and vertigo have been reported.[35] Treatment of atrial myxomas is surgical resection.

DIAGNOSTIC APPROACH AND MANAGEMENT

A through history and clinical examination will give a clue toward the diagnosis of vasculitis or its mimics. A history of ongoing fever, significant lymphadenopathy, or fleeting cardiac murmurs in addition to the pointers in the foregoing discussion favor a diagnosis of vasculitic mimics. Cytopenias or altered coagulation parameters (of disseminated intravascular coagulation) are usually not seen in patients with PSVs. Blood cultures, viral serologies, and autoantibodies (may be falsely positive in case of drug induced vasculitis) need to be routinely considered. Tissue biopsy, wherever feasible, should be done. However, no single investigation will help in identifying either of these conditions.

Identifying the underlying cause will help in the successful management of vasculitic mimics. Treatment of the underlying conditions will usually abate the symptoms of vasculitis.

CONCLUSION

Identifying vasculitis mimics is often a challenge in multisystemic presentations, as no single feature defines this group of conditions. The management of each of these conditions poses a challenge in clinical practice, as the choice between institution of immunosuppressive therapy or otherwise has a direct bearing on the successful treatment of the patient.

KEY POINTS

- Vasculitis mimics should be excluded in any suspected case of vasculitis.
- Red flag signs such as atypical presentations, extremes of age, or underlying other systemic illness should always lead to a suspicion of vasculitis mimics.
- The word "MEDICAL" may be helpful in remembering some of the causes of vasculitis mimics: *m*alignancy, *e*ndocarditis, *d*rugs, *i*nfections, *c*ollagen disorders, and *a*ntiphospho*l*ipid antibody syndrome.
- No single investigation is enough for the diagnosis of systemic vasculitis.

REFERENCES

1. Puett DW. Vasculitis. Bull Rheum Dis. 1995;44:4-8.
2. Naides SJ. Known infectious causes of vasculitis in man. Cleve Clin J Med. 2002;69:SII15-9.
3. Witort-Serraglini E, Del Rosso M, Lotti TM, et al. Endothelial injury in vasculitides. Clin Dermatol. 1999;17:587.
4. Millikan LE, Flynn TC. Infectious etiologies of cutaneous vasculitis. Clin Dermatol. 1999;17:509-14.
5. Tervaert JW, Popa ER, Bos NA. The role of superantigens in vasculitis. Curr Opin Rheumatol. 1999;11:24-33.
6. Brusch JL. Infective endocarditis and its mimics in the critical care unit. Infect Dis Ther Ser. 2006;40:221.
7. Karchmer AW. Infectious endocarditis. Braunwald's Heart Disease: A Textbook of Cardiovascular Medicine, 8th edition. St Louis, Mo: WB Saunders; 2007.
8. Choucair J. Infectious Causes of Vasculitis, in Updates in the Diagnosis and Treatment of Vasculitis, Prof. Lazaros Sakkas (Ed.), 2013, pp 131-160. ISBN: 978-953-51-1008-8, InTech, DOI: 10.5772/55189. Available from: http://www.intechopen.com/books/updates-in-the-diagnosis-and-treatment-of-vasculitis/infectious-causes-of-vasculitis. http://dx.doi.org/10.5772/55189.
9. Biswas JS, Lyons OT, Bell RE, et al. Extra-aortic mycotic aneurysm due to group a streptococcus after pharyngitis. J Clin Microbiol. 2013;51:2797-9.
10. Jenckes GA 3rd. Aspergillus aortitis. J Thorac Cardiovasc Surg. 1990;99:375-6.
11. Vyas SK, Law NW, Loehry CA. Mycotic aneurysm of left subclavian artery. Br Heart J. 1993;69:455-6.
12. Walker DH, Cain BG, Olmstead PM. Laboratory diagnosis of Rocky Mountain spotted fever by immunofluorescent demonstration of rickettsia in cutaneous lesions. Am J Clin Pathol. 1978;69:619-23.
13. Davi G, Giammarresi C, Vigneri S, et al. Demonstration of Rickettsia Conorii-induced coagulative and platelet activation *in vivo* in patients with Mediterranean spotted fever. Thromb Haemost. 1995;74:631-4.
14. George F, Brouqui P, Boffa MC, et al. Demonstration of Rickettsia Conorii-induced endothelial injury *in vivo* by

measuring circulating endothelial cells, thrombomodulin, and von Willebrand factor in patients with Mediterranean spotted fever. Blood. 1993;82:2109-16.

15. Allins AD, Wagner WH, Cossman DV, et al. Tuberculous infection of the descending thoracic and abdominal aorta: case report and literature review. Ann Vasc Surg. 1999;13:439-44.

16. Strnad BT, McGraw JK, Heatwole EV, et al. Tuberculous aneurysm of the aorta presenting with uncontrolled hypertension. J Vasc Interv Radiol. 2001;12:521-3.

17. Tuder RM, Renya GS, Bensch K. Mycobacterial coronary arteritis in a heart transplant recipient. Hum Pathol. 1986;17:1072-4.

18. Whitaker DC, Lynch PJ. Erythema nodosum and coccidioidomycosis. Ariz Med. 1979;36:887-9.

19. Dearaujomartins-Romeo D, Garcia-Porrua C, Gonzalez-Gay MA. Cutaneous vasculitis is not always benign. Rev Rhum. 1999;66:240.

20. Garcia-Patos V, Barnadas MA, Domingo P, et al. Cutaneous vasculitis during bacteremia caused by meningococcus serogroup B. Rev Clin Esp. 1992;190:311-3.

21. Beddhu S, Bastacky S, Johnson JP. The clinical and morphologic spectrum of renal cryoglobulinemia. Medicine (Baltimore). 2002;81:398-409.

22. Agnello V, Abel G. Localization of hepatitis C virus in cutaneous vasculitic lesions in patients with type II cryoglobulinemia. Arthritis Rheum. 1997;40:2007-15.

23. Buisson GG, Vernant JC. Neurologic pathology and HTLV-I virus. Rev Prat. 1990;40:2124-6.

24. Mochizuki M, Tajima K, Watanabe T, et al. Human T lymphotropic virus type 1 uveitis. Br J Ophthalmol. 1994;78:149-54.

25. Mochizuki M, Watanabe T, Yamaguchi K, et al. HTLV-I uveitis: a distinct clinical entity caused by HTLV-I. Jpn J Cancer Res. 1992;83:236-9.

26. Adelman HM, Wallach PM, Gutierrez F, et al. Scurvy resembling cutaneous vasculitis. Cutis. 1994;54:111-4.

27. Wiik A. Drug-induced vasculitis. Curr Opin Rheumatol. 2008;20:35-9.

28. Ravindran V, Anoop P. Rheumatologic manifestations of benign and malignant haematological disorders. Clin Rheumatol. 2011;30:1143-9.

29. Kramann R, Brandenburg VM, Schurgers LJ, et al. Novel insights into osteogenesis and matrix remodelling associated with calcific uraemic arteriolopathy. Nephrol Dial Transplant. 2013;28:856-68.

30. Michaud M, Pourrat J. Cryofibrinogenemia. J Clin Rheumatol. 2013;19:142-8.

31. Merhoff GC, Porter JM. Ergot intoxication: historical review and description of unusual clinical manifestations. Ann Surg. 1974;180:773-9.

32. Mendoza CE, Rosado MF, Bernal L. The role of interleukin-6 in cases of cardiac myxoma. Clinical features, immunologic abnormalities, and a possible role in recurrence. Tex Heart Inst J. 2001;28:3-7.

33. Park J, Song JM, Shin E, et al. Cystic cardiac mass in the left atrium: hemorrhage in myxoma. Circulation. 2011;123:e368-9.

34. Sakamoto H, Sakamaki T, Kanda T, et al. Vascular endothelial growth factor is an autocrine growth factor for cardiac myxoma cells. Circ J. 2004;68:488-93.

35. Smith MJ, Chaudhry MA, Humphrey MB, et al. Atrial myxoma and bone changes: a paraneoplastic syndrome? J Card Surg. 2011;26:375-7.

CHAPTER 42

Secondary Vasculitis

Varun Dhir

INTRODUCTION

Secondary vasculitis refers to vasculitis in which a cause is apparent or obvious, i.e., either vasculitis has manifested in a chronic illness or there is a near simultaneous onset of vasculitis with another illness. The pathogenesis of secondary vasculitis is thought to be due to an immune reaction against either self-antigens or exogenous antigens leading to immune-complex deposition and damage. Secondary vasculitis must be excluded before making a diagnosis of primary vasculitides, as the therapy in the former is also directed against the primary process, i.e. infection or neoplasm.

This chapter will cover vasculitis secondary to rheumatoid arthritis, systemic lupus erythematosus (SLE), paraneoplastic vasculitis, and infection-associated vasculitis.

RHEUMATOID VASCULITIS

The simplest definition of rheumatoid vasculitis is vasculitic manifestations occurring in the presence of rheumatoid arthritis, with no other obvious etiology apparent. In general, rheumatoid vasculitis refers to systemic vasculitic manifestations. However, from a purist's point of view it also includes subclinical vasculitis (found on histopathology of autopsy specimens) and cutaneous vasculitis (typically small-vessel vasculitis).

Prevalence

The prevalence of rheumatoid vasculitis varies from 1 to 5% in different series.[1-3] There is some evidence to suggest that the prevalence of rheumatoid vasculitis is declining. A retrospective register-based study, from a homogeneous English population, found that the prevalence of rheumatoid vasculitis had declined from 11.6 per million to 3.6 per million over 10 years. The authors contrasted the declining prevalence of rheumatoid vasculitis with the stable (or increasing) prevalence of other systemic vasculitides over the same period, to emphasize that there was a true decline of rheumatoid vasculitis.[4] A hospital-(record) based study from the United States of America also found a decline in the rate of hospital admissions for rheumatoid vasculitis from 170 per 100,000 to 99 per 100,000 over 20 years, representing a decrease of almost 30%. As rheumatoid vasculitis invariably requires hospitalization, this offers a reasonable estimate of the burden of disease.[5] However, some studies have not found a decline in the prevalence of rheumatoid vasculitis.[6]

On autopsy, the presence of rheumatoid vasculitis (subclinical in most of the patients) has been reported to vary from 15 to 31%. However, the criteria used for defining vasculitis in some of these series have been questioned, and some reviews have suggested that the presence of vasculitis may have been overestimated by including mild or chronic lesions.[7-10]

Pathology and Pathogenesis

The sine qua non or essential histopathological feature of rheumatoid vasculitis is the presence of fibrinoid necrosis in a vessel accompanied by transmural inflammatory cell accumulation and the presence of leukocytoclasis (presence of nuclear fragments or debris of polymorphonuclear cells). The pathogenesis is believed to be immune-complex mediated, i.e. due to the deposition of immune complexes containing the rheumatoid factor in the vessel wall leading to inflammation and consequent damage to the vessel.[10] The risk factors for rheumatoid vasculitis include smoking, male gender, coexisting vascular disease, severe rheumatoid disease, high titer RF, erosions, nodules, nail fold lesions, and low C_4. In addition, treatment-related factors have also been shown in some studies. This includes the use of biologics, higher number of DMARDs used in the past in a patient (a marker of severity of disease), and association with Azathioprine or D-pencillamine.[11-13]

Clinical Manifestations

Most of the series have reported an equal predilection in males and females. The age of onset is typically around the sixth decade of life, with a disease duration of 10 years or more. The most commonly involved organs are the skin and nerves (Table 42.1). Most of the series have reported high prevalence of a positive-rheumatoid factor, usually in high titers. In the skin, a distinction must be made between leukocytoclastic and small-vessel vasculitis that manifests as nail bed infarcts or purpura and occurs without any systemic features, and skin involvement occurring as a part of systemic rheumatoid vasculitis. The manifestations of systemic rheumatoid vasculitis in the skin include digital gangrene and deep ulcers (typically on the legs in sites such as the calf and dorsum of foot).

Table 42.1 The major series on patients with rheumatoid vasculitis (most recent first).

Series (Author, center, year of publication)	Duration	Number of patients (% male)	Age, years (mean)	Disease duration, years (mean)	Common clinical manifestations	Risk factors
Makol A, Mayo Clinic, USA, 2014[11]	10 years (2000–2010)	86 (42%)	63	10.8	Cutaneous, neuropathy	Smoking, coexisting vascular disease, severe RA, CVA, use of biologics
Ntatsaki, London, United Kingdom 2014[33]	10 years (2000–2010)	18 (55%)	72	15.6	Cutaneous, pulmonary, neuropathy	
Nishimura, Brazil, 2012[34]		17 (11.8%)	57.8	13.1	Only included deep ulcers (cutaneous)	
Guignard S, Paris, France, 2008[35]	1997–2004	6 on anti-TNF 12 on DMARDs	66.5 5.3	12.2 13.8	Cutaneous, neuropathy, visceral	
Watts RA, United Kingdom 2004[4]	1988–2002	51 (47%)	61	16.8	Cutaneous, neuropathy, pulmonary	
Voskuyl, leiden, Netherlands, 1996[12]	1980–1993	69	66	12		Male, high titer RF, erosions, nodules, no. of DMARDs ever, Azathioprine or D-pen therapy, nail fold lesions
Puechal, 1995 (only on patients with nerve involvement)[14]	7.2 years	32 (28%)	59	16	Mononeuritis multiplex (51%), cutaneous (38%), cardiac involvement (12.5%)	
Bely M, Hungary, 1992 (Autopsies)[8]		36 (Clinically overt in 7)			Heart, skeletal muscle, peripheral nerves	
Geirsson AJ, Lund, Sweden 1987[13]	10 years	16 (62%)	64–69	7.5–8.0	Mononeuritis multiplex, cutaneous ulcers, digital gangrene, bowel ulcerations	High titer RF, low C4
Schneider 1985[36]	10 years	13 (54%)			Sensory neuropathy, mononeuritis multiplex, felty's, leg ulcers	
Scott DG, Bath, United Kingdom 1981[31]	5.5 years	50 (50%)	59.5	13.6	Cutaneous, neuropathy, cardiac, pulmonary	

The neuritic manifestations include mononeuritis multiplex and polyneuropathy. Mononeuritis multiplex typically manifesting as motor weakness and foot or wrist drop is perhaps the most well recognized manifestation of rheumatoid vasculitis. This is caused by axonal loss secondary to vasculitic involvement of the vasa vasorum that supply the nerves. Sensory loss or paresthesias are present in the areas supplied by that particular nerve. Polyneuropathy, especially if rapid in onset, can be part of a confluent mononeuritis multiplex and a detailed analysis and nerve conduction study can help to clarify the diagnosis. In some cases, true polyneuropathy may be a manifestation of systemic vasculitis. A distinction must be made from the chronic polyneuropathy, which is a typically insidious in onset, and is a common accompaniment of rheumatoid arthritis. In that case, a variety of etiologies have been implicated in different patients including drugs and vasculopathy rather than vasculitis. In a series on 32 patients with biopsy proven rheumatoid vasculitis of the nerves, the most common presentation was as mononeuritis multiplex (51%), followed by mononeuritis (14%) and distal sensory or motor neuropathy (34%).[14]

In the eye, presence of retinal vasculitis has been documented to be fairly high (up to 18% by fluorescein angiography) in some series.[15] However, the presence of clinically apparent retinal vasculitis is less common. Peripheral ulcerative keratitis or corneal melt is an important manifestation of systemic rheumatoid vasculitis and needs to be managed aggressively even in the absence of other systemic manifestations. There are numerous reports on involvement of different organs like the heart, central nervous system, and gastrointestinal (GI) system. Involvement of the heart has been reported in the form of coronary arteritis, whereas involvement of the central nervous system in the form of granulomatous meningitis and vasculitis leading to infarcts.[16-27] Gastrointestinal involvement typically presenting as bowel gangrene has been reported.[28-30]

Diagnosis

The diagnosis of rheumatoid vasculitis is often straightforward when vasculitic manifestations are recognized in the context of an established diagnosis of rheumatoid arthritis. A common mistake may be to confuse a systemic vasculitis like Wegener's granulomatosis (granulomatosis with polyangiitis) that begins as polyarthritis that may precede the vasculitic manifestations by some months as rheumatoid vasculitis. In that case, the absence of any erosions and the presence of antineutrophil cytoplasmic antibody (ANCA) may help to clarify the diagnosis. Classically, rheumatoid vasculitis occurs

Table 42.2 Scott and Bacon's criteria for the diagnosis of systemic rheumatoid vasculitis[6,31]
Either of
• Mononeuritis multiplex or
• Peripheral gangrene or
• Typical digital or nail-fold infarcts in a patient with systemic features or
• Deep cutaneous ulcers
With
Histological evidence of vasculitis

A pleuritis, pericarditis, and scleritis.

in a long-standing case of rheumatoid arthritis, generally with apparent deformities. A diagnostic criterion has been proposed by Scott and Bacon (Table 42.2) and it has been used for classification by some studies.[6,31] It emphasizes the presence of common manifestations in the skin and nerves, as well as histological features and constitutional symptoms. An important site that provides histological evidence of vasculitis is the sural nerve, when it is found to be involved by nerve conduction studies.

Laboratory Tests

There is no specific-laboratory test for rheumatoid vasculitis. In general, high titers of rheumatoid factor and markers of acute inflammation including a high erythrocyte sedimentation rate are seen. In addition, leukocytosis and high globulin levels may also be seen as part of the inflammatory response. Although a variety of autoantibodies have been described, none has established itself as being specific or sensitive for this diagnosis.

Treatment and Prognosis

The treatment of rheumatoid vasculitis is based on the same principles as the management of any systemic vasculitis. The bedrock of management remains corticosteroids in combination with other immunosuppressives, typically cyclophosphamide (Table 42.3). High-dose oral corticosteroids are usually continued for 1–2 months and then tapered off slowly over the next 6–12 months. In severe and life- or organ-threatening disease, pulses steroid therapy is often given for the initial few days to bring rapid control and then oral steroids are initiated. Cyclophosphamide is commonly given as IV bolus, typically monthly, in a dose that can vary from 15 mg/kg to 1 g/m^2 of body surface area.

In the milder manifestations of vasculitis, typically cutaneous, azathioprine, or methotrexate have been used

Table 42.3 Therapy and prognosis as reported in various series of rheumatoid vasculitis (most recent first)

Series	N, follow-up	Treatment	Remission rates	Relapse rates	Mortality rates
Makol A, Mayo Clinic, USA, 2014[11]	86 Median FU 16 months (2.4–59)	Oral cyclophosphamide 69 (83%) Oral and IV cyclophosphamide 12 (14%) IV cyclophosphamide 2 (2%) Anti-TNF 12 Rituximab 6	38% (6 months)	36% (5 years)	26% (5 years)
Ntatsaki, United Kingdom, 2014[33]	18	IV cyclophosphamide (17/18) IV methylprednisolone	N/A	N/A	12% (1 year) 60% (5 years)
Puechal, Paris, France 2012[37]	17 33.1 months (6–69)	IV rituximab	71% (6 months) 82% (12 months)	33% (no RTX maintenance) 0% (on RTX maintenance)	
Puechal, Paris, France 2008[38]	9 (CYC refractory)	Anti-TNF	55% (6 months)		
Puechal 1995[14]	32 7.2 years	Corticosteroids +/– immunosuppressive			43% (5 years) 55% (10 years)
Heurkens, Leiden, Netherlands 1987[39]	9	Oral prednisolone + azathioprine	All improved at 3, 9 and 18 months	0	11%
Scott DG, United Kingdom 1984[40]	21	IV cyclophosphamide + methyprednisolone versus others (azathioprine or steroids or D-pen or chlorambucil)	Early responses (0–4 months) more with IV CYC + MP	IV CYC + MP 24% Others 54%	IV CYC + MP 24% Others 29%

successfully. In refractory cases, biological typically anti-TNF (generally infliximab) or rituximab (anti-CD20) have been resorted to, with fairly good results.

A review of the various series shows that, with treatment, the remission rate at 6 months varies from 30 to 70%. The long-term outcome in the various series is fair, with mortality at 5 years varying from 20 to 45% (Table 42.3). It has been estimated that the mortality of rheumatoid vasculitis patients is increased compared to that of rheumatoid arthritis.[32]

LUPUS VASCULITIS

Vasculitic manifestations occurring in a patient with SLE is referred to as lupus vasculitis. This chapter will first focus on lupus vasculitis *in general* and then discuss specific-organ vasculitis in lupus namely lupus mesenteric vasculitis (GI vasculitis) and CNS vasculitis.

Prevalence

The prevalence of lupus vasculitis has been reported to vary from 11 to 20% in large series on lupus patients.[41-43] However, nearly 90% of patients have only cutaneous vasculitis, without any systemic involvement.

Clinical Features

In a large series on 670 patients of lupus, 76 (11%) had vasculitis. In a majority (89%) it limited to the skin and occurred as a small-vessel vasculitis.[41] Common cutaneous lesions in lupus vasculitis are erythematous lesions on the fingertips and palms, palpable purpura, and ulcerations. Systemic vasculitis manifests as involvement of the nerves, kidney, muscle, and lungs in patients with SLE. Involvement of the nerves is typically in the form of mononeuritis multiplex as a part of medium-vessel vasculitis and is the most common manifestation of a systemic vasculitis in lupus patients. Involvement of the kidney is often unsuspected, and detected with lupus nephritis on renal biopsy. In addition, there are a number of reports describing lupus vasculitis to involve different sites like the gallbladder, the appendix, coronary arteries,[44] the liver,[45] and the uterus.[46,47] Arterial occlusions of the medium arteries supplying the extremities has been reported. In a series of six patients of gangrene of the extremities in lupus, the diagnosis was suggested by a good response to immunosuppression.[48] The manifestations included fingertip or toe gangrene to gangrene of the forefoot requiring amputation. The prevalence of digital or distal limb gangrene was reported to be 1.3% from a large series of 520 lupus cases.[49]

Diagnosis

The diagnosis of vasculitis in lupus requires an exclusion of antiphospholipid-associated vascular occlusion or embolic vascular occlusion. However, this differentiation is difficult and often artificial, as both can occur simultaneously and antiphospholipid antibodies are commonly found in patients with lupus vasculitis. Thus, the diagnosis is often clinical and in some cases histopathological. The diagnosis may be suggested by the presence of active disease and hypocomplementemia.

Management

The management of lupus vasculitis is similar to any primary systemic vasculitis, and involves the use of steroids. In case of cutaneous vasculitis, the use of low or moderate dose of steroids may be adequate. Additional drugs for cutaneous vasculitis include hydroxychloroquine, methotrexate, and azathioprine. In case of systemic involvement, the therapy is usually more aggressive and includes pulse steroids along with cytotoxic drugs such as cyclophosphamide.

Lupus Mesenteric Vasculitis (GI Vasculitis due to Lupus)

Lupus mesenteric vasculitis has also been referred to commonly as lupus enteritis or GI vasculitis due to lupus.[50]

Prevalence

The prevalence of lupus mesenteric vasculitis has been reported to vary from 0.2 to 9.7%.[41,51-55] Importantly, in a patient of lupus who presents with an acute abdomen, the prevalence of lupus mesenteric vasculitis can range from 29% to as high as 65%.[53,54,56] Lupus mesenteric vasculitis is commonly suspected and diagnosed in rheumatological centers dealing with patients of SLE. However, it is relatively uncommon in unselected patients with SLE.

Clinical Features

Lupus mesenteric vasculitis typically presents as an acute abdomen. There may be absence of bowel movements or exaggerated bowel movements that manifest as diarrhea, vomiting, hematochezia, or extensive bleed.[50,57] Lupus mesenteric vasculitis typically occurs in the presence of active lupus manifestations in other organs.[54,56,58] Studies have found a higher prevalence of lupus mesenteric vasculitis in active compared to inactive patients of SLE presenting with abdominal pain. Similarly, it has been found that, patients who present with lupus mesenteric vasculitis as the cause of abdominal pain, are more likely to have received high-prednisolone doses in the previous months, again, pointing to ongoing disease activity. Some patients have a tendency to have recurrent episodes of lupus mesenteric vasculitis.

Diagnosis and Laboratory Tests

The diagnosis of lupus mesenteric vasculitis is primarily based on the clinical setting of high disease activity and the exclusion of other causes, with some radiological tests that may suggest this diagnosis. The investigation of choice is a computed tomographic study of the abdomen that may reveal signs of bowel ischemia.[50] These signs are not specific for lupus *per se*, and can be found in a variety of other vasculitic diseases like Henoch–Schönlein purpura and polyarteritis nodosa. In addition, other pathologies like embolic and atherosclerotic disease giving rise to bowel ischemia may have a similar picture. These signs include bowel wall thickening (symmetrical), halo sign, engorgement of mesenteric vessels, mesenteric edema, and ascites.[50,59] Bowel wall thickening can be focal or diffuse and involve either or both of the small and large intestines. The bowel wall may show a "halo" sign, which occurs due to enhancement of the inner and outer parts of the bowel wall, with a hypodense center, due to edema, or hemorrhage.

Management and Prognosis

The treatment of lupus mesenteric ischemia involves immunosuppression. Steroids are the anchor drugs for management, with initial parenteral administration (dose of 1 mg/kg/day prednisolone equivalent) or high-dose pulse therapy. In addition, cyclophosphamide is often used in monthly pulses or in some centers as oral therapy till the patient stabilizes followed by monthly IV pulses. The requirement for surgical exploration becomes mandatory in case of signs of frank peritonitis or bowel perforation. However, in other cases, a wait-and-watch policy is often employed, with immunosuppression given as the first line, with a surgical back up if required.

The prognosis of this condition varies with its severity, with a recent series reporting a mortality rate of 13.4%. Recurrence in that series occurred in 22.8%, and was associated with severe thickness of bowel wall (>8 mm) and was negatively associated with cyclophosphamide therapy.[55] Another study that compared patients who had a recurrence compared to those without a recurrence suggested that if the bowel was markedly thickened the chances of recurrence seem to be higher.[58]

CNS Vasculitis in SLE

True CNS vasculitis in SLE relatively uncommon, and, other more common etiologies need to be excluded before making this diagnosis.[60] Common causes of CNS dysfunction in SLE include metabolic causes, infections, and finally thrombotic occlusions secondary to antiphospholipid syndrome or cardioembolism. Although CNS lupus in general can present as a variety of syndromes, CNS lupus vasculitis should be suspected in cases of acute unexplained loss of consciousness, features suggesting multiple infarcts and focal deficits.[61]

Imaging

Magnetic resonance imaging with contrast is the standard investigation of choice in CNS vasculitis. A classical presentation would be with multiple infarcts in different territories occurring acutely. These will be picked up depending on their age by different MRI protocols.[62] In addition, angiographic studies can reveal focal abnormalities of vessels in the form of stenosis or dilatations.

Although brain biopsy is the gold standard, it carries a high chance of giving a false negative result, due to sampling from an unaffected area, and carries a risk of leading to focal deficits.

Management

The management of CNS vasculitis in SLE follows the principles of management of any severe life-threatening manifestation and consists of steroids with cyclophosphamide. A variety of other agents have been used including azathioprine and cyclosporine.

PARANEOPLASTIC VASCULITIS

Paraneoplastic vasculitis, i.e. vasculitis associated with a malignant disease is uncommon. Indeed, many centers do not routinely screen patients of vasculitis for a malignancy. This seems to be reasonable, considering that the most common malignant diseases that could present as a vasculitis, would involve the lymphoreticular and hematologic system, and thus would be picked up on a routine examination (lymph nodes) and blood tests (cytopenias).

Prevalence

One study found that among all cases of cutaneous vasculitis, nearly 4% were associated with malignancy.[63]

Pathogenesis

The pathogenesis of paraneoplastic vasculitis has been proposed to be tumor antigen-induced autoantibody production and subsequent deposition of immune complexes containing these antigen-antibody complexes in vessels. Another theory invokes the production of certain cytokines or toxic substances that lead to changes in the permeability or damage the vessels.[64]

Clinical Features

Cutaneous vasculitis and polyarteritis nodosa seem to be the most common manifestations of malignancy associated with vasculitis. Cutaneous vasculitis is typically a small-vessel vasculitis, and this has been estimated to account for 50–60% of all paraneoplastic vasculitis.[64]

The most common neoplasms include lympho-proliferative malignancies including Hodgkin's disease, non-Hodgkin's lymphoma, multiple myeloma, and hairy cell leukemia. Although solid neoplasms are much less associated than lymphoproliferative diseases, there are reports with squamous cell bronchogenic carcinoma, renal, prostatic and colon carcinoma, and head/neck carcinoma.[65] In some cases of lymphoproliferative diseases, the vasculitis may be related to cryoglobulinemia. It is estimated that 6–15% of cryoglobulinemia may be related to malignancies.[64] The common associated malignancies with cryoglobulinemic vasculitis include Waldenström's macroglobulinemia, non-Hodgkin's lymphoma, and chronic lymphocytic leukemia.

In a study of 421 adult-cutaneous vasculitis patients, 16 patients (3.8%) with a paraneoplastic cause were identified. The mean interval from the onset of vasculitis to the diagnosis of malignancy was approximately 2 weeks. In this series, important clues in the form of cytopenias or immature cells on the peripheral smear were present in a majority of the cases. Nine of the cases were associated with a hematological malignant condition, most commonly myelodysplastic syndrome, and Waldenström's macroglobulinemia.[63] In this study, a solid organ malignancy was the cause/associated with vasculitis in seven cases, the most common being breast carcinoma. Another study looked at 15 patients diagnosed with vasculitis and solid tumors within 12 months of the onset of either disease. In seven cases the diagnosis of vasculitis was prior to detection of malignancy, in six cases both malignancy and vasculitis were detected simultaneously, and in two patients, vasculitis was detected after diagnosis of cancer. The most common vasculitis associated with neoplastic process is cutaneous-leukocytoclastic vasculitis (60%). Other vasculitides that may present as a paraneoplastic manifestation are Henoch–Schönlein purpura, polyarteritis nodosa, and giant cell arteritis. The most common malignancies in this series on solid tumors was carcinomas of urinary organs (40%), lung (26.7%), and GI tract (26.7%).[66] Although ANCA-associated vasculitis can occur as a paraneoplastic syndrome, this is relatively rare (<5%).[64]

Management and Prognosis

The management of paraneoplastic secondary vasculitis includes therapy of the malignancy and treatment of the vasculitis (if needed). In case of the cutaneous vasculitis, the therapy includes corticosteroids, hydroxychloroquine, and dapsone. Immunosuppressive such as cyclophosphamide, cyclosporine, and azathioprine may be used in cases with systemic involvement.

INFECTION-ASSOCIATED VASCULITIS

A variety of infections have been associated with secondary vasculitis. The infections associated include infective endocarditis,[67,68] tuberculosis, syphilis,[69] hepatitis B and C virus-associated cryoglobulinemic vasculitis, hepatitis B-associated polyarthritis nodosa, invasive fungal infections,[70] *Borrelia burgdorferi*, rickettsial infections,[71] *varicella zoster* infection,[72,73] and human immunodeficiency virus. The pathogenesis could involve the complementarity of the infectious antigen with a self-antigen or a type III reaction due to immune complexes.[74,75]

A variety of reports have found HIV to be associated with vasculitis. Over a 5-year-period, 34 patients with HIV were documented to have inflammatory vascular disease on biopsy of the muscle, nerve, or skin. The most common was mononuclear inflammatory vascular disease occurring in 17 patients, and necrotizing arteritis that occurred in three patients.[76] A polyarteritis nodosa like clinical presentation was the clinical correlate of the necrotizing arteritis that was found in biopsy. Indeed, polyarteritis nodosa like presentation with HIV has been reported in other case reports as well.[77,78] In a series of nine patients of stroke with HIV, five of these were found to be secondary to varicella-zoster vasculitis.[79] Another series on four patients with HIV and severe stroke, found

improvement with corticosteroids suggesting a vasculitic etiology of the stroke in some of these cases.[80]

Management

The management of infection-associated vasculitis is first and foremost directed to the inciting agent, i.e. the infection. However, in case of life-threatening manifestations or refractoriness to therapy, corticosteroids, and immunosuppression is used.

CONCLUSION

Secondary vasculitis includes a variety of syndromes, ranging from rheumatoid arthritis-associated vasculitis to HIV-associated vasculitis. The management of secondary vasculitis follows the same principles as in a primary vasculitis, i.e. the treatment is dictated by the severity of the vasculitic manifestation in case of rheumatic disease-associated vasculitis. In secondary vasculitis due to infections or neoplasms, the treatment of the underlying condition is important, and that may take care of the vasculitic manifestations. It is important to be aware of secondary vasculitis, to suspect it, to investigate accordingly and finally to manage optimally.

KEY POINTS

- Secondary vasculitis in rheumatoid arthritis is most commonly an isolated cutaneous vasculitis in the form of nail bed infarcts and purpura and may not require any specific treatment.
- Systemic rheumatoid vasculitis typically occurs in patients having rheumatoid arthritis of around 10 years duration and having a severe deforming disease requiring the use of multiple DMARDs (past or present). It commonly presents as deep cutaneous ulcers or mononeuritis multiplex (wrist or foot drop) and requires aggressive treatment.
- Lupus vasculitis is commonly cutaneous, however, can involve any organ like rheumatoid vasculitis.
- Lupus mesenteric vasculitis (also called lupus enteritis or GI vasculitis) should be suspected in a patient of SLE presenting with acute abdomen and having active disease in other organs.
- The most common cause of paraneoplastic vasculitis is lymphoproliferative diseases. The most common manifestation is as a small-vessel cutaneous vasculitis. However, this is rare and most centers do not routinely

screen for neoplasms in patients with vasculitis. A physical examination for lymph nodes and blood counts (cytopenias) are probably enough to pick up most of these cases. Although, less common, vasculitis have been associated with solid-organ malignancies as well.

- Infection-associated vasculitis can occur in association with a variety of infections. In HIV-associated vasculitis, in cases of stroke varicella zoster-induced vasculitis has been found in some series. A polyarteritis nodosa like presentation has also been found in HIV.

REFERENCES

1. Salvarani C, Macchioni P, Mantovani W, et al. Extra-articular manifestations of rheumatoid arthritis and HLA antigens in northern Italy. J Rheumatol. 1992;19:242-6.
2. Kaye O, Beckers CC, Paquet P, et al. The frequency of cutaneous vasculitis is not increased in patients with rheumatoid arthritis treated with methotrexate. J Rheumatol. 1996;23:253-7.
3. Wattiaux MJ, Kahn MF, Thevenet JP, et al. Vascular involvement in rheumatoid polyarthritis. Retrospective study of 37 cases of rheumatoid polyarthritis with vascular involvement and review of the literature. Ann Med Interne (Paris). 1987;138:566-87.
4. Watts RA, Mooney J, Lane SE, et al. Rheumatoid vasculitis: becoming extinct? Rheumatology (Oxford). 2004;43:920-3.
5. Ward MM. Decreases in rates of hospitalizations for manifestations of severe rheumatoid arthritis, 1983–2001. Arthritis Rheum. 2004;50:1122-31.
6. Turesson C, Mcclelland RL, Christianson TJ, et al. No decrease over time in the incidence of vasculitis or other extra-articular manifestations in rheumatoid arthritis: results from a community-based study. Arthritis Rheum. 2004;50:3729-31.
7. Suzuki A, Ohosone Y, Obana M, et al. Cause of death in 81 autopsied patients with rheumatoid arthritis. J Rheumatol. 1994;21:33-6.
8. Bely M, Apathy A, Beke-Martos E. Cardiac changes in rheumatoid arthritis. Acta Morphol Hung. 1992;40:149-86.
9. Kemper JW, Baggenstoss AH, Slocumb CH. The relationship of therapy with cortisone to the incidence of vascular lesions in rheumatoid arthritis. Ann Intern Med. 1957;46:831-51.
10. Genta MS, Genta RM, Gabay C. Systemic rheumatoid vasculitis: a review. Semin Arthritis Rheum. 2006;36:88-98.
11. Makol A, Crowson CS, Wetter DA, et al. Vasculitis associated with rheumatoid arthritis: a case-control study. Rheumatology (Oxford). 2014;53:890-9.
12. Voskuyl AE, Zwinderman AH, Westedt ML, et al. Factors associated with the development of vasculitis in rheumatoid arthritis: results of a case-control study. Ann Rheum Dis. 1996;55:190-2.
13. Geirsson AJ, Sturfelt G, Truedsson L. Clinical and serological features of severe vasculitis in rheumatoid arthritis: prognostic implications. Ann Rheum Dis. 1987;46:727-33.
14. Puechal X, Said G, Hilliquin P, et al. Peripheral neuropathy with necrotizing vasculitis in rheumatoid arthritis. A clinicopathologic and prognostic study of thirty-two patients. Arthritis Rheum. 1995;38:1618-29.
15. Giordano N, D'ettorre M, Biasi G, et al. Retinal vasculitis in rheumatoid arthritis: an angiographic study. Clin Exp Rheumatol. 1990;8:121-5.
16. Akrout R, Bendjemaa S, Fourati H, et al. Cerebral rheumatoid vasculitis: a case report. J Med Case Rep. 2012;6:302.
17. Caballol Pons N, Montala N, Valverde J, et al. Isolated cerebral vasculitis associated with rheumatoid arthritis. Joint Bone Spine. 2010;77:361-3.
18. Guadalupe Loya-De La Cerda D, Aviles-Solis JC, Delgado-Montemayor MJ, et al. Isolated rheumatoid arthritis-associated cerebral vasculitis: a diagnostic challenge. Joint Bone Spine. 2013;80:88-90.
19. Kurne A, Karabudak R, Karadag O, et al. An unusual central nervous system involvement in rheumatoid arthritis: combination of pachymeningitis and cerebral vasculitis. Rheumatol Int. 2009;29:1349-53.
20. Mrabet D, Meddeb N, Ajlani H, et al. Cerebral vasculitis in a patient with rheumatoid arthritis. Joint Bone Spine. 2007;74:201-4.
21. Ohno T, Matsuda I, Furukawa H, et al. Recovery from rheumatoid cerebral vasculitis by low-dose methotrexate. Intern Med. 1994;33:615-20.
22. Ohta K, Tanaka M, Funaki M, et al. Multiple cerebral infarction associated with cerebral vasculitis in rheumatoid arthritis. Rinsho Shinkeigaku. 1998;38:423-9.
23. Pedersen RC, Person DA. Cerebral vasculitis in an adolescent with juvenile rheumatoid arthritis. Pediatr Neurol. 1998;19:69-73.
24. Ramos M, Mandybur TI. Cerebral vasculitis in rheumatoid arthritis. Arch Neurol. 1975;32:271-5.
25. Singleton JD, West SG, Reddy VV, et al. Cerebral vasculitis complicating rheumatoid arthritis. South Med J. 1995;88:470-4.
26. Spath NB, Amft N, Farquhar D. Cerebral vasculitis in rheumatoid arthritis. QJM. 2012.
27. Watson P, Fekete J, Deck J. Central nervous system vasculitis in rheumatoid arthritis. Can J Neurol Sci. 1977;4:269-72.
28. Babian M, Nasef S, Soloway G. Gastrointestinal infarction as a manifestation of rheumatoid vasculitis. Am J Gastroenterol. 1998;93:119-20.
29. Pagnoux C, Mahr A, Cohen P, et al. Presentation and outcome of gastrointestinal involvement in systemic necrotizing vasculitides: analysis of 62 patients with polyarteritis nodosa, microscopic polyangiitis, Wegener granulomatosis, Churg-Strauss syndrome, or rheumatoid arthritis-associated vasculitis. Medicine (Baltimore). 2005;84:115-28.
30. Parker B, Chattopadhyay C. A case of rheumatoid vasculitis involving the gastrointestinal tract in early disease. Rheumatology (Oxford). 2007;46:1737-8.
31. Scott DG, Bacon PA, Tribe CR. Systemic rheumatoid vasculitis: a clinical and laboratory study of 50 cases. Medicine (Baltimore). 1981;60:288-97.

32. Wolfe F, Mitchell DM, Sibley JT, et al. The mortality of rheumatoid arthritis. Arthritis Rheum. 1994;37:481-94.

33. Ntatsaki E, Mooney J, Scott DG, et al. Systemic rheumatoid vasculitis in the era of modern immunosuppressive therapy. Rheumatology (Oxford). 2014;53:145-52.

34. Nishimura WE, Costallat LT, Fernandes SR, et al. Association of HLA-DRB5*01 with protection against cutaneous manifestations of rheumatoid vasculitis in Brazilian patients. Rev Bras Reumatol. 2012;52:366-74.

35. Guignard S, Gossec L, Bandinelli F, et al. Comparison of the clinical characteristics of vasculitis occurring during anti-tumor necrosis factor treatment or not in rheumatoid arthritis patients. A systematic review of 2707 patients, 18 vasculitis. Clin Exp Rheumatol. 2008;26:S23-9.

36. Schneider HA, Yonker RA, Katz P, et al. Rheumatoid vasculitis: experience with 13 patients and review of the literature. Semin Arthritis Rheum. 1985;14:280-6.

37. Puechal X, Gottenberg JE, Berthelot JM, et al. Rituximab therapy for systemic vasculitis associated with rheumatoid arthritis: Results from the AutoImmunity and Rituximab Registry. Arthritis Care Res (Hoboken). 2012;64:331-9.

38. Puechal X, Miceli-Richard C, Mejjad O, et al. Anti-tumour necrosis factor treatment in patients with refractory systemic vasculitis associated with rheumatoid arthritis. Ann Rheum Dis. 2008;67:880-4.

39. Heurkens AH, Westedt ML, Breedveld FC. Prednisone plus azathioprine treatment in patients with rheumatoid arthritis complicated by vasculitis. Arch Intern Med. 1991;151:2249-54.

40. Scott DG, Bacon PA. Intravenous cyclophosphamide plus methylprednisolone in treatment of systemic rheumatoid vasculitis. Am J Med. 1984;76:377-84.

41. Ramos-Casals M, Nardi N, Lagrutta M, et al. Vasculitis in systemic lupus erythematosus: prevalence and clinical characteristics in 670 patients. Medicine (Baltimore). 2006;85:95-104.

42. Estes D, Christian CL. The natural history of systemic lupus erythematosus by prospective analysis. Medicine (Baltimore). 1971;50:85-95.

43. Vitali C, Bencivelli W, Isenberg DA, et al. Disease activity in systemic lupus erythematosus: report of the consensus study group of the European workshop for rheumatology research. I. A descriptive analysis of 704 European lupus patients. European consensus study group for disease activity in SLE. Clin Exp Rheumatol. 1992;10:527-39.

44. Caracciolo EA, Marcu CB, Ghantous A, et al. Coronary vasculitis with acute myocardial infarction in a young woman with systemic lupus erythematosus. J Clin Rheumatol. 2004;10:66-8.

45. Alanazi T, Alqahtani M, Al Duraihim H, et al. Hepatic vasculitis mimicking liver abscesses in a patient with systemic lupus erythematosus. Ann Saudi Med. 2009;29:474-7.

46. Massasso D, Cheruvu C, Joshua F, et al. Ovarian vasculitis in an adult with fatal systemic lupus erythematosus. Lupus. 2009;18:364-7.

47. Pereira RM, De Carvalho JF, De Medeiros AC, et al. Ovarian necrotizing vasculitis in a patient with lupus. Lupus. 2009;18:1313-5.

48. Da Rocha MC, Vilar MJ, Freire EA, et al. Arterial occlusion in systemic lupus erythematosus: a good prognostic sign? Clin Rheumatol. 2005;24:602-5.

49. Dubois EL, Tuffanelli DL. Clinical manifestations of systemic lupus erythematosus. Computer analysis of 520 cases. JAMA: The Journal of the American Medical Association. 1964;190:104-11.

50. Ju JH, Min JK, Jung CK, et al. Lupus mesenteric vasculitis can cause acute abdominal pain in patients with SLE. Nat Rev Rheumatol. 2009;5:273-81.

51. Sultan SM, Ioannou Y, Isenberg DA. A review of gastrointestinal manifestations of systemic lupus erythematosus. Rheumatology (Oxford). 1999;38:917-32.

52. Drenkard C, Villa AR, Reyes E, et al. Vasculitis in systemic lupus erythematosus. Lupus. 1997;6:235-42.

53. Lee CK, Ahn MS, Lee EY, et al. Acute abdominal pain in systemic lupus erythematosus: focus on lupus enteritis (gastrointestinal vasculitis). Ann Rheum Dis. 2002;61:547-50.

54. Lian TY, Edwards CJ, Chan SP, et al. Reversible acute gastrointestinal syndrome associated with active systemic lupus erythematosus in patients admitted to hospital. Lupus. 2003;12:612-6.

55. Yuan S, Ye Y, Chen D, et al. Lupus mesenteric vasculitis: clinical features and associated factors for the recurrence and prognosis of disease. Semin Arthritis Rheum. 2013.

56. Medina F, Ayala A, Jara LJ, et al. Acute abdomen in systemic lupus erythematosus: the importance of early laparotomy. Am J Med. 1997;103:100-5.

57. Chen SY, Xu JH, Shuai ZW, et al. A clinical analysis 30 cases of lupus mesenteric vasculitis. Zhonghua Nei Ke Za Zhi. 2009;48:136-9.

58. Kim YG, Ha HK, Nah SS, et al. Acute abdominal pain in systemic lupus erythematosus: factors contributing to recurrence of lupus enteritis. Ann Rheum Dis. 2006;65:1537-8.

59. Byun JY, Ha HK, Yu SY, et al. CT features of systemic lupus erythematosus in patients with acute abdominal pain: emphasis on ischemic bowel disease. Radiology. 1999;211:203-9.

60. Nikolov NP, Smith JA, Patronas NJ, et al. Diagnosis and treatment of vasculitis of the central nervous system in a patient with systemic lupus erythematosus. Nat Clin Pract Rheumatol. 2006;2:627-33; quiz 34.

61. Rizos T, Siegelin M, Hahnel S, et al. Fulminant onset of cerebral immunocomplex vasculitis as first manifestation of neuropsychiatric systemic lupus erythematosus (NPSLE). Lupus. 2009;18:361-3.

62. Acioly MA, Farina EM, Dalmonico AC, et al. Severe cerebral vasculitis in systemic lupus erythematosus: from stroke to multiple fusiform aneurysms. Eur Neurol. 2012;67:352-3.

63. Loricera J, Calvo-Rio V, Ortiz-Sanjuan F, et al. The spectrum of paraneoplastic cutaneous vasculitis in a defined population: incidence and clinical features. Medicine (Baltimore). 2013;92:331-43.

64. Park HJ, Ranganathan P. Neoplastic and paraneoplastic vasculitis, vasculopathy, and hypercoagulability. Rheum Dis Clin North Am. 2011;37:593-606.

65. Buggiani G, Krysenka A, Grazzini M, et al. Paraneoplastic vasculitis and paraneoplastic vascular syndromes. Dermatol Ther. 2010;23:597-605.

66. Solans-Laque R, Bosch-Gil JA, Perez-Bocanegra C, et al. Paraneoplastic vasculitis in patients with solid tumors: report of 15 cases. J Rheumatol. 2008;35:294-304.

67. Park JH, Jang HR, Lee JE, et al. Infective endocarditis with multiple mycotic aneurysms mimicking vasculitis: a case report. Can J Infect Dis Med Microbiol. 2012;23:e67-8.

68. Zaki SA, Shanbag P, Gokhale YA. Infective endocarditis in a child masquerading as vasculitis: case report. Ann Trop Paediatr. 2010;30:141-5.

69. Jo J, Heo ST, Kim JW, et al. Secondary syphilis with nodular vasculitis mimicking Behçet's disease. Infect Chemother. 2013;45:451-4.

70. Mearelli F, Occhipinti A, Altamura N, et al. Invasive filamentous fungus infection with secondary cerebral vasculitis in a patient with no obvious immune suppression. Int J Infect Dis. 2014;19:91-2.

71. Nickerson A, Marik PE. Life-threatening ANCA-positive vasculitis associated with rickettsial infection. BMJ Case Rep. 2012;2012.

72. Poonyathalang A, Sukavatcharin S, Sujirakul T. Ischemic retinal vasculitis in an 18-year-old man with chickenpox infection. Clin Ophthalmol. 2014;8:441-3.

73. Yaramis A, Herguner S, Kara B, et al. Cerebral vasculitis and obsessive-compulsive disorder following varicella infection in childhood. Turk J Pediatr. 2009;51:72-5.

74. Rodriguez-Pla A, Stone JH. Vasculitis and systemic infections. Curr Opin Rheumatol. 2006;18:39-47.

75. Belizna CC, Hamidou MA, Levesque H, et al. Infection and vasculitis. Rheumatology (Oxford). 2009;48:475-82.

76. Gherardi R, Belec L, Mhiri C, et al. The spectrum of vasculitis in human immunodeficiency virus-infected patients. A clinicopathologic evaluation. Arthritis Rheum. 1993;36:1164-74.

77. Libman BS, Quismorio FP Jr, Stimmler MM. Polyarteritis nodosa-like vasculitis in human immunodeficiency virus infection. J Rheumatol. 1995;22:351-5.

78. Sambatakou H, Tsiachris D, Stamouli S, et al. Systemic vasculitis with gastrointestinal involvement in an HIV-infected adult. Am J Med Sci. 2008;335:237-8.

79. Gutierrez J, Ortiz G. HIV/AIDS patients with HIV vasculopathy and VZV vasculitis: a case series. Clin Neuroradiol. 2011;21:145-51.

80. Melica G, Brugieres P, Lascaux AS, et al. Primary vasculitis of the central nervous system in patients infected with HIV-1 in the HAART era. J Med Virol. 2009;81:578-81.

CHAPTER 43

Cogan's Syndrome

Tommy CY Chan, Vishal Jhanji

INTRODUCTION

Cogan's syndrome is characterized by the presence of bilateral sensorineural hearing loss, vestibular symptoms, and inflammatory ocular manifestations, particularly interstitial keratitis.[1] David Glendenning Cogan, an ophthalmologist, first described the classic form of the disease in 1945 as nonsyphilitic interstitial keratitis with audiovestibular symptoms. More than 100 cases of Cogan's syndrome have been reported in the literature. The etiology and pathogenesis are unknown, but are believed to involve autoimmunity to the inner ear, cornea, and vascular endothelium.[2-4] The presence of autoantibodies against inner ear, corneal, and endothelial antigen, and others including the antineutrophil cytoplasmic antibodies, rheumatoid factor, antinuclear antibodies, and reduced complement levels suggests that immune mechanisms are involved.[5] Since Cogan's syndrome is often preceded by a viral-like illness, it is thought that infectious antigens may sensitize this autoimmunity through molecular mimicry.[2,6] Pathologic studies have shown lymphocytes and plasma cell infiltration of corneal stroma and cochlea, suggestive of a cell-mediated immune response rather than direct pathogen invasion.[7] Several human leucocyte antigens (HLA) such as HLA-A9, HLA-Bw17, HLA-Bw35, and HLA-Cw4 have been correlated with an increased incidence of Cogan's syndrome.[8] However, Cogan's syndrome is not believed to have hereditary transmission.

EPIDEMIOLOGY

Cogan's syndrome has been reported mostly in young Caucasian adults.[3,4] The peak of incidence occurs in the third decade of life, and the full range encompasses both pediatric and geriatric populations. There is no known gender predominance.

Typical Cogan's Syndrome

Typical Cogan's syndrome is encountered in two-thirds of patients with Cogan's syndrome.[3,9] This is defined by the following conditions: (i) nonsyphilitic interstitial keratitis; (ii) audiovestibular symptoms similar to those of Meniere's syndrome with sudden onset of tinnitus and vertigo, accompanied by hearing loss that usually progress to deafness in 1–3 months; and (iii) an interval between the onset of ocular and audiovestibular manifestations of <2 years.

Atypical Cogan's Syndrome

Atypical Cogan's syndrome is characterized by the following presentations according to the criteria suggested by Haynes et al.:[3,9] (i) inflammatory ocular manifestations, with or without interstitial keratitis, (ii) audiovestibular symptoms mostly different from Meniere-like symptoms, and (iii) a delay of >2 years between the onset of ocular and audiovestibular manifestations.

CLINICAL FEATURES

The diagnosis of Cogan's syndrome is mainly based upon the characteristic involvement of both eye and inner ear. They are equally likely to be the cause of presenting symptoms. Only 5% of the patients initially present with interstitial keratitis, cochlear, and vestibular dysfunction, while up to 85% develops both eye and ear symptoms within 2 years.[3,4,6] In addition to ocular and audiovestibular dysfunctions, about 50% of patients have an underlying systemic disease associated with vasculitis of any vessel size. Systemic manifestations are much more frequent in atypical Cogan's syndrome, and less than 5% of patients have systemic manifestations as the initial presentation.[3,9] Patients may describe a history of fever, headache, arthralgia, myalgia, or preceding upper respiratory infection. The disease course of Cogan's syndrome varies from monophasic episodes, multiple recurrent attacks to chronic active inflammation. If not managed promptly and adequately, visual loss secondary to corneal scarring and permanent hearing loss may occur in Cogan's syndrome.[10]

OCULAR MANIFESTATIONS

The predominant ocular feature of Cogan's syndrome is interstitial keratitis, which typically causes eye redness, pain, photophobia, and blurred vision. It occurs in 80% of cases, and it is mostly bilateral, with great variability in symptoms from one eye to the other. Slit-lamp examination demonstrates a patchy, deep, granular corneal infiltrate. Cases of early interstitial keratitis may produce a faint peripheral, anterior stromal, subepithelial keratitis.[11-13] Rarely, uncontrolled corneal inflammation may lead to neovascularization and corneal clouding, resulting in permanent visual loss. Late findings include stromal scarring and ghost vessels.[14] Other ocular manifestations mainly observed in patients with atypical Cogan's syndrome include conjunctivitis, scleritis, episcleritis, iritis, posterior uveitis, vitritis, retinitis, optic neuritis, tendonitis, and orbital inflammation. Cataract, glaucoma and vascular occlusion are complications associated with those ocular manifestations.[12,13,15] A moderate and transient visual impairment is not uncommon, but blindness may also occur.

AUDIOVESTIBULAR MANIFESTATIONS

The inner ear manifestations of Cogan's syndrome are Meniere's-like attacks consisting of vertigo, ataxia, nausea, vomiting, tinnitus, and hearing loss.[9] Hearing loss has been reported to be sudden, bilateral, fluctuating, and progressive. Recurrent episodes of inner ear disease frequently result in profound hearing loss. Progression to complete bilateral hearing loss was detected in audiometric assay in almost 50% of patients, whereas permanent hearing loss in one ear was observed in 20% of patients.[3,4] Recurrent episodes of inner ear disease may also result in cochlear hydrops.[4] This may be associated with down fluctuations in hearing because of changes in the cochlear pressure independent of inflammation. Sensorineural hearing loss, preferentially involving the low- and high-range frequencies, is reported upon audiometry testing.

Vestibular dysfunction may cause oscillopsia, a perception of objects jiggling back and forth after abruptly turning the head to one side or the other.[10,16,17] At least 20% of patients have spontaneous or gaze-induced nystagmus. Bilateral weak or absent vestibular responses to caloric testing may be noticed in up to 40% of cases. Most clinical symptoms of vestibular dysfunction are transient or episodic that last for days or weeks from the time of onset.

SYSTEMIC MANIFESTATIONS

About half of the patients with Cogan's syndrome have features of systemic manifestations, the mechanism of which in most cases is considered to be vasculitis.[2-4,9,18] The systemic vasculitis associated with Cogan's syndrome mainly involves the medium- and large-sized vessels. Aortitis with aortic insufficiency are the most serious complications associated with Cogan's syndrome. The large-vessel vasculitis associated with Cogan's syndrome may resemble Takayasu's arteritis, causing an occlusion of the aortic arch vessels with resultant limb claudication or renal artery stenosis.[19,20] However, Takayasu's arteritis does not routinely involve the eyes and ears.

Cogan's syndrome has also been associated with a number of rheumatologic diseases, including polyarteritis nodosa, Wegener's granulomatosis, rheumatoid arthritis, Crohn's disease, relapsing polychondritis, giant cell arteritis, and spondyloarthritis. The disease can rarely associate with sarcoidosis, HIV infection, mastocytosis, and pregnancy.

DIAGNOSTIC APPROACH AND INVESTIGATIONS

The diagnosis of Cogan's syndrome is mainly clinical and is based on ocular inflammation, audiovestibular symptoms, and nonreactive serologic tests for syphilis in the presence of vasculitis. There is a lack of specific laboratory tests to confirm the diagnosis. The diagnosis of Cogan's syndrome is often based on the good response to corticosteroid treatment.

The differential diagnoses of Cogan's syndrome include polyarteritis nodosa, Wegener's granulomatosis, rheumatoid arthritis, and sarcoidosis. These diseases may indeed coexist as systemic manifestation of Cogan's syndrome. Other diagnostic possibilities include congenital syphilis, tuberculosis, chlamydial infection, and viral infection including measles, mumps, and herpes zoster.

Important investigations include vestibular function, audiometry testing, radiographic studies, and serological assay. Complete blood count with differential, erythrocyte sedimentation rate, C-reactive protein, creatinine, urinalysis, treponemal test, complement levels, antineutrophil cytoplasmic antibodies, rheumatoid factor, antinuclear antibodies, and tuberculin test should be considered. Leukocytosis, eosinophilia, elevated erythrocyte sedimentation rate can be found in Cogan's syndrome. Most patients have normal or mildly reduced complement levels as well as a negative antinuclear antibodies results. Cranial computed tomography and magnetic resonance imaging are often normal, but calcification or obliteration of the vestibular labyrinth and the cochlea are sometimes observed in patients of Cogan's syndrome.

TREATMENT

Anterior segment inflammation in Cogan's syndrome is usually treated with topical corticosteroids with or without mydriatics. Prednisolone acetate 1% one drop per affected eye may be administered four times per day or even hourly depending upon the severity of the inflammation.[21] Rarely, treatment of interstitial keratitis or anterior uveitis may require systemic glucocorticoid therapy, if topical treatments are ineffective after 2 weeks. Other forms of anterior ocular inflammation, including conjunctivitis, scleritis, and episcleritis, should also be treated with topical glucocorticoid therapy. Topical or systemic nonsteroidal anti-inflammatory drug therapy may benefit some patients with episcleritis and scleritis. Nodular scleritis or scleritis unresponsive to topical glucocorticoids and oral nonsteroidal anti-inflammatory drug therapy may require treatment with systemic glucocorticoids at a dose of prednisolone of 1 mg/kg/day.[21,22] Cataract extraction may be needed to improve visual acuity. Secondary glaucoma due to prolonged corticosteroid use can be managed with topical or occasionally oral antiglaucoma agents. Progressive corneal opacification or scarring may require corneal transplantation.

Posterior ocular inflammation is treated with systemic corticosteroids beginning at a dose of prednisone of 1 mg/kg/day.[21,22] In cases that does respond to corticosteroids, other immunosuppressive drugs, including methotrexate, azathioprine, cyclosporine A or cyclophosphamide may be used.[23] When used together with another immunosuppressive agent, the glucocorticoid dose should be tapered to the lowest possible dose or should be discontinued, as tolerated, over

the subsequent 3–4 months. If the patient remains free of active disease for 6–9 months, tapering the additional agent over the next 3–4 months should be considered.

The audiovestibular dysfunction always requires rapid initiation of high-dose systemic corticosteroids (prednisone 1–2 mg/kg/day) for 2–6 months duration.[2,4,22] Audiometry may be used to determine the degree of hearing loss and to monitor the treatment effect. Steroid taper may begin when auditory and vestibular functions are stable. Some patients may require long-term systemic corticosteroids therapy because of recurrent hearing loss during attempts to reduce the dosage.[21,22] Steroid sparing therapy should be considered in patients where excessive amounts of steroids are required to prevent hearing loss or if significant steroid-related side effects result. This consists of methotrexate, azathioprine, cyclosporine A, tacrolimus or cyclophosphamide.[24,25] Hearing loss is sometimes associated with cochlear hydrops. A trial of diuretic therapy such as hydrochlorothiazide and furosemide can be used for 4–7 days, along with systemic immunosuppressants. In patients with profound hearing loss, cochlear implant surgery is often indicated with satisfactory outcome. Acute vestibular dysfunction may be treated with antihistamines or benzodiazepines and bed rest. Recurrent vestibular dysfunction is always accompanied by hearing loss and should be treated with systemic immunosuppressive therapy.

Active rheumatologic disease and systemic vasculitis associated with Cogan's syndrome must be treated with prompt and prolonged immunosuppressive therapy starting with prednisone 1 mg/kg/day.[21,22] For the treatment of large-vessel vasculitis, weekly methotrexate is used as an additional immunosuppressive agent.[26] Azathioprine or mycophenolate mofetil may be used when response to methotrexate is poor. Alternatively, oral cyclophosphamide given for 4–6 months can be used as an alternative immunosuppressant. Treatment with additional immunosuppressive agents is generally continued for 6–12 months after all evidence of disease activity has resolved. Unfortunately, some cases associated with an underlying systemic vasculitis progress despite immunosuppressive therapy and lead to significant morbidity. Other novel immunotherapies including antibodies against tumor necrosis factor-alpha (Etanercept, Infliximab), interleukin-6 receptor (Tocilizumab), and lymphocyte CD20 surface antigen (Rituximab), offer encouraging results in patients with Cogan's syndrome refractory to the conventional immunosuppressive therapy.[27,28] Plasmapheresis is another treatment option in patients resistant to or intolerant to high level of immunosuppression. Surgical bypass grafting or aortic valve replacement may be required in some patients with severe ischemic symptoms or heart failure. Such procedures should be preferably performed during periods of disease quiescence.

KEY POINTS

- Cogan's syndrome is an inflammatory disorder that affects young adults.
- Clinical manifestations include ocular and inner ear inflammation.
- Associations between Cogan's syndrome and systemic vasculitis are important indicating an autoimmune pathogenesis.
- Cogan's syndrome is a diagnosis of exclusion.
- Collaborative management by ophthalmologists, otorhinolaryngologists, and rheumatologists is crucial.
- Mild corneal or anterior segment diseases can be treated by topical corticosteroids, while systemic immunosuppressive therapy is the mainstay of treatment for majority of patients with severe inflammation.
- If medical treatment fails, corneal transplant and cochlear implant can be considered for corneal opacity and hearing loss, respectively.

REFERENCES

1. Cogan DG. Syndrome of nonsyphilitic interstitial keratitis and vestibuloauditory symptoms. Arch Ophthal. 1945;33:144-9.
2. St Clair EW, McCallum RM. Cogan's syndrome. Curr Opin Rheumatol. 1999;11:47-52.
3. Haynes BF, Kaiser-Kupfer MI, Mason P, et al. Cogan syndrome: studies in thirteen patients, longterm follow-up, and a review of the literature. Medicine (Baltimore). 1980;59:426.
4. Vollertsen RS, McDonald TJ, Younge BR, et al. Cogan's syndrome: 18 cases and a review of the literature. Mayo Clin Proc. 1986;61:344.
5. Lunardi C, Bason C, Leandri M, et al. Autoantibodies to inner ear and endothelial antigens in Cogan's syndrome. Lancet. 2002;360:915.
6. Gluth MB, Baratz KH, Matteson EL, et al. Cogan syndrome: a retrospective review of 60 patients throughout a half century. Mayo Clin Proc. 2006;81:483.
7. Fisher ER, Hellstrom HR. Cogan's syndrome and systemic vascular disease. Analysis of pathologic features with reference to its relationship to thromboangiitis obliterans (Buerger). Arch Pathol. 1961;72:572.
8. Migliori G, Battisti E, Pari M, et al. A shifty diagnosis: Cogan's syndrome—A case report and review of the literature. Acta Otorhinolaryngol Ital. 2009;29:108-13.
9. Grasland A, Pouchot J, Hachulla E, et al. Study Group for Cogan's Syndrome. Typical and atypical Cogan's syndrome: 32 cases and review of the literature. Rheumatology (Oxford). 2004;43:1007-15.
10. Greco A, Gallo A, Fusconi M, et al. Cogan's syndrome: an autoimmune inner ear disease. Autoimmun Rev. 2013;12:396-400.
11. Cobo LM, Haynes BF. Early corneal findings in Cogan's syndrome. Ophthalmology. 1984;91:903.
12. Witcup SM, Smith JA. Nonsyphilitic Interstitial Keratitis. In: Krachmer JH, Mannis MJ, Holland EJ (Eds). Cornea, 2nd edition, Vol. 1. Philidelphia: Elsevier Mosby; 2005. pp. 1161-7.
13. Chynn EW, Jakobiec FA. Cogan's syndrome: ophthalmic, audiovestibular, and systemic manifestations and therapy. Int Ophthalmol Clin. 1996;36:61-72.
14. Cogan DG, Kuwabara T. Late corneal opacities in the syndrome of interstitial keratitis and vestibuloauditory symptoms. Acta Ophthalmol Suppl. 1989;192:182.
15. Shah P, Luqmani RA, Murray PI, et al. Posterior scleritis: an unusual manifestation of Cogan's syndrome. Br J Rheumatol. 1994;33:774.
16. Kessel A, Vadasz Z, Toubi E. Cogan syndrome: pathogenesis, clinical variants and treatment approaches. Autoimmun Rev. 2014;13:351-4.
17. Pagnini I, Zannin ME, Vittadello F, et al. Clinical features and outcome of Cogan syndrome. J Pediatr. 2012;160:303-7.
18. Cheson BD, Bluming AZ, Alroy J. Cogan's syndrome: a systemic vasculitis. Am J Med. 1976;60:549-55.
19. Cochrane AD, Tatoulis J. Cogan's syndrome with aortitis, aortic regurgitation, and aortic arch vessel stenosis. Ann Thorac Surg. 1991;52:1166.
20. Raza K, Karokis D, Kitas GD. Cogan's syndrome with Takayasu's arteritis. Br J Rheumatol. 1998;37:369.
21. McCallum RM, Haynes BF. Cogan's syndrome. In: Pepose JS, Holland GN, Wilhelmus KR (Eds). Ocular Infection & Immunity, 1st edition, Mosby: St. Louis; 1996. p. 446.
22. McCallum RM. Cogan's syndrome. In: Franunfelder FT, Hampton R (Eds). Current Ocular Therapy, 4th edition. Philadelphia: WB Saunders; 1993. p. 410.
23. Dev S, McCallum RM, Jaffe GJ. Methotrexate treatment for sarcoid-associated panuveitis. Ophthalmology. 1999;106:111.
24. Riente L, Taglione E, Berrettini S. Efficacy of methotrexate in Cogan's syndrome. J Rheumatol. 1996;23:1830.
25. Matteson EL, Tirzaman O, Facer GW, et al. Use of methotrexate for autoimmune hearing loss. Ann Otol Rhinol Laryngol. 2000;109:710.
26. Unizony S, Stone JH, Stone JR. New treatment strategies in large-vessel vasculitis. Curr Opin Rheumatol. 2013;25:3-9.
27. Shibuya M, Fujio K, Morita K, et al. Successful treatment with tocilizumab in a case of Cogan's syndrome complicated with aortitis. Mod Rheumatol. 2013;23:577.
28. Allen NB, Cox CC, Cobo M, et al. Use of immunosuppressive agents in the treatment of severe ocular and vascular manifestations of Cogan's syndrome. Am J Med. 1990;88:296.

CHAPTER 44

Malignancy-associated Vasculitis

Narendra Kumar, Pankaj Kumar, Rupali Agarwal, Shabab Lalit Angurana

INTRODUCTION

Vasculitides are characterized by inflammation and damage of blood vessel walls, leading to lumen compromise, resulting in ischemia of tissues supplied by the involved vessel. The clinical spectrum of disease is varied with diverse etiologies and can be the consequence of infections, allergy, rheumatologic and/or autoimmune diseases, or drugs. A broad group of syndromes may result from this process, since any type, size, and location of blood vessel may be involved. Vasculitis and its consequences may be the primary or sole manifestation of the disease or it may be secondary component of another primary disease. Certain vasculitis syndromes are predominantly systemic in nature and can lead to irreversible organ system damage and even death if untreated, while others are usually localized to skin and rarely result in irreversible dysfunction of vital organs.

The primary systemic vasculitis is associated with circulating autoantibodies directed against certain proteins in cytoplasm of human neutrophil [antineutrophil cytoplasmic antibody (ANCA)]. The presence of ANCA has led this group of conditions to be considered as autoimmune diseases, but the nature of triggering antigen remains unknown. These conditions include granulomatosis with polyangiitis [GPA, previously Wegener's granulomatosis (WG)], microscopic polyangiitis (MPA), and eosinophilic granulomatosis with polyangiitis (EGPA, previously Churg-Strauss syndrome). Classic polyarteritis nodosa (PAN) is often considered a part of this group because it involves vessels of similar size but is not ANCA associated.

Predominantly, cutaneous vasculitis or cutaneous leukocytoclastic vasculitis is a group of diseases characterized by involvement of small vessels of skin and present as palpable purpura or nonspecific lesions: papules, nodules, bullae, ulcerations, and/or necrotic lesions. This syndrome is presumed to be associated with an aberrant hypersensitivity reaction to an exogenous antigen such as an infectious agent, or a drug, or an endogenous antigen, such as vasculitis associated with neoplasms, connective tissue diseases, or congenital deficiencies of complement system. In these conditions, skin involvement generally dominates the clinical picture, but skin is not always the exclusive organ involved. Any organ system can be involved with this type of vasculitis; however, the extracutaneous involvement is usually much less severe than that of systemic vasculitis. Systemic manifestations usually include fever, arthralgias and arthritis and, less commonly, renal, neurological, or gastrointestinal compromise.[1,2]

ASSOCIATION OF VASCULITIS AND MALIGNANCY

Vasculitis occasionally develops secondarily to malignancy. The relationship between vasculitis and malignancy remains unclear. It can be *true malignancy-associated vasculitis* or *malignancy induced by immunosuppressive drugs* prescribed to treat vasculitis.

The *malignancy-associated vasculitis* syndrome can be grouped under three categories:[3]

1. Vasculitis-associated malignancies or true paraneoplastic syndrome.
2. Malignancies masquerading as vasculitis; failure to respond appropriately to therapy should prompt a search for malignancy with biopsy of suspicious lesions even if diagnosis of vasculitis has been histologically proven.
3. Vasculitis masquerading as malignancies. A large mass of inflammatory tissue associated with constitutional symptoms may be misdiagnosed as a malignancy, like the

differentiation between lymphoma and WG of the upper airways can be particularly difficult, biopsies of lesion usually rule out malignancy.

Malignancy-associated vasculitis has been described with lymphoid and myeloid cancers, myelodysplasia, and a broad spectrum of solid tumors.[2,4-8] Malignancy-associated vasculitis is rare, constituting 0.4–4.2% of all vasculitis cases in some investigations; malignancy may not be clinically obvious at presentation.[1,7,9] Vasculitis frequency during cancer has been estimated at 1 in 1,800 for hemopathies and 1 in 80,800 for solid tumors.[10] The hematological malignancies most frequently described are myelodysplastic syndrome (MDS) and lymphoproliferative diseases such as hairy cell leukemia and lymphomas.

Over an 18.5-year period, Hutson and Hoffman reviewed the records of 2,800 patients with vasculitis and 69,000 patients with cancer, and could identify only 69 patients with both vasculitis and cancer (2.5% of patients with vasculitis and 0.1% of those with cancer). There were 12 patients (17%) in whom the cancer and vasculitis occurred within 12 months. Six patients had solid organ tumors, four had lymphoma, and one each had leukemia and multiple myeloma. The most common type of vasculitis was cutaneous leukocytoclastic vasculitis (seven patients), followed by giant cell arteritis (two patients), PAN (two patients), and GPA (one patient). The authors concluded that vasculitis is rarely the presenting manifestation of malignancy, and the close temporal relationship of cancer and vasculitis in their patients adds to circumstantial evidence of vasculitis at times being a paraneoplastic condition. Failure of vasculitis to respond to conventional therapy should raise questions about underlying malignancy. Effective treatment of the cancer enhances the likelihood of improvement in vasculitis.[7] In 1987, the American Cancer Society found 41 cases of vasculitis among 75,000 patients with hematological malignancies versus 11 cases of vasculitis in all other malignancies.[11] Sanchez-Guerrero et al.[12] reviewed 222 patients with malignancies, 11 of whom had vasculitis, and Castro et al.[13] found seven patients with cutaneous vasculitis in 162 patients with MDS.

Fain et al. retrospectively analyzed the characteristics and outcomes of vasculitis associated with malignancies in 60 patients. The inclusion criterion for this 10-year study was development of vasculitis in patients with a progressing malignancy; malignancies secondary to immunosuppressants used to treat vasculitis were excluded. Vasculitis was diagnosed concurrently with malignancy in 38% of the cases. Vasculitis was cutaneous leukocytoclastic in 45%, PAN in 36.7%, GPA in 6.7%, MPA in 5%, and Henoch-Schönlein purpura (HSP) in 5% patients. Malignancies

were distributed as hematological in 63.1%, MDS in 32.3%, lymphoid in 29.2%, and solid tumor in 36.9% patients.[5]

Cutaneous leukocytoclastic vasculitis: It is the most frequently observed paraneoplastic vasculitis; this clinicopathological type constitutes nearly 30–40% of all paraneoplastic vasculitis.[1,14] The majority of individuals with leukocytoclastic vasculitis secondary to hematological disorders suffer from lymphoid neoplasms, most commonly lymphoproliferative (nearly 20% of cases) or MDS (3–5% of cases).[2,15] Other authors have also reported cutaneous leukocytoclastic vasculitis as the most common form of vasculitis associated with hematological malignancies.[9,10,16-18] Systemic vasculitic syndromes have also been observed in cancer patients, with PAN being the predominant disease phenotype.[5]

RISK FACTORS AND PATHOGENESIS OF MALIGNANCY-ASSOCIATED VASCULITIS

A close temporal relationship between diagnosis of cancer and onset of vasculitis suggests that inflammatory responses provoked by the underlying neoplasm contribute to the pathogenesis of malignancy-associated vasculitis.[2,4,5,7,8] In addition, some cases of vasculitis may occur in patients with previous or concomitant cancer because of risk factors predisposing to both conditions.[19] However, the relationship between vasculitis and hematological conditions still remains a matter of controversy. In patients with hematological malignancies, manifestation of vasculitis may be secondary either to the malignancy itself or to many frequent events in these patients such as infections, drug intake, or cryoglobulin deposition that are known to be responsible per se for the development of vasculitis and may be responsible for biases in the interpretation of the association between vasculitis and hematological malignancies. Drawing precise conclusions about the true relationship between these diseases is therefore still mandatory. The frequent implication of underlying lymphoproliferative disorders in vasculitis is expected as these conditions are frequently responsible for various autoimmune diseases, such as hemolytic anemia, thyroiditis and subepidermal bullous diseases,[20,21] and cryoglobulinemia.[22] These factors are detected in 39% of the patients who develop cutaneous vasculitis during the course of hematological malignancies. The pathogenic events that cause vasculitis in cancer patients remain though incompletely understood and real paraneoplastic syndromes are rarely observed. If the parallelism between neoplasia and target organ manifestations was indeed fully requested for considering a disease as paraneoplastic, vasculitis should therefore not be considered as truly paraneoplastic but rather as "associated" to hematological malignancies. Indeed, cancer appears more such as a vasculitis-triggering factor, and the outcomes of the two diseases are not strictly chronologically parallel.[4] Therefore, a careful exclusion of other triggering factors for vasculitis is mandated before assessing a link between an underlying disease and vasculitis. In a series dealing only with hairy cell leukemia (HCL) and vasculitis, the ratio of infections was very high, reaching 88%.[23] In a study by Paydas et al., 28 patients had cutaneous vasculitis and leukemia. They considered that only 39% of their patients had "true" paraneoplastic vasculitis while 61% would have drug-induced vasculitis. The culprit drugs were antibacterial therapy given for febrile neutropenia, chemotherapy including ATRA, hydroxyurea, methotrexate, aracytine, interferon, and G-CSF. Of note, the precise criteria for attributing vasculitis to drugs were not given in detail, and the role of underlying infection in patients treated with antibiotic therapy could also be hypothesized rather than the drugs.[24]

In 1986, Longley et al. first suggested that malignant neoplasms might produce antigens and can cause paraneoplastic vasculitis.[25] In the same year, McLean established two necessary criteria to define paraneoplastic vasculitis: first, the simultaneous appearance of both vasculitis and neoplasms; and second, their parallel course.[26] From that date to 1993, Kurzrock and Cohen identified a total of 200 patients with both cancer and paraneoplastic vasculitis reported in the world literature, of whom 88 presented with cutaneous leukocytoclastic vasculitis.[1] Most of these cases of vasculitis occurred in patients with hematological malignant neoplasms (two-thirds of the total number of cases of paraneoplastic vasculitis).[1,2,14] The pathogenetic mechanisms for the development of paraneoplastic vasculitis in malignancy and the significantly stronger association between vasculitis and hematological malignancies as compared with solid tumors, as well as the different tendency for each hematological disorders to develop vasculitis, is poorly understood. The suggestions for pathogenic link include a common genetic susceptibility, abnormal production of proteins that bind to endothelial walls, chronic stimulation of the immune system, generation of autoantibodies against various autoantigens, and defective apoptosis.[27,28]

In the *pathogenesis of leukocytoclastic vasculitis*, the dynamic nature of the infiltrate as well as the upregulation of vascular adhesion molecules have been well documented.[29,30] Most authors consider that immune complex deposition in the vessel walls is the initial step in the development of the disease.[30] Immune complexes would activate complement components that attract polymorphonuclear neutrophils.

While these cells attempt to phagocytize immune complexes, lysosomal enzymes would be released leading to vessel wall destruction. In this view, the immune complexes would correspond to tumor antigens together with antibodies directed against these. However, other mechanisms than immune complex deposition could also lead to vasculitis in the context of hematological malignancies. Antineutrophil cytoplasmic antibody—upon their deposition within vessel walls—may also trigger neutrophilic infiltrate migration at this site.[31] Alternatively, aberrant properties of polymorphonuclear neutrophils in some myeloid malignancies may lead to the abnormal adhesion of these cells to vessel walls. However, such a mechanism could not explain the cases developing in patients with lymphoid malignancies. Also, the production of various cytokines by tumor cells may modify polymorphonuclear neutrophil properties and stimulate the adhesion of these cells to the endothelium.[29,32] All these possible mechanisms illustrate the various pathways that may be responsible for the development of vasculitis in malignancies.

Thus, cutaneous vasculitis constitutes a symptom developing in association with hematological malignancies. However, since, other known triggering factors for vasculitis frequently develop with such conditions, the re-evaluation of the prevalence of vasculitis in hematological malignancies, once other causes are excluded and stringent histopathological criteria of vasculitis are applied, would bring contributive information to this field.

CLINICAL PRESENTATION AND PROGNOSIS

In general, the signs and symptoms of paraneoplastic vasculitis are similar to those in patients who do not suffer from an underlying cancer. The main features that may raise suspicion about the possible presence of a neoplasm in individuals with vasculitis are decline in general health,[14] loss of weight, or a chronic relapse course of the skin purpura.[15,33] Patients having chronic or recurrent vasculitis may harbor an underlying malignancy. More importantly, the appearance of vasculitis can suggest recurrence or progression of a tumor. Laboratory studies do not usually show specific alterations suggesting underlying neoplasm; however, sometimes an increased erythrocyte sedimentation rate, anemia, or lymphocytosis can be seen. Positive tests for rheumatoid factor or decrease in complement levels can also be detected.[14]

In apparently idiopathic cutaneous leukocytoclastic vasculitis, especially in patients aged over 50 or with some of the referred symptoms, a screening examination should be performed to detect any underlying neoplasm. In these patients, preliminary studies should include an exhaustive history and physical examination, complete blood count, serum chemistries (including antinuclear factors, rheumatoid factors, cryoglobulinemia, and tumor markers), and chest X-ray.[14]

Histological features of leukocytoclastic paraneoplastic vasculitis do not differ from those identified in different etiological vasculitis. Direct immunofluorescence studies disclose immunoglobulins (IgM, IgG, or IgA in HSP) and/or complement deposits in vessel walls in most of the leukocytoclastic vasculitis. Nevertheless, the percentage of positive biopsies for direct immunofluorescence declines considerably in later lesions, especially when more than 24 hours have elapsed since the beginning of the purpura.[1]

The overall outcomes for patients with severe vasculitis and malignancy are poor, with the most important predictor of a better prognosis being availability of effective treatment and the response of the underlying malignancy to treatment. As expected for a paraneoplastic syndrome, cutaneous lesions heal after surgical removal or radiation therapy of the cancer.[14] When a curative treatment of the neoplasm is not possible, paraneoplastic vasculitis responds to treatment with glucocorticoids alone or in combination with immunosuppressive agents.[2] Antineutrophil cytoplasmic antibody-associated vasculitis is more difficult to treat in patients with malignancy, as the vasculitis may be refractory to standard therapy. In the majority of the cases, deaths are due to metastatic or recurrent tumor rather than to vasculitis complications.[2,14]

Fain et al. in their retrospective study observed fever (41.7%), cutaneous involvement (78.3%), arthralgias (46.7%), peripheral neuropathy (31.7%), renal involvement (23.3%; 11.7% glomerulonephritis, 11.7% microaneurysms, and 6.7% renal insufficiency), and ANCA (20.4%) as the manifestations of vasculitis. Vasculitis treatments were corticosteroids (78.3%) and immunosuppressant(s) (41.7%). Vasculitis was cured in 65% of patients, but 58.3% died, with one death secondary to vasculitis. Independent of subtype, patients with vasculitides associated with MDS more frequently had renal manifestations ($p = 0.02$) and steroid dependence ($p = 0.04$) and achieved complete remission less often ($p = 0.04$) than patients with vasculitis associated with other malignancies. Patients with vasculitis associated with a solid tumor more frequently had peripheral neurological involvement ($p = 0.05$). Patients with vasculitis associated with lymphoid malignancy had less frequent arthralgias ($p = 0.01$) and renal involvement ($p = 0.02$). The authors concluded that vasculitis occurring during malignancies present distinctive features according to the vasculitis subtype and nature of the malignancy.[5]

SPECIFIC MALIGNANCY-ASSOCIATED VASCULITIS

Myelodysplastic syndromes: It comprises a heterogeneous group of hematological diseases, characterized by cytopenia and the presence of dysplastic blood cells. According to the World Health Organization classification of the myeloid neoplasms, chronic myelomonocytic leukemia (CMML) is classified as an overlap syndrome of MDS and myeloproliferative neoplasms, since it can present with both myelodysplastic symptoms such as cytopenia and proliferative features such as remarkable leukocytosis and splenomegaly.[34] The combination of MDS especially CMML with autoimmune manifestations have been described before in a number of case reports, with a reported prevalence of autoimmune manifestations of 10–18% in CMML.[16] Pirayesh et al. in the review of literature on the combination of MDS and vasculitis found that the majority of patients had leukocytoclastic cutaneous vasculitis and more rarely PAN.[35] Other reports also state that the autoimmune manifestations seen in MDS largely concern cases of mild rheumatological symptoms or cutaneous leukocytoclastic vasculitis, but also various types of systemic vasculitis.[36-39] A wide spectrum of autoimmune abnormalities has been reported in patients with MDS including systemic vasculitis, such as giant-cell arteritis, aortitis, and medium- and small-sized vessel vasculitis.

The pathogenesis of vasculitis in MDS is still largely unknown. In patients with CMML, high numbers of circulating monocytes and related cytokines are found that may lead to vascular inflammation. At the same time phagocytic clearance is impaired, leading to prolonged circulation of immune complexes with subsequent activation of inflammatory mediators.[40,41] Furthermore, the presence of interferon regulatory factor-1 (IRF-1) has been associated with the development of autoimmune deregulation in MDS.[42] Interferon regulatory factor-1 also plays a role in the induction of immune responses. Interferon regulatory factor-1 is usually low in MDS patients when compared with healthy individuals. This decrease probably plays a role in the pathogenesis of MDS and in the transformation to acute leukemia.[43]

Previous reports about the prognosis of patients with hematological malignancies in combination with autoimmune disorders have shown conflicting results. In some retrospective reports, a worse outcome in MDS patients with immunological manifestations or with systemic vasculitis was demonstrated when compared with other MDS patients.[44] However, in a prospective study by Giannouli et al. including

13 patients, no influence on median survival was reported. But in this study patients with various types of autoimmune manifestations of variable severity were included; only two of the studied patients had systemic vasculitis.[45]

Bilateral perirenal hemorrhage has also been described in PAN associated with CMML. Refractory anemia with excess blasts, CMML, or MDS during the period around transformation into acute leukemia appears to trigger vasculitis onset. Indeed, vasculitis often appeared to be a sign preceding transformation, and treatment of vasculitis itself with corticosteroids with or without immunosuppressive medications can improve symptoms. In this context, immunosuppressive drugs should be used prudently and reserved for uncontrolled vasculitis or severe involvement because they increase the risk of fatal infections in the long term, especially for patients who have previously been treated with etoposide or hydroxyurea for MDS, and accelerate transformation into acute leukemia. In the study by Fain et al., nine patients died of infectious complications; four of them had received immunosuppressants for PAN. The authors found that vasculitis associated with MDS was more severe and development of systemic vasculitis was associated with worse outcome in MDS patients.[5]

In conclusion, comparison with the general population, systemic vasculitis is more prevalent in patients with MDS and in particular CMML, with a particular risk of bilateral renal hemorrhage. The prognosis of MDS patients with systemic vasculitis is worse than similar patients without vasculitis, because of the risk of both vasculitis- and treatment-related complications.

Hairy cell leukemia: It is a rare lymphoproliferative disease characterized by the presence of mononuclear cells with hair-like cytoplasmic projections in peripheral blood, bone marrow, spleen, and liver. Affected patients are susceptible to infection, especially by intracellular pathogens, possibly as a consequence of impaired monocyte function or reduced numbers of monocytes and granulocytes.[46] Hairy cell leukemia has been strongly associated with systemic necrotizing vasculitis, especially PAN, and cutaneous leukocytoclastic vasculitis.[6] Direct infiltration of the vessel walls by hairy cells has been seen in some cases. The association between HCL and PAN was first noted by Hughes et al. in 1976.[46] This work and later studies found that the coincidence of the two diseases was highly unlikely caused by chance, and it is hypothesized that an etiological relationship exists between the two conditions. In the majority of cases, the leukemia is diagnosed first and the interval between the two diagnoses may be several years. The vasculitis is not usually the cause of

death, which is usually due to complications of leukemia and its therapy.

Non-Hodgkin's lymphoma: As discussed, vasculitis has been described in association with various hematological malignancies, but it seems to be very uncommon among lymphomas. Non-Hodgkin's lymphoma (NHL) is more often associated with vasculitis (leukocytoclastic vasculitis, lymphocytic, cutaneous granulomatous, PAN, and HSP) than Hodgkin's disease.[36] A condition of immunodysregulation is known to underlie both vasculitis and NHL development. Hence, it might be hypothesized that vasculitis and NHL could be found in the same patient as the result of a common facilitating factor, without the need for a direct pathogenetic relationship between the two diseases. In a study by Milone et al., it was found that if vasculitis appeared late during the clinical course of NHL, an aggressive phase or an impending relapse of the lymphoid neoplasia may be expected, and a possible histological conversion should also be actively pursued, whereas when vasculitis precedes the lymphoid neoplasia, it may not signal a poor prognosis.[47] Fain et al. detected cryoglobulins in 22% of patients with vasculitis–NHL and considered them to be the origin of the vasculitis rather than lymphoma. Vasculitis and lymphoma were diagnosed simultaneously in 70% of the reported cases, but the responses of the two diseases to treatment showed no parallelism. Regarding treatment in these patients, corticosteroids and/or chemotherapy were often found to be effective.[36]

Multiple myeloma: The incidence of paraneoplastic vasculitis in patients with multiple myeloma is very low, approximately 0.8%.[1] Monoclonal gammopathies are detected in cryoglobulinemic vasculitis and other cutaneous vasculitis (leukocytoclastic, erythema elevatum diutinum), mostly monoclonal IgA type. There is tendency of IgA to act as a chemotactic factor of polymorphonuclear cells, which can explain that the IgA myeloma has been the most frequent type reported in association with paraneoplastic cutaneous leukocytoclastic vasculitis. Indeed, 66% of multiple myelomas associated with vasculitis reported by Sanchez et al. were of the IgA type; vasculitis was always cutaneous, and the outcome was favorable in all cases, either spontaneously or with treatment of the myeloma.[48] Some authors have suggested that paraprotein in myelomas may act as an antigenic factor and precipitate the immune response, but these theories are not completely proved as the existence of immunocomplexes, the decrease in complement levels, or the immunoglobulins deposits in affected vessels have not always been observed, because they depend on the time when the biopsy is performed.[49]

Solid tumor-associated vasculitis: Solid tumors, predominantly lung, colon, and renal, are more rarely associated with vasculitis. Polyarteritis nodosa and HSP are reported more frequently than leukocytoclastic vasculitis or GPA. Vasculitis can appear as early as 25 months before cancer is diagnosed.[36] Pertuiset et al. compared HSP patients with and without malignancy, those with malignancy (solid tumor in two thirds of the cases) were more likely to be older and male, and have more joint involvement and fewer preceding infections. It is worth noting that HSP is characteristically a disease of younger people, so if it presents in the elderly a coexisting malignancy should be considered.[50] Granulomatosis with polyangiitis and renal cancer have been reported simultaneously in 60% of the 23 cases described by Tatsis et al. and the cancer seemed to be a triggering factor. Granulomatosis with polyangiitis outcome thereafter was independent of the malignancy.[51] Magyarlaki et al. observed that renal cancer developed significantly more frequently in patients with GPA than those with rheumatoid arthritis. A pathogenetic link was not clear because proteinase 3 was not detected in the tumors. However, a pathogenic role of IgA was suggested for cancers associated with HSP, which could also explain the connection between IgA multiple myeloma and vasculitis, and renal cancer and IgA nephropathy.[52] In those settings, IgA1 had an *O*-linked glycosylation deficiency (sialic acid deficient) that activates the complement pathway and favors mesangial deposits.[53]

Interestingly, other rheumatological conditions associated with vasculitis have also been linked with malignancy, including rheumatoid arthritis with an increased risk of lymphoma.[54]

Nerve and muscle microvasculitis: These are defined as mononuclear cell infiltrations into the walls of small arteries whose calibers are < 70 mm, but without leukocytoclastic or fibrinoid necrosis. Their association with cancer, mainly a solid tumor, was reported in 10–28% of cases.[55] Clinical manifestations were primarily peripheral neuropathies: mononeuropathy multiplex or sensorimotor polyneuropathy. Cutaneous signs or muscle lesions were rare. Outcomes varied widely: remission after cancer treatment or under corticosteroid treatment, or disease progression.

Digital ischemia: It has also been associated with cancer (mostly solid tumors rather than hematological malignancies) in 0.07% of the cases.[56] Vasculitis is only one of the mechanisms

and other factors are also involved: sympathetic nerve hyper-reactivity, enhanced viscosity, or coagulability, tumor secretion of vasoactive substances, bleomycin chemotherapy, etc. A cancer of the digestive tract (esophagus, stomach, small intestine, or colon) was found in one-third of the reported patients. Digital ischemia disappeared after cancer therapy in > 50% of patients who achieved complete remission of cancer.[36]

ANCA-ASSOCIATED VASCULITIS AND MALIGNANCY

Antineutrophil cytoplasmic antibody-associated vasculitis (AAV), which includes the subentities GPA and MPA, is an organ- and life-threatening chronic inflammatory small-vessel vasculitis. This therapy is based on glucocorticoids combined with an immunosuppressive agent tailored to disease severity. But relapse risk remains high and some patients require prolonged immunosuppressive therapy. To circumvent and reduce therapy related toxicity, AAV therapy is split into remission-induction and maintenance phases, which limits the use of cyclophosphamide, a pivotal drug used in AAV. There is also recent evidence of the benefit of targeted biological treatment with rituximab as a substitute for conventional immunosuppressive drugs.[57,58]

Presently, research is focused on survivor prognosis as short-term efficacy of therapy might be compromised by untoward long-term outcomes such as cardiovascular and cancer morbidity.[57] Cancer development is a significant problem and adequate identification of this association is important for prevention and screening measures.[59] Cancer has also been linked with AAV as a potential causal or disease-triggering factor. Understanding the link between cancer and AAV development is crucial for understanding AAV pathogenesis and for clinical practice.

AAV and cancer risk: Many chronic primary autoimmune and/or inflammatory diseases have been associated with increased risk of development of cancer.[60-64] Several pathways are implicated in cancer development in chronic autoimmune and inflammatory diseases.
- Immunosuppressive therapy decreases the immune system's ability to recognize and eliminate malignant cells and it may have direct mutagenic properties.
- Long-standing immune activation, per se, may be oncogenic and is thought to explain the increased rate of lymphoma seen in a number of chronic autoimmune and inflammatory rheumatisms[54] and the increased risk of lung cancer in autoimmune and inflammatory

diseases commonly manifesting with pulmonary involvement.[65]

- Also, the association of chronic autoimmune or inflammatory conditions with cancer may be confounded by shared exogenous risk factors or genetic susceptibility.

In a study by Heijl et al., cumulative overall cancer incidence rates in patients diagnosed with AAV (mainly GPA) at 5 and 8 years were 8 and 13%, respectively, and 12% of recorded deaths were attributed to malignancies.[66] Cancer incidence may have decreased over time because of the availability of less cyclophosphamide-intensive treatment regimens. The potential effect of specific therapeutic agents on cancer incidence in AAV is highlighted by the highest reported incidence rates observed in a multicenter clinical trial of GPA among patients receiving etanercept that is a soluble fusion protein designed to inhibit tumor necrosis factor (TNF); this finding led to the suggestion of an association of cancer with etanercept use in AAV.[67] The specific cancer-types associated with AAV are urinary tract cancer;[68,69] leukemia, mostly acute myeloid leukemia[70] and skin cancer particularly nonmelanoma skin cancer.[66]

The relative carcinogenicity of specific immuno-suppressive agents varies across compounds because of their particular pharmacological properties. In present day AAV therapy, multiple immunosuppressive agents are commonly given sequentially or in combination, so determining the hazards of single agents in cancer development is difficult. The main agents implicated are cyclophosphamide,[68,69] etanercept,[67] azathioprine, methotrexate, mycophenolate mofetil, or Rituximab.[71] Patient care in AAV should include preventive measures and screening in view of the increased risk of treatment related malignancies.

CONCLUSION: WHEN AND HOW TO RULE OUT UNDERLYING MALIGNANCY IN A PATIENT OF VASCULITIS?

The association between malignancy and vasculitic diseases is complex. Vasculitis often presents with a systemic illness including fever, weight loss and sweats, which can represent symptoms of a malignancy. The diagnosis of vasculitis requires a search for cancer, as well as other potential etiologies. When vasculitis is initially diagnosed, a complete and careful physical examination with standard biological and radiological examination is required to make the differential diagnosis. Tissue biopsy may be required to exclude malignancy, particularly if there is a solitary mass lesion in, for example, the chest. Suspicious lesions should always be biopsied, even if the diagnosis of vasculitis has

been confirmed. But the search for a cancer is particularly mandatory when the vasculitis becomes chronic, treatment is no longer effective, or the disease escapes control. An inappropriate response to therapy should also prompt a reassessment for the presence of malignancy. Tumor relapse or cytological transformation should come to mind when vasculitis develops in a patient followed for a malignancy. Vasculitis occurring during malignancy, usually present with distinctive features according to the vasculitis subtype, and also the nature of the malignancy. In conclusion, vasculitis may be the presenting feature of malignancy, although this is uncommon and the strongest link is between cutaneous vasculitis and hematological malignancies. Further large-scale studies are required to evaluate the associations and interactions between vasculitis and malignancy.

The magnitude of cancer incidence in patients undergoing treatment for ANCA-associated vasculitis has become better understood. More data are needed to determine whether reducing exposure to immunosuppressive agents can reduce the cancer risk.

KEY POINTS

- Malignancy-associated vasculitis is rare.
- The hematological malignancies most frequently described are myelodysplastic syndrome (MDS) and lymphoproliferative diseases.
- The pathogenic link between malignancy and vasculitis is unclear.
- The overall outcomes for patients with severe vasculitis and malignancy are poor.

REFERENCES

1. Kurzrock R, Cohen PR. Vasculitis and cancer. Clin Dermatol. 1993;11:175-87.
2. Kurzrock R, Cohen PR, Markowitz A. Clinical manifestations of vasculitis in patients with solid tumors. A case report and review of the literature. Arch Intern Med. 1994;154:334-40.
3. Fortin PR. Vasculitides associated with malignancy. Curr Opin Rheumatol. 1996;8:30-3.
4. Bachmeyer C, Wetterwald E, Aractingi S. Cutaneous vasculitis in the course of hematologic malignancies. Dermatology. 2005;210:8-14.
5. Fain O, Hamidou M, Cacoub P, et al. Vasculitides associated with malignancies: analysis of sixty patients. Arthritis Rheum. 2007;57:1473-80.
6. Hasler P, Kistler H, Gerber H. Vasculitides in hairy cell leukemia. Semin Arthritis Rheum. 1995;25:134-42.

7. Hutson TE, Hoffman GS. Temporal concurrence of vasculitis and cancer: a report of 12 cases. Arthritis Care Res. 2000;13:417-23.

8. Podjasek JO, Wetter DA, Pittelkow MR, et al. Cutaneous small-vessel vasculitis associated with solid organ malignancies: the Mayo Clinic experience, 1996 to 2009. J Am Acad Dermatol. 2012;66:e55-65.

9. Blanco R, Martinez-Taboada VM, Rodriguez-Valverde V, et al. Cutaneous vasculitis in children and adults. Associated diseases and etiologic factors in 303 patients. Medicine (Baltimore). 1998;77:403-18.

10. Greer JM, Longley S, Edwards L, et al. Vasculitis associated with malignancy. Medicine (Baltimore). 1988;67:220-30.

11. Cancer Facts and Figures. New York: American Cancer Society; 1987.

12. Sanchez-Guerrero J, Gutierrez-Urena S, Vidaller A, et al. Vasculitis as a paraneoplastic syndrome. Report of 11 cases and review of the literature. J Rheumatol. 1990;17:1458-62.

13. Castro M, Conn DL, Su WP, et al. Rheumatic manifestations in myelodysplastic syndromes. J Rheumatol. 1991;18:721-7.

14. Hayem G, Gomez MJ, Grossin M, et al. Systemic vasculitis and epithelioma. A report of three cases with a literature review. Rev Rhum Engl Ed. 1997;64:816-24.

15. Martin Oterino J, Sánchez Rodríguez AS, Chimpén Ruiz VA, et al. Hypersensitivity vasculitis as a paraneoplastic manifestation of an acute monocytic leukaemia. Med Clin (Barc). 1997;109:238-9.

16. Hamidou MA, Derenne S, Audrain MA, et al. Prevalence of rheumatic manifestations and antineutrophil cytoplasmic antibodies in haematological malignancies. A prospective study. Rheumatology (Oxford). 2000;39:417-20.

17. Gran JT, Sund S, Langholm R. Small cell pleomorphic T-cell lymphoma presenting with cutaneous vasculitis. Clin Rheumatol. 1994;13:628-30.

18. Ng JP, Murphy J, Chalmers EM, et al. Henoch–Schönlein purpura and Hodgkin's disease. Postgrad Med J. 1988;64:881-2.

19. Knight A, Askling J, Granath F, et al. Urinary bladder cancer in Wegener's granulomatosis: risks and relation to cyclophosphamide. Ann Rheum Dis. 2004;63:1307-11.

20. Duhrsen U, Augener W, Zwingers T, et al. Spectrum and frequency of autoimmune derangements in lymphoproliferative disorders: analysis of 637 cases and comparison with myeloproliferative diseases. Br J Haematol. 1987;67:235-9.

21. Aractingi S, Bachmeyer C, Prost C, et al. Subepidermal autoimmune bullous skin diseases associated with B-cell lymphoproliferative disorders. Medicine (Baltimore). 1999;78:228-35.

22. Dispenzieri A, Gorevic PD. Cryoglobulinemia. Hematol Oncol Clin North Am. 1999;13:1315-49.

23. Farcet JP, Weschsler J, Wirquin V, et al. Vasculitis in hairy-cell leukemia. Arch Intern Med. 1987;147:660-4.

24. Paydas S, Zorludemir S, Sahin B. Vasculitis and leukemia. Leuk Lymphoma. 2000;40:105-12.

25. Longley S, Caldwell JR, Panush RS. Paraneoplastic vasculitis. Unique syndrome of cutaneous angiitis and arthritis associated with myeloproliferative disorders. Am J Med. 1986;80:1027-31.

26. McLean DI. Cutaneous paraneoplastic syndromes. Arch Dermatol. 1986;122:765-7.

27. Mody GM, Cassim B. Rheumatologic manifestations of malignancy. Curr Opin Rheumatol. 1997;9:75-9.

28. Nowack R, Flores-Suarez LF, van der Woude FJ. New developments in pathogenesis of systemic vasculitis. Curr Opin Rheumatol. 1998;10:3-11.

29. Swerlick RA, Lawley TJ. Role of microvascular endothelial cells in inflammation. J Invest Dermatol. 1993;100:111S-5S.

30. Callen JP. Cutaneous vasculitis: what have we learned in the past 20 years? Arch Dermatol. 1998;134:335-7.

31. Ballieux BE, Hiemstra PS, Klar-Mohamad N, et al. Detachment and cytolysis of human endothelial cells by proteinase 3. Eur J Immunol. 1994;24:3211-5.

32. Sais G, Vidaller A, Jucgla A, et al. Adhesion molecule expression and endothelial cell activation in cutaneous leukocytoclastic vasculitis. An immunohistologic and clinical study in 42 patients. Arch Dermatol. 1997;133:443-50.

33. Zehnder P, Jenni W, Aeschlimann AG. Systemic vasculitis and solid tumors (epitheliomas). Rev Rhum Engl Ed. 1998;65:442.

34. Vardiman JW, Thiele J, Arber DA, et al. The 2008 revision of the World Health Organization (WHO) classification of myeloid neoplasms and acute leukemia: rationale and important changes. Blood. 2009;114:937-51.

35. Pirayesh A, Verbunt RJ, Kluin PM, et al. Myelodysplastic syndrome with vasculitic manifestations. J Intern Med. 1997;242:425-31.

36. Fain O, Guillevin L, Kaplan G, et al. Vasculitis and neoplasms: 14 cases. Ann Med Interne (Paris). 1991;142:486-504.

37. Saif MW, Hopkins JL, Gore SD. Autoimmune phenomena in patients with myelodysplastic syndromes and chronic myelomonocytic leukemia. Leuk Lymphoma. 2002;43:2083-92.

38. Espinosa G, Font J, Muñoz-Rodríguez FJ, et al. Myelodysplastic and myeloproliferative syndromes associated with giant cell arteritis and polymyalgia rheumatica: a coincidental coexistence or a causal relationship? Clin Rheumatol. 2002;21:309-13.

39. Hamidou MA, Boumalassa A, Larroche C, et al. Systemic medium-sized vessel vasculitis associated with chronic myelomonocytic leukemia. Semin Arthritis Rheum. 2001;31:119-26.

40. Lopez FF, Vaidyan PB, Mega AE, et al. Aortitis as a manifestation of myelodysplastic syndrome. Postgrad Med J. 2001;77:116-8.

41. Voulgarelis M, Giannouli S, Ritis K, et al. Myelodysplasia-associated autoimmunity: clinical and pathophysiologic concepts. Eur J Clin Inv. 2004;34:690-700.

42. Thielen N, Ossenkoppele G, Schuurhuis GJ, et al. New insights in the pathogenesis of chronic myeloid leukemia: towards a path to cure. Neth J Med. 2011;69:430-40.

43. Pinheiro RF, Metze K, Silva MR, et al. The ambiguous role of interferon regulatory factor-1 (IRF-1) immunoexpression in myelodysplastic syndrome. Leuk Res. 2009;33:1308-12.

44. de Hollanda A, Beucher A, Henrion D, et al. Systemic and immune manifestations in myelodysplasia: a multicenter retrospective study. Arthritis Care Res (Hoboken). 2011;63:1188-94.

45. Giannouli S, Voulgarelis M, Zintzaras E, et al. Autoimmune phenomena in myelodysplastic syndromes: a 4-yr prospective study. Rheumatology (Oxford). 2004;43:626-32.

46. Hughes GR, Elkon KB, Spiller R, et al. Polyarteritis nodosa and hairy-cell leukemia. Lancet. 1979;1:678.

47. Milone G, Stagno F, Guglielmo P, et al. Cutaneous vasculitis in non-Hodgkin's lymphoma. Haematologica. 1995;80:529-31.

48. Sanchez NB, Canedo IF, Garcia-Patos PE, et al. Paraneoplastic vasculitis associated with multiple myeloma. J Eur Acad Dermatol Venereol. 2004;18:731-5.

49. Lucas Guillen E, Martínez Ruiz A, Guerao Ramirez M, et al. Hypersensitivity vasculitis as the first manifestation of a multiple myeloma. An Med Interna. 1997;14:374-5 (in Spanish).

50. Pertuiset E, Liote F, Launay-Russ E, et al. Adult Henoch–Schönlein purpura associated with malignancy. Semin Arthritis Rheum. 2000;29:360-7.

51. Tatsis E, Reinhold-Keller E, Steindorf K, et al. Wegener's granulomatosis associated with renal cell carcinoma. Arthritis Rheum. 1999;42:751-6.

52. Magyarlaki T, Kiss B, Buzogany I, et al. Renal cell carcinoma and paraneoplastic IgA nephropathy. Nephron. 1999;82:127-30.

53. Saulsbury FT. Alterations in the O-linked glycosylation of IgA1 in children with Henoch–Schönlein purpura. J Rheumatol. 1997;24:2246-9.

54. Ekstrom K, Hjalgrim H, Brandt L, et al. Risk of malignant lymphomas in patients with rheumatoid arthritis and in their first-degree relatives. Arthritis Rheum. 2003;48:963-70.

55. Vincent D, Dubas F, Hauw JJ, et al. Nerve and muscle microvasculitis: 50 cases. Rev Neurol (Paris). 1985;141:440-6 (in French).

56. Taylor LM Jr, Hauty MG, Edwards JM, et al. Digital ischemia as a manifestation of malignancy. Ann Surg. 1987;206:62-8.

57. Berden A, Goceroglu A, Jayne D, et al. Diagnosis and management of ANCA associated vasculitis. BMJ. 2012;344:e26.

58. Bosch X, Guilabert A, Espinosa G, et al. Treatment of antineutrophil cytoplasmic antibody associated vasculitis: a systematic review. JAMA. 2007;298:655-69.

59. Mahr A, Heijl C, Le Guenno G, et al. ANCA-associated vasculitis and malignancy: current evidence for cause and consequence relationships. Best Pract Res Clin Rheumatol. 2013;27:45-56.

60. Gridley G, McLaughlin JK, Ekbom A, et al. Incidence of cancer among patients with rheumatoid arthritis. J Natl Cancer Inst. 1993;85:307-11.

61. Smitten AL, Simon TA, Hochberg MC, et al. A meta-analysis of the incidence of malignancy in adult patients with rheumatoid arthritis. Arthritis Res Ther. 2008;10:R45.

62. Bernatsky S, Boivin JF, Joseph L, et al. An international cohort study of cancer in systemic lupus erythematosus. Arthritis Rheum. 2005;52:1481-90.

63. Olesen AB, Svaerke C, Farkas DK, et al. Systemic sclerosis and the risk of cancer: a nationwide population-based cohort study. Br J Dermatol. 2010;163:800-6.

64. Theander E, Henriksson G, Ljungberg O, et al. Lymphoma and other malignancies in primary Sjögren's syndrome: a cohort study on cancer incidence and lymphoma predictors. Ann Rheum Dis. 2006;65:796-803.

65. Hemminki K, Liu X, Ji J, et al. Effect of autoimmune diseases on risk and survival in histology-specific lung cancer. Eur Respir J. 2012;40:1489-95.

66. Heijl C, Harper L, Flossmann O, et al. Incidence of malignancy in patients treated for antineutrophil cytoplasm antibody-associated vasculitis: follow-up data from European Vasculitis Study Group clinical trials. Ann Rheum Dis. 2011;70:1415-21.

67. Silva F, Seo P, Schroeder DR, et al. Solid malignancies among etanercept-treated patients with granulomatosis with polyangiitis (Wegener's): long-term follow up of a multicenter longitudinal cohort. Arthritis Rheum. 2011;63:2495-503.

68. Travis LB, Curtis RE, Glimelius B, et al. Bladder and kidney cancer following cyclophosphamide therapy for non-Hodgkin's lymphoma. J Natl Cancer Inst. 1995;87:524-30.

69. Westman KW, Bygren PG, Olsson H, et al. Relapse rate, renal survival, and cancer morbidity in patients with Wegener's granulomatosis or microscopic polyangiitis with renal involvement. J Am Soc Nephrol. 1998;9:842-52.

70. Pedersen-Bjergaard J, Specht L, Larsen SO, et al. Risk of therapy-related leukaemia and preleukaemia after Hodgkin's disease. Relation to age, cumulative dose of alkylating agents, and time from chemotherapy. Lancet. 1987;2:83-8.

71. Tarella C, Passera R, Magni M, et al. Risk factors for the development of secondary malignancy after high-dose chemotherapy and autograft, with or without rituximab: a 20-year retrospective follow-up study in patients with lymphoma. J Clin Oncol. 2011;29:814-24.

CHAPTER 45

Pregnancy and Vasculitis

Shankar Naidu, Susmita Sharma, Aman Sharma, Surjit Singh

INTRODUCTION

Primary systemic vasculitides are uncommon disorders characterized by inflammation and tissue necrosis within the blood vessel wall. The symptoms vary from mild to life-threatening manifestations, and the clinical course can vary from one of self-limiting disease to life-threatening manifestations. Although vasculitis can cause significant morbidity and mortality, the use of immunosuppressive drugs such as cyclophosphamide, azathioprine, mycophenolate mofetil, and biological agents such as rituximab have improved the survival of these patients. This has led to reports of successful pregnancy outcomes amongst these patients. The frequencies of pregnancy outcomes are different in different vasculitides due to their predilection for age and gender. Vasculitides such as the Takayasu's arteritis (TA) and Behçet's disease (BD) predominantly affect younger aged females, and hence more number of pregnancies has been reported among these vasculitides. The various cytotoxic drugs, such as cyclophosphamide and methotrexate, used in the management of vasculitis also have a negative impact on fertility and also have teratogenic effects on the fetus and can lead to various congenital anomalies, miscarriages, or preterm deliveries.

The outcome of pregnancies in vasculitis is good when vasculitis is diagnosed before pregnancy and remission is achieved before conception. Most maternal complications observed during pregnancy are due to the damage caused by vasculitic process on maternal organs such as accelerated hypertension in TA, renal dysfunction, or lung involvement in ANCA-associated vasculitis. The main obstetrical complications seen are pregnancy loss, preterm births, growth retardation, and risk of cesarean section. Hence, pregnancy in vasculitis patients should be considered as high-risk pregnancy and should be managed by close coordination by the obstetricians and rheumatologists with expertise in dealing with such conditions.

FERTILITY CONCERNS

Fertility issues are of significant concern among young men and women who are diagnosed with vasculitis. Because of the initial life-threatening or organ-threatening manifestations of vasculitis, fertility issues may not be of immediate concern to the patients. However, these issues should be identified and discussed with the patients and family at an early stage and before therapy with potentially cytotoxic drugs is initiated. The various factors that have an impact on the fertility, such as age, fertility status of the patient, drugs used in management, need to be identified and discussed with the patient.

Vasculitis is a systemic inflammatory condition that can cause a transient functional neuroendocrine dysregulation of the hypothalamic–pituitary–ovarian axis leading to infertility.[1] Direct involvement of female reproductive organs is rare in vasculitis such as granulomatosis with polyangiitis (GPA), polyarteritis nodosa (PAN), or BD.[2-5] Involvement of male reproductive organs causing orchitis or epididymo-orchitis is classically seen in PAN but can also be seen in GPA, BD, or Henoch–Schönlein purpura (HSP).[6-9] However, the intratesticular inflammation is usually reversible, but can rarely cause testicular necrosis.[10]

Cyclophosphamide is the most potent drug used in the treatment of vasculitis. However, it has a high risk of causing infertility among men and women. Depending on the patient's age and the cumulative dose of cyclophosphamide used in that particular patient, about 20–85% of women can develop infertility.[11] The cumulative dose of cyclophosphamide causing premature ovarian failure in women decreases with increasing age as the ovarian reserve of viable oocytes decreases with advancing age. Clowse et al. have shown that the anti-Müllerian hormone levels can be used as a marker of ovarian reserve in women with subfertility.[11] Cyclophosphamide also has an impact on the fertility of men. Sterility, oligospermia, or azoospermia have been observed in about 50–90% of men who received cyclophosphamide.[12] As in women, men younger than 40 years are more likely to recover from oligospermia or azoospermia after discontinuation of cyclophosphamide.

Among the other drugs used in the treatment of vasculitis, only methotrexate has been reported to induce reversible oligospermia and impact fertility.[13] Other drugs used in the treatment of vasculitis, such as azathioprine, mycophenolate mofetil, leflunomide, corticosteroids, colchicine, TNFα blockers, and rituximab, have not been shown to cause infertility or subfertility in men or women.[12,14,15]

Gonad preservation prior to use of cytotoxic drugs can help the patients in maintaining fertility. Cryopreservation of sperm in male patients is an easy and cost-effective procedure and should be suggested before initiation of cyclophosphamide. Cryopreservation of oocytes, ovarian tissue, or embryos can be suggested for women, but these procedures are expensive and available in few specialized centers. However, the practice of these procedures in both men and women is not always possible due to the urgent and life-threatening indications to initiate therapy with cyclophosphamide.

Various drugs have been studied to decrease and prevent the effects of cytotoxic drugs on the ovaries so as to decrease the chances of infertility.[16-18] Progesterone, in the form of depot medroxyprogesterone acetate and as combined oral contraceptive pill, has been used during the initial treatment phases to decrease the ovarian activity and thus the exposure of cytotoxic drug to oocytes. Gonadotropin-releasing hormone (GnRH) analogues such as leuprolide acetate and GnRH antagonists such as cetrorelix have also been used to decrease ovarian stimulation and decreasing the exposure of oocytes to cytotoxic drugs.

CONCEPTION AND PRECONCEPTION COUNSELING

Ideally, pregnancy should be planned when the vasculitic activity is in sustained remission for at least 6 months on pregnancy-safe medications. It has been seen that patients with active vasculitis have organ dysfunctions and complications due to the vasculitic process, such as uncontrolled hypertension, renal dysfunction, cardiac insufficiency, or respiratory failure, which are contraindications for pregnancy or act as risk factors for complicated pregnancy.

The drugs used in the treatment of vasculitis can alter the chances of conception and also have teratogenic effects on the embryo and fetus. Cyclophosphamide, methotrexate, mycophenolate mofetil can cause miscarriages and fetal malformations, and these drugs need to be stopped 3–6 months before conception.[19] Leflunomide has been found to cause fetal malformations when given during pregnancy, but no adverse effects on fetus were seen when used prior to pregnancy.[20]

A complete baseline assessment should be done, the organ damage due to vasculitic process should be assessed prior to conception, and the couple should be counseled regarding the complications anticipated during pregnancy and the potential effects of the drugs on pregnancy and outcomes.

PREGNANCY OUTCOMES

More number of pregnancies has been reported from patients with TA and BD, as these diseases affect young women, with an average age at disease onset being 20–30 years. The treatment of these diseases primarily consists of corticosteroids that are safe during pregnancies. Diseases such as GPA, microscopic polyangiitis (MPA), eosinophilic GPA (EGPA), and PAN usually affect women around 50 years of age, and these patients usually receive strong immunosuppression, mostly cyclophosphamide, hence few pregnancy outcomes have been reported in these patients. Even though pregnancy is not a known trigger for vasculitis, few cases of TA, PAN, ANCA-associated vasculitis, anti-glomerular basement membrane (anti-GBM) antibody disease, IgA-associated vasculitis, and cryoglobulinemic vasculitis, who had disease onset during pregnancy or postpartum period, have been reported.[21-26] These patients had poor outcomes when compared to those with a diagnosis of vasculitis prior to conception. The risk of vasculitis flare during pregnancy appears low, especially in TA and PAN where it is <5%.[27] The risk of vasculitis flare during pregnancy is about 10–40% in GPA, 25–50% in EGPA, and <50% in MPA.[21-24] In BD, 60% have improvement during pregnancy and 30% can have a relapse, which tends to be severe.[28]

LARGE-VESSEL VASCULITIS

Takayasu's Arteritis

Takayasu's arteritis is a large-vessel vasculitis involving aorta, its branches, and the pulmonary arteries. It typically affects women of childbearing age. More than 200 pregnancies have been reported in patients with TA.

Severe hypertension and/or pre-eclampsia were the most common maternal complications in these patients, and it has been seen in 18–63% of patients. Other less commonly seen maternal complications are congestive heart failure, aortic regurgitation, aortic dissection, pulmonary artery involvement, and stroke, seen in about 5–22% of patients. The risk of disease flare was very low, seen in about 3% of patients. With regard to fetus, low birth weight and intrauterine growth retardation were the most common complications seen in about 22–47% of pregnancies. Preterm delivery was seen in about 16–27% pregnancies and fetal loss was present in 9–27%. Cesarean section was performed to deliver baby in about 30–83% of pregnancies.[22,29,30]

Giant Cell Arteritis

Giant cell arteritis is a large-vessel vasculitis that is classically associated with jaw and arm claudication, headache, and visual loss. It usually effects older adults, with mean age of onset of disease >55 years. Hence, no pregnancy outcome has been reported in patients with giant cell arteritis. However, there is some evidence that previous pregnancy may be protective against development of giant cell arteritis.[31]

MEDIUM-VESSEL VASCULITIS

Polyarteritis Nodosa

Polyarteritis nodosa is a disorder characterized by necrotizing inflammation of medium-to-small-sized arteries leading to renal infarction, mesenteric ischemia, and mononeuritis multiplex. Polyarteritis nodosa affects men more frequently than women, with predominant age group being affected, i.e. 45–65 years. Hence, very few pregnancies have been reported in literature till now. The most important maternal complications observed were uncontrolled hypertension and renal failure. The maternal outcome was poor when PAN was diagnosed during pregnancy as compared to patients who were diagnosed prior to conception and were in remission. Concerning the fetus, premature rupture of membranes leading to preterm deliveries was the most common complication seen in about 50–100% of patients in various reports.[22,29,30,32]

Kawasaki Disease

Kawasaki disease (KD) is a medium-vessel vasculitis predominantly affecting infants and young children, but it rarely affects adults also. Kawasaki disease is characterized by fever, polymorphic exanthemas, conjunctival injection,

oral mucosal involvement and nonsuppurative cervical lymphadenopathy. The major maternal complications seen in patients with KD are related to pre-eclampsia and postpartum hemorrhage. Few patients had myocardial infarction or stroke during pregnancy.[33-38]

SMALL-VESSEL VASCULITIS

Granulomatosis with Polyangiitis

Granulomatosis with polyangiitis is an uncommon small-vessel necrotizing vasculitis that usually involves upper respiratory tract, lungs, and kidneys. The average age of onset of disease is around 40 years, hence, very few pregnancies have been reported in patients with GPA. Till date, only 48 pregnancies have been reported in patients of GPA. The flare up of vasculitis during pregnancy was seen in 10–40% of patients who were in remission during conception and 75–100% of patients who had active disease at the time of conception. Pre-eclampsia was seen in about 15–20% of patients. Other maternal complications noted were mainly due to damage in kidneys, heart, and lungs due to vasculitis. Fetal loss was seen in 10–33% of pregnancies. Growth retardation with low birth weight was observed in 10–25% of pregnancies and preterm birth was seen in 10–30% pregnancies. Cesarian section was done for delivery in around 30–50% of patients.[22-24,29,30]

Microscopic Polyangiitis

Microscopic polyangiitis is another form of ANCA-associated vasculitis loosely related to GPA but differentiated by the absence of upper respiratory tract involvement. Very few data of MPA with pregnancy are available, as MPA was initially considered as a subset of PAN. Disease flare was seen in <50% of patients and the maternal and fetal complications noted were similar to those of GPA.[22,25,30]

Eosinophilic Granulomatosis with Polyangiitis

Eosinophilic GPA is an ANCA-associated vasculitis characterized by pulmonary and systemic small-vessel vasculitis, extravascular granulomas, eosinophilia, and asthma. Flare-up of vasculitis was seen in about 26% of patients. Pre-eclampsia was seen in about 5% of patients. Other commonly observed maternal complications were related to cardiac insufficiency and asthma exacerbations. Fetal complications, such as fetal loss in about 19%, IUGR in 8%, preterm delivery in 23%, were noted. Cesarean section was performed in 15–40% among various series.[22,30,32]

Henoch–Schönlein Purpura (IgA Vasculitis)

Henoch–Schönlein purpura is an IgA-mediated small-vessel necrotizing vasculitis characterized by palpable purpura, arthritis/arthralgia, and gastrointestinal involvement. It predominantly affects children and hence infrequently observed during pregnancy. Most of the cases of HSP associated with pregnancy had developed features of HSP *de novo* during pregnancy. Pregnancy outcomes were good among patients who had developed HSP during childhood compared to those who had *de novo* disease during pregnancy. Pre-eclampsia or eclampsia was seen in 17% of pregnancies. Spontaneous abortions, preterm delivery, and IUGR were reported in few patients. Cesarian section was performed in 28% of pregnancies.[22,39]

Essential Mixed Cryoglobulinemic Vasculitis

Very few case reports of pregnancy with mixed cryoglobulinemic vasculitis have been reported, and the maternal and fetal outcomes appear to be good. Few case reports of transient minor skin erythematous lesions in newborns due to transplacental transfer of cryoglobulins have been published in literature.[40,41]

Anti-GBM Antibody Disease

Very few cases of anti-GBM antibody disease associated with pregnancy have been reported till now with variable maternal and fetal outcomes. Most of the patients developed features of anti-GBM disease, either during pregnancy or close to pregnancy. Maternal complications were defined by the severity of renal involvement.[26,42]

VARIABLE-VESSEL VASCULITIS

Behçet's Disease

Behçet's disease is chronic, relapsing, inflammatory disease involving small, medium, and large vessels. It is characterized by recurrent oral and genital ulcers, ocular, gastrointestinal, neurological involvement, and thrombosis. It predominantly affects young women in childbearing age. More than 200 pregnancies have been reported among patients with BD. Disease relapse was seen in 8–56% of patients during pregnancy. In various case series, 38–92% of patients had improvement in symptoms during pregnancy. Thromboembolic complications, such as deep venous thrombosis, Budd–Chiari syndrome, pulmonary thrombosis, and cerebral venous thrombosis, were less common, seen in about 3% of patients during pregnancy. Fetal loss was seen in 4–21% of pregnancies, more commonly in patients with severe BD. Preterm deliveries and IUGR were seen in less than 5% of patients. Cesarean section was performed in around 5–15% of pregnancies.[22,28,43]

Cogan's Syndrome

Cogan's syndrome is characterized by interstitial keratitis and vestibuloauditory involvement. Only three cases of pregnancy were reported among patients with Cogan's syndrome, with two showing disease flare during pregnancy while the third patient remained in remission. However, the overall maternal and fetal outcomes appear to be good in these patients.[44]

Primary CNS Vasculitis

Primary CNS vasculitis is a fulminant vasculitis presenting as severe headache and multiple neurologic deficits affecting multiple vascular territories. Even though this disease is less commonly seen among women, few reports of primary CNS vasculitis have been reported during pregnancy and postpartum period. This entity should be differentiated from reversible cerebral artery vasoconstrictive syndrome that is more commonly associated with pregnancy and present with similar clinical features. Among the limited data available, the pregnancy outcomes seem to be poor due to the fulminant nature of the disease itself.[45,46]

KEY POINTS

- The frequencies of pregnancy outcomes are different in different vasculitides due to their predilection for age and gender.
- The various cytotoxic drugs used in the management of vasculitis have a negative impact on fertility and also have teratogenic effects on the fetus.
- Cyclophosphamide is the most potent drug used in the treatment of vasculitis and it has a high risk of causing infertility among men and women.
- Gonad preservation prior to use of cytotoxic drugs can help the patients in maintaining fertility.
- Pregnancy should be planned when the vasculitic activity is in remission for at least 6 months on pregnancy-safe medications.
- The risk of vasculitis flare during pregnancy appears low in TA and PAN where it is <5%.
- The risk of vasculitis flare during pregnancy is about 10–40% in GPA, 25–50% in EGPA, and <50% in MPA.
- In BD, 60% have improvement during pregnancy and 30% can have a relapse, which tends to be severe.

REFERENCES

1. Edozien LC. Mind over matter: psychological factors and the menstrual cycle. Curr Opin Obstet Gynecol. 2006;18:452-6.
2. Lombard CM, Moore MH, Seifer DB. Diagnosis of systemic polyarteritis nodosa following total abdominal hysterectomy and bilateral salpingo-oophorectomy: a case report. Int J Gynecol Pathol. 1986;5:63-8.
3. Kaya E, Utas C, Balkanli S, et al. Isolated ovarian polyarteritis nodosa. Acta Obstet Gynecol Scand. 1994;73:736-8.
4. Kariv R, Sidi Y, Gur H. Systemic vasculitis presenting as a tumor like lesion. Four case reports and an analysis of 79 reported cases. Medicine. 2000;79:349-59.
5. Tan JW, Howe HS, Chng HH. Ovarian vein thrombosis in Behçet disease. J Clin Rheumatol. 2012;18:89-91.
6. Pagnoux C, Seror R, Henegar C, et al. Clinical features and outcomes in 348 patients with polyarteritis nodosa: a systematic retrospective study of patients diagnosed between 1963 and 2005 and entered into the French vasculitis study group database. Arthritis Rheum. 2010;62:616-26.
7. Dufour JF, Le Gallou T, Cordier JF, et al. Urogenital manifestations in Wegener granulomatosis: a study of 11 cases and review of the literature. Medicine (Baltimore). 2012;91:67-74.
8. Pektas A, Devrim I, Besbas N, et al. A child with Behçet's disease presenting with a spectrum of inflammatory manifestations including epididymoorchitis. Turk J Pediatr. 2008;50:78-80.
9. Davol P, Mowad J, Mowad CM. Henoch–Schönlein purpura presenting with orchitis: a case report and review of the literature. Cutis. 2006;77:89-92.
10. Barber TD, Al-Omar O, Poulik J, et al. Testicular infarction in a 12-year-old boy with Wegener's granulomatosis. Urology. 2006;67:846e9-10.
11. Clowse ME, Copland SC, Hsieh TC, et al. Ovarian reserve diminished by oral cyclophosphamide therapy for granulomatosis with polyangiitis (Wegener's). Arthritis Care Res (Hoboken). 2011;63:1777-81.
12. Langford CA, Klippel JH, Balow JE, et al. Use of cytotoxic agents and cyclosporine in the treatment of autoimmune disease. Part 2: inflammatory bowel disease, systemic vasculitis, and therapeutic toxicity. Ann Intern Med. 1998;129:49-58.
13. Martinez Lopez JA, Loza E, Carmona L. Systematic review on the safety of methotrexate in rheumatoid arthritis regarding the reproductive system (fertility, pregnancy, and breastfeeding). Clin Exp Rheumatol. 2009;27:678-84.
14. Ostensen M, Lockshin M, Doria A, et al. Update on safety during pregnancy of biological agents and some immunosuppressive anti-rheumatic drugs. Rheumatology (Oxford). 2008;47:iii28-31.
15. Hyrich KL, Verstappen SM. Biologic therapies and pregnancy: the story so far. Rheumatology (Oxford). 2014;53:1377-85.
16. Chen H, Li J, Cui T, et al. Adjuvant gonadotropin-releasing hormone analogues for the prevention of chemotherapy induced premature ovarian failure in premenopausal women. Cochrane Database Syst Rev. 2011;11:CD008018.
17. Somers EC, Marder W, Christman GM, et al. Use of a gonadotropin-releasing hormone analog for protection against premature ovarian failure during cyclophosphamide therapy in women with severe lupus. Arthritis Rheum. 2005;52:2761-7.
18. Henes JC, Henes M, von Wolff M, et al. Fertility preservation in women with vasculitis: experiences from the FertiPROTEKT network. Clin Exp Rheumatol. 2012;30:S53-6.
19. Dawson AL, Riehle-Colarusso T, Reefhuis J, et al. The National Birth Defects Prevention Study. Maternal exposure to methotrexate and birth defects: a population based study. Am J Med Genet A. 2014;9999:1-5.
20. Cassina, M, Johnson DL, Robinson LK, et al. (For the Organization of Teratology Information Specialists Collaborative Research Group). Pregnancy outcome in women exposed to leflunomide before or during pregnancy. Arthritis Rheum. 2012;64:2085-94.
21. Pagnoux C, Le Guern V, Goffinet F, et al. Pregnancies in systemic necrotizing vasculitides: report on 12 women and their 20 pregnancies. Rheumatology (Oxford). 2011;50:953-61.
22. Gatto M, Iaccarino L, Canova M, et al. Pregnancy and vasculitis: a systematic review of the literature. Autoimmun Rev. 2012;11:A447-59.
23. Tuin J, Sanders JS, de Joode AA, et al. Pregnancy in women diagnosed with antineutrophil cytoplasmic antibody-associated vasculitis: outcome for the mother and the child. Arthritis Care Res. 2012;64:539-45.
24. Koukoura O, Mantas N, Linardakis H, et al. Successful term pregnancy in a patient with Wegener's granulomatosis: case report and literature review. Fertil Steril. 2008;89:457. e1-5.
25. Milne KL, Stanley KP, Temple RC, et al. Microscopic polyangiitis: first report of a case with onset during pregnancy. Nephrol Dial Transplant. 2004;19:234-7.
26. Hatfield T, Steiger R, Wing DA. Goodpasture's disease in pregnancy: case report and review of the literature. Am J Perinatol. 2007;24:619-21.
27. Hidaka N, Yamanaka Y, Fujita Y, et al. Clinical manifestations of pregnancy in patients with Takayasu arteritis: experience from a single tertiary center. Arch Gynecol Obstet. 2012;285:377-85.
28. Marsal S, Falga C, Simeon CP, et al. Behçet's disease and pregnancy relationship study. Br J Rheumatol. 1997;36:234-8.
29. Seo P. Pregnancy and vasculitis. Rheum Dis Clin North Am. 2007;33:299-317.
30. Pagnoux C, Mahendira D, Laskin CA. Fertility and pregnancy in vasculitis. Best Pract Res Clin Rheumatol. 2013;27:79-94.
31. Duhaut P, Abert MC, Le Page L, et al. Giant cell arteritis and polymyalgia rheumatic: influence of past pregnancies? The GRACG multicenter case–control study. Rev Med Interne. 2004;11:792-800.
32. Langford CA, Kerr GS. Pregnancy in vasculitis. Curr Opin Rheumatol. 2002;14:36-41.
33. Gordon CT, Jimenez-Fernandez S, Daniels LB, et al. Pregnancy in women with a history of Kawasaki disease: management and outcomes. BJOG. 2014. doi: 10.1111/1471-0528.12685. Epub ahead of print.
34. Kanno K, Sakai H, Nakajima M, et al. An adult case of Kawasaki disease in a pregnant Japanese woman: a case report. Case Rep Dermatol. 2011;3:98-102.

35. Tsuda E, Ishihara Y, Kawamata K, et al. Pregnancy and delivery in patients with coronary artery lesions caused by Kawasaki disease. Heart. 2005;91:1481-2.

36. Nolan TE, Savage RW. Peripartum myocardial infarction from presumed Kawasaki's disease. South Med J. 1990;83:1360-1.

37. Tsuda E, Kawamata K, Neki R, et al. Nationwide survey of pregnancy and delivery in patients with coronary arterial lesions caused by Kawasaki disease in Japan. Cardiol Young. 2006;16:173-8.

38. Fason JT, Fry YW, Smith D. Kawasaki disease in a postpartum patient. J Natl Med Assoc. 2004;96:1499-502.

39. Tayabali S, Andersen K, Yoong W. Diagnosis and management of Henoch–Schönlein purpura in pregnancy: a review of the literature. Arch Gynecol Obstet. 2012;286:825-9.

40. Gupta A, Gupta G, Marouf R. Cryoglobulinemic vasculitis in pregnancy. Int J Gynaecol Obstet. 2008;103:177-8.

41. Laugel V, Goetz J, Wolff S, et al. Neonatal management of symptomatic transplacental cryoglobulinaemia. Acta Paediatr. 2004;93:556-8.

42. Vasiliou DM, Maxwell C, Shah P, et al. Goodpasture syndrome in a pregnant woman. Obstet Gynecol. 2005;106:1196-9.

43. Bang D, Chun YS, Haam IB, et al. The influence of pregnancy on Behçet's disease. Yonsei Med J. 1997;38:437-43.

44. Currie C, Wax JR, Pinette MG, et al. Cogan's syndrome complicating pregnancy. J Matern Fetal Neonatal Med. 2009;22:928-30.

45. Singh S, Soloman T, Chacko G, et al. Primary angiitis of the central nervous system: an ante-mortem diagnosis. J Postgrad Med. 2000;46:272-4.

46. Ducros A, Boukobza M, Porcher R, et al. The clinical and radiological spectrum of reversible cerebral vasoconstriction syndrome. A prospective series of 67 patients. Brain. 2007;130:3091-101.

CHAPTER 46

Prevention and Management of Infections

Gaurav Prakash, Subhash Varma, Pankaj Malhotra

INTRODUCTION

Treatment of vasculitis is often a challenging task, and equally challenging is the prevention and management of various opportunistic infections that may arise following immunosuppressive therapy used for the treatment of various forms of vasculitis. Infections are one of the major causes of deaths from vasculitis. In various series, 13–20% patients with vasculitis died due to infective complications. Infection in an immunocompromised host is often a race against time. Timely identification and prompt treatment of infections are of paramount importance in order to have a satisfactory outcome in a patient being treated for vasculitis. Since infections are a potential cause of morbidity and mortality in an immunocompromised host, an understanding of their patterns and outcome is essential for optimum management.[1] Prevention of these infections by various pharmacological and nonpharmacological means is even more desirable.

This chapter deals with various aspects of prevention and management of infections in an immunocompromised host suffering from vasculitis. The suggested investigation in a vasculitis patient on immunosuppressive therapy is showing in Table 46.1.

DEFINING IMMUNOCOMPROMISED HOST

Any patient with alteration of phagocytic, cellular, or humoral immunity arising out of basic disease or due to drugs used for the treatment of the illness is at increased risk of infections. Few key points about the pattern and characteristics of infections in an immunocompromised host are as follows:

- Common infective pathogens present in severe form and often in an atypical manner

Table 46.1 Suggested investigation in a vasculitis patient on immunosuppressive therapy
Investigations in most patients
• Complete blood counts
• Blood biochemistry
• Blood cultures
• Urine microscopic examination/culture
• Chest X-ray
• HRCT chest
Investigation needed in a select group of patients
• Stool examination
• Sputum gram stain and ZN stain
• CECT scan chest and abdomen
• MRI brain
• Cerebrospinal fluid analysis
• Bronchoalveolar lavage
• Biomarkers for cytomegalovirus, herpes, *Aspergillus*, mycobacterium
• Aspiration/biopsy from suspected site of infection

- Organism of low virulent potential can cause severe infection
- Commensal bacteria in oral cavity and gastrointestinal tract can become pathogenic
- Higher risk of infections from environmental fungi
- Higher risk of reactivation of latent infections in a patient's body.

Unlike other rheumatological disorders, vasculitis is peculiar with common involvement of skin and mucosal surfaces, often leading to formation of small ulcers. Mechanical breach in skin and mucosa, permits microorganisms to produce local infections. This infection may remain contained to skin and subcutaneous tissue, but as most of the patients with vasculitis are on immunosuppressive therapy, it is not uncommon for such infections to gain access to the systemic circulation and resulting in septicemia.

COMMON MEDICATIONS IN THE TREATMENT OF VASCULITIS THAT CAUSE IMMUNOSUPPRESSION

Treatment of vasculitis primarily comprises glucocorticoids, cytotoxic chemotherapeutic drugs, and lately targeted biological therapies such as anti-CD20 rituximab and anti-TNF agents.

Corticosteroids

Glucocorticoids are nonspecific suppressors of the immune system, and always lead to downregulation of both humoral and cellular immune system. These are among the most potent immunosuppressive agents. Dose >1 mg/kg or high-dose pulse steroid therapy or dose of prednisolone 20 mg/day for more than 2 weeks is considered as highly immunosuppressive.

Cytotoxic Agent

These drugs are commonly used for granulomatosis with polyangiitis (GPA), microscopic polyangiitis (MPA), and eosinophilic GPA. Due to their use in cancer chemotherapy, infection risks associated with them are well known. Cyclophosphamide is an alkylating agent, which leads to DNA damage, and is widely used as a potent anticancer agent. Among various chemotherapeutic agents this drug has high immunosuppressive effect due to its impact on lymphocytic and neutrophilic function. Azathioprine and methotrexate belong to antimetabolite group of anticancer drugs, and they lead to inhibition of various enzymes involved in nucleotide synthesis. Calcineurin inhibitors mainly inhibit cell-mediated immunity and target T-cell function.

Monoclonal Antibodies

Anti-CD20 monoclonal antibody rituximab has emerged as one of the treatment options for GPA (previously Wegener's granulomatosis) and MPA.

Majority of the experience with this molecule has emerged from its use in B-cell lymphoid malignancies. In the pooled, placebo-controlled studies, 39% of patients in the rituximab group experienced an infection of any type compared to 34% of patients in the placebo group. The most common infections in rituximab-treated patients were in the respiratory system such as sinusitis, pharyngitis, and laryngotracheobronchitis.[2] The second most common site of infection was urinary tract. In the experience from the cohort of rheumatoid arthritis patients, the rate of serious infections was 4.31 per 100 patient-years. The most common serious infections (≥0.5%) were pneumonia, urinary tract infections, and severe cellulitis. Infections leading to death in this group included pneumonia, sepsis, and colitis.

In a study on rituximab use in patients with Wegener's granulomatosis and MPA, 22% patients developed rituximab-related adverse events. Seven percent of these patients had infection related serious adverse event (grade 3 or more). An interesting observation in this study was that the incidence of serious infection was equal in patients treated with rituximab versus cyclophosphamide. This finding shows that the targeted therapies such as rituximab can predispose a patient for infection to an extent, which is not lesser than conventional chemotherapeutic agents used in the management of vasculitis.[3] Though this might be related to the concomitant use of corticosteroids also.

Some peculiar infections emerged in phase IV studies of rituximab such as increased incidence of progressive multifocal leukoencephalopathy with JC polyoma virus and higher incidence of reactivation of hepatitis B virus (HBV) in carriers. Reactivation of hepatitis B in recipients of rituximab is likely to have higher extent of hepatocellular injury and liver failure. Therefore, it is highly recommended to test for hepatitis B carrier state before starting rituximab therapy in any patient.

Biological agents such as infliximab, adalimumab, and tocilizumab mainly lead to alteration in cytokine profile. As a result, these agents produce an indirect yet profound suppression of the immune system. Apart from increased overall susceptibility to various serious infections, activation of latent mycobacterial infection is an important risk involved with the use of these biological agents. This risk is much more pronounced in the populations with higher prevalence of mycobacterial infection.

PREVENTION OF INFECTIONS IN THE PATIENT TREATED FOR VASCULITIS

Personal Hygiene

- This is the most inexpensive yet effective method of preventing cross transmission of infection to an immunocompromised host from environment. Patients, particularly those who have received chemotherapy agents or biologic agents for treatment of vasculitis, should avoid close contact with any person having symptoms suggestive of an infection.

- Adequate hand hygiene is recommended and it includes thorough cleaning with soap and water for 2 minutes. Use of anti-infective alcohol-based hand rubs is useful, but these agents should be used as an adjuvant to hand washing not as a replacement of it. Adequate amounts (2–3 mL) of alcohol-based disinfectants should be rubbed in both hands for not less than 30 seconds or till the hands get dried.
- Raw food and salads should be avoided.

Vaccination

Most vasculitic illnesses present acutely. Therefore there is less than sufficient time to plan an immunization strategy for this group of patients. However, vaccination done in a timely manner can immensely help in preventing or reducing the incidence of various vaccine preventable illnesses.

Most remarkable point about vaccination in immunocompromised host is contraindication for live vaccines as they have potential risk of infection from reactivation of live attenuated strains. Vaccines that may be given include antipneumococcal, meningococcal, anti-*Haemophilus influenzae* B, and influenza vaccination. Since, immunosuppressive effect of medications used for vasculitis can last for years, it is recommended that these patients should be vaccinated every year against influenza and every 5 years for pneumococci. CDC, epidemiology, and prevention of vaccine preventable diseases recommend that patients vaccinated during the phase of immunosuppressive therapy should be reimmunized after 3 months of cessation of medications as immunization done in immunosuppressed phase is suboptimal and short lasting.

The recommendation of vaccination is showing in Table 46.2.

Chemoprophylaxis

Chemoprophylaxis is one of the important medical interventions in order to prevent infections in patients being treated for vasculitis. The basic premise of chemoprophylaxis is that these anti-infective agents should be well-tolerated, easy to administer, and effective in preventing emergence of specific infection. The recommendations for anti-infective prophylaxis in patients of vasculitis on immunosuppressive therapy are showing in Table 46.3.

Table 46.2 Recommendation for vaccination

Antipneumococcal	Polyvalent vaccine at the time of diagnosis of vasculitis. To be repeated every 5 years.
Anti-influenza	Annual immunization as per regional variation in influenza strain.
Diphtheria, purtusis, tetanus	Immunization against these infections is not mandatory. Must be offered to unimmunized patients or to the patients at increased risk.

Table 46.3 Recommendation for anti-infective prophylaxis in patients of vasculitis on immunosuppressive therapy

Specific pathogen	Recommendation
Pneumocystis jirovecii	Cotrimoxazole • 400/80 mg daily once • 800/160 mg alternate day once For sulfonamide allergy • Daily atovaquone OR • Monthly pentamidine aerosol
Antifungal prophylaxis	Not routinely recommended, advised for a patient with the past history of fungal infection • Fluconazole 200–400 mg/day • Voriconazole 200–400 mg/day
Herpes zoster	Not routinely recommended, advised for a patient with the past history of herpetic infection • Acyclovir 400 mg BD • Valacyclovir 500 mg BD

Pneumocystis Jirovecii

This infection most commonly presents in the form of severe pneumonia with rapid course. It carries high risk of mortality if detected late or not treated promptly.[4,5] Among vasculitis, *P. jirovecii* pneumonia (PJP) is frequently described in GPA patients. Administration of prophylactic doses of cotrimoxazole helps in containing such infective episodes. In a meta-analysis of 12 large randomized trials in oncology patients, cotrimoxazole prophylaxis reduced the risk of occurrence of PJP by 91%. There are no such data in treatment of vasculitic disorders. However, vasculitis patients on various immunomodulatory agents are equally immunocompromised and should be started on PJP prophylaxis along with main therapy. Risk of *P. jirovecii* persists even after cessation of immunosuppressive therapy until restoration of the immune system. Therefore, it is recommended to continue cotrimoxazole prophylaxis for at least 4–8 weeks after stopping immunosuppressive therapy.

Commonly used prophylactic dose schedules for cotrimoxazole are as follows:

- Tablet cotrimoxazole (800/160), twice in a day, on two days per week
- Tablet cotrimoxazole (800/160), once in a day, on alternate days
- Tablet cotrimoxazole (400/80), once in a day, daily.

Fungal Infections

These infections are less common but have high-case fatality rate. Patients with vasculitis are at increased risk of candida and filamentous fungi like *aspergillous*. Routine antifungal prophylaxis of all patients being treated for vasculitis is not recommended. However, patients who have had a fungal infection previously should be given antifungal prophylaxis in all subsequent courses of immunosuppressive therapy. On the basis of published data from randomized clinical trials, azoles group of agents (fluconazole, itraconazole, voriconazole, etc.) are the most effective and relatively well-tolerated agents for antifungal prophylaxis in an immunocompromised host.

Tuberculosis

Patient being treated with anti-TNF therapy should be screened for tuberculosis before starting these agents. This is much more relevant in patients living in areas with higher prevalence of mycobacterial infection. Guidelines recommend this screening in the patients suffering from rheumatoid arthritis. This recommendation can be applied in patients on anti-TNF therapy for vasculitis as well. Oral rifampicin and isoniazid can be used in patients at high risk of acquiring mycobacterium from the surrounding or in the patients who have high risk of its reactivation. Routine use of these drugs for prophylaxis of tuberculosis is not indicated.

Bacterial Infections

Patients with vasculitis are at increased risk of various bacterial infections. However, the spectrum of various possible bacterial infections is very diverse. A single prophylactic agent often does not prevent against most of them. Besides, there is risk of emergence of resistance with prolonged antibacterial prophylaxis. Therefore, routine prophylaxis of all vasculitis patients with oral antibiotics is not recommended.

Viral Infections

There are no clear guidelines regarding antiviral prophylaxis. However, patients treated with steroids and rituximab are at increased risk of herpes zoster and hepatitis B reactivation. It is recommended that all the patients who have had herpes zoster in the past should be on antiviral prophylaxis throughout the phase of immunosuppressive therapy. Acyclovir or Valacyclovir are preferred agents for prophylaxis against herpes infection. All the patients who are planned for rituximab therapy should be screened for latent HBV infection and carrier state.

Care for Breaks in Natural Barriers due to Vasculitis and its Treatment

Vasculitic lesions over skin and mucosa often lead to breach in epithelial/mucosal barrier. A cytotoxic agent such as cyclophosphamide can further complicate this situation by causing mucositis leading to mucosal ulceration in the digestive tract. This may lead to local invasion by pathogenic organism on skin as well as in mucosal surfaces mainly in the oro-anal region. Daily self inspection by the patient or by a healthcare provider for any sign of infection is advised. Regular chlorhexidine-based mouth washes after each meal and sitz bath with betadine-containing solution should be advised to all the patients receiving cytotoxic chemotherapy for systemic vasculitis.

TREATMENT OF VASCULITIS IN SPECIFIC INFECTIONS

- *Hepatitis B:* Patients with concomitant HBV infection should be started on anti-HBV therapy. HBV viral load monitoring should be done at a regular interval.
- *Hepatitis C:* Systemic antiviral therapy is usually not required for concomitant latent hepatitis C infection. However, it is recommended to periodically check for hepatitis C virus RNA copies and liver function test to detect reactivation of this infection.
- *HIV:* All newly diagnosed patients of systemic vasculitis should be tested for HIV. Those who are positive for HIV should be given antiretroviral therapy before initiating immunosuppressive therapy.

CLINICAL FEATURES AND EVALUATION OF INFECTIONS IN AN IMMUNOCOMPROMISED HOST

The biggest challenge in successfully treating infection in a patient on immunosuppressive therapy is its early detection. Lack of classical signs of infection and variation in their presentation in an immunocompromised host makes this task of early detection of infection further demanding. Fever, a most common sign of infection can be frequently absent in patients on corticosteroid therapy. Such patients may present with tachycardia, altered sensorium, and hypotension or organ dysfunction. High index of suspicion is recommended for any new sign or symptom in these patients and a possibility of an infective etiology should be kept. It is not uncommon to have a fungal etiology for a newly developed lung nodules in a patient on therapy for GPA.

A comprehensive history regarding contacts to any potential source of infection, past history on infections, and nature of treatment taken must be recorded. Close examination of oral cavity, paranasal sinuses, vascular access site, skin folds like axilla, groin area, and perianal area should be done at admission and then at frequent intervals.

Investigation strategy is based on the clinical clues obtained from history and systemic examination. In a febrile immunocompromised (mainly neutropenic) patient, besides complete blood counts and biochemical parameters, blood culture must be drawn from a peripheral vein. In patients with a central venous catheter paired sample from central line port and one from a peripheral vein should be taken before starting antibiotics. Baseline chest radiograph should be obtained promptly. There is evidence that in a neutropenic patient, high-resolution CT scan (HRCT) of chest has better sensitivity in detecting pulmonary infection. Therefore, in any patient with features localizing to the respiratory system but with an apparently normal chest X-ray, a HRCT of chest should be advised.

Various CNS infections may present subtly with only headache or behavioral changes. CNS imaging and cerebrospinal fluid examination may be needed in some cases even in the absence of meningeal signs. Emerging biomarkers of infections such as serum galactomannan and beta D-glucan for invasive fungal infection, procalcitonin for bacterial infections, gamma interferon, and gene-expert molecular diagnostic test for mycobacterial infections are often helpful in deciding treatment for patients with overlapping presentation.

MANAGEMENT

The cornerstone of management of infection in an immunocompromised host is early initiation of treatment. If fever occurs following cytotoxic agents given for vasculitis and the patient is in the neutropenic phase, then the treatment with intravenous antibiotics should be started promptly after drawing blood cultures. Choice of antibacterial agent depends on the local sensitivity pattern. Studies suggest that selected antibiotics should have a broadspectrum with cover for pseudomonas infection. If a patient is having coexisting shock, mucositis, or suspected central catheter-related

infection, then gram-positive coverage with vancomycin or teichoplanin is warranted from the beginning. Close collaborations between treating rheumatologist, infectious disease specialist, and clinical microbiologist are of paramount importance in management of these cases.

Invasive fungal infections are notorious for their cryptic nature of presentation and aggressive course. In case of non-resolution of fever or infection with in few days of antibacterial therapy, empirical antifungal agents should be started. Granulocyte colony stimulating factors are useful adjunct to antibacterial therapy in a neutropenic patient as the single most important factor in recovery from infection is recovery of neutrophil counts.

Patients on steroid therapy often develop oropharyngeal candidiasis that can progress to painful esophageal candidiasis or candidemia. Local infection can be treated with oral fluconazole therapy. However, painful conditions that preclude oral therapy (like esophageal candidiasis) and systemic infection requires parenteral antifungal agents. Amphotericin B is a broad spectrum antifungal agent; however, its toxicity often limits in use in therapeutic doses. Recently echinocandins such as caspofungin, micafungin, and anidulafungin have emerged as equally efficacious yet less toxic alternative of amphotericin B for systemic candidial infection.

Reactivation of herpes zoster can be treated with oral acyclovir in therapeutic doses. However, there should be high index of suspicion for systemic viral infection that should be treated with IV acyclovir therapy. Reactivation is always a possibility in seropositive patients for cytomegalovirus (CMV). There is recommendation of periodic testing for CMV copies by RQPCR in postallogeneic transplant patients, but there is no such policy for patient treated for vasculitis. Therefore, high index of suspicion for CMV infection should be kept for any patient presenting with pneumonia, gastrointestinal tract involvement, and cytopenias.

KEY POINTS

- Infections in an immunocompromised host are common yet preventable cause of morbidity and mortality.
- Commoner sites of infection in these patients are respiratory tract, skin/subcutaneous tissue, and genitourinary tract.
- Infections in these immunocompromised patients can have subtle presentation. Therefore, high index of suspicion and aggressive approach for evaluation and treatment of any possible focus of infection holds the key for a successful outcome.

- Personal hygiene, cleaning and hand washing techniques, and simple dietary modifications are inexpensive ways of preventing infections, and these should be recommended to all patients of vasculitis on immunosuppressive therapy.
- Vaccinations as per recommendations discussed in this chapter are helpful in preventing certain infections. However, live attenuated vaccines are contraindicated during immunosuppressive therapy.
- An understanding of the underlying condition, use of an appropriate preventive strategy with vaccination or chemoprophylaxis, and use of appropriate empiric antimicrobial drugs are the keys to manage these patients successfully.

REFERENCES

1. Pizzo PA. Fever in immunocompromised patients. N Engl J Med. 1999;341:893-900.
2. Kelesidis T, Daikos G, Boumpas D, et al. Does rituximab increase the incidence of infectious complications? Int J Infect Dis. 2011;15:e2-16.
3. Stone JH, Merkel PA, Spiera R, et al. Rituximab versus cyclophosphamide for ANCA-associated vasculitis. N Engl J Med. 2010;363:221-32.
4. Waite S, Jeudy J, White CS. Acute lung infections in normal and immunocompromised host. Radiol Clin North Am. 2006;44:295-315.
5. Donnelly JP, De Pauw BE. Infections in immunocompromised host: general principles. In: Mandell GL, Bennet JE, Dolin R (Eds). Principles and Practice of Infectious Disease, 6th edn. New York: Churchil Livingstone; 2005. pp. 4321-31. (A comprehensive overview on the subject.)

Index

Page numbers followed by *f* refer to figure and *t* refer to table